THE ROUTLEDGE INTERNATIONAL HANDBOOK OF COUPLE AND FAMILY THERAPY

The Routledge International Handbook of Couple and Family Therapy is a comprehensive text that promotes innovative frameworks and interventions in couple and family therapy from a cross-cultural perspective.

A diverse range of international contributors explore the role that demography, regionality, cultural and political crises, and policy have on the issues faced by couples and families. Collectively, the chapters articulate unique ideas in conceptualizing the needs of families with international backgrounds, adapting the current models and frameworks to work with this population most effectively. The text is split into four sections covering: personal voices and philosophical perspectives, theory and models, specific applications with international populations, and emerging perspectives.

This handbook is essential for individual practitioners, researchers, psychotherapists, and related mental health professionals as well as academics with an interest in working with couples and families.

Katherine M. Hertlein, Ph.D. (she/her) is Professor in the Couple and Family Therapy Program in the Department of Psychiatry and Behavioral Health, School of Medicine, University of Nevada, Las Vegas (UNLV). She received her master's degree in marriage and family therapy from Purdue University Calumet and her doctorate in human development with a specialization in marriage and family therapy from Virginia Tech. Across her academic career, she has published over 90 articles, 12 books, and over 50 book chapters. She is currently the Editor-In-Chief of the *Journal of Couple and Relationship Therapy*. She was a 2018–2019 Fulbright Core Scholar, and in this role, served as a Visiting Lecturer and Guest Researcher at the University of Salzburg in Salzburg, Austria. She lectures nationally and internationally on technology, couples, and sex. Hertlein maintains a private practice in Las Vegas, Nevada.

ROUTLEDGE INTERNATIONAL HANDBOOKS

ROUTLEDGE INTERNATIONAL HANDBOOK OF MULTIDISCIPLINARY
PERSPECTIVES ON DESCENDANTS OF HOLOCAUST SURVIVORS
Edited by Judith Tydor Baumel-Schwartz and Amit Shrira

ROUTLEDGE INTERNATIONAL HANDBOOK OF VISUAL-MOTOR SKILLS,
HANDWRITING, AND SPELLING
Edited by Yanyan Ye, Tomohiro Inoue, Urs Maurer, and Catherine McBride

ROUTLEDGE HANDBOOK OF ENVIRONMENTAL POLICY
Edited by Helge Jörgens, Christoph Knill and Yves Steinebach

THE ROUTLEDGE HANDBOOK OF SOFT POWER
(2nd **Edition**)
Edited by Naren Chitty, Lilian Ji, Gary D Rawnsley

THE ROUTLEDGE HANDBOOK OF URBAN LOGISTICS
Edited by Jason Monios, Lucy Budd and Stephen Ison

THE ROUTLEDGE HANDBOOK OF COMPARATIVE
GLOBAL URBAN STUDIES
Edited by Patrick LeGalès and Jennifer Robinson

THE ROUTLEDGE HANDBOOK OF TRANSATLANTIC RELATIONS
Edited by Elaine Fahey

THE ROUTLEDGE INTERNATIONAL HANDBOOK OF DISABILITY
HUMAN RIGHTS HIERARCHIES
Edited by Stephen J. Meyers, Megan McCloskey and Gabor Petri

THE ROUTLEDGE HANDBOOK OF PUBLIC SECTOR ACCOUNTING
Edited by Tarek Rana and Lee Parker

THE ROUTLEDGE INTERNATIONAL HANDBOOK OF COUPLE AND FAMILY THERAPY

Edited by Katherine M. Hertlein

R Routledge
Taylor & Francis Group

NEW YORK AND LONDON

Designed cover image: © Getty Images

First published 2024
by Routledge
605 Third Avenue, New York, NY 10158

and by Routledge
4 Park Square, Milton Park, Abingdon, Oxon, OX14 4RN

Routledge is an imprint of the Taylor & Francis Group, an informa business

© 2024 selection and editorial matter, Katherine M. Hertlein; individual chapters, the contributors

Library of Congress Cataloging-in-Publication Data
Names: Hertlein, Katherine M., editor.
Title: The Routledge international handbook of couple and family therapy /
edited by Katherine M. Hertlein.
Description: New York, NY : Routledge, 2024. | Series: Routledge international handbooks |
Includes bibliographical references and index. |
Identifiers: LCCN 2023018954 (print) | LCCN 2023018955 (ebook) |
ISBN 9781032286617 (hardback) | ISBN 9781032286631 (paperback) |
ISBN 9781003297871 (ebook)
Subjects: LCSH: Couples therapy–Handbooks, manuals, etc. |
Marital psychotherapy–Handbooks, manuals, etc. |
Family psychotherapy–Handbooks, manuals, etc.
Classification: LCC RC488.5 .R678 2024 (print) |
LCC RC488.5 (ebook) | DDC 616.89/1562–dc23/eng/20230622
LC record available at https://lccn.loc.gov/2023018954
LC ebook record available at https://lccn.loc.gov/2023018955

ISBN: 978-1-032-28661-7 (hbk)
ISBN: 978-1-032-28663-1 (pbk)
ISBN: 978-1-003-29787-1 (ebk)

DOI: 10.4324/9781003297871

Typeset in Sabon
by Newgen Publishing UK

To Adam, the Ultimate Human/Genius! You are the most amazing person I have ever known.

I am so grateful to be your mom. I love you!

CONTENTS

Contents

SECTION II
Theories and Models in an International Context   **81**

Contents

Contents

ABOUT THE EDITOR

Katherine M. Hertlein, Ph.D. (she/her) is Professor in the Couple and Family Therapy Program in the Department of Psychiatry and Behavioral Health, School of Medicine, University of Nevada, Las Vegas (UNLV). She received her master's degree in marriage and family therapy from Purdue University Calumet and her doctorate in human development with a specialization in marriage and family therapy from Virginia Tech. Across her academic career, she has published over 90 articles, 12 books, and over 50 book chapters. She is currently the Editor-In-Chief of the *Journal of Couple and Relationship Therapy*. She was a 2018–2019 Fulbright Core Scholar, and in this role, served as a Visiting Lecturer and Guest Researcher at the University of Salzburg in Salzburg, Austria. She lectures nationally and internationally on technology, couples, and sex. Hertlein maintains a private practice in Las Vegas, Nevada.

ABOUT THE CONTRIBUTORS

Elena Angelkova, M.S., is a graduate of the Couple and Family Therapy Master's program at the University of Nevada, Las Vegas (UNLV), and is expected to graduate in December of 2022. She received her bachelor's degree in Psychology, with a minor in Couple and Family Therapy from UNLV. Elena immigrated from Macedonia to Las Vegas, Nevada in 2009, and is the second one from her family to have attended college. Elena was a Vice President of Membership for the International Marriage and Family Honors Society, Delta Kappa Zeta (DKZ) Chapter at UNLV. She also received her Graduate Research and Teaching Certificate.

Ronald Asiimwe, PhD., is an Assistant Professor in the Couple and Family Therapy Program at the University of Minnesota. He grew up in Uganda and is currently a doctoral candidate in Human Development and Family Studies specializing in Couple and Family Therapy at Michigan State University. He holds a master's degree in Marriage and Family Therapy from Oklahoma Baptist University – Shawnee, Oklahoma. Prior to moving to the United States, Ronald attended Makerere University in Kampala, Uganda where he received his bachelor's degree in Community Psychology. Ronald has research and clinical experience practicing in the States of Oklahoma and Michigan in the U.S.A., and in his home country of Uganda. His current research focuses on parenting and systemic/relational interventions grounded in context and culture. Ronald believes that healthy human relationships are the foundation for a healthy and fulfilled life. With this, he has special interest in the development, adaptation, and implementation of relational/systemic interventions in Africa. He spends much time reading and writing about this topic, and if invited, enjoys presenting on family therapy in Africa. He has published articles in top tier journals, including the *Journal of Marital and Family Therapy* and *Family Process Journal*. Additionally, he has won several awards, including a 2020–2021 national leadership development award from the American Association for Marriage and Family Therapy (AAMFT); https://ronschol arlyhub.com/

Saliha Bava, Ph.D., LMFT, is a professor of marriage and family therapy at Mercy College (New York), Taos Institute advisory board member and associate, and founding board member of the International Certificate in Collaborative-Dialogic Practices. She focuses on expanding relational intelligence for an inclusive world by harnessing the power of play and dialogue. Partnering with individuals and organizations worldwide, she combines inter-disciplinary ideas and methodologies to create generative, inclusive change. Performative methodologies, hyperlinked thinking, and dialogue guide her academic and social activism, which aims to unsettle dominant discourses regarding research, social justice, and identity. She co-authored *The Relational Workplace* and *The Relational Book for Parenting* with her partner Mark Greene; and is a co-editor of the forthcoming *Routledge International Handbook of Postmodern Therapies*. Based in New York City, she consults with couples, companies and communities. Learn more at SalihaBava.com | Email: drbava@gmail.com. Follow @ThinkPlay.

J. Maria Bermudez, Ph. D., LMFT, is an associate professor at the University of Georgia in the Department of Human Development and Family Science and the Ph. D. program in Marriage and Family Therapy. She is a Clinical Fellow and Approved Supervisor of the American Association for Marriage and Family Therapy. Her work focuses on feminist informed and strength-based approaches to research and service for Latinx immigrant families. She is on the editorial board of seven peer-reviewed journals, has published over 60 peer-reviewed articles and book chapters, and presented over 100 professional presentations in family therapy. Bermudez has recently published two books- *Socioculturally Attuned Family Therapy: Guidelines for Equitable Theory and Practice* with her colleagues Teresa McDowell and Carmen Knudson Martin, and *Intersectionality and Context across the Lifespan: Readings for Human Development*.

Barbara Bräutigam, Prof. Dr. phil. habil., professor at the University of Applied Sciences Neubrandenburg for psychology, counseling and psychotherapy, psychological psychother-apist, teaching therapist for systemic therapy and systemic supervisor.

Andres Larios Brown (They/He/Elle) is a Queer & Non-Binary Mescla (mixture) bella (beautiful) of a Guatemalan Immigrant Father and an American citizen from Western European roots mother. They are a licensed Marriage and Family Therapist and graduated from the University of Oregon's Couple and Family Therapy program in 2017. They are the current Director of Cultural Engagement and Assistant Clinical Director at Encircle Therapy (non-profit that works with LGBT+ youth and families from religiously conserva-tive cultures). They study queer identity development and trauma healing among collect-ivist and community-focused cultures. With experience working in a wide range of settings (Non-profits, College counseling centers, community centers, and training clinics), Andres also focuses a large part of their work on teaching, training, and education. They believe that we are truly whole when in connection and community and seeks to bridge the gap between research and clinical practice.

Jakub Caha (1996) has his bachelor in psychology from the Ruprecht Karls Universität Heidelberg and currently studies master degree psychology at the Faculty of Social Studies, Masaryk University, Brno.

Ruth Casabianca, Ph.D., is the Director of the Family and Brief Therapies Institute, Santa Fe, Argentina; President of the Catholic University of Santa Fe, Argentina (2004–2019); President of the International Family Therapy Association (2015–2017) and author of books, articles, and researches in the psychosocial field.

Connor Callahan, MS, is a Family Social Science and Couple and Family Therapy Doctoral Student at the University of Minnesota. He has received a Master of Science in Marriage and Family Therapy from Northwestern University. He is a practicing therapist who has worked in both community and private practice settings. His research and clinical interests focus on bridging the gaps in the way school, and family systems provide support for sexual and gender minority youth.

Zamzam Dini, MA, is a licensed associate marriage and family therapist (LAMFT) in the state of Minnesota. Zamzam is also a doctoral student at the University of Minnesota in the Department of Family Social Science, specializing in Couple and Family Therapy. Zamzam's clinical work focuses on Complex PTSD and trauma in individuals and families. In her research, she seeks to understand refugee trauma, specifically the intergenerational transmission of trauma in refugee families and how trauma manifests in generations beyond the first. Zamzam has developed clinical and research-specific training about immigrant and refugee families, cultural awareness in practice, and increasing diversity in the field of marriage and family therapy.

Nicole Feno received her M. S. from the University of Nevada, Las Vegas Couple and Family Therapy program. She is a state intern working toward licensure who specializes in sex therapy, relationship issues, and trauma and PTSD.

Benjamin T. Finlayson (he/him), Ph.D, MFTC, recently joined Regis University as Assistant Professor in the Division of Counseling and Family Therapy. He graduated from Texas Tech University after successfully defending his dissertation, The moderating roles of hope and emotion regulation between minority stress and negative social media experiences on psychological distress and help-seeking behaviors for LGBTQIA adult individuals. Benjamin's research on LGBTQIA identity, solution focused therapy, suicide, and medical family therapy (MedFT) has been published and presented in academic spaces across the United States. His current projects center on LGBTQIA experiences of obtaining and receiving healthcare and solution-focused teletherapy practices. He spends additional time offering workshops in both academic and clinical spaces on topics ranging from crisis intervention, identity, to religion/spirituality.

Nesteren Gazioglu is a psychologist, family psychotherapist and an academic. She is a certified Satir and EMDR Therapist and has been applying systemic transformational model to her counseling and projects. Since 2009, Nesteren has been working as a facilitator in TOÇEV's (an educational NGO) domestic violence, adolescence and family projects. She is also a board member and general secretary of Turkish Couple and Family Therapy Association. Nesteren is a member of Satir Global, IFTA and APA. She is working as a family therapist at a private practice and has established an organization called PSIEO, where keynote speakers around the world on IPV and Well-being are invited to give seminars and workshops in Turkey. She is also a professional speaker, speaking at schools, municipalities and public. In her public speeches, she generally prefer creating awareness about IPV and domestic violence. Besides fieldwork, Nesteren is an assistant professor at Maltepe University Department of Psychology. She also gives supervision classes at Bilgi University Couple and Family Therapy Clinical Psychology Graduate Program. Her research interests are domestic violence, internet addiction, middle adulthood and positive psychology. Her doctoral thesis is on internet use and well-being in middle adulthood. She is particularly interested in integrating Satir Model perspective in couple therapy and Family Therapy. She has written several book chapters and translated two books into Turkish on family therapies.

Norma Gomez received her M. S. from the University of Nevada, Las Vegas Couple and Family Therapy program. She is a state intern working toward licensure who specializes in relationship issues, parenting, and child issues.

Dumayi Gutierrez, Ph.D., LMFT, LMHP, is an assistant professor at Alliant International University. Gutierrez has a passion for working with multiple diverse communities. She centers minority stress, the intersectionality of self and family systems, resiliency, and intersectional culturally competent care through an experiential, narrative, and feminist lens.

Nicole Sabatini Gutierrez, PsyD, LMFT, is an associate professor in the Couple and Family Therapy Department at Alliant International University, Irvine. She is also a Licensed Marriage and Family Therapist in the state of California and an AAMFT Approved Supervisor. She has a private group practice and specializes in providing trauma-informed, social justice-oriented therapy for individuals, couples and other intimate relationship structures, families, and groups. She primarily works with clients that have experienced interpersonal trauma (IPV, sexual trauma), transgenerational trauma, and/or substance misuse.

Cheri L. Hausmann is a Ph.D. student in marriage and family therapy at Texas Woman's University in Denton, Texas. Her dissertation research orientation is in the psychoanalytic and philosophical perspectives of relational psychotherapy and psychoanalysis, specifically involving, existential crises, grief, and death. Uncovering specifically, mourning and melancholia in the death drive theory, the work of Melanie Klein, Sabina Spielrein, Sigmund Freud, Carl Jung; and in association with the Socratic philosophers of Greece, and 17th century Europe. Currently a licensed marriage and family therapist associate and licensed chemical dependency counselor, Cheri integrates relational psychotherapy with that of Eastern and Western philosophy and psychoanalytic thought. She has a private practice in Denton, Texas, and is a mom of one son. You can learn more about her and her research at: www.cherihausmann.com

Marwa W. Ibrahim, M.A., is a counseling psychology doctoral student at the University of St. Thomas, Minnesota, where she also received her Master of Arts in Counseling Psychology. She is also a psychotherapist at a group practice in Minneapolis, Minnesota, where she provides psychotherapy services in Arabic and English to clients from diverse backgrounds. Many of her clients identify as immigrants or refugees; hence, acculturation, adjustment, and trauma issues have been prominent aspects of her work.

Sara Smock Jordan, Ph.D, a licensed marriage and family therapist, is a professor, graduate coordinator, and program director of UNLV's Couple and Family Therapy Program. Dr. Jordan's research focuses on recognizing solution-focused brief therapy (SFBT) as an evidence-based practice. Her work on applying SFBT with substance abusers has been nationally recognized by the Substance Abuse and Mental Health Health Services Administration's National Registry of Evidence-based Programs and Practices. A co-founding member of the International Microanalysis Associates, Dr. Jordan's expertise lies in microanalysis of face-to-face dialogue, which is the systematic, moment-by-moment examination of specific observable behaviors in face-to-face dialogue, focusing on their immediate communicative functions. Dr. Jordan has received national and international recognition for her research efforts.

Carmen Knudson-Martin, Ph.D., LMFT, is professor of Marital, Couple, and Family Therapy Program at Lewis & Clark College, Portland OR, USA. She has published over 80 articles and book chapters on the influence of the larger sociocultural context in couple and family relationships and the political and ethical implications of therapist actions on marital equality, relational development, and couple therapy. She is the developer of Socio-Emotional Relationship Therapy, which addresses the micro-processes by which societal power processes play out in couple relationships. Carmen is editor/author of three books: *Socio-Emotional Relationship Therapy–Bridging Emotion, Societal Context, and Couple Interaction; Couples, Gender, and Power–Creating Change in Intimate Relationships;* and *Socioculturally Attuned Family Therapy: Guidelines for Equitable Theory and Practice.* She was the 2017 recipient of the Distinguished Contribution to Family Therapy Theory and Practice award from the American Academy of Family Therapy.

Michelle Karume, Ph.D., received her bachelor's degree in Psychology from the University of Houston-Main, her Masters in Marriage and Family Therapy from the University of Houston-Clear Lake, and a Doctorate in Marriage and Family Therapy with a concentration in Medical Family Therapy from Loma Linda University. When Michelle Karume started teaching at the United States International University – Africa, it became very clear that her expertise and passion would collide in very diverse ways. As an assistant professor, teaching, psychotherapy, training, and research are ways in which she intrinsically imparts knowledge and restores relationships. With a belief that the family unit is the training ground for life and that healthy relationships; professional or otherwise are the cornerstone for success, she is passionate about; Marriage and Family Therapy, Medical Family Therapy, Collaborative Care, and Program Development. All of which afford her the platforms of doing psychotherapy in Nairobi, and teaching Undergraduate, Masters, and Doctorate level students at the University. With extensive clinical experience, teaching, and training experience Karume has worked with clients, students, and individuals from exceptionally diverse backgrounds. It is this diversity that gives her the appreciation for culture, difference, education, and awareness. Her current clinical, research, and development interest are: (1) examining the associations between experiences of early childhood trauma, adult disease, and impacts on relationships; (2) development of accredited Marriage and Family Therapy (MFT) training programs in Kenya; (3) improving MFT-student training outcomes by producing the caliber of students that are proficient and competent mental health professionals. Clinically, her practice integrates the bio-psychosocial-spiritual (BPSS) frameworks to heighten the importance of emotional care and improve relationships in families.

Rosco Kasujja, Ph.D., is an alumna and the current Director of the Department of Mental Health and Community Psychology at Makerere University. He serves as the President of the Uganda Clinical Psychology Association and has extensive experience and professional expertise on national mental healthcare and policymaking efforts in Uganda. Kasujja is a leading clinical psychologist and professional leader in the community mental health field in Uganda. He is widely consulted by both local and international agencies in the field of mental health in Uganda. Kasujja has published scholarly articles on clinical supervision, culturally tailored training, trauma, and the adaptation of both psychological interventions and measures for both Ugandans and refugees in Uganda. He has maintained a private practice since 2010 maintaining a systemic view in his practice.

Vaida Kazlauskaite, Ph.D., LMFT-I, is Assistant Professor in the Couple and Family Therapy Program at the University of Nevada, Las Vegas (UNLV). She received her Ph.D. in Family Social Science at the University of Minnesota, Twin Cities and her master's degree in Marriage and Family Therapy at UNLV. Dr. Kazlauskaite's research lies within Medical Family Therapy and integrated behavioral health care. Specifically, her research focuses on communication between parents and children, when a parent is diagnosed with a chronic or terminal illness. As well as how medical and mental health professionals can be better trained within this foci. Dr. Kazlauskaite is a Pre-Clinical Fellow with the American Association for Marriage and Family Therapy (AAMFT) and currently working on her Approved Supervisor Designation.

Pei-Fen Li, Ph.D., is a full-time faculty member in a COAMFTE accredited program in the United States. She is a licensed Marriage and Family Therapist and AAMFT-approved supervisor. She has clinical experiences in Taiwan and the U.S. Her research interests include enhancing individual and relational well-being in different social/cultural contexts, informed by general systems, stress processes, and life course theories. She has done research projects that examined reentry experiences of international students in Taiwan, dyadic analysis of couple dynamics and cultural characteristics associated with relationship quality, solution-focused brief therapy with parents of children on the spectrum, and application of MFT models in Eastern cultures.

A. H. Lohrasbi Nejad born and raised in Iran. He has a bachelor's degree in psychology from Iran and a master's degree in counseling from Germany. He is working in the project "Support offers KiJuFa-Integration work with children, young people and families in refugee accommodations" at the Diakonie Munich and Upper Bavaria.

Reihaneh Mahdavishahri, M.A., AMFT, is a doctorate candidate in Marriage and Family Therapy at Alliant University. Her expertise lies in addressing the gaps across systems of care and the well-being of marginalized populations, particularly immigrant women and communities of color. Serving marginalized populations through the application of culturally informed Emotionally Focused Therapy (EFT), Accelerated experiential dynamic psychotherapy (AEDP) and EMDR are among the focus of her work.

Teresa McDowell, Ed.D., is professor emerita and past department chair at Lewis & Clark Graduate School of Education and Counseling in Portland, Oregon. Her work has focused on applying critical social theory to the practice of family therapy, which resulted in a book published in the AFTA Springer Series in 2015. She also aims to center social justice in family therapy education. Teresa's most recent contributions include introducing third order thinking and third order change to the field of family therapy. McDowell co-authored *Socioculturally Attuned Family Therapy: Guidelines for Equitable Practice* along with her colleagues, Carmen Knudson-Martin and Maria Bermudez.

John K. Miller, Ph.D., LMFT, is a former full professor in the School of Social Development and Public Policy at Fudan University in Shanghai, China, an Adjunct Professor in the Department of Psychology at the Royal University of Phnom Penh in Cambodia, and the Director of the Sino-American Family Therapy Institute (SAFTI) in China. He is a former Fulbright Senior Research Scholar to China (2009–2010) and the Associate Editor for International Initiatives for the Journal of Marital and Family Therapy (JMFT).

Jonathan Molina received his M. S. from the University of Nevada, Las Vegas Couple and Family Therapy program. He is a state intern working toward licensure who specializes in relationship issues, anxiety, and self esteem. He also teaches undergraduate courses at University of Nevada Las Vegas.

Carmen V. Neito was born and Raised in Las Vegas, Nevada. She graduated from University of Nevada, Las Vegas with her Bachelor of Arts degree in Psychology with minors in Family Studies and Neuroscience. She is currently working through the M.S. in Couple and Family Therapy program within UNLV's Kirk Kerkorian School of Medicine. She is interested in early social, cultural, and family influences that impact cognition & development, and plans to focus on that through her graduate studies. Ultimately, she hopes to work towards the expansion of accessibility for mental health resources within underrepresented communities.

Sreevidya Nibhanupudi is a current senior at the University of Wisconsin-Madison, graduating with a Bachelor of Science in Psychology.

Rajeswari (Raji) Natrajan-Tyagi, Ph.D., is a professor and Branch Director in the Couple and Family Therapy Program (CFT) at Alliant International University, California. She graduated with her Ph.D. in Child Development and Family Studies with a specialization in Marriage and Family Therapy (MFT) at Purdue University, Indiana. She also earned her Master's in Social Work from Madras School of Social Work, India. Her research interests are in the area of Immigration, bicultural parenting, cross-cultural training, cross-cultural relevance of family therapy, cultural competency, self-of-therapist training and supervision, qualitative research and systemic training & evaluation. She is a licensed Marriage and Family Therapist and in her private practice she works mainly with couples and families with children, specifically of South Asian descent.

Maxine Notice, Ph.D., LMFT, LMHC, NCC, is a core faculty in the Marriage and Family Therapy Online Program at Abilene Christian University-Dallas. Maxine received her doctorate in Applied Psychology with a specification in Marriage and Family Therapy from Antioch University New England and a master's degree in Clinical Mental Health Counseling from CUNY City College. She is an AAMFT Clinical Fellow and Approved Supervisor, as well as an Advisory Committee Member for the AAMFT Minority Fellowship Program (MFP). Maxine is passionate about the education and training of marriage and family therapists and hopes to grow the field towards higher levels of cultural competency. Her current research interests include evaluating therapy with interracial couples and multiracial families; multicultural supervision; medical family therapy; and clinician training and development.

Matthias Ochs, Prof. Dr. (1968), is a psychologist, psychotherapist (certified by the German psychotherapy law), systemic family therapist, trainer for systemic therapy and counseling (certified by the German systemic associations) and a Gestalt therapist. He is a professor for Psychology and Counseling at a department for Social Work at the Fulda University of Applied Sciences in Germany and a professor member of the Ph.D. center for social work of the Hessian State Universities of Applied Sciences. He is the president of the German Association for Systemic Therapy, Counseling and Family Therapy, General Board member of the European Family Therapy Association (EFTA) and chair of the research committee of EFTA. His current topics of interest are systemic practice and research, epistemology of psychotherapy and systemic work, dialogism in systemic work, systems theory of professional networks, multi- and interprofessional cooperation, risks and side-effects of systemic therapy.

Rachael A. Dansby Olufowote, Ph.D., LMFT, is the online MA Branch Director and Assistant Professor of Marital and Family Therapy in the department of Couple and Family Therapy at Alliant International University. She received her doctorate in couple, marriage, and family therapy from Texas Tech University. Dansby Olufowote's research and clinical interests center around attachment theory, couple relationships, and interracial couples, and the intersections of these with faith, learning, and mental health. She won the 2020 AAMFT Education and Research Foundation's Outstanding Research Publication Award with her dissertation article entitled, "How Can I Become More Secure? A Grounded Theory of Earning Secure Attachment." Her current research focuses on longitudinal dyadic attachment change and resilience among couples raising an autistic child. She is licensed as a Marriage and Family Therapist and an AAMFT Approved Supervisor.

Werner Pfab, Prof. (i.R.), is a psychologist in Communication Research
University of Applied Science, Fulda.

Bernhild Pfautsch (Germany) is a psychologist, family therapist and trauma counselor working with families, children, and young people for years. As peace worker with the Civil Peace Service of the German Corporation for International Cooperation (GIZ) in 2015–2018, she initiated systemic family therapy training in collaboration with the Royal University in Phnom Penh, Cambodia. Still connected in an advisory capacity with the

Southeast-Asian university, she is now pursuing her Ph.D. in international social work in Germany beside teaching trauma-sensitive social work for practitioners from various contexts.

Jason James Platt´s educational, research and clinical focus has been aimed at internationalizing mental health services and training. His professional interests have been aimed at exploring the effectiveness of alternative educational and training modalities, particularly on the use of critical pedagogy and theater of the oppressed. Dr. Platt has been based in Mexico City, Mexico since 2005 and has facilitated immersion programs in Mexico, India, Cuba, Costa Rica, El Salvador, Belize, and Cambodia. He served as a program director of a master's program in International Psychology for fourteen years. Currently he is primarily engaged in clinical work with bi-national couples and with humanitarian aid workers around the globe.

Shruti Singh Poulsen, Ph.D., received her master's degree in Child, Family, and Community Services, and Ph.D. in Couple and Family Therapy from Purdue University. Currently she is an associate professor in the Couple and Family Therapy online program at Alliant International University. She is also the Branch Director of the online PsyD in MFT program. Poulsen is an AAMFT Clinical Fellow and Approved Supervisor, and has been in the field of CFT as a clinician and academic since 1994. Poulsen's research focuses on cultural responsiveness in CFT clinical supervision and training, and clinical work, topics such as interracial relationships, multicultural families, and immigration and its impact on families, couples, and individuals. Poulsen is currently clinically active in a small private practice providing therapy to individuals, couples, and families.

Afarin Rajaei, Ph.D., LMFT, is an assistant professor at Alliant International University in San Diego, CA. She is specifically trained in couples therapy based on Gottman Method and has vast experience in working with couples nationally and internationally. She has published various peer-reviewed articles, book reviews, book chapters, and presented in various national and international conferences. Her research interests include various aspects of couples' relationships ranging from biopsychosocial-spiritual (BPSS) stressors in conflicted intimate relationships, romantic relationship quality, couples, and online social networks and media, disclosure of romantic challenges, marital conflicts, sexual and relationship satisfaction, divorce and remarriage to relationship recovery and repair. She maintains a private practice in San Diego. She loves experiencing nature, traveling, and spending time with her husband, family, and friends.

Teri Raven is an M.S. student in the Couple and Family Therapy program at the University of Nevada, Las Vegas. She also has an interest in music and was a professional musician and singer prior to embarking on her career as a marriage and family therapist.

Tomáš Řiháček, Ph.D. (1978), is a psychologist and psychotherapist. He works as an associate professor at the Faculty of Social Studies, Masaryk University, Brno, where he teaches several research- and methodology-oriented courses. His research interests include psychotherapist development, psychotherapy integration, psychosomatics, assessment of psychotherapeutic change, outcome and process monitoring, and negative effects of psychotherapy.

Karrison A. Rimon was born and raised in Queens, New York. He graduated with his Bachelors of Arts in Criminal Justice and developed a passion for serving the community during his undergrad while working with a youth court in Nevada, Las Vegas. Helping children navigate their way through some of their challenges and life experiences became meaningful and very important to him. Karrison is currently pursuing his Masters Degree in Couples and Family Therapy at the University of Nevada Las Vegas. His passion, commitment and experience are what qualify him to write on the subject of Children and behavioral telehealth. Within the field of CFT, Karrison has an interest in helping to make long lasting change for couples, families and individuals in his community.

Alysha Robinson graduated in 2018 with her Bachelor's in Sociology and minor in Couples Family Therapy from University of Nevada, Las Vegas as well as obtained her Master's in Couples Family Therapy in 2021. She also has Degrees in Dance and Fine Arts. She has a passion for working with couples and families to help others learn to communicate in healthy ways and creating a safe space for mental health.

Parmida Safavi is a graduate student at Alliant International University in Irvine, CA. Parmida is passionate about couple therapy based on Gottman Method and is currently using that method in working with couples including Iranian couples. She has vast experience in working with couples and families with various cultural backgrounds. She also loves to be in nature, exercise, write, travel, and spend time with her loved ones.

Sarah K. Samman, Ph.D., LMFT is an associate professor in the masters and doctoral Couple and Family Therapy Program at Alliant International University, San Diego, United States. She earned her masters degree in Marriage and Family Therapy from Lewis & Clark College and her post-masters certificate in Medical Family Therapy and doctoral degree in Marital and Family Therapy from Loma Linda University. She has presented at national and international conferences on issues of internationalism and interculturalism, spirituality, and gender and power on couple and family relationships. Samman utilizes a biopsychosociospiritual approach to therapy based on a strong interdisciplinary background and a deep commitment to diversity issues and interpersonal and social justice. She also has an interest in student clinical/therapeutic and research preparedness and qualitative research. She is licensed as a Marriage and Family Therapist and an AAMFT Approved Supervisor.

Mona El Roby Saleh, MA, is a doctoral student in the Couple and Family Therapy Program at Alliant International University, San Diego, United States. El Roby Saleh earned several masters degrees including Counseling Psychology from the American University in Cairo (AUC) in Egypt and in Marital and Family Therapy from Alliant International University in San Diego. She has clinical experience in a primary healthcare facility, non-profit organization, educational institute, and the Psychological Counseling Services and Training Center at AUC. She currently provides hospice related care in the San Diego area. El Roby Saleh's research interests include the exploration of Egyptian and Arab couples' relational struggles and the role both socio-cultural and religio-spiritual discourses play in developing and reinforcing these struggles. She is currently an AAMFT Supervisor in Training.

Senem Zeytinoğlu Saydam is an assistant professor at Ozyeğin University's Department of Psychology and the program director of its couple and family therapy master's program in İstanbul, Turkey. She is a licensed marriage and family therapist; an AAMFT-app supervisor. She is a certified EFT supervisor and trainer. Aside from her faculty position, she holds a private practice where she sees individuals, couples, and families and provides clinical supervision to graduate students. Senem received her Masters' degree from Columbia University Teachers College in counseling psychology and her doctorate from Drexel University in couple and family therapy. Her research and clinical interests include person of the therapist, couple's issues, medical family therapy, and coping with illness and trauma. She is the co-founder and the president of the Turkish Emotionally Focused Individual, Couple, and Family Therapies Association. She is currently serving on the board of the International Family Therapy Association.

Gita Seshadri, Ph.D., received her master's degree and doctoral degree in Marital and Family Therapy, from Loma Linda University. Currently she is an associate professor in the Couple and Family Therapy program at Alliant International University. She is also the Branch Director of the Sacramento campus for the CFT program. Seshadri is an AAMFT Clinical Fellow and Approved Supervisor and has been working in the field of CFT since 2003. Seshadri's research focuses on interracial couples and families, diversity, intersectionality, process based qualitative research, mentoring, and emotion management. Seshadri is currently clinically active in a small private practice.

K. Loette Snead, MA, AMFT, Loette is a registered Associate Marriage and Family Therapist in the state of California and a doctoral candidate in the Couple and Family Therapy Department at Alliant International University, Irvine. She works in an agency that provides therapeutic services to clients that have experienced chronic, complex, interpersonal trauma. She is passionate about working with clients that are exploring their ethnic-racial identities and coping with race-based traumatic stress.

Yudum Söylemez has a Masters's degree from the University of Massachusetts Boston MFT program and a Ph.D. in MFT from Antioch University New England. She is currently the coordinator of the CFT Track in Clinical Psychology Masters Program. She is a licensed Marriage and Family Therapist in Massachusetts, USA. Yudum is the past president of the Couple and Family Therapy Association of Turkey (ÇATED), vice president of the Turkish Psychological Association Istanbul branch, and a board member of the Emotionally Focused Individual, Couple and Family Therapy Association (DOÇAT). Her research interests are the effectiveness of family therapy, intergenerational transmission of family values, community work with disadvantaged populations in Turkey, technology, gender, culture, and family relationships.

Eman Tadros, Ph.D., is an assistant professor and the Marriage and Family Counseling Track Leader at Governors State University in the Division of Psychology and Counseling. She is a licensed marriage and family therapist, MBTI certified, and an AAMFT Approved Supervisor. She is the Illinois Family TEAM leader advocating for MFTs and individuals receiving systemic mental health services. Her research focuses on incarcerated couples and families.

Umberta Telfener, clinical psychologist with a degree in Philosophy and one in Psychology, has been a adjunct professor at the Ph.D. Course in Health Psychology of the University La Sapienza of Roma from 1998 till 2018. She has worked in a Public Health Center for ten years, is in private practice from 1980 and supervises the work of professionals both in private and public settings. She is a teacher of the Milan Family Therapy School (Boscolo & Cecchin), has edited many books and articles among which Sistemica, voci e percorsi nella complessità, a systemic dictionary built as a dialogical hypertext that she edited with the supervision of Heinz von Foerstert (Bollati Boringhieri, Torino 2003); Apprendere i contesti (Cortina Editore Milano 2011) on working in larger systems and institutions; Ricorsività in psicoterapia (Recursion in psychotherapy, Bollati Boringhieri, Torino 2014) on second order reflexive operations common to every form of psychotherapy. In the field of hypermodern relationships she has published Letti sfatti (Undone beds, Giunti 2018), Ho sposato un narciso (I married a narcissus/ daffodil, 2006) e Le forme dell'addio (Shapes of goodbye, 2007), La manutenzione dell'amore (Manutention of love, 2014) the last three by Castelvecchi publisher, Roma. She published many scientific articles both in Italian and foreign journals among which Becoming through belonging, the spiritual dimension in psychotherapy in the Australian and New Zeeland Journal of Family Therapy (Vol 38, N°1 pp. 206–220); Community Work and Psychotherapy as Two Sides of the Same Cooperative Practice in I. McCarthy, G. Simon Systemic Therapy as Transformative Practice, Everything Connected Pub 2016; she has co-edited a book on the evolution of the Milan school that has come out in Italian in may 2019: P.Barbetta, U.Telfener, Complexity and psychotherapy, the legacy of Boscolo and Cecchin, Cortina Editore, Milano.

Jia-Xin (Kailey) Teo was born in Singapore and moved to America with her family at a young age. Jia-Xin completed her Bachelor of Arts degree in Psychology with a minor in neuroscience from the University of Nevada, Las Vegas (UNLV). She is currently pursuing her Master's degree in Couple and Family Therapy at UNLV together with her husband. Jia-Xin is passionate to bring evidence-based practices to help individuals, couples and families in her clinical work and to broaden the utilization of mental health services in Asian communities and various faith communities.

Chi-Fang Tseng, PhD., is an assistant professor in the Couple and Family Therapy Doctoral Program in the Department of Human Development and Family Studies at Michigan State University. She is a native Taiwanese who holds a master's degree in Marriage and Family Therapy from the Purdue University Northwest. Before moving to the U.S., Chi-Fang also received a master's degree in Counseling Psychology from the National Taipei University of Education in Taiwan. She is also licensed as a Counseling Psychologist in Taiwan and worked with Taiwanese couples and families for five years. Chi-Fang's research interests include the cultural adaptation of evidence-based couple and family interventions, couple and family therapy outcome research, and Asian and immigrant couples and families.

Kimberly N. Usbeck was born and raised in Ecuador and graduated from the University of Nevada, Las Vegas with a bachelor's degree in Psychology along with a minor in Couples and Family Therapy. She is currently enrolled in the graduate program at Kirk Kerkorian School of Medicine at UNLV pursuing a master's degree in Couple and Family Therapy. As an undergraduate, Kimberly was a research assistant, worked at an emergency shelter for youth, served as the Chapter Public Relations Coordinator for Psi Chi, and held many other rewarding positions in organizations such as Alpha Xi Delta and Silver State Service Dogs. In her spare time, Kimberly enjoys painting, traveling and trying new things.

Alexis N. Washington is currently a 22 year old undergraduate student seeking a degree in psychology and a minor in MFT at University of Nevada, Las Vegas, and is an aspiring Marriage and Family Therapist. Her purpose is to support people in the way she wishes she could have been helped when she was younger. She has always wanted to help people in an impactful way, and continuing her education and challenging herself is a start.

Tabitha N. Webster, Ph.D., LMFT, a proud neurodivergent, is an Associate Professor for Alliant International University who loves experiential therapies. While Webster's clinical and research interests are many, they all center around the "hub" of trauma, its neurobiological and socio-cultural impacts on diverse individuals, couples, families, and children, and the systems they live in.

Lisa Werle, M.A. Counselling, was born in 1993 in Heidelberg, Germany. After graduating from high school, she worked at a psychiatric hospital while earning her Bachelor's Degree in Healthcare Economics through an integrated degree program. Having spent some time abroad, she then studied Counselling at Hochschule Neubrandenburg in Neubrandenburg, Germany. She now lives in Cologne, Germany and works with people who suffer from chronic mental illness or addictions as a social worker.

Elizabeth Ann Willems is a clinical psychologist, public speaker, and director of the hybrid virtual-in-person clinic Intercultural Psychological Services. She offers psychotherapy and neuropsychological assessment to adolescents and adults. She has served as an adjunct faculty member at Schiller International University. Additionally, she has trained, volunteered, and worked from bases in Mexico, Spain, Chile, and Czech Republic intermittently during short and long-term periods for more than ten years in total. Her work and training have taken place in association with various institutions such as University of Wisconsin in Milwaukee, Lesley University, and Harvard University in the USA as well as Tecnológico de Monterrey and Alliant international University in Mexico, Universidad de Valladolid, Spain, as well as Harvard's David Rockefeller Center for Latin American Studies, Chile.

Dai ("Daisy") Xing, BS, is a psychotherapist and counselor at the Neiguan Counseling Center in Shanghai, China. She has worked with the Institute since 2016. She is an honors graduate of Sino-American Family Therapy Institute (SAFTI) post-degree program.

Hu ("Yaoyao") Yaorui, BS, is a private practice therapist focusing on dance and movement therapy as well as family therapy in Shanghai, China. She has worked with the institute since 2016. She is an honors graduate of Sino-American Family Therapy Institute (SAFTI) post-degree program.

Melissa M. Yzaguirre (She/Her/Ella) is an assistant professor in the Department of Counseling and Marital and Family Therapy at the University of San Diego. She is a cisgender, heterosexual female, bilingual second-generation Mexican American, and first-generation college graduate. As a family therapist, Melissa has experience providing individual, couple, and family therapy for clients of diverse backgrounds (e.g., gender, sexual orientation, race/ethnicity, and language), including services for English and Spanish-speaking Latino populations. Additionally, Melissa is a three-time recipient of the SAMHSA Minority Fellowship Program. Melissa's program of research is based on her specified interest to advance culturally relevant practices among family therapists working with Latino families through an inclusive systemic application. Specifically, she is interested in understanding the translation of ethnic-racial socialization practices into the therapeutic context. She believes therapists can serve as social agents to support Latino families from the effects of ethnic-racial discrimination.

Ingo Zimmermann, Professor Dr., was born in 1971 in Münster, Germany, studied educational science, psychology, sociology and philosophy, holds a doctorate in health and nursing science and is a professor for social work and social sciences. He worked for 15 years in psychiatric clinics, especially child and adolescent psychiatric clinics, as well as youth welfare institutions. He is the training director of one of the largest institutes for the training of systemic consultants and therapists and family therapists in Germany and head of Dr. Zimmermann Consulting and carries out supervision, coaching, mediation and organizational development as well as couple and family therapy in his own practice. Education: Social therapist, systemic and family therapist (DGSF), systemic and family teaching therapist (DGSF), supervisor (DGSv), teaching supervisor (IFS, DGSv), coach (DCV), senior coach (DCV), teaching coach (DCV) and (business) Mediator (DTM). Certificate for value orientation in further education. Further training in: change management, Conflict Transformation and TRANSCEND by Johan Galtung, Motivational interviewing, Social ethics, Sexual Therapy, Hypnotherapy, Intercultural mediation, NLP, Psychodrama, Clinical study management, Sand play therapy according to D.Kalff, Qigong, Spiritual guidance etc.

FOREWORD

This text is one in which I hope you will find hope and clarity about what it means and looks like to be a systemic psychotherapist (often called family therapist or relational counselor) around the world. As a white, cisgender, educated male from the United States, I find I simultaneously have a lot and very little to offer an international community on the world of family therapy. The privilege to converse with and learn from so many of the giants in our field who authored these texts does give me the opportunity to think about it all as a whole.

My experience is one of feedback loops, interactive cycles, homeostasis, and the biopsychosocialspritual model. It is one of integrating theory and practice, of insurance and evidence-based models, of academic pressures and publication requirements that so few people in the field actively engage but is so vital in moving the Overton window of clinical excellence. I especially appreciated the historical nature of some chapters to deepen the thoughtful reflection of each culture's experiences. My work as a clinician both in private practice and in interdisciplinary group settings have taught me the importance of the common factors model to look beyond any one set of ideas or diagnostics. This text is full of generalizable tools and techniques. My work in hospitals and school settings have taught me the versatility of family resilience and the importance of social and economic infrastructure to support the amazing human beings we care about and want to support. Chapters in this text consistently point out the power dynamics in each context. Even those of you with varied professional backgrounds will find nuances within these pages to enhance both your perspective of the whole and specific.

In the pages and chapters of this textbook, you will find insights and wisdom, humor and pain, opportunities to grow and reminders that so many of you are already on the right path. Stories from all over the world round out the discourse often dominated with American ideology regarding medical treatment and clinical conceptualization. It is of course still in an academic format, in English, with editors and organizations entrenched in the Western world, but it does demonstrate truth and process beyond the borders of the US. Each chapter in this book offers an occasion to peek through a window with which you may not be familiar. Ideally, you will find nuggets of astuteness and clinical suggestions that have been distilled from the waters of each setting and personal story. Some of the chapters are meant to help understand and work in culturally diverse situations, others look at a particular model or idea in multiple contexts, while yet others dive deeply into a particular phenomenon in a particular location.

When one looks at systemic psychotherapy around the world from the global perspective, an important takeaway is that the field is and has always been wrestling with how to think about and interact with healing and growth from a relational perspective. The majority of countries and cultures where psychotherapy is practiced is based on an individual psychology, exacerbated by the medical model of individual health and healing. If you happen to be fortunate enough to talk to any of the truly systemic and dynamic thinkers in our field, they understand no person is isolated and alone. They use this fundamental truth to understand health and well-being as a dynamical and interactional reality. They understand and conceptualize disease and dysfunction from a lens that allows for the biological as well as the social. This text is full of authors sincerely and fervently reminding us to think in ways that align the abstract and the concrete.

The history of systemic psychotherapy is in many ways the intersection of paradigms of medical training, social work and human services, and spiritual healers. Different chapters in this text elucidate the ways in which practical and ancient wisdom are in dialogue with the technical and the political. Part of what I hope you get out of this book, and I certainly have, is a reminder that we are all trying to figure out life and ways to get through it together. And it is my belief, and so well-articulated throughout this book, that the notion of togetherness can be summed up and maintained through four core virtues of patience, respect, humility, and curiosity. As you read and engage these texts, continue to hold in your mind and heart these virtues. The stories of the authors, as well as the clinical situations they talk about come to life as the human element of diagnosis and treatment becomes an artistic and colorful expression of the human condition.

Since most places where systemic psychotherapy is done as a profession also have powerful and privileged arenas of hospitals and medical practices regulated by university training programs and governmental oversight bodies, the paradigm of regulation and license is also pervasive for relational therapy. Differences of training and scopes of practice and regulation are not comprehensively outlined in this text, but it is useful to remember each situation has different ways of creating and maintaining mental health professionals. Licensure or certification in most places that have such a designation is typically done at the graduate level, and typically takes two to four years. There are some exceptions where one can claim to be a family therapist or systemic psychotherapist with only weeks of specialized training, but even these places typically have requirements of experience and education to provide mental health services. The majority of these regulations have been put in placed in order to protect the public from charlatans and professional abuse, and as a whole, they are effective at reducing the amount of harms done by professionals. Globalization and international collaboration have also ensured countries and associations improve their codes of ethics that guide and hold accountable the actions of its professionals.

Currently, the global field is also in the midst of a reawakening around the art of psychotherapy from the rigidity of the science of psychotherapy. Europe in particular is attempting to find professional and academic ways to demonstrate that practice-based evidence is a valuable epistemology toward clinical excellence in ways the evidence-base practice movement was often so dismissive. Clinicians and helping professionals in more collectivist cultures have known the importance of interactive healing and growth since the beginning, of the value of the phrase "when in doubt, expand the system." This pushback and ethical resistance to some of the medical model hegemony has inspired clinicians and even training programs to reengage experiential and inductive learning. The dangers of capitalism and optimizing people as commodities for productivity have been thoroughly revealed to those who have paid attention, and postmodern deconstruction has facilitated us to questioned why the human being has been pressured into becoming a human doing.

Systemic psychotherapy has become a vessel for change by reminding people when they slow down, check their assumptions, and engage each other with those four core relational virtues, we can be seen and loved and valued. People can be reminded their trauma and their suffering is not because they are "crazy" or "broken," but rather that their reactions are normal and understandable responses to unhealthy situations and social dynamics. It is the belief and hope of family systemic psychotherapists around the world (and authors throughout this text) that when we engage people in their communication and connections, all kinds of change become available. This text reveals how to think about clinical situations you may be familiar with, but from a different cultural lens. This text beckons us to come to the larger table with our recipes to share. This text has something to offer any professional in any mental health field around the world, and I hope you find it as comprehensively engaging and inspiring as I did.

Daniel Stillwell, Ph.D., LMFT – United States

PREFACE

This addition to Routledge's series on International Handbooks is a special one for me. The invitation came shortly after I returned from my Fulbright experience and had a renewed appreciation for the practice of therapy (and education) across the globe. The mission of Fulbright is simple: it is to increase mutual understanding across people in the world through education. With this mission firmly in mind, I set out to fashion this book in a similar image: to educate couple and family therapy professionals across the world to who we are as a field and to understand what connects us as professionals, no matter where we live. In this text, my vision was to present different practice strategies, perspectives, and worldviews to encourage cooperation and conversation to generate more interventions.

Another goal for this text, however, is to teach how to embrace difference. In this trying political time, the global landscape is changing. New lines and new territories are being drawn as we speak with little knowledge about what is to come. It is this time when we need to demonstrate more empathy, connection, and compassion than ever.

This book is one of the several texts within Routledge's International Handbook series. Routledge's International Handbooks are prestige reference works providing an overview of a whole subject area or sub-discipline, and which survey the state of the discipline including emerging and cutting-edge areas. The aim of the series is to produce a comprehensive, up-to-date, definitive work of reference that can be cited as an authoritative source about Couple and Family Therapy on a global scale. The objective in the *Routledge International Handbook of Couple and Family Therapy* is to add on to the distinguished legacy of the those in the series that have come before it. We aim to present a highly focused and comprehensive text that promotes innovative frameworks and interventions in couple and family therapy from a cross-cultural perspective. In this text, the authors will be exploring the role that demography, regionality, cultural and political crises, and policy have on the issues faced by couples and families. Collectively, the chapters articulate unique ideas in conceptualizing the needs of families with international backgrounds, adapting the current models and frameworks to work with this population most effectively. In short, this text is designed to assist systemic therapists in critically reviewing their approaches to working with those from international backgrounds as well as to advance research with an international focus in our discipline.

The book is divided into four sections: Personal Voices and Philosophical Perspectives, Theory and Models in an International Context, Specific Applications with International Populations, and Emerging Perspectives. In addition, for continuity between the chapters and sections, each author was asked to include the following in their chapter:

- Clinical examples/application
- Reflection on where the research agenda is likely to advance in the future
- Resources and Further Reading (a brief list; these can be electronic links, library resources, online journals, etc.)
- "Three Key Takeaways" section: what are the three key points the reader should take away from your chapter?

We hope you enjoy the book!

ACKNOWLEDGMENTS

I want to acknowledge the many people who have contributed to this book. Our editors at Taylor & Francis were always available and extremely helpful. Thank you to Sarah Gore and the amazing staff at Taylor & Francis, who always made time for me and my questions and ideas. I also thank my husband, Eric, who showed infinite patience and support when working on this project. I am also indebted to my wonderful editorial assistant, Mr. Ricky Raphael, who kept on top of correspondence to contributors, drafts, and my schedule. He has a keen eye for editing, and I look forward to his successful career. I am sure I speak for all the contributors when I say that we are very humbled by the clients who have been vulnerable with us in sharing their struggles, feelings, and successes. This book would not be possible without you.

SECTION I

Personal Voices and Philisophical Perspectives

1

THE STATE OF COUPLE AND FAMILY THERAPY INTERNATIONALLY

Katherine M. Hertlein and Alexis N. Washington

Introduction

As Helen Keller once said, "Although the world is full of suffering, it is full also of the overcoming of it." As therapists, we are on the front lines of hearing the suffering from clients all over and working with them to overcome that suffering. The suffering Keller referenced seems to be growing. We are in a global mental health crisis. (Patterson et al., 2018). Depression and anxiety are increasing in prevalence at alarming levels, even for young people (Phillips & Yu, 2021). Mainstream news reports war, disease, shootings, climate disasters, and human atrocities, which serves to surround us with negative and distressing content that can negatively impact our psychological state (Chao et al., 2020). At the same time, the resources to manage these serious issues are limited due to access challenges, personnel shortages, disparity in treatment, and disrespect toward patients with mental health diagnoses (Larrier et al., 2017). Depression and anxiety are also associated with increases in physical disability, a finding that is especially true for those in low- to middle-income countries (Ma et al., 2023; World Health Organization, 2017). In addition, the rise in social media usage worldwide has also ushered in a new era of challenges in socialization, which has resulted in its own physical and psychological problems. From cyberbullying to catfishing to sexting, all the way to sleep and posture problems, social media usage and advances in technology have had a profound effect on our well-being (Hertlein & Twist, 2019; Hertlein & Ancheta, 2014; Hertlein & van Dyck, 2018). Each of these issues increases the need for effective intervention to return to a healthy state of being, both personally and globally.

Couple and family therapists are uniquely positioned to address the burgeoning need introduced by our contemporary world. The evaluation of the multiple factors responsible for our constraints and conditions can be attended to by systems therapists who are trained to see how the interaction between the multiple factors also might contribute to a symptom, condition, or maladaptive pattern.

DOI: 10.4324/9781003297871-2

History of Couple and Family Therapy

Anyone desiring a historical reference as to the development of family therapy need to look no further than Ng's (2005) article and Ng's (2003) book about the development of family therapy across global markets. In the United States, the story might begin in New York in the early 1940s when a group of interdisciplinary scholars met to discuss communication in both machines and non-machines. Gregroy Bateson, an attendee at this meeting, brought the ideas discussed in the meeting about information, communication, control, and feedback (termed "cybernetics") into a burgeoning new field of family therapy (Piercy et al., 1986). From Bateson's ideas on the cybernetic principles of communication as well as Bateson's relationships came the emergence of specific models who each sought to change family patterns in different ways. Meanwhile, in Italy, the Milan school of therapy's focus was on helping families identify problems within their interactions sequences to direct change in their family system (Borsca et al., 2013; Piercy et al., 1986). Each of these perspectives pushed us to really examine the way in which individual elements of communication evolved in relationships and what meanings were made as a result of interactions with one another.

And the world kept turning. The family therapy of the 1950s and 1960s, chiefly provided by psychiatrists, gave way to new professional identities and ideas in the 1970s through evolving sociopolitical contexts, global events, and the changing needs of the families served. The original view that family therapy was rooted in theories that "used a unidirectional, reductionist analysis emphasizing the role of family relationships in mental health problems" (Wampler et al., 2019, p. 7) was challenged. As Salvador Minuchin astutely put it in an interview with Celia Falicov at the International Family Therapy Association Conference in 2013, "We started family therapy by denying that the individual existed. We all agreed. We agreed that the past wasn't important...we were wrong." (Minuchin, 2013). We learned more. We shifted how we thought to incorporate what we found worked and what did not.

Similarly, couple therapy also endured transformational phases. Gurman and Fraenkel (2002) trace these traditions across four phases: atheoretical marital counseling formation, psychoanalytic experimentation, family therapy incorporation, and refinement, extension, diversification, and integration. While the authors define couples therapy, for the purposes of their writing, as "the prototypic case that focuses primarily on dyadic relational elements," (p. 202), the spirit of the text demonstrates the ever-changing nature of who was included in the conjoint therapy process as well as evolution to frameworks and models.

Couple and family therapy both had to adapt and welcome new ideas about the etiology of problems in relationships and develop effective strategies to treat them. This included widening the lens to incorporate a biopsychosocial model with emphasis on interpersonal relationships that affect an individual (Wampler et al., 2019, p. 7). In other words, the system was expanded to include more than the people in the room; it was also to include the context supporting the individual and family, which included their biology. It was this system that had to be added in the conceptualizations of couple and fanily therapy to maintain positive change in the family system will allow the patient to succeed in their treatment. Developing solutions to problems within the couple and family facilitates how clients carry out change long term while shaping a more supportive environment to maintain improvements and growth.

The Role of a Therapist

Just as the field of couple and family therapy has changed over time, so has the role of the therapist. For those following a Milan practice toward the origins of systemic therapy, the role of the therapist is distant; it is an observer, who is tasked with describing and understanding what transpires in the family system (Piercy et al., 1986). As treatment models evolved, the role of the therapist also exists on a continuum. At one extreme, it is more akin to the observer; at the other end, it can be highly directive. For many apporoaches, the role of the therapist is somewhere in the continuum.

As it pertains to this text, the role of a therapist can mean different things in different cultures. Therapists are critical change agents in the process and their relationships with clients. Therapists who continue to study and apply the knowledge in treatment settings are more effective (Blow & Karam, 2017). In addition, effective therapists should have a talent for therapy. The role of the therapist is also affected by the layers in which the therapist and clients are embedded. For example, the role of a therapist in open litigation in high conflict divorce cases is often to stay in one role and not serve the family in multiple and confusing roles (Knapp & Mapes, 2017). It may be that there are some cultural contexts where the role of the therapist is more direct and other cases where the role of the therapist is indirect.

The role of a therapist may also be compromised by a general misunderstanding about the role from the public and other professional entities. While couple and family therapists do see couples and families, to limit our work to only seeing couples and families does not fully and accurately describe the role a couple and family therapist has in our current healthcare system (Thoburn & Sexton, 2016; Wampler et al., 2019). Fot example, in countries such as India therapy may be handled in an informal fashion by relatives, friends, or priests. It is these differences that set the field apart from other healthcare professions, but also lend to some of the misunderstandings about the nature of couple and family therapy.

Practice Pattern Differences

People go to couple and family therapy for many different reasons, both articulated and unarticulated. Common issues cited by therapists for their clients include substance use, communication issues, role shifts, lack of loving feelings, sexuality problems, money, and parenting discord. Members of the professional association, the American Association for Marriage and Family Therapy, cite the most common problems they treat in marriage and family sessions are depression and anxiety, marital-couple issues, sexual abuse, and parent-adolescent conflicts, anger management, ADD, and school issues (Christner et al., 2007; Doherty & Simmons, 1996; Palmer, 2017). It is also noted that about 42% of clinicians' time is spent on couples and family therapy while the rest is spent on individual therapy (Palmer, 2017, p. 51). Additionally, couples or families who participate in therapy together might also wish to participate in individual therapy.

In European countries, the reasons for going to couples and family therapy may be the result of how families are affected by or respond to social change. It might also be an attempt to resolve issues related to families' transitions, such as roles, rules, and gender. In a study done by Giovanna Gianesini (2014) on European family structures, it was found

European families face a number of different political, social, and cultural challenges. They might include:

> the redefinition of gender roles, the need for reconciliation between family and work, the presence of immigrants taking up the role of caregivers and a second demographic transition have caused tensions and conflicts due to inequalities in access to social services and inadequate negotiations among genders and generations.
>
> (p.1)

In sum American households seem to be centered around the married couple, and topics of infidelity or individual psychological issues like depression and anxiety. European nations are more focused on how large transitions affect the family, including social transitions such as the aging of children, new marriages, gender roles, and careers.

Theoretical Emphases in Different Regions

Couples and families as well as individuals go to therapy for many different reasons. As noted earlier, U.S. citizens report seeking services for depression and anxiety; on the other hand, European families seek services related to transitions within the families. As a result, there are a vast number of theories therapists use to be able to treat these issues. To address the changing needs of the couples and families served, long-standing models are being applied in unique and innotiave ways. For example, frameworks that originated in the early phase of theory development in family therapy were criticized for not attending to current contexts and sitautions (i.e., Hare-Mustin's 1978 critique of structural family therapy). As the field began to adopt more postmodern perspectives, these theories shifted away from the core systemic principles such as hierarchy and family structure (Wampler et al., 2019).

While it is not the purpose of this chapter to present and review each of the models and frameworks for couple and family therapy, the point is to recognize that different models and frameworks may vary in popularity depending on the region. In part, this is due to differences in how constructs in couple and family therapy vary based on culture. For example, the definition of intimacy differs culturally, thus resulting in unique experiences, meanings, and presenting problems (Abele et al., 2020). The region itself may have a prominent set of frameworks used the interventions used might also be shaped by the political context of the region. In cultures affected by war, for example, some therapists have used scaling questions and reflecting teams to address the specific needs of that population (Charles, 2010).

No matter what type of therapeutic model a therapist uses, the client-to-clinician relationship is key, because "patients are more likely to drop out from treatment when there is lack of congruence between patients' and therapists' expectations of potential treatment interventions" (McIntosh et. al., 2016). The therapist and the client need to be on the same page about the expectations they have that the client will succeed in treatment. The client also needs to be motivated in their recovery. Whether it is CBT or IFT, the client–therapist relationship is essential to growth.

Licensure Processes and Credentials for Professional Organizations

To be a couples and family therapist anywhere there are credentials that must be met to practice. In the United States two of the top organizations that paved the way for couple and family therapy are the American Association of Marriage and Family Therapists (AAMFT) and the Council on Accreditation for Marriage and Family Education (COAMFTE). AAMFT began as a way to separate the practice of MFT from social work, psychology, and psychiatry (Erikson, 1999, p. 9). MFT professionals wanted to emphasize the effect of family on an individual's mental health. The AAMFT advocated for specific training and standards for couple and family therapists. The COAMFTE recognizes that couple and family therapy is a separate practice from other mental health practices, and created certain accreditations state by state for licensure for couples and family therapy including "course requirements, supervision requirements, required hours of supervised experience, and required hours of direct client contact" (Erikson, 1999, p. 9) that must be completed to become licensed. In addition, the professional association itself is evolving. Recently they have dropped the annual conference name from "Marriage and Family Therapy" to "Systemic Therapy" in a shift back to their roots and to promote greater inclusivity.

The Institute of Family Therapy (IFT) is an organization started in the 1970s that emphasizes training and therapy nationally and internationally, and is now the largest training organization in the United Kingdom (Singh, 2005, p. 289). The IFT noticed that refugees and immigrants were coming into countries that were unfamiliar with their family struggles because of the lack of education on their cultural background, making it difficult for couple and family therapists to deliver appropriate treatment. The IFT began The Refugee Program in London, England that provides training to couple and family therapists centered on: "basic counseling and family work skills, and hence promote the access of black and minority ethnic families to culturally appropriate training and mental health services" (Singh, 2005, p. 290). The programs offered include skills workshops, discussion, and lectures, with emphasis on topics like language barriers, diversity, case consultations, the strengths of refugees, and beyond (Singh, 2005, pp. 290–291).

Finally, telehealth has established itself as a bonafide manner in which to treat individuals, couples, and families. The licensing laws in the United States, however, vary from state to state and change frequently. Readers are encouraged to check with their state licenseing boards and online resource to determine the current status of licenses for telehealth. One option is reading the telehealth certification website (https://telementalhealthtraining.com/states-rules-and-regulations) where a listing of updated state regulations is posted.

So Where Does That Leave Us?

The professional associations for couple and family therapy have also become involved in the politics of day-to-day living. Cloud (1997) summarizes the broad work of therapists by connecting the ideas of understanding the sociopolitical context in which our couples and families are embedded as being based on the work of founders such as Bateson. She encourages therapists to consider the roles they may play in cases of highly politicized contexts, deprivation, racism, and other social issues that contribute to the issues families have (Mirkin, 1990).

Today, in a world of difference, we find it unthinkable to describe anything with-out including the subject involved in the description. Equally unthinkable for us is the belief that an experience could be replicated or applied to another, let alone to claim universal standing. We find it unthinkable to assert these three pillars of theCartesian scientific model. Instead, today we think that, in order to describe, we must assume that our concepts are inadequate for translating the concepts of others. It is thus necessary to integrate both proposals – the other and ours – in a new shared assemblage, not as a synthesis of both but as a way to "contain the difference." This is the sense and the value we see in Bateson's concept of double description (Bateson,1982, p. 82).

(Cavagnis, p. 265)

Final Thoughts

The evolution of couple and family therapy is not over. To effectively grow as a field – globally – we need to "develop an appropriate, widely accepted and comprehensive framework for articulating the identity of CMFT and the extensive scholarship that underlies both the practice and profession" (Wampler et al., 2019, p. 15). In our view, family therapy as a story of creativity, as a story of science, and as a story of innovation.

Family Therapy is a Story of Innovation and Creativity

As a science based on systems, communication, and context, as the world changes, therapists must come to the table with new ways to intervene in contemporary problems. Part of how we might be nimble in adapting to shifting circumstances and problems is through our theory development and refinement. Wampler et al. (2019) summarize the theoretical trends and shifts in the theory utilization. The theoretical frameworks – or at least the way in which we develop and evaluate the effectiveness of our theories and approaches – need revision (Wampler et al., 2019). The field has to be innovative in creating new approaches grounded in the systemic foundations and conceptualizations.

In her article describing the development of family therapy around the world, Ng (2005) noted that creativity is one of the foremost distinctive characteristics of Italian family therapy. and has also translated into psychotherapy and family therapy and other regions. For example, a lot of the training programs had to be quite creative in the early days of family therapy as people began to understand that providing family therapy made more impressive outcomes.

Family Therapy is a Story Of Science

Maturana, a legend in cybernetic thought and general systems theory, was convinced that cybernetics was both science and art of understanding. In today's managed care environment, family therapy must also emphasize the importance of measurement and effectiveness (Wampler et al., 2019). We can develop contemporary methods to more effectively measure progress in treatment, including relevant and unique approaches from an evidence-based perspective. In short, we must ensure we are employing the most effective practices in our work, and teaching our trainees to do the same. At the same time it is important to be able to measure the characteristics and qualities of a skillful therapist. As Blow and Karam (2017) remind us, it is not just about the evidence-based practice but also about the talent of the therapist delivering the treatment: good therapists have both. As therapists attempt to identify one's talents in therapy in a more formal manner, it should result in more cohesive and appropriate treatments. This may be characterized by a well-developed research agenda testing the different types of models/frameworks and interventions that we have come to know. It also may involve developing new ones in pursuit of knowledge and as a way to address the continuing new problems facing families.

Family Therapy is a Story of How to Reinvent Yourself

Finally, family therapy is a story of how to reinvent ourselves in both in the issues we take on and the ways in which we measure our effectiveness. One primary example of this is the way in which family therapy had to reinvent itself to provide treatment during the pandemic. The field of family therapy had not fully embraced online practice. The emphasis and the value placed on in-person meetings may have made prevented us from fully embracing telebehavioral health. This left many practitioners and training programs scrambling when the pandemic hit. In addition, therapists had to reinvent ways to evaluate whether teletherapy practices were effective. As Wampler et al. (2019) suggests, measurement of our effectiveness is a cornerstone to moving forward. Hertlein et al. (2021) also notes the importance of having a plan moving forward to ensure that the strategies that were developed in isolation during the pandemic are being executed in effective and appropriate ways. This might require a encouraging supervisors and clinicians to adopt the perspective that they are still learners. This also corresponds with what Blow and Karam (2017) discussed about the lifelong student perspective, which ultimately makes therapists more effective (Hertlein et al., 2021a; 2021b).

In short, we look back to the advice of Wampler et al. (2019):

> To be leaders, we must be informed. As such, it would be valuable to incorporate more training on systemic evidence-based models into our curriculum. There are a number of barriers, however, to doing so. Training costs tied to some of these models pose a significant obstacle. In academic contexts in which shrinking budgets are a reality, we, as a discipline, must determine which training costs are priorities.
>
> (p. 15)

As a discipline, we need to get back to our roots by embracing the way in which family therapy is practiced worldwide and continue to learn from each other.

References

Abela, A., Vella, S., & Piscopo, S. (2020). *Couple relationships in a global context understanding love and intimacy across cultures*. Springer.

Bateson, G. (1982). *Espíritu y Naturaleza*. Buenos Aires: Amorrortu.

Blow, A., & Karam, E. A. (2017). The therapist's role in effective marriage and family therapy practice: The case for evidence based therapists. *Administration and Policy in Mental Health and Mental Health Services Research*, 44(5), 716–723. https://doi.org/10.1007/s10488-016-0768-8

Cavagnis, M. E. (2021). An ethno-eco-systemic perspective: The coming into being of a family therapy institution in Argentina – politics, practices, and experiences. *Australian and New Zealand Journal of Family Therapy*, 42(3), 261–275. https://doi.org/10.1002/anzf.1463

Chao, M., Xue, D., Liu, T., Yang, H., & Hall, B. J. (2020). Media use and acute psychological outcomes during COVID-19 outbreak in China. *Journal of Anxiety Disorders*, 74, 102248–102248. https://doi.org/10.1016/j.janxdis.2020.102248

Charles, L. (2010). Family therapists as front line mental health providers in war-affected regions: using reflecting teams, scaling questions, and family members in a hospital in Central Africa. *Journal of Family Therapy*, 32(1), 27–42. https://doi.org/10.1111/j.1467-6427.2009.00481.x

Christner, R. W., Stewart, J. L., & Freeman, A. (2007). *Handbook of cognitive-behavior group therapy with children and adolescents: specific settings and presenting problems.* Routledge.

Cloud, D. L. (1997). *Control and Consolation in American Culture and Politics: Rhetoric of Therapy.* New York: Sage Publications.

Doherty, W. J., & Simmons, D. S. (1996). Clinical practice patterns of marriage and family therapists: a national survey of therapists and thier clients. *Journal of Marital and Family Therapy, 22*(1), 9–25. https://doi.org/10.1111/j.1752-0606.1996.tb00183.x

Eriksen, K. (1999). Marriage and family licensing, state by state. *The Family Journal, 7*(1), 7–17. https://doi-org.ezproxy.library.unlv.edu/10.1177/1066480799071002

Gianesini, G. (2014). European families: structures, policies and social trends.

Gurman, A. S., & Fraenkel, P. (2002). The history of couple therapy: A millennial review. *Family Process, 41*(2), 199–260. https://doi.org/10.1111/j.1545-5300.2002.41204.x

Hare-Mustin, R. (1987). The problem of gender in family therapy theory. *Family Process, 26*(1), 15–27. https://doi.org/10.1111/j.1545-5300.1987.00015.x

Hertlein, K. M., & Ancheta, K. (2014). Advantages and disadvantages of technology in relationships: findings from an open-ended survey. *Qualitative Report, 19*(11), 1–11. https://doi.org/10.46743/2160-3715/2014.1260

Hertlein, K. M., Drude, K. P., & Jordan, S. S. (2021a). "What Next?": Toward telebehavioral health sustainability in couple and family therapy. *Journal of Marital and Family Therapy, 47*(3), 551–565. https://doi.org/10.1111/jmft.12510

Hertlein, K. M., Drude, K. P., Hilty, D. M., & Maheu, M. M. (2021b). Toward proficiency in telebehavioral health: applying interprofessional competencies in couple and family therapy. *Journal of Marital and Family Therapy, 47*(2), 359–374. https://doi.org/10.1111/jmft.12496

Hertlein, K. M., & van Dyck, L. (2020). Predicting engagement in electronic surveillance in romantic relationships. *Cyberpsychology and Behavior, 23*(9), https://doi.org/10.1089/cyber.2019.0424.

Hertlein, K. M., Twist, M. L. C. (2019). *The internet family: Technology in couple and family relationships.* Routledge.

Knapp, S., & Mapes, B. (2017). Boundaries for forensic and treating psychologists. *The Pennsylvania Psychologist, 77*(1), 1-5.

Larrier, Y., Allen, M. D., & Larrier, I. M. (2017). The role of stigma in the global mental health crisis: A literature review. *Journal of Global Engagement and Transformation, 1*(1). https://doi.org/10.52553/10001a

Lebow, J., Chambers, A. L., Christensen, A., & Johnson, S. M. (2012). Research on the treatment of couple distress. *Journal of Marital and Family Therapy, 38*(1), 145–168. https://doi.org/10.1111/j.1752-0606.2011.00249.x

Ma, R., Romano, E., Vancampfort, D., Firth, J., Stubbs, B., & Koyanagi, A. (2023). Association between physical activity and comorbid anxiety/depression in 46 low- and middle-income countries. *Journal of Affective Disorders, 320*, 544–551. https://doi.org/10.1016/j.jad.2022.10.002

Masters, W. H., & Johnson, V. (1966). *Human sexual response.* Boston: Little Brown.

Masters, W. H., & Johnson, V. (1970). *Human sexual inadequacy.* Boston: Little, Brown.

McIntosh, V. V. W., Jordan, J., Carter, J. D., Frampton, C. M. A., McKenzie, J. M., Latner, J. D., & Joyce, P. R. (2016). Psychotherapy for transdiagnostic binge eating: A randomized controlled trial of cognitive-behavioural therapy, appetite-focused cognitive-behavioural therapy, and schema therapy. *Psychiatry Research, 240*, 412–420. https://doi-org.ezproxy.library.unlv.edu/10.1016/j.psychres.2016.04.080

Minuchin, S. (2013, February 20). *An Encounter Between Two Old Friends:Salvador Minuchin and Celia Falicov.* Workshop at the International Family Therapy Association Congress, Orlando, CA, USA.

Mirkin, M. P. (Ed.). (1990). *The social and political contexts of family therapy.* Allyn & Bacon.

Ng, K. S. (2003). *Global perspectives in family therapy: development, practice, and trends.* Brunner-Routledge.

Ng, K. S. (2005). The development of family therapy around the world. *The Family Journal, 13*(1), 35–42. https://doi.org/10.1177/1066480704270264

Palmer, Thane R., "A Profile of Professional Activities and Practice Patterns for Marriage and Family Therapists in Utah" (1998). All Graduate Theses and Dissertations. 2545. https://digitalcommons.usu.edu/etd/2545

Patterson, J., Edwards, T. M., & Vakili, S. (2018). Global mental health: A call for increased awareness and action for family therapists. *Family Process*, 57(1), 70–82. https://doi.org/10.1111/famp.12281

Piercy, F. P., Sprenkle, D. H., & Wetchler, J. (1986). *Family therapy sourcebook*. Guilford Press.

Phillips, S. P., & Yu, J. (2021). Is anxiety/depression increasing among 5–25 year-olds? A cross-sectional prevalence study in Ontario, Canada, 1997-2017. *Journal of Affective Disorders*, 282, 141–146. https://doi.org/10.1016/j.jad.2020.12.178

Singh, R. (2005). Therapeutic skills for working with refugee families: an introductory course at the Institute of Family Therapy. *Journal of Family Therapy*, 27(3), 289–292.

Thoburn, J. W., & Sexton, T. L. (2016). *Family psychology: Theory, research, and practice*. Santa Barbara, CA: Praeger.

Wampler, K., Blow, A. J., McWey, L. M., Miller, R. B., & Wampler, R. S. (2019). The profession of Couple, Marital, and Family Therapy (CMFT): Defining ourselves and moving forward. *Journal of Marital and Family Therapy*, 45(1), 5–18. https://doi.org/10.1111/jmft.12294

World Health Organization. (2017). *Depression and other common mental disorders: global health estimates* (No. WHO/MSD/MER/2017.2). World Health Organization.

Wynne, L. C., McDaniel, S. H., & Weber, T. T. (1987). Professional politics and the concepts of family therapy, family consultation, and systems consultation. *Family Process*, 26(2), 153–166.

2

ADDRESSING EXISTENTIAL CONCERNS IN FAMILIES AMONGST CONTEMPORARY SHIFTS

A Psychoanalytic, Object Relations Perspective

Cheri L. Hausmann

Introduction

In this chapter, I draw from various philosophical, historical, and psychoanalytic sources to gain insight and epistemic benefit for the assistance of families dealing with the loss of a family member through death, and the potential corresponding existential crises. I also present psychoanalytic thought and historical reference to point to the universality of its application, which presupposes a relevance for clinical work in the field of marriage and family therapy for an international audience.

I use the terms client, patient, and family unit interchangeably in association with direct treatment from a clinical lens. I also to some degree use the terms psychotherapy, family therapy, and relational therapy as synonymous in this chapter. While I make the distinction between relational psychoanalysis, systems therapy, and traditional psychoanalysis, I seek to find their common identifiers corresponding with psychoanalytic thought, philosophy, family systems, and the presenting universal concerns of loss and grief that may arise in a clinical space.

The discussion provided in this chapter can open up further research and insight into how family therapists can effectively view treatment modalities concerning existential crises and death. In that, I argue for a more philosophical focus in viewing therapeutic cases informed by Socratic thought and drawing on the work of Sigmund Freud and Melanie Klein.

Case examples are also presented in relation to death and bereavement applicable to modern concerns for family therapists.

Phenomenology of Death in Families

Within the psychotherapy space, particularly when working with families experiencing grief, loss, and questions of death, conversations involving the meaning of life and the nature of

DOI: 10.4324/9781003297871-3

suffering may arise. Depending upon the level of association with a lost family member and the variables of cultural expectations in the processing of grief, systems therapists help clients navigate their emotional response and find appropriate ways to deal with grief.

Coming to terms with the loss of a loved one may involve questions about mortality. In the United States, in particular, death is not typically explored in a public manner. The dead lie underground in cushioned caskets or are cremated and kept tucked away in urns. Loved ones seek to quickly mourn or may potentially deny themselves the space to grieve the departed. But eventually, the living may come to acknowledge the fragility of life as they contemplate the memories of the deceased.

The concept of death can vary among cultures according to spiritual, religious, cultural, and anthropological contexts. Family units are largely influenced by the cultural context in which they find themselves; children identify with the religion of their parents. The church, temple, or holy place can be a common place of refuge of for questions such as the meaning of life and death. This may be especially true in societies where death is a taboo and avoided. The lack of insight concerning death in areas contemporary society may lead to a systemic denial: an underlying perpetuating anxiety with no outlet for release or objective reflection.

On the other hnd, there are some scoieties who have a different relationship with death than avoiding it. The river Ganges, for example, are known to theHindu population to be sacred and used publicly as a funeral pyre where the dead are set ablaze bearing flowers and ornaments (Bhagirath, 2014). In some parts of India, both death and life are intergrated into religious and spiritual traditions.

A Historical Shift in Family Dynamics Due to War

During the early 1940s in the United States, the progression of the Second World War began to create a shift in the dynamics of traditional family life. Women were called to fill the roles of the men brought into battle. Propaganda such as "Rosie the Riveter" bearing messages of "We Can Do It" were driven into the minds of American culture (Fussell,1989).

With casualties topping 60 to 70 million, the entire world was shaken by loss (Vagts, 1945). Scenes of atrocity haunted those who remained alive. Even after multiple generations have lived and died, the effects of grief, post-traumatic stress, substance abuse, suicide, and physical impairments as a result of injury remain in the genealogy of families.

The war during the early 1940s would dominate all aspects of life for countries of the axis and allied alike. The significant loss of life that impacted men, women, and children in Europe, Japan, China and the United States, created an environment of near to global mourning. Grief-stricken families relied heavily upon community to restore and heal from the impacts of loss that would affect families for generations. Due to the significant impact of government involvement in the lives of citizens and the millions of men, women, and children who lost their lives, religious centers and family homes if still standing, were turned into places of solace and mourning in most places directly impacted in Europe, Japan, and beyond (Vagts, 1945).

Freud and Death in Psychoanalysis

Before family therapy as a branch of psychotherapy fully developed, Freud oriented admits to psychoanalytic training to administer applications for the relief of neurosis as the primary presenting concern in early 19th century Europe. Starting initially through applications of hypnotherapy, psychoanalysis began as a derivative of Freud's work with hypnosis (Rieff, 1977). With little consideration for treating the entire family system at the time, hypnotherapy would eventually come to be utilized by Jay Haley's mentor, Milton Erickson. Jay Haley, an American family systems pioneer, developed strategic family therapy out of his work with Dr. Erickson (Haley, 1973).

In Plato's *Phaedo*, Socrates asserts, "those who pursue philosophy aright study nothing but dying and being dead." (p. 64a). Freud also asserted something similar when he said in *Beyond the Pleasure Principle*, "the goal of all life is death" (p. 30). Freud sought to define the human condition based on mechanisms of objective reasoning. Specifically, many threads in orientation can possibly link Freud's assertion about death to logical positivism. According to a chapter titled *Psychoanalysis and Logical Positivism*, by Phillipp Frank, there is a degree of scientific confirmation:

> Since the second quarter of our twentieth century the principal advocate of strict criteria for admission has been the school of Logical Positivism which originated from the "Vienna Circle." The psychoanalytic doctrines called "meaningless" or "tautological," as representatives of Logical Positivism have often and gladly branded the doctrines of "school philosophy" like Platonism... according to the usage of terms in modern science, a theory is "scientifically confirmed" if, firstly, all facts which are derived from the theory are in agreement with actual observation.
>
> (Frank, 1990)

Freud postulated that all persons fluctuate between the reality principle and the pleasure principle. That is, the reason an individual, couple, or family might seek psychotherapy treatment can be derived to a large degree from a need to release psychological pain and suffering personally and relationally (Levi, 1959).

The school of psychoanalysis initially evolved out of the structural drive model; Freud sought to define the human condition as first emanating from a biological basis and its associations to that of Darwinian theory (Levi, 1959). Although Freudian analysis is primarily focused on the analyst treating an individual, the content arising in the analysis is typical of a relational basis. Davies (2010) uncovers the following about Freud in the use of psychoanalytic concepts:

> Freud's work was influential in moving professional thinking from a focus on symptoms to an emphasis on the central importance of primary family relationships and, in analysis, on the relationship between analyst and patient.
>
> (p. 6)

Psychoanalysis at its origin derives from a relational unfolding within the therapeutic space itself. Largely, there is a focus on the polarity between the libidinal and anti-libidinal instincts. Synonymously, the libidinal is the sex drive and one's procreative factors, whereas the anti-libidinal is likened to the death drive and one's aggressive components (Segal, 1964). The death drive was based on the work of Sabina Spielrein, a former patient and herself an analyst. Acknowledged by a footnote in Freud's *Beyond the Pleasure Principle*, Spielrein's work in *Destruction and the Cause of Coming into Being* became popular and would play a role in the preliminary basis of the death drive theory in psychoanalysis (Skea, 2016).

Object Relations Psychoanalysis

Transference conditions are a key focus in the applications of psychoanalytic therapy (Horner, 1991). Klein asserted that the transference dynamic is based on nuances derived from birth in relational interactional patterns. With a key focus on the role of the mother, Klein brought recognition to maternal importance within psychoanalysis during a time when the mother's role was not as explicitly recognized.

Although not without a degree of contention, Klein was a highly influential member of the British Psychoanalytic Society (Grosskurth, 1986). She dealt with existential crises when considering the possibility of her work becoming lost and left intimate family letters behind as an ode to her personal legacy (Grosskurth, 1986). Her work in the death drive theory provided an avenue for psychoanalytic conversations involving the nature of aggression and loss.

The response of grief and mourning derives from an attachment to the sensation the object of association gives, a universal sadness that may bring about early memories of childhood disappointment. Klein emphasized in her work, *Love, Guilt and Reparation*, that suffering is not an occurrence taking place in mere adulthood. Suffering exists even as a child, something she discovered in the applications of psychoanalysis:

Although psychology and pedagogy have always maintained the belief that a child is a happy being without any conflicts, and have assumed that the sufferings of adults are the results of the burdens and hardships of reality, it must be asserted that just the opposite is true. What we learn about the child and the adult through psychoanalysis shows that all the sufferings of later life are for the most part repetitions of these earlier ones, and that every child in the first years of life goes through an immeasurable degree of suffering.

(p. 307)

A Psychoanalytic, International Lens

Although a Western philosophical orientation is primarily addressed concerning object relations and psychoanalytic therapy in a historical context, the underlying links of association to that of India starting in the early 1900s could be applied on a global level. Concurrently in the year 1910, Sigmund Freud and Carl Jung established the International Psychoanalytic Association at the advising of Hungarian psychoanalyst, Sándor Ferenczi (Klett, 2014). Ferenczi is known to be the founder of all relationship-based psychoanalysis and worked in pioneering efforts to collaboratively develop object relations theory.

The clinical relevance of families inquiring into the nature of individual and relational experiences after facing a death provides a phenomenological advantage to the work of marital and family therapists in a global way. These experiences affect us all, no matter where we live. The ambiguity of existential crises that may arise grants the opportunity for both therapist and client to face the deeper questions of life. When working with families, a therapist is recognizing that the time is used effectively by guiding clients to a deeper level of processing (Twenge et al., 2016).

However, the nature of life in that it ends in death remains to be, despite religious orientation or in regard to the myriad number of changes, bound to occur within societal systems. Object relations recognizes the need for the processing of grief in order to heal psychologically. Those who hold religious backgrounds might find those relevant in their healing. As societal norms and traditions changes over time, dynamics of cultural associations with religion, and structural changes within the family, are requiring family therapists to provide near-to clergy work in areas once nurtured by the church, religious affiliations, or closely knit family relations.

These contemporary shifts open the need for marital and family therapists to play a role in supporting end-of-life transitions and grief. Philosophic, psychoanalytic psychotherapy treatments for individuals and families are a means for dialogue and in-depth pondering of the meaning of life after a family loss.

From an international perspective, it can be observed that regardless of relational or cultural associations, family therapists must help clients address grief, loss, and meaning of life within the axioms of psychoanalytic thought, Socratic discourse, and diverse religious orientations.

Future Developments and Implications

The consideration of the equal role that women played in the engagement of philosophical discourse in Plato's Academy of Athens, opens dialogue with recognition to a feminist lens applicable to contemporary relations in a psychotherapy space (Brisson, 2012). Upon the establishment of higher education in the form of the Athens Academy established by Plato, women were given the advancement to access of knowledge and engagement of discourse.

Unifying the presence of women to that of men during a time when even in Europe, women were not typically allowed to engage in philosophical discourse or study (Brisson, 2012). Although greatly unrecognized, many female philosophers did exist during the Socratic age, and were seen to be equal in areas of intellect and access to knowledge:

> "Therefore, if the male sex is seen to be different from the female with regard to a particular craft or way of life, we'll say that the relevant one must be assigned to it. But if it's apparent that they differ only in this respect, that the females bear children while the males beget them, we'll say that there has been no kind of proof that women are different from men with respect to what we're talking about, and we'll continue to believe that our guardians and their wives must have the same way of life." differs from men in respect of the sort of education she should receive.

> (Plato, 1992 p.5)

Plato recognized the propensity for women to engage in the same level of education as men. With mere variation in roles concerning biological constructs, Plato and Socrates were ahead of their time in the recognition of the value of knowledge. However, when considering a philosophical lens from an international scope, this would also require that a family therapist remain sensitive to a multicultural perspective. Recognizing the variants in culture that can arise in terms of family roles and expectations.

Working to find a certain level of satisfaction in philosophical discourse and the nuances of previous unconscious material that can arise, family units sort through the technical-ities that can emerge after the death of a family member. Presuppositions in family affairs concerning the handling of funeral arrangements, items of the departed, grief reactions, and unexpected wishes contained in a will; can arise to be addressed in session. A certain level of facilitation is oriented in a largely experiential case of a blended family unit.

Case Study: The Case of a Blended Family

A family of five seeks therapy after the parting of a beloved grandmother. The family is a culturally diverse, blended family unit of varying ages ranging from 2 years old to 45 years old. The male and female couple were previously married to other spouses now divorced. This is both the husband and wife's second marriage, with one 2-year-old daughter that is of their union. The family deals with significant grief after the unexpected passing of the grandmother (wife's mother) who operated as the primary caregiver of her daughter's children from a previous marriage. The wife is of first generation Mexican-American, and her mother was living in the family home as a caretaker of her daughter's teenage children ranging from 13, 16, and 18 years old. The husband, a second-generation native of Germany, was closely bonded with her and found his grandmother-in-law to be of pertinent assistance. Since her death 3 months ago, the family no longer spends time together as they used to. The daughters stay in isolation in their rooms and do not assist mom with household chores. The family is in a state of mourning over the loss of their grandmother.

Case Conceptualization

The family therapist in this case first recognizes the cultural dynamics and family backgrounds of the parents. The therapist seeks to understand the unique family perspective from a relational lens utilizing insight with a multicultural sensitivity. The therapist invites each member of the family to share their perspectives in relation to the deceased grandmother. The therapist comes to understand the presenting cultural variances from an object relations perspective. The therapist recognizes the transference arising and shifts from reflection to inquiry. The therapist recognizes any counter-transference as a result of the presenting material. Ultimately, the family's object cathexis towards that of the grandmother led to a family homeostasis that has now fallen out of alignment. The therapist makes space for the family to grieve and work through conflicts without immediately providing a solution or behavioral intervention. As the level of trust finds root in the space, the therapist invites conversations of spiritual and philosophical relevance.

Future of Treatment for Family Therapists

The work of Melanie Klein and those in association with the school of and those in association with the development of object relations broadened the horizon of psychoanalytic thought for psychotherapists engaged in family therapy applications. The integration of philosophy, psychoanalysis, and family systems opens the door for clinical options for psychotherapists working from both a relational and individual perspective. Explicitly and implicitly with a focus on grief, death, and existential crises, clients have the space to ponder the meaning of their lives after experiencing a death.

The therapist provides empathetic reflection and refrains from judgment or persecutory remarks if the inquiry should be contrary to religious ideology. Therapists can engage a family's need for applications of meaning and utilize their clinical skills in assessing the most favorable interventions with a degree of psychoanalytic insight and depth. Recognizing the universality of death, family therapists that seek a preponderance for grief work are embracing depth utilization for an international framework.

Cheri L. Hausmann

Three Key Points for Clinical Research and Practice

1. The changing dynamics of cultural associations with religion, as well as the corresponding structural changes within the family, are requiring family therapists to provide near-to clergy work with regard to areas once nurtured by the church, religious affiliations, or closely knit family relations. These shifts require marital and family therapists to play a role in end-of-life transitions and the grief experienced by family members as a result of death.
2. The universality of death and loss opens the door for further research into the most applicable psychotherapy treatments during a time when religious life is not as widely recognized or practiced (Twenge, Sherman, Exline, & Grubbs, 2016). Psychoanalytic, philosophically oriented psychotherapy along with family systems provides a means for addressing grief, and the uncovering of human agency where community, church, and family support may be lacking. The integration of psychoanalysis and philosophy could lead to a revolutionary treatment modality for use in family therapy worldwide.
3. Psychoanalytic applications in family systems involve the object relations schools most popularly known by the work of Melanie Klein and the school of object relations. The work of Melanie Klein and those in association with relational psychoanalysis began with intimate, professional encounters with Sigmund Freud. Freud's work in philosophy, anthropology, and psychoanalysis led to the development of psychoanalysis (Levi, 1959).

References

Brisson, Luc. (2012). *Women in Plato's Republic*. OpenEdition Journals.
Davies, H. (2010). *The Use of Psychoanalytic Concepts in Therapy with Families: For All Professionals Working with Families*. Taylor & Francis Group.
Dhar, A. (2018). Girindrasekhar Bose and the history of psychoanalysis in India. *Indian Journal of History of Science, 53*(4).
Frank, P. (1990) *Psychoanalysis Scientific Method and Philosophy, Psychoanalysis and Logical Positivism*. Routledge.
Freud, S. (2015). *Beyond the Pleasure Principle*. Dover Publications.
Fussell, P. (1989). *Wartime*. Oxford University Press, Incorporated.
Grosskurth, P. (1986). *Melanie Klein Her World and Her Work*. Jason Aronson Inc.
Haley, J. (1973). *Uncommon Therapy; The Psychiatric Techniques of Milton H. Erickson,*. M.D. W. W. Norton.
Hook, S. (1959). *Psychoanalysis, Scientific Method, and Philosophy: A symposium*. New York University Press.
Horner, A. (1991). *Psychoanalytic Object Relations Therapy*. Jason Aronson Inc.
Klein, M. (1998). *Love, Guilt and Reparation: And Other Works 1921–1945*. Vintage.
Klett, S. (2014). *Sándor Ferenczi's legacy: His influence on my work with difficult patients. Psychoanalytic Inquiry*. 34(2), 171–177.
Levi, A. (1959). *Philosophy and The Modern World*. Indiana University Press.
Majmudar, B. (2014). *Cremation Rites in Hinduism: death, after death, and thereafter', in Ellen L. Idler (ed.), Religion as a Social Determinant of Public Health*. Oxford Academic.
Noone, R. J. (2021). *Family and Self: Bowen Theory and the Shaping of Adaptive Capacity*. Lexington Books.
O'Reilly, D., & Rosato, M. (2015). Religion and the risk of suicide: Longitudinal study of over 1 million people. *British Journal of Psychiatry, 206*(6), 466–470.
Plato. (1911). *Plato's Phaedo*. Oxford: Clarendon Press.
Plato. (1992). *Republic (2nd ed.)*. Hackett Publishing Company, Inc.
Rieff, P. (1977). *Sigmund Freud Therapy and Technique*. Collier Books New York

Scharff, D. E. & Scharff, J. S. (1987). *Object Relations Family Therapy*. Aronson.

Segal, Hanna. (1988). *Introduction to the Work of Melanie Klein*. Karnac Books.

Skea, B. R. (2006). Sabina Spielrein: out from the shadow of Jung and Freud. *Journal of Analytical Analysis, 51*, 527–552.

Twenge, J. M., Sherman, R. A., Exline, J. J., & Grubbs, J. B. (2016). Declines in American Adults' Religious Participation and Beliefs, 1972–2014. *SAGE Open, 6* (1).

Vagts, A. (1945). Battle and Other Combatant Casualties in the Second World War, II. *Journal of Politics, 7*(4), 411–438.

3

MILAN SCHOOL OF FAMILY THERAPY

Umberta Telfener

Introduction

I desire to introduce myself to the reader. I am an Italian systemic professional, teacher of the Milan school of family therapy, the one organized around Luigi Boscolo e Gianfranco Cecchin – unfortunately both dead – that was one of the leading theoretical outposts in the 1980s and 1990s of the last century. The school has continued to evolve, and this chapter will propose some ideas we are very keen about.

As a systemic thinker I don't consider myself only a psychotherapist nor do I pay attention mainly to families; I also do not subdivide therapy according to the people I see: the unit of observation is not families as groups united by a history, nor individuals or nets but rather relational processes, transversal to social units. I choose who to consider, the system as a whole or parts of it, according to the request received and the contract we have made; I intervene in many contexts with processes that are specialized as psychotherapy (second-level interventions) or as consultants with contributions in the social domain as in a hospital, a court, or many other possible institutions (first-level involvements). Systemic therapy obliges us to work with the observing system – a concept suggested by von Foerster (1984), representative of the constructivist epistemology – that includes us and other healthcare professionals around the issue treated where the professionals are integral part of the game and try to help transform symptoms by treating systems.

I will start with a case to illustrate what I mean.

Mara calls me to ask for an appointment with her husband Franco. She is 41, he is 55, they have been together for 15 years and their relationship has deteriorated since the birth of their son, Angelo, now three years old; it has worsened in this last year due to COVID. Mara feels heaviness, and too much responsibility for the household and the son; he feels peripheral and depressed; sex has stopped. It seems to me they are looking for an external judge that specifies who is wrong and who is right. I investigate their role as parents in order to keep the child uninvolved in the situation as soon as possible: quite immediately it looks like Angelo is keeping them glued together through his frequent tantrums and his lack of autonomy. They have been sent by a colleague, friend of the couple and former student of mine, who has told them I work with couples and am quite direct and nonjudgmental.

DOI: 10.4324/9781003297871-4

Systems theory emerges within the distinctive operations we perform together with our clients. When we identify a system it generally includes the significant others, who can take in a physician, other professionals, relatives and friends of the subject(s) who make us the request, our colleagues and supervisors and many other contacts: the problem-determined system of which Goolishian and Andersen speak about (1986). Altogether, we come to share meanings and actions around the problem. As professionals we are responsible for the actions that occur during the therapeutic process since we are invested socially as "experts of change" and we have a social mandate; families and individuals, on the other hand, are "experts" of their own life. We could say that the relationship between us is equal but asymmetrical.

When intervening, the aim is neither to acquire new techniques, nor to invent new theories. We need to think about our practices and about the operations we organize and suggest, in order to build an evolutive, processual, and responsible therapeutic space. The therapeutic practice should emerge and be maintained as an act of possibilities and creation, as a self-organizing system in which disorder and order dance interactively. The image of a self-organizing system is that of a murmuration where the birds act according to internal laws and there is not one in charge.

Doing therapy means creating inquiries in a recursive loop, taking the design turn, exploring the mutual influence of the poetic interactions we have co-created. Not everything that we propose is right: there are different levels of plausibility, topics make sense for some people but not for others; sometimes they are the right ones in the right moment, but may not make sense before or after. We respond to stimuli and work on the feedback we receive. Focused attention is dedicated to adherence to one's epistemology, which is the frame that gives meaning both to the daily behaviors and to all the therapeutic "actions" in the different contexts. Premises – Boscolo used to say – are like the soles of your feet: you can't see them because you are resting on them.

The analysis of the services request with Mara and Franco takes one session and creates a suspended space – nonjudgmental, jointly shared – to organize the generative practice to be proposed (Telfener, 2011). It is useful to become an observing system and to understand what is requested from us, why now, what has been already tried, what are the expectations for treatment and resources. I ask them which is their view of their problem: they have just set apart more and more, they expect to become friends again and the view of the problem is quite different among them: Mara says she feels too responsible and that she can't count on Franco for help; she also feels she needs to take full charge since he doesn't help and feels bolted to the relationship. Franco says she sets the rules in the household, and he feels he has no say; their son is also mother-centric, and he perceives himself as useless.

I redefine their request since every request for therapy is done within the same premises that have created the symptom and the professional needs not to enter into that specific logic in order not to collude (Ugazio, 1989). I restate that in couple's therapy I work with both of them together and singularly, always having in mind the destiny of their relationship.

Complexity is Our Mandate

Complexity is our epistemological mandate. Every hypothesis, every explanation we propose is an emergence of many situations that relate to us heavily. I am proposing a multiple positioning, not so much of different kinds of [1]capta, but rather a manifold point of view that combines a) the consideration of the context in which we are acting; b) the observation on the asymmetrical but equal relationship established between the client and the professional and their reference systems; c) an analysis of the observed system, the client and their significant relationships; and d) a reflection on the generativity of the process, on the poetics that emerge from what has been proposed, said and done.

There is not an one "cause" of a clinical problem that can be discovered. There is no etiopathogenetic theory that stands out as a strong theory. Attention comes back on the process: as clinicians we need to manage the explanations of the current situation – pathology included – since this is our specific responsibility.

We must remember that society and language tend to simplify "reality" and that we need to maintain multifold hypothesis and lenses, remaining open to possibilities that are all around us. We must be aware that with our blind spots we build and create what is missing. The album cover of Pink Floyd's *The Dark Side of the Moon* shows a ray of light (information) that crosses a prism (the setting) and separates in its fundamental frequencies (different shades of meaning), becoming something else. It becomes a series of colors that were present but hidden. A plane of immanence that shows its complexity. This is similar to the process in therapy in that at first glance the nuances that lie underneath are not apparent.

Psychotherapy as philosophy, art, and science is a discipline that creates and invents. It creates and invents concepts, connections, imagines of thought, actions, possibilities, and potentialities that do not exist already. In order for them to emerge new connections must emerge, consonances found, hypothesis determined, common goals set, alternatives found, in order to to create change. While clients bring with them a narrative of their reality, the professional proposes an alternative hypothesis and acts as an active agent in a non-instructive process, working on the here and now, careful not to simplify and to remain generative. Many are the layers of curiosity: the present, the future, the past, three-generation interchanges, the individual, the family domains. We act on a "strategic," a relational, and a contextual level; we propose double descriptions; we bring into play a technical, a contextual, and a relational competence (Fruggeri, 1992); we operate on different levels of understanding, on different levels of responsibility, a fundamental attitude about which we will discuss in the conclusions of this chapter.

As soon as Franco enters the second session he states that he is aggressive, grumpy, and unpleasant, authoritarian with Angelo, and impatient than his wife. What is he signaling? What does this negativity towards himself mean? I react immediately, sharing some thoughts that come to mind: *"Are you signaling that you exist in the picture while Mara only has eyes for Angelo? Is it the only way to be heard? Are you trying to push her away in order not to take responsibility for the breakup? Are you stating your depression that usually implies seeing everything negatively, including oneself, and asking Mara for help? Are you unable to recharge and are you throwing the negative energy on the whole system, on us in the here and now? Who are you punishing with this self-accusation?"* As can be seen, I make an explicit hypothesis of the game he could be playing, a hypothesis that involves both partners, both positively and negatively.

"How could you re-build your complicity? Let's create a ping pong tournament in which each states what each person expects from the other." Mara asks him to recuperate some enthusiasm, to be less fussy, not *"to simmer in negativity that lowers energy."* At the beginning Franco has done his usual simmering. I did not answer as usually Mara does, participating in the accusation and involving him instead in the challenge to understand.

Franco asks her to be less judgmental and not to consider him "the destructor" of their life. I end the session asking them to work on their complicity as a predictive sign of the state of their relationship. That is, each one of them should try and organize/propose actions that bring them together, not necessarily with ease, just on the same tentative team (*compassion comes from cum-passio, vibrate together*, I tell them).

A hypothesis needs to consider new questions, so new connections emerge. We need to multiply interactions and emotions, to free them from old presuppositions, without being afraid to enter the unknown. This attitude doesn't imply looking for novelty in itself, but rather maintaining an evolutive stance and knowing what to look for (Mariotti et al., 2001) and considering what comes back to us, the feedback we receive. To perturb in therapy means to create events, make things happen, utilize words, actions, and space. As therapists we need to produce something not expected, not recognized in order to evoke change.

Following Bateson, we need to transcend the dichotomy between social and individual by accessing the ability to describe individuals as observers and authors of their narratives and to connect ideas to the immanent mind of the system. This includes attention to the set of actions, feedbacks, assumptions, and behaviors of the expanded system, which includes all the subjects involved and their context, the professional and her connections.

The duty of systemic professionals is to combine emotional, biological, and social aspects with the "contextual knowledge," so that dialogue through actions and words becomes the only way out. This is the core positioning of the Milan school clinicians. Once again, we propose a repudiation of neutrality, objectivity, and Truth with a capital T.

Therapy as a Construction

Therapy is an act of creation, a poetical construction in which people are asked to invent themselves, answering questions and taking distance from the usual blueprints. The specificity of each meeting takes life from the common dance and is not predictable in advance; the dialogue brings forward experiences, ideas, emotions, and actions of all the participants. We know that when people have common tasks, they are pushed to find a common path, to have the same frequency: a morphogenic field emerges (Sheldrake, 2009) in which intuition and heart vibrate together.

When we refer to the constructive lenses we utilize as therapists we put forward a viewpoint combining the cognitive and social aspects of understanding, as two sides of the same coin. The idea that reality is constructed modifies the process of knowledge. In a cybernetic epistemology, the therapist doesn't know better and more than the client: her theories, her hypothesis, her comments are not true nor false, they are as plausible as those of the client. Clients bring us an explicit and repetitive narrative that makes them suffer; it is our job to propose an alternative hypothesis through a self-organizing process that includes everyone. The difference is that the professional's hypotheses are in a different logical order, not at the content level of the client. They are interwoven in the processes that build how we think, perceive, and decide: not at the first-order level of "understanding" but rather at the second-order level of "understanding our understanding" and "knowing about knowing." The professional positions herself at a different level from the client: she needs a broader awareness, not about herself but about the relational aspects in connection with the other(s). The clinician asks questions to get information about the system she is dealing with the aim is – through questions – to perturb everyone included in the new born observing system. The clinical work has to do with defining problems over and over again in order to try and dissolve them. If usually what was not known was the solution of a problem – the problem being clear and stated – in a constructive cybernetic epistemology also the definition of a problem is questioned and needs redefining and specification. Problems and their possible solutions originate from the specific viewpoint of the one posing them. The therapeutic context gives these problems and possible solutions new meaning.

It is from this co-creative process that an evolutive process emerges. The constructionist professional can't avoid values, she needs to take a political positioning and assume responsibility for her actions. Working with the other's subjectivity and her own, the therapeutic job is no longer a technical one, since therapy implies an ethical, an esthetical as well as a political stance.

Therapy is an act of creation, in the middle between the ax and the tree of Bateson, between the orchid and the bee of Deleuze, a poetry contest where people have to answer our questions, taking a distance from their usual script. One "arrives in the middle of something – as Deleuze states (1983) – and only in the middle one creates, giving new directions, bifurcations to pre-existing lines." It is a morphogenetic space organized by resonance, an instinct to enlarge conscience to include more and more elements, considering inside and external elements as strictly connected.

The sessions with the couple continue with our explicit agenda to find a new way for them to be together. I don't have a defined idea of how they should act together, nor do I wish to control their conduct. I need to remain generative, to consider their interaction as evolutive and to maintain my perturbative energy, my curiosity, without the need to control them (it would be impossible!). I therefore utilize every occasion they give me to enhance the positive and softly underline the alternatives to their negative dynamics. They need to put energy and attention into every step of their interaction instead of taking it for granted and therefore acting as usual. We discover together the need for clear boundaries and some space for themselves, however they want to utilize it.

Therapy as a Second-order Reflexive Process

Systemic psychotherapy is a recursive practice in which we reflect on our reflection, interpret our interpretations; it is considered the ability of a system to turn to itself and to become the object of its own observation. It is the ability to use oneself to investigate oneself in relation to others and what they bring to us: knowledge as an operation on knowledge. Therapy is a self-monitoring activity that implies moments of time-out to reflect on the ongoing processes that include us. The process involves taking multiple positions at the same time, observing oneself and one's behavior and using this observation to calibrate interventions. This requires many levels of presence: contextual, relational, "strategic," and reflective. We assume at least a triple positioning, i.e., we access news of difference and consider ourselves an integral part of the ongoing process, observing our participation in it to calibrate the interventions and the relationship. We are therefore inside and outside; we are in the therapy room to connect to clients and to have an internal conversation (Rober, 2005), a negotiation between the self and the role, to monitor how the process is taking place, but we also take moments of suspension to perform a self-monitoring activity that involves moments of time out to stop, reflect on the ongoing process that includes us. We question the relationship that has been built and how. How was my theory built, my understanding and consequently my actions? How does my being in the situation and the use of myself become the tool in understanding the dynamics taking place. The therapist actively utilizes herself and her abilities to connect, bringing with herself the bits and pieces of her own existence and acting with the aim to create a morphogenetic field in which to share an unconscious and a common intent, that is, "change." This field is made of all the people that interact within it, their intentions and their desires, a common unconscious.

As von Foerster argues, the situations we are confronted with as clinicians are indeterminable and the problems unpredictable (1984); no problem setting, and consequent solution can be right in an absolute way. We don't know the solutions to the questions posed to us. For the clinic to become a good practice, it is necessary to take care of the treatment process and establish a second-order recursive process. The clinician doesn't ask questions to get information about the system she is dealing with; the aim instead is to generate an encounter and perturb everyone included in the newborn observing system which includes the professional (von Foerster). The ability to act/think/operate in an ethical manner requires reflexivity, understood as a turning back of one's own experience on oneself, in order to think and reflect on the actions of others. It is the ability to use oneself to investigate oneself in relation to others, to explore the concepts that have been used and how others have understood and reacted to them. Reflexivity is considered the ability of a system to address itself and become the object of its own observation, where knowledge becomes an operation on knowledge. At any time, the observer relates to the system through her own understanding of the system, which modifies the relationship with it (Fruggeri, 1992). Operations on operations lead us to talk about knowledge of our knowledge, diagnosis of the diagnosis, change in the process of change.

I interrogate constantly the process that involves me in the sessions. How is it going? What could I do differently? My ongoing curiosity is a sign that the process is staying evolutive. I can also ask them to give me feedback on the process, as a way to make them feel responsible as co-therapists of the "client" that is their relationship. Am I too active? Do I care? That is, if the relationship level seems ok, if we respect each other, if we are interested in what others say, and we take turns and feel respected. The "strategic" attitude is safe, I try to feel the purpose of our encounters, to monitor the changes in process, to look for isomorphisms between what happens with me and what is their relationship. Within the reflective stance I ask myself if I could act differently and if there are areas I am blind to.

The Importance of Relationship

Following von Foerster (1984), if one adopts the relativity principle, neither oneself nor the other can be at the center of the universe. As in the heliocentric system a third must exist who constitutes the central point of reference. This third is the relation among I and you, and this relationship constitutes the identity from which the dance emerges: reality is embedded in community. We can only be born in the encounter which is not just being present: intuition, hypnotization, connecting, exploring become important actions as well. Therapy is an interactive, dialogical, performative second-order, recursive process in which we explore present, past, and future without goal-directed planning.

The clinical work has to do with defining problems over and over again, deconstructing premises that have led to them, exploring emotions and expectations, these being the ways to make the unexpected appear, the context giving it meaning. The question we pose ourselves is which lines are present and can be built. The possible solutions to problems originate from the specific and not always rational choices of who is posing the questions; they arise from the dance performed between professional and clients, keeping in mind significant others. Changes of state and disintegration of usual ways of behaving are not determined by the properties of the disturbing agent with which the system interacts (according to Maturana there are no instructive interactions) (Maturana, 1988). I am speaking of therapy as a co-evolutionary process where transparency, irreverence, curiosity, and openness are fundamental, where responsibility becomes the way to act ethically. An inquiring pathway.

Paraphrasing Sartre, we could say that the therapist is organized by paths towards freedom, and must therefore give access to the presence of other possible worlds using pathos, curiosity, and desire. The therapist uses herself and her skills to connect. She brings with her the resources and learning of her own existence and acts with the aim of creating a field in which to share a common intent, which is "change." This field is made up of the people who interact with it, their desires, their intentions (an unconscious and a shared pre-conscious). Therapy relies on the construction of a space "between" values and ideas, new and old scripts, between the stories that are brought and the specific themes of people, between all the interactive spaces and family history, and much more. This includes a space in which hypothesis are made and changed if they do not resonate with others. Ours is an active discipline to be curious, act irreverent towards problems, and maintain the perspective that evolution is possible.

When the therapeutic process with Franco and Mara goes well, I have the feeling we dance together, that the discourse emerges quite naturally from our interactions, from the questions and hypothesis we all have. It is the relationship I establish with both of them that allows for new ways of behaving; it is the trust we have in each other that keeps the conversation going. This flow would be impossible if I felt judgmental towards one of the two, if I did not think they were each doing their best, if I thought their interaction was hopeless, and if I did not see both their desire to change and to remain the same.

Where Body and Movement Stand

Body and movement are instead active resources to create realities worthy of meanings. "We prefer to talk from the body," as noted by Brenda Farnell and Charles Varela (2008) and Francisco Varela (1979) speaks about the emotional and relational co-emergence, a sensory experience and perception, a non-linguistic and pre-reflexive mode of experiencing the world (*knowing how* instead of *knowing that*). The therapist becomes a moving agent in a spatially organized world of meanings, who considers human action as a dynamically embodied discursive practice, signifying units of movement, repositioning the moving body.

According to von Foerster (1984) action and language are neither necessarily simultaneous nor two overlapping concepts. He describes objects as symbols of self-behaviour generated by motor actions and asserts the primacy of action over nominalization: "If you wish to know learn how to act, as the way you act determines what you see." Von Foerster suggests that language is made up of two "tracks": the linguistic definition and the social relationship aspect. While verbal language creates labels, definitions, names, and denotations, the social dance is a connotative process of lived embodied experiences, only partially translatable into words, based on common doing. He underlines the impossibility of separating the two processes – the linguistic from the affective, the private/emotive aspect of language sharing from the public/social one – in that together they allow the always completely social construction of the world. Denying the corporeal, biological, non-verbal, processual aspects would lead to a "disembodied" world and to a coldly rationalistic vision of it. As clinicians we are well aware that the verbal description of behaviour or intentions is by no means always "accessible" and anything but at our disposal, deriving rather from a sometimes contradictory set of possible descriptions not always aware to the subject. Commonly people with traumas don't have the words to tell us what is bothering them, and we need to access through actions to their memories. In addition to language games, I therefore suggest also taking into consideration the presence of emotional and relational games within the couple's treatment, understood as independent and parallel processes that jointly constitute the exclusively social game of the construction of "reality" (Telfener, Casadio, 2003).

The body becomes a dynamic source of meaning making in a life shared with others. I suggest embodied actions, actions as imbricated in biology, body movement as a fundamental component of social actions. An active "fight" against the mainstream thinking, the already digested blueprints, the idea that people arrive to us with well-organized plots. Therapy becomes a praxis; to perturb in therapy means to create events, make things happen. To access pre-cognitive and pre-verbal events and feelings we need to inspire action in therapy. At Milano we speak about active techniques: postcards, writing, dramatizing, sculptures, role-playings, etc.

One day in a session I feel that too many words have been spent. I therefore ask each one of them to choose some characters that represent them among a shelf full of transitional objects in my office. "*Which object would you choose to represent you? Which one do you feel like? Choose among the puppets in my room a figure that represents you as you feel usually.*" Franco chooses a naïve peasant that looks nice, spaced out and immobile, while Mara chooses a superhero female figure in a fighting posture. "*Now choose another figure: how would you like to feel and to be seen by others?*" She chooses a big relaxed red cat, he chooses Captain Hook. I myself have chosen a puppet that represents in my heart their relationship: a small car too filled up that could go faster if lighter. We discuss together what our choices in objects mean and what it would imply to become what they would like to be. Mara seems amused by the game, and goes to the shelf and picks her image of their relationship, an angry small figure shouting. She encourages Franco to do the same. Franco picks some dice, commenting that he never understands if what he does is right or wrong. "*What would they prefer their relation to look like?*" She proposes a group of mice that communicate very well together and perform as a team; Franco a basket of fruit: "*different fruits that seem comfortable one next to the other,*" he comments. We spend the whole session making propositions on how to act differently in order to reach their wishes.

Two Last Keywords: Ethics and Aesthetics

In general, we still need to apply the systemic paradigm in its full potentiality, we need constantly to revolutionize it since the people who come to us are influenced by the society they live in and do not act always the same. It is from this co-creative process – which involves ALL the entities who rotate around a life script consciously aware of the dance or just aware of the others with no intention to collaborate – that an evolutive process emerges. The constructivist professional can't avoid values; she needs to take a political position and assume responsibility for her actions. Working with the other's subjectivity and with her own, with the ideas and relationships personified in the dance, which is an active action.

Ethics within this frame is not "you must," "you must not": we take responsibility for the decisions that emerge from the dance, for the diagnosis that emerged; responsibility is necessarily explicit, ethics becomes an esthetic implicit stance. Ethics becomes a positioning that implies 1. The epistemological stance we assume (a complex view that holds both the point of view of the clinician and the one of the client in a complementary positioning) and 2. the posture we utilize (von Foerster, 1990). It means allowing words and actions to flow in the underground river of ethics, without making ethics explicit in order not to become moralistic. Responsibility deals with patterns that favor or restrain the co-construction of shared meanings and the making of a generative, evolutionary reality.

Therapy with this proposal is not a question of content but of attitude and style. To act in a responsible manner means to build an esthetic process, to open up one's heart and feel connected. New is always unforeseen. Therapy works on being present, without proposing a beginning or an end. The process allows the clinician to explicit what she was able to see. Experimenting instead of affirming, problematizing, carto-graphing, designing temporary maps, making connections emerge, etc.

When I meet the two individuals alone, I look for specific individual topics. I have stated to clients in advance that they can't propose any secret since this would create an unwanted and impossible coalition with the person who has shared it with me. With Mara we talk about her irrational need to be parented: *"Who can perform as my mother since – as you say – I am constantly the mother of Angelo, of my old parents, of my colleagues at work, and even of Franco?"* She tells me that already in 2011 Franco, during a trip together, had come up with the possibility of having a child together and she had freaked out and panicked. We talk about her need to let go of one of the Mara's, the one existing before giving birth that was selfish and full of self-reference energy, while the new one is oppressed by responsibilities. She will need to find stimuli that re-fill her emotionally and become her own source of energy, meeting friends, organizing social activities that she likes.

With Franco we talked about his autonomy and his low-key way of functioning: he looks like a Jeko that can remain still for days and only if incited may move in order then to become still again, as soon as possible. *"I love Jekos –* I tell him in order to sweeten the pill *– do you?"* He continues telling me that he feels guilty if he listens to Marta without solving her problems and that's the reason he closes up, in order not to feel a failure. It is unthinkable for him to listen without intervening, since his father used to do so.

He agrees that it is he who decided to be in a relationship and to participate in the child's project, but now he is acting as if he had been forced to become a parent. He admits that many of his actions are not organized for the well-being of Angelo but to get on Mara's nerves, that he feels substituted and has lost his companion.

In a subsequent session Mara asks for some space for herself without Franco nor Angelo, while Franco asks for some time as a couple. They contract their specific needs and try to go toward each other.

Conclusions

I appreciate the systemic approach as it is a flexible and complex model that involves not acquiring new techniques, or inventing new theories to read systems and contexts, but reflecting more and more on the actions we already know/implement, in order to build an evolutionary and responsible practice. This is not a solipsistic operation, all in our heads, but something that emerges from the relationships we share.

In a cybernetic epistemology nothing is good or harmful in itself. It can be defined either one or the other way only within a relationship and a context. Successes or failures do not depend unilaterally on the clinician or on the client, but are generated within the story of their relationship and of their reciprocal encounter. Successes and failures emerge from the coordination of actions and meanings. The clinician has no unidirectional power on what is happening; rather, the responsibility of the creation of an evolutive setting where an asymmetry of roles takes place within a human and personal equality. The therapist asks questions, and the dance that ensues determines the content and the process.

The clinician also shares a second-order responsibility: a responsibility regarding the very modalities according to which one's professional responsibility is understood. This implies giving oneself a co-responsibility that is shared with those we meet.

References

Anderson, H., Goolishian, H. A., & Windermand, L. (1986). Problem determined systems: Towards transformation in family therapy. *Journal of Strategic & Systemic Therapies, 5*(4), 1–13.

Bateson G. (1972). *Steps to an echology of mind.* San Francisco: Chandler Publishing Company.

Buber M. (1937). *I and Thou.* Edinburgh: T. & T. Clark.

Deleuze, G. (1983). *Che cos'è l'atto di creazione?* Napoli: Cronopio edizioni, 2003.

Farnell B., Varela C. (2008). The second somatic revolution. *Journal of the Theory of Social Behaviour, 38*(3), 215–240.

Foerster H. (von) (1984). *Observing Systems.* Seaside: Intersystems.

Foerster, H. (von) (1990). *Ethics and second order Cybernetics.* Plenary Session at the Congress: Systémes, Etique, Perspectives en thérapie familiale, Paris, 4–6 October.

Fruggeri L. (1992). Therapeutic process as social construction of change, in S. McNamee & K. J. Gergen (Eds.), *Therapy as social construction.* (pp. 40–53). Newbury Park, California: Sage.

Mariotti M., Bassoli F., Frison R. (2001). *Manuale di psicoterapia sistemica e relazionale.* Roma: Ed. Sapere.

Maturana H. (1988). Ontology of Observing, The biological foundations of self-consciousness and the physical domain of existence. Conference Workbook: *Texts in Cybernetics, American Society For Cybernetics Conference.* Felton, CA. 18–23 October.

Pietro, B., Cavagnis, M. E., Krause, I., & Telfener, U. (2022). *Ethical and Aesthetic Explorations of Systemic Practice: New Critical Reflections.* London: Routledge.

Rober P. (2005). The therapist's self in dialogical family therapy: Some ideas about not-knowing and the therapist's inner conversation,. *Family Process, 44*(4), 477–495.

Sheldrake R. (2009). *Morphic Resonance: The Nature of Formative Causation.* Rochester, VT: Park Street Press.

Telfener U. (2011). *Apprendere I contesti.* Milano: Cortina editore.

Telfener U., Casadio L. (2003). *Sistemica, voci e percorsi nella complessità.* Torino: Bollati Boringhieri.

Treacher, A. (1988). The Milan method-a preliminary critique*. *Journal of Family Therapy, 10*(1), 1–8. https://doi.org/10.1046/j..1988.00295.x

Ugazio V. (1989). L'indicazione terapeutica: una prospettiva sistemico-costruttivista. *Terapia Familiare, 31,* 27–40.

Varela F. (1979). *Principles of Biological Autonomy.* North Holland, Amsterdam.

4

A NARRATOLOGICAL STUDY OF A FAMILY-THERAPEUTIC CASE HISTORY

Werner Pfab

OUR STORY BEGINS ...

The "Disguised" Problem: Writing Case Histories

In the year 2018 one of the most acclaimed journalists of the German political magazine, Der Spiegel, was fired after it was discovered that some of his reportages were faked. He is not the only one who could make the public believe that his fictious texts were stories about real events. The most spectacular case probably was that of US-American journalist Janet Cooke who in 1981 was honored with the Pulitzer Prize for journalism for a story about an eight-year-old heroin-addicted boy from Washington – a story she made up.

How does an author succeed in making a story credible in the eyes of his readers? How does he succeed in attracting his readers?

These questions are relevant in writing stories for magazines, but they are also relevant for scientific texts too, although not for all of them. While these questions are not relevant for scientific texts that argue for or against a certain position (i.e., for theoretical explanations) – in those texts it is a matter of sound reason – these questions, however, are relevant for scientific texts that have features of reports or stories – and therefore they are relevant for psychotherapeutic case studies too.

The question of how a scientific case history gains its persuasive power is strongly emphasized by anthropologist Clifford Geertz (1988). Geertz discussed this question with regard to ethnographic reports and case studies. He finds that in anthropology the question is treated in a "disguised" way:

> Disguised, because it has been generally cast not as a narratological issue, a matter of how best to get an honest story honestly told, but as an epistemological one, a matter of how to prevent subjective views from coloring objective facts.
>
> (1988, p. 9)

Geertz finds the cause for this – in his eyes misleading – position in a fear of subjectivity. From this position follows a severe conclusion: "If the relation between observer and

DOI: 10.4324/9781003297871-5

observed (rapport) can be managed, the relation between author and text (signature) will follow – it is thought – of itself" (1988, p. 10). Faced with the fundamental problem of how to understand the other in the encounter with the researcher the problem "of facing the page" (p. 10) disappears. By that however "the oddity of constructing texts ostensibly scientific out of experiences broadly biographical, which is after all what ethnographers do, is thoroughly obscured" (p. 10). The question of the peculiar rhetorical or even poetical quality of scientific texts is met with defensiveness: To deal with such a question (not being related to the subject of scientific inquiry but to the – narcistic – person of the author) is not typically the way to behave in the scientific community, the question

Furthermore, the question is deemed not worth considering as scientific texts are scientific texts not artificially poetic texts. Above all the questions presuppose the assumption that scientific insights can be fabricated arbitrarily. The assumption that all scientific insights are nothing but the result of verbal constructions leads "to a corrosive relativism in which everything is but a more or less clever expression of opinion" (p. 2). Geertz, however, holds that it is necessary to deal with the strategies and mechanisms of writing reports and stories. One reason is that the most commonly mentioned criterion for the convincing power of a text – richness of facts – does not stand the test – at least for ethnographic texts. Some ethnographers succeed better than others "in conveying in their prose the impression that they have had close-in contact with far-out lives... In discovering how, in this monograph or that article, such an impression is created, we shall discover, at the same time, the criteria by which to judge them" (p. 6).

It would be misleading, however, to regard the question of persuasive power only as a question of textual qualities. Each text is socio-culturally contextualized: Where is the text published? How is the relation of the text to recent socio-cultural topics and debates? etc.

How the Problem Emerged

The importance of accurately and effectively writing case histories becomes relevant when the social domain of science emerges and is separated from literature. According to scholars such as historian Foucault and literary critic Eagleton this separation took place within the 17th century in Europe. When Michel de Montaigne wrote his "Essays" he was not yet confronted with this question. The separation of literature and science occurred within a broader cultural change and with the establishment of a new cultural frontline, which can be characterized by the following competing concepts:

- fact – fiction
- objectivity – subjectivity
- observation – rhetoric
- description – narration
- truth – deception
- reality – illusion

Yet scholars and researchers, especially those who innovatively changed their disciplines, also changed the way scientific writing was done, such as in the case of Charles Darwin the writings of Charles Dickens (cf. Levine, 1989). According to his own remark Sigmund Freud was inspired by the writings of Ephrahim Lessing (cf. Mahony, 1989, S. 145).

Contributions to the Problem in Several Social Sciences

Case histories play a role in social and cultural studies although in different ways. In this section a short (and selective) overview is given on how the problem of writing case stories is discussed in anthropology, history, and sociology. It is striking that the debate on writing case histories comes along with disciplinary crises in the respective scientific domains, anthropology (Clifford & Marcus, 1986), history (Evans, 2000), and psychoanalytic psychotherapeutic research (Stuhr & Deneke, 1993). It is also noteworthy that most of the contributions to the problem of writing case stories were published in the interval 1980–2000. It is an open question if the debates ended by "exhaustion" as Gottowik (2007, p. 124) suspects for anthropology, or what other causes might be relevant. It can be suspected, however, writing using common literary features present in scientific texts may be seen as an outrage in scientific communities. Above that respective evidences to support this create a feeling of demystification and disappointment. Geertz compares this disappointment to that which occurs when the trick of the "lady sawed in half" is uncovered: "Exposing how the thing is done is to suggest that, like the lady sawed in half, it isn't done at all" (1988, p. 2).

The following is a critical reflection of how family-therapeutic case stories can be developed from them.

Ethnography: The Writing-culture Debate

In anthropology the discussion of the literary quality of ethnographic texts was a reaction to a methodological crisis of the discipline, a crisis of representation. The discussion mainly occurred in the writing-culture debate triggered by the text "Writing Culture," edited by James Clifford and George Marcus in 1986. According to Gottowik, this volume is "one of the most relevant publications in Anthropology within the last twenty or thirty years" (2007, p. 121). On the one hand, the writing-culture debate is aimed at ways to write ethnographic texts ("dialogical ethnography"). On the other hand, it aimed at critical reflections of ethnographic descriptions. This critical reflection focused on the textual rhetorical means and strategies and the socio-cultural frames of description and interpretation by which ethnographers bestowed their texts credibility and authority. An important activity was to investigate in what way the power relations in ethnographic research found its way into ethnographic texts.

This form of critical reflection can be illustrated by a text Renato Rosaldo published in the abovementioned "Writing Culture" where he refers to the "anatomy of ethnographic rhetoric" (1986, p. 77) and elaborates on two classical works in anthropology: one written by one of the most influential anthropologists of the 20th century, E.E. Evans-Pritchard, about the Nuer, and the other about the everyday life of South-French peasants in the Middle Ages, written by E. LeRoi Ladurie. In both cases the data were highly influenced by aspects of power: Evans-Pritchard gained his data in a context of colonialization; Ladurie took them from the files of an inquisition process. Rosaldo is especially interested in how this aspect of power is reflected in these two texts. His research questions illustrate the scientific interests the participants of the writing-culture debate were interested in:

- How do these texts gain their authoritative power?
- How are the main figures of the reported events verbally construed?
- How are the power relations reflected?

- In what kind of "mode" are the texts written?
- What kind of relation exists between the respective mode and the aspects of power?
- How is the relation defined between the author of the text, the narrator of the stories, and the acting figures within the stories?

History: The case of Hayden White

The debate on the literal, poetic quality of historical stories has a long tradition in history, as historian Evans reminds us, referring among others to the work of historian Trevelyan (2000, p. 20 ff.). One of those who stress this quality in writing historical stories, was historian Hayden White. White was interested in the methodological foundations of history. His research question is "What are the possible *forms* of historical representation and what are their bases?" (1987, p. 81). White's main thesis is that scholars in history take archetypes of literary narrations as a pattern for their descriptions of historic events. From that he concludes that writing in history is "essentially a literary, that is to say fiction-making, operation" (1987, p. 85), a finding scholars in history suppress by the opposition of fact and fiction. Keeping this opposition in mind, they are able to work in the "space between" (1987, p. 83).

In fact, history – the real world as it evolves over time – is made sense of in the same way that the poet or novelist tries to make sense of it, i.e., by endowing what originally appears to be problematic or mysterious with the aspect of a recognizable, because it is a familiar, form. It does not matter whether the world is conceived to be real or only imagined; the manner of making sense of it is the same (1987, p. 98).

In his definition of these archetypes of literary White refers to the work of historian Northrop Frye. Frye distinguished between tragedy, comedy, romance, and satire as the basic forms of narration. White works with these concepts in his study of classical works in history, and shows that these works corresponded to these basic forms of narration. He stresses that it is not a question of stylistics but instead a question of narrative structure used in a historical study because it is only the narrative structure that creates a coherent context for a single historical "fact."

"Considered as potential elements of a story, historical events are value-neutral. Whether they find their place finally in a story that is tragic, comic, romantic, or ironic to use Frye's categories depends on the historian's decision to configure them according to the imperatives of one plot structure or mythos rather than another" (1987, p. 84).

Moreover, the narrative structure not only creates a coherent context but the perception and labeling of a single fact too. As White noted, "…it tells us in what direction to think about the events and charges out thought about the events with different emotional valences" (1987, p. 91).

A further aspect of course is that the plot structure works as a selective filter deciding what is a "fact" and what is not. Using archetypical structure the scholar adds authority to his story, which leads to rapport between his text and his readers. It depends on the respective structure. According to White: "In my view, we experience the fictionalization of history as an explanation for the same reason that we experience great fiction as an illumination of the world that we inhabit with the author. In both, we recognize the forms by which consciousness both constitutes and colonizes the world it seeks to inhabit comfortably" (1987, p. 99). White stresses that working with poetic writing strategies does not lessen the scientific quality of a historical text but allows a scholar to reflect his own rhet-orical strategies critically.

Reportage As a Prototype for Doing Sociology

The topic of literary writing is not discussed much in sociology – at least not in German sociology: "The sociological discourse shows a tendency to marginalize the relevance of writing a text" (Przyborski & Wohlrab-Sahr, 2008, p. 353), adding in their handbook the admonition: "Impressionistic descriptions' are at the frontier to literary formats and should find a place only rarely on single selective spots in scientific presentations" (p. 358).

It seems at first glance that literary forms of writing have no significant place in such disciplines. . But there are some exemptions. For example, a paper by sociologist Paul Atkinson on "Goffman's poetic" (1989), and a special branch of sociology called the "Chicago school."

As Atkinson finds in his study of Goffman's poetic, "His appeal seems to rest on the usual criteria for 'good' sociology or social psychology. Rather, it derives from the distinctive, not to say unique, persuasive style of his writing. Perhaps more than any other modern soci-ologist, Goffman's analysis was *rhetorical*, in that it depends so much upon the persuasive power of his written style, the elegance of his use of figures and tropes, and the wit with which he used those resources" (1989, p. 61). Relying on the work of other sociologists Atkinson finds "that the persuasive and pleasing force of Goffman's texts derived from his use of *metaphor* and *irony* or *perspective by incongruity*" (p. 62). Atkinson's thesis is that Goffman's style "is a direct embodiment of [his] subject-matter... Goffman's texts represent his sociology throughout their modes of writing" (p. 74 f.).

With regard to the "Chicago school" there exists a strong relation between literary forms and science in sociology. The so-called Chicago school, had its origin and its base in a form of non-scientific writing: the journalistic reportage (c.f. Lindner). In this case a literary form (reportage) and the corresponding professional stance ("be there, keep your eyes open") became the prototype for engaging in sociology as a research program of "social worlds" with first-hand knowledge (city quarters, social places, social groups. Relevant methodological principles were adopted from journalistic professional working procedures. The sociological field-worker "is nothing as a 'reporter-in-depth'" (Lindner, p. 141).

> For if the novelist was analogous to the sociologist, so he was to the journalists, the city room reporter or the crusading investigator of social facts, the man who walked in the city, observed, explored, the man who had been there, in the place of experience – the ghetto, the stockyard, the apartment block, the battlefield, the social jungle.
>
> (Bradbury, 1983, p. 8)

Not surprisingly, the spiritus rector of this tradition, Robert Ezra Park, worked for more than ten years as a police reporter himself. Again, we find the ambivalent attitude against literary features of scientific texts in sociology too: Although the results of this sociological tradition are highly praised in sociology the journalistic heritage of its founder is typically "forgotten" in his biographies, as Lindner remarks:

"The scholarly community undoubtedly took note of the journalistic influence on Park's sociology, and yet the systematic import of his influence has hitherto scarcely been considered. The space taken up by the years of journalistic experience in the Park biographies is itself symptomatic of the 'oblivion' to which this less prestigious background has been consigned" (1996, p. 98 f.).

Contributions to the Problem in Psychoanalytic Psychotherapeutic Research

In contrast to the above discussed disciplines in psychoanalysis case studies have sacral status. In psychoanalysis they are seen as the cornerstone of the discipline (cf. Stuhr, 1993), and have an important didactive function in the socializing process of becoming a psychoanalyst. These texts also contribute to the development of psychoanalytic tradition and professional identity. They served Freud as programmatical declarations against his opponents in the psychoanalytic community, and were engraved in the textual shape of his case stories.

It was Freud himself (with colleague Joseph Breuer) who "spoke of his discomfort with the report" (Michels, p. 356) that his case studies were considered as literary products: "it still strikes me myself as strange that the case histories I write should read like short stories and that, one might say, they lack the serious stamp of science" (Breuer & Freud, SE 2, p. xxiv). Freud stated the reason for the literary quality of his case histories: "the nature of the subject is evidently responsible for this, rather than any preference of my own" (SE 2, p. xxiv). Psychoanalyst Stuhr adds: "It is peculiar for the subject of psychoanalytic study that its relevant aspects due to the psychic often unconscious action of defense are latent, dynamic and overdetermined" (Stuhr, 2007, p. 953) and later on: "Some aspects we can describe only narratively, and I don't mean 'the unconscious' only but the whole aspects of paradoxa which cannot be grasped by formal logic" (p. 957).

After Freud's work, the literary quality of case histories was mainly regarded from a didactical point of view as material for education, with the recommendation that they should be written as a "vivid description of our work" (Stein, 1988, p. 115). Michels (2000) states their poetic quality in a pointed manner:

"As a result, most of the classic case histories used in analytic teaching are like reconstructed histories of childhood or like grammar school textbooks of history – as dramatic and engaging as possible, telling a story that makes a point, whether it be the textbook account of the grandeur of the Founding Fathers and the nation they constructed, the psychoanalytic reconstruction of the burdens of childhood and the heroic struggle to overcome them, or the teacher's report of the provocative and challenging problems of transference and resistance, the initial entanglement with them, and the eventual recognition, understanding, final escape, and simultaneous liberation of the patient. We all know that the real events of history, childhood, or analysis may not have happened quite that way, but the good teacher tells a story that is designed to be vivid and useful for the student's education, not to replicate exactly the experience of being present at the real event. Can anyone recall Freud's describing a dream he was unable to understand or interpret, or a case that failed to 'make a point'?..."

As Tuckett (1983) notes, "the more a narrative is intellectually, emotionally and aesthetically satisfying, the better it incorporates clinical events into rich and sophisticated patterns, the less space is left to the audience to notice alternative patterns and to elaborate

	Objects of study	*Aspects of study*	*Studied authors*
History	Stories of historical events plot-structures	Socio-cultural genres, narrative archetypes	Michelet, Ranke, Burkardt
Anthropology	Ethnographic descriptions, strategies, power-relations	Socio-cultural patterns of Mead, reception, textual	Geertz, Evans-Pritchard, Levi-Strauss, Malinowsky
Sociology	Descriptions of social worlds as reportages	Sociological descriptions, modes of writing	Park, Goffman
Psychoanalytic	Therapeutic case-studies	Features of short novels	Freud
Psychotherapy		Features of novels	
Research			

Figure 4.1 Debates on the poetic nature of scientific texts in several disciplines and their subjects.

alternative narratives' (p. 1183). A story that is too well told conceals the uncertainty and ambiguity of the real world" (p. 362 f.).

One peculiar aspect which must be considered in writing psychotherapeutic case studies is the aspect of confidentiality. Considering this aspect "we run a risk of essentially writing fiction if we become firm protectors of confidentiality" (Goldberg, 1997, p. 438).

According to Wegner (1998) and others (Meyer, 1984) the main focus of psychoanalytic case stories changed from symptomatological features of the patient to the patient-therapist-relationship, stressing aspects of transference and countertransference. "It is not surprising that case histories almost disappeared from our literature during an era in which analysts disavowed ever trying to influence anyone, and that the genre is coming back into fashion as analysts have begun to discuss their inevitable influence on the patient" (Michels, 2000, p. 372). Case stories become "histories of interaction" ("Interaktionsgeschichten") which "portray the process of relation-building and understanding" (Wegner, p. 36). between patient and therapist. It goes without saying that such an alignment requires an even richer vivid narration.

Although some forms of experimental writing resulted from these debates (see Figure 4.1), they had altogether no major impact on the disciplines. The challenging of the literal quality of scientific texts was too often misunderstood as a claim that scientific texts were fake, false and fraud, and the reaction to that was governed by anxiety, resulting in ignorance and paralysis. The position of historian Nancy Partner is typical for this stance:

> The theoretical destabilizing of history achieved by language-based modes of criticism has had no practical effect on academic practice because academics have had nothing to gain and everything to lose by dismantling their special visible code of evidence-grounded reasoning and opening themselves to the inevitable charges of fraud, dishonesty and shoddiness.
>
> (Partner, cited in Evans, 2000, p. 4)

A Case Story

In this section I analyze the narrative, poetic strategies of a family-therapeutic case history using the insights discussed above with the help of some literary-stylistic categories.

The case story is a well-known text written by an author-team led by the famous Italian family-therapist Mara Selvini Palazzoli. It was published in 1977 in one of the most relevant journals in the family-therapeutic field, *Family Process*. The title of the text is: "Family Rituals. A Powerful Tool in Family Therapy." A remarkable, literarily rich text it is a case story divided into four paragraphs with the following headings:

- The Structure of a Family Myth
- The Family Begins the Therapy
- A Ritual Against a Deadly Myth
- How to Define a Family Ritual

The authors tell the story of a family-therapeutic treatment of a family with the index-client Nora. Besides her, the youngest daughter, the family consists of mother Pia, father Siro, and the elder daughter Zita. Nora had sought medical treatment on grounds of bulimia and had been transferred to the family-therapeutic center. However, the reader learns about this treatment later. Instead, the text begins as a narration of the history of the family. The first sentence begins with the words *Our story of the Casanti family begins*.

In the following I retell this story (i.e., the history of the family and the therapeutic process) in some detail (quotations in italics). After that I analyze the rhetorical strategies used in this narration. The first sentence of the text sounds *Our story of the Casanti family begins during the year 1900 on a large and isolated farm in a depressed area of Central Italy*. What follows can be read as an ethnographic description of an isolated, traditional culture reigned by authoritarian power: *The head of the family was the Capoccia, an iron-fisted worker who based his uncontested authority upon a large tradition of patriarchal rules ... His wife could have stepped from the pages of The Book of the Family, written by Leon Battista Alberti at the end of the fifteenth century*. An ethnologically inspired reading is already suggested by the heading *The Structure of a Family Myth* and indicated by the expression *clan* for the larger family. This isolated small world is then described as being endangered by modern times and their seductions:

- Isolation: *the isolated farm* vs. *the outside world*
- Tradition: *For these people to be born a peasant was to die a peasant* vs. modern times: *They... were amazed when they saw elegant women who smoked and even drove cars!*
- Authority: *no protest on the parts of the sons were tolerated* vs. rebellion: *They began to complain about these restrictions.*

To restore their own world against these seductions and dangers, the authors explain to us, solidarity within the family increases/intensifies/mounts to an undisputable conviction *But the Casanti brothers, still led by the Old Capoccia, were suspicious. These were all signs of a world gone mad. Their strength was always the old one – to work hard and to be united. To stay together, they had to create a myth, a collective product whose very existence and persistence would be able to reinforce the homeostasis of the group against any disruptive influence*. This myth persists, the authors go on, even when the clan eventually leaves home and moves into town, all together in the same block of flats. This new urban surrounding is described as stamped by competition, rivalry, and jealousy. It is said to stress the stability of the myth so that it became *rigidified to the extreme. Even the Casanti cousins were true brothers, they shared their joys and sorrows. Together they suffered the failure of another, together they rejoiced in the good luck of another. The unmentioned iron rule* not only forbade them to speak, but also did not permit any gesture or comment whatever that would be said to be motivated by jealousy, envy, or competition.

At this point the story focuses on the family with the index client Nora who is said to change dramatically when she turns 13 years old and becomes beautiful. While her father is proud of his beautiful daughter, she herself is not pleased and *she reacted nervously to any compliments on her beauty… urged to go on outings or to dances… [s]he nearly always returned home depressed… In school things started going badly.* The pre-history of the therapy ends with mentioning that Nora stopped eating, *was reduced to a skeleton.* Individual psychotherapy did not help. Then she was – together with father, mother, and sister – referred to the family-therapeutic center.

The portrayal of the adjacent family-therapeutic process is divided into two parts: *The Family Begins the Therapy* and *A Ritual Against the Deadly Myth*. The first phase is said to have been stamped by *outstanding factors* consisting on the one hand of assessments, mistaken diagnosis, and other failures of the therapeutic team and a remarkable recovery of the index client Nora on the other. This recovery is interpreted by the therapists as an effort by Nora to maintain the stability of the clan system. The therapists at this point decide to interrupt the therapeutic process. *We wanted to sound out the family.* The situation remains open until the team is informed that Nora committed a – failed – suicide. Then the therapy resumes.

The second part, *A Ritual Against the Deadly Myth*, starts with a portrayal of confessions and revelations made by father and sister that reveal the real quality of relations within the clan. Although these revelations are withdrawn immediately by family members and the clan is defended, *the therapists refused to take the carrot offered to them… It was urgent that we invent and prescribe a ritual.* At the same time the therapists urged the family to stick to the family's myth thereby putting the family in a paradoxical situation. Then the ritual is described in some detail and the therapeutic considerations for the ritual are elucidated. Then the text goes on and says *The family carried out the ritual and two weeks later presented itself greatly changed.* The members of the family are described as being able to talk openly about the pressures and hostile feelings they experienced from other members of the clan, especially Nora from cousin Luciana. *[T]he rule was broken… The therapy had finally touched the system's nerve center…Once the field was cleared of the myth, it became possible to work on the family's internal problems.* A footnote informs the reader that Nora became a successful model in the fashion industry later on.

The following research questions arise in this analysis:

- How do the authors succeed in holding the reader spellbound during the reading process?
- What bestows the text authoritative power?
- Whose voices are priviledged in the narration – and whose are not?
- What kind of narrative plot underlies the narrative?
- How does the text deal with the aspect of power-relations between clients and therapists?

For the persuasive power of a text, the author succeeds in enthralling the reader and to include him into the story. One strategy to make a story vivid is to make the text "polyphonic," i.e., to people the text with voices. "Polyphony" is a typical feature of novels, and was first described by Russian literary critic Michael Bachtin in his analysis of Dostojevsky's novels (Bachtin, 1981). A text that is composed of different voices (what Bachtin calls "hybrid construction," 1981, p. 304 f.) engages the reader in a peculiar way because the reader feels she gets "to be there" and be involved in a more intense way than in a typical monologic text. At the same time a mixture of different voices creates a "carnival of voices," fascinating and confusing the reader at the same time especially when he is uncertain about whose voice he is reading ("concealed speech of another," 1981, p. 306). In the Palazzoli text the speed in which the voices change is remarkable as illustrated in Figure 4.2.

The question of who authorizes the text is quickly answered: names are listed in the first lines. The question however *whose* story is told is more complex. The very first word of the text – *our* – shows this complexity.

Who does *our* refer to?

- Is it *our* history – the history which we, the Casanti family, told the therapists (or the authors?) – supposed that all members of the family told the story in an identical way? And would other members of the Casanti clan (e.g., Luciana) tell a different story – different from *our* story in contrast to the stories of these other members?
- Or is it *our* history – the history which we, the therapeutic team, construed from what we heard the Casanti family saying, i.e. our history in contrast to that the family had said (or perhaps would have said?)?
- Or is it *our* history – the history which we, the authors, wrote about the Casanti family and the therapeutic team, i.e., *our* history, a history about the family and the team as figures in a story?
- Or is it *our* history in the sense that the readers of the text are included and – by what whatever – participate in the story?
- And who authorizes the story, who is responsible? And who speaks in whose name, and in whose name not?

Rivalry was unthinkable – the children of one were the children of all.	Clan's voice
Thus was born the family myth of	Therapists' voice
"one for all and all for one,"	Clan's and socio-
a myth	cultural voice
also shared by whoever had contact with the family	Therapists' voice
"No other family in the region gets along like the Casantius … such a big family and everybody loves one another … no fighting, no bickering…"	Narrator's voice / Neighborhood's voice (with fictious direct speech)
But the Casanti brothers, still led by the Old Capoccia, were suspicious.	Narrators' voice
These were all signs of a world gone mad.	Clans' voice
Their strength was always the old one –	Clans' or narrator's voice
To work hard and to be united.	Casanti-moral voice
To stay together they had to create a myth, a collective product whose very existence and persistence would be able to reinforce the homeostasis of the group against any disruptive influence.	Therapists' voice

Figure 4.2 Storyteller.

Note: Author – author-icy: Who tells the story?

Voices and Silent Voices: Who Has His Say and Who Not?

Stories are animated by figures who stand in relation to each other. Stories become vivid by the way the figures are sketched and how they are animated. One strategy to animate them is to give them voices by direct speech. Seen from this perspective the following picture emerges: The first figure which is endowed with a voice is the index-client Nora. However, before her voice is heard (or *read*) her voice is contextualized in what Bachtin calls "character zones" (1981, 316). At first her behavior is clinically labeled: *her behavior was psychotic.* After that her interactive presence resp. non-presence is established: *Completely removed from what was going on during the session.* Her forthcoming voice is characterized as a typical form of catatonia, not interactionally related speaking: *she limited herself to moaning, repeating a stereotyped phrase every once in a while.* The reader, so prepared, is presented with Nora's utterance itself in direct speech: *"You should make me put on weight without making me eat"* – a paradoxical request that characterizes the confused state of the index client.

The main focus of this account is on a list of failures of the therapeutic team and an account of their considerations for interrupting the therapeutic process. This is the only voice in the account of the first phase of therapy. Nobody else is given a voice. The considerations of the team are presented as insights of the team: *We learned that for months she had only left her bed in order to indulge in bulimic orgies, which were inevitably followed by bouts of vomiting that reduced her to prostration.*

In the account of the second phase of the therapeutic process (after Nora's failed suicide) father Siro and sister Zita are endowed voices, characterized as *confession* and *revelation*: *The father confessed that in September the clan had shown itself hostile to the idea of the family's return to therapy… Zita, the sister, made an important revelation.* Zita is then described as immediately depreciating her revelation. This is presented to the reader in direct speech: *Maybe all this is just an impression that Nora has.* Nora is said to be silent in this exchange while her parents defend Luciana.

The Narrative Plot of the Story – What Is Really Told?

A story that aims to hold the reader spellbound must meet two requirements: it must rise suspense or at least interest, and it must be plausible and familiar. The second requirement can be fulfilled by using a narrative structure that makes sense for the reader and that is familiar to him. Then he is able to follow the story in its sequential process and its logicIt is possible to get on the track of the plot by paraphrasing the story in a condensed way as follows:

An originally helpful but later on destructive attitude establishes itself within a family and causes harm. Initial efforts to get rid of it fail. The destructive attitude intensifies and causes even more harm. It is only when the healers apply a ritual that the attitude vanishes and the family recovers.

In this condensed paraphrase you can see the narrative plot of an exorcism story. The therapeutic story turns out to be structurally the story of an exorcism with its characteristic components:

- the demon creeps into the family
- the demon dominates the family

- the demon is attacked
- the demon restrains
- the demon is driven out
- the family is freed from the demon and all is well

In this plot the therapists take the figure of an exorcist. One of the characteristic emotional features of this plot, creeps, is induced when Nora is described as *a frightening skeleton.*

Narrative Plot and Relations of Power: The Power of the Therapists is Veiled/Disguised

In the writing culture debate one relevant question relates to how the interactional contexts for gaining data and power relations of these contexts are textually represented. This question can be applied to family-therapeutic case stories too. Due to the institutional context of therapy and the role-relations between therapist and client, there is an asymmetrical power in the therapist-client relationship. In the case story at hand, the exorcism plot can distract away from this aspect to the relation of the therapists and the demon which is to be exorcized and which resists. By this distraction the therapist-client relation can be textually constructed free of power aspects. There are some passages in the text where the aspect of power could have been a topic. But this can be done unobtrusively – almost in the shadow of the therapists-demon relationship. The basic themes are:

- *The family accepted.*
- *The family, duly impressed, agreed to do so.*
- *The family carried out the ritual.*

These descriptions of moments in the therapeutic process are lapidary.

Key Takeaways

This chapter started with a quotation from Clifford Geertz: in conveying in their prose the impression that they have had close-in contact with far-out lives... In discovering how, in this monograph or that article, such an impression is created, we shall discover, at the same time, the criteria by which to judge them (1988, p. 6).

As can be seen, the above narratological analysis of the Palazzoli case history should not be classified as impure verbal, poetic means in a scientific report with the admonition: "See, this is not how it should be done!" Just the opposite: the analysis shows by what verbal means a case story can convince the reader "that this is how it happened."

At the same time such an analysis can be understood as a critical instrument for the reader. Therefore, the conclusion is twofold: It is a plea for a poetic, carefully verbally constructed composition of verbal means to make a case story as convincible as possible, using rhetorical strategies and poetic means that emphasize the version of the author of "what happened" (cf. Pfab & Klemm, forthcoming). At the same time, it is a plea for a literary critic stance against such a case story allowing for questions put on such a text, detecting the very strategies and means, and putting weight on open questions which remained unanswered by the text of the case story itself.

A narratological text like this would be incomplete if it didn't include a self-critical reconsideration of the own writing strategies and stylistic means used, and the interpretative patterns suggested. I list here brief three elements:

1. The selective adaptation of the Palazzoli story: Every adaptation is tacitly governed by the interests, aims, and attitudes of the one who writes the adaptation. Each adaptation is a text itself with its peculiar wording, thematic stress, and its own plot.
2. The "condensed paraphrase" of the text: The "condensed paraphrase" (c.f. 5.4) is of course only one way to read and understand the text resp. the story. It is questionable
3. "The reader": "The reader" is a literal construction used to cement a peculiar interpretation of a text as the only possible one. The article is decisive. It's not *a* reader (among others). "*The* reader" excludes other readers and their alternative readings.

Resources and References

Atkinson, P. (1989). Goffman's poetics. *Human Studies, 12*, p. 59–76.

Bachtin, M. (1981). Discourse in the Novel. In: Holmquist, M. (ed.). *The Dialogic Imagination.* (p. 259–422). Austin: University of Texas Press.

Bradbury, M. (1983). *The Modern American Novel.* Oxford: Oxford University Press.

Breuer, J., & Freud, S. (2001). Studies on hysteria. *Standard Edition* Vol 2. London: Vintage.

Clifford, J., & Marcus, G. (eds.) (1986). *Writing Culture. The Poetics and Politics of Ethnography.* Berkeley: University of California Press.

Darnton, R. (1984). *The Great Cat Massacre.* New York: Basic Books.

Davis, N. (1984). *The Return of Martin Guerre.* Cambridge: Harvard University Press.

Devereux, G. (1967). *From Anxiety to Method in the Behavioral Sciences.* Paris: Mouton.

Eagleton, T. (1983). *Literary Theory.* Oxford: Oxford University Press.

Eason, D. (1986). On journalistic authority: The Janet Cooke Scandal. *Critical Studies in Mass Communication, 3*, p. 429–447.

Evans, R. (2000). *In Defense of History.* New York: Norton.

Foucault, M. (1973). *The Order of Things.* New York: Vintage.

Frye, N. (1957). *Anatomy of Criticism. Four Essays.* Princeton: Princeton University Press.

Geertz, C. (1988). *Works and Lives. The Anthropologist as Author.* Stanford: Stanford University Press.

Goldberg, A. (1997). Writing case histories. *International Journal of Psycho-Analysis, 78*, p. 435–438.

Gottowik, V. (2007). Zwischen dichter und dünner Beschreibung: Clifford Geertz' Beitrag zur *writing-culture*-Debatte. In: Därmann, J. & Damme, C. (eds.) *Kulturwissenschaften.* (p. 119–142). München: Fink.

Latour, B. (1993). *We have never been modern.* Cambridge: Harvard University Press.

Levine, G. (1988). *Darwin and the Novelists. Pattern of Science in Victorian Fiction.* Chicago: University of Chicago Press.

Lindner, R. (1996). *The reportage of urban culture. Robert Park and the Chicago school.* Cambridge: Cambridge University Press.

Luria, A. (1968). *The Mind of a Mnemonist: A Little Book About a Vast Memory.* Cambridge: Harvard University Press.

Mahony, P. (1987). *Freud as a writer.* New Haven: Yale University Press.

Marcus, G. & Cushman, D. (1982). Ethnographies as Text. *Annual Review of Anthropology 11*, p. 25–69.

Marcus, S. (1985). Freud and Dora. In Bernheimer, C., Kahane, C. (eds.) *Dora's case: Freud, hysteria, feminism.* (p. 56–91). London: Virago.

Michels, R. (2000). The case history. *Journal of the American Psychoanalytic Association, 48(2)*, p. 355–375.

Nothdurft, W. (2006). Gesprächsphantome. *Deutsche Sprache, 34*, p. 32–43.

Overbeck, G. (1993). Die Fallanalyse als literarische Verständigungs- und Untersuchungsmethode – Ein Beitrag zur Subjektivierung. In Stuhr, U. & Deneke, F. (eds.) *Die Fallgeschichte. Beiträge zu ihrer Bedeutung als Forschungsinstrument.* (p. 43–60). Heidelberg: Asanger.

Palazzoli, M. S., Boscolo, L., Cecchin, G. F., Prata, G. (1977). Family rituals. A powerful tool in family therapy. *Family Process, 16*, p. 445–453.

Pfab, W., & Klemm, M. (forth). Einführung in den Kommunikativen Realismus. (Ms.).

Przyborski, A. & Wohlrab-Sahr, M. (2008). *Qualitative Sozialforschung. Ein Arbeitsbuch.* München: Oldenbourg.

Rosaldo, R. (1986). From the door of his tent: The fieldworker and the inquisitor. In: Clifford, J. & Marcus, G. (eds.) (1986). *Writing Culture. The Poetics and Politics of Ethnography.* (p. 77–97). Berkeley: University of California Press.

Rüsen, J. (2020). A turning point in theory of history: The place of Hayden White in the history of metahistory. *History and Theory, 59*, p. 92–102.

Sacks, O. (1995). *An Anthropologist on Mars.* New York: Knopf.

Stein, M. (1988). Writing about psychoanalysis: I. Analysts who write and those who do not. *Journal of the American Psychoanalytical Association, 36*, p. 105–124.

Stoller, R. (1988). Patients' responses to their own case reports. *Journal of the American Psychoanalytic Association, 36*, p. 371–391.

Stuhr, U., & Deneke, F. W. (1993). *Die Fallgeschichte* [The case story]. Heidelberg: Asanger.

Stuhr, U. (2007). Die Bedeutung der Fallgeschichte für die Entwicklung der Psychoanalyse. *Psyche 61.* p. 943–965.

Tuckett, D. (1993). Some thoughts on the presentation and discussion of clinical material of psychoanalysis. *International Journal of Psycho-Analysis 74.* p. 1175–1188.

Vann, R. (2002). The reception of Hayden White. *History & Theory 37.* p. 143–161.

Weber, K. (2009). Das Schreiben der (Fall-)Geschichte. Was französische Analytiker von Fallgeschichten erwarten. In Kächele, H. & Pfäfflin, F. (eds.) *Behandlungsberichte und Therapiegeschichten. Wie Therapeuten und Patienten über Psychotherapie schreiben.* (p. 111–136). Gießen: psychsozial.

Wegner, P. (1998). Die Fallgeschichte als Instrument psychoanalytischer Forschung. In Kimmerle, G. (ed.) *Zur Theorie der psychoanalytischen Fallgeschichte.* (p. 9–44). Tübingen: edition discord.

White, H. (1987). *Tropics of Discourse. Essays in Cultural Criticism.* 3th print. Baltimore: Johns Hopkins University Press.

White, H. (1992). *The Content of the Form.* 2nd print. Baltimore: Johns Hopkins University Press.

White, H. (1997). *Metahistory. The historical imagination in nineteenth-century Europe.* Baltimore: Johns Hopkins University Press.

5

FAMILY RITUALS

Carmen V. Nieto, Kimberly N. Usbeck, Jia-Xin (Kailey) Teo, and Karrison A. Rimon

Defining Rituals

What does a ritual mean to you? No matter who you are, or what part of the world you reside in, rituals are all around us. When glancing behind the door of any home, it would not take long to identify distinct customs and patterns of interaction conducted by groups of people. These acts we call rituals are often routinely conducted and practiced by a wide array of races, ethnicities, and cultural backgrounds. Despite our religious beliefs, or where geographically our family of origin is from, the concept of a ritual is something we all share in common even though it looks different across cultures and time. This chapter will focus on defining what a family ritual means, the development of rituals in systems, how rituals are maintained or broken, the importance of recognizing family rituals, and strategies for how to re-design rituals all under the critical consideration of cultural sensitivity.

Wolin and Bennet (1984) define family ritual as "a symbolic form of communication that, owing to the satisfaction that family members experience through its repetition, is acted out in a systematic fashion overtime." It is via the family's unique meaning and their nature that rituals can have a significant impact on the foundation and preservation of a family's identity. Furthermore, "family rituals involve communication with symbolic meaning, establishing and perpetuating the understanding of what it means to be a member of the group" (Spagnola and Fiese, 2007). In other words, rituals serve as a window to a family's identity, and are shaped by the family's behavioral and emotional patterns across generations. It is important to note, and later discussed, how these emotional connections made over time can be either positive or negative exchanges. The importance of family rituals will also be discussed.

Routines vs. Rituals

A ritual in itself is an ambiguous concept. A ritual can be noticeably clear and explicit in its appearance, yet perplexing and confounding when it comes to its boundaries and the effects it has on the individuals involved. Many injunctively defined concepts of a ritual lack clear

DOI: 10.4324/9781003297871-6

distinction of the meaning and merge with similar notions such as traditions, customs, or routines. It is understandable as to why people would often use these terms interchangeably as both terms, family routines and rituals, entail repeated practices that involve two or more members in a family system (Spagnola & Fiese, 2007). Even though some would consider their everyday routines to be a part of their ritualistic experience, it should be noted that when using these words in reference to family systems, there is a distinct difference between the two. Routines and rituals contrast along the dimensions of communication, commitment, and continuity (Fiese et al., 2002).

As previously mentioned, we define family rituals as distinct customs and patterns of interaction conducted by groups of people. Celebrations (such as a graduation), customs (such as yearly birthday parties), and structured interactions (such as a family dinner) are examples of family rituals (Wolin & Bennett, 1984). On the other hand, family routines are distinguished by instrumental communication, a brief time investment, and frequent repetition with no special significance (Spagnola & Fiese, 2007). Family rituals do not signify anything unique. These are the exchanges that take place every day. However, family customs have a symbolic component.

Dr. Mary Spagnola and Dr. Barbara H. Fiese suggest that another method to distinguish between routines and rituals is to think about how the disruption of these two activities might affect the family. Routine disruptions might be inconvenient, but ritual disruptions put the cohesiveness of the family at risk. Therefore, both routines and rituals can play significant roles in upholding the emotional environment and structure of everyday family life.

It must be noted that even though these two terms are different, they do coexist in daily life. Dinnertime, for example, is neither a routine nor a ritual, but has elements of both. There are certain practices that may occur during a meal that may not have a special meaning and others that do. Setting the table, bringing the plates, or cleaning the dishes, for example, may not have any particular meaning; nonetheless, important symbolic features may include saying a prayer, inquiring about everyone's day, or eating only certain foods on specific days. Dinnertime thus reflects both routines and rituals.

Development of Rituals in Systems

There are several components that influence the development of rituals across cultures. To begin to understand how rituals come to be, clinicians must consider client backgrounds and explore their concept of intersectionality. By obtaining insight into a client's identity and experiences shaped through culture, race, class, and gender, clinicians can further understand the impact of rituals thereafter. Prior to delving into the impact of rituals, clinicians must understand how an individual's rituals are first developed, and then, in turn, how they affect the client's lives. Through understanding the foundational components of rituals clinicians can note the influence of rituals on the client's symptoms to provide the best level of care and services necessary.

Influences: Rituals Across Generations

As individuals grow and differentiate from their families of origin, they have the decision to either keep, modify, and/or create their own, or leave behind the traditions, rituals, and practices they grew up with. Wolin and Bennett (1984) note that:

[At] the start of the family career, a young couple may rely heavily on their families of origin as a model for their own ritual occasions, while remaining open to novel events. Rituals can be initially adopted in one form, to be later adapted to their changing needs and interests.

(p. 10)

That is, as families adapt, evolve, and grow within their family cycles, so can their rituals to maintain a position within a family system. As children are introduced within a family system, family rituals are adjusted to include the new family members within their practice. Through the inclusion of children within family rituals, families create a sense of "familiarity, family cohesiveness, and continuity" for their children to "thrive in" (Wolin & Bennett, 1984). Family bonds are strengthened through their shared quality time, and rituals enforce the consistency of those relationships for all members of the family.

From the perspective across generations, clinicians can note the development of rituals over time, beginning as traditions and growing into rituals through repetition and structure implemented by families. Throughout the various stages of families, rituals may require more or less involvement from family members, and expectations can shift and fluctuate. In the beginning stages of family development, the adult family members may lead rituals, modeling important behaviors for their children to learn how to become involved in the ritual. Parents and older relatives may share stories and experiences with older children to emphasize the importance and the meanings behind their rituals. In each of these stages, the adult family members seek the same goal in teaching their children to appreciate, follow, and respect their family rituals. As newer generations grow, families may step back from the "rigid adherence" of rituals, allowing them to form their own meanings and develop their own versions of the family rituals (Wolin & Bennett, 1984). The involvement of all generations within family rituals promotes continuity and the development of legacies, thereafter, eventually forming traditions, which will be discussed further in the chapter.

Due to the immense social nature of humans, it is important to note the impact of migration across generations as it relates to ritual development. Migrating between countries may also lead to families facing shifts within culture, which will further be examined later in the chapter. However, the influence on rituals from migration itself, specifically in terms of the connections developed between family members, should also be explored by clinicians. An ethnographic study conducted by Meng Li (2018) examined "forms and functions of ritualizing" in migrant Chinese families. Li examines rituals in terms of integration for families as part of their migration experience to "bring geographically dispersed kin into proximity and provide them with opportunities to reinvigorate relational bonds" (p. 289). This research further highlights the function of rituals to strengthen "kinship ties," communal interaction, and cultural celebration to enhance senses of belonging within new "host societies" of migrant families (Li, 2018). As families undergo permanent relocations, whether they are in search of new opportunities, seeking refuge, or for any other reason, rituals allow them to maintain ties to their families and places of origin. Ultimately, considering the geographical changes for families could lead to greater insight into the formation of rituals as families adapt to new environments.

Influences: Traditions

Wolin and Bennett explain that "family traditions, as a group, are less culture-specific and more idiosyncratic for each family" (1984, p.3). That is, family traditions differ from rituals in terms of their inherent organization. While rituals are attached directly to specific moments in time (i.e., birthdays, holidays, rites of passage, or milestones, etc.), traditions relate closely to the behaviors associated with those celebrations. Traditions are defined through the actions of a family to perform their rituals. For example, if birthdays are categorized in rituals as explained previously in the chapter, how a family celebrates the birthday (e.g., having cake, singing, dancing, and so on) will form their traditions. In this aspect, child participation within traditions, and in turn, rituals, is further seen. On the other hand, it is also by the guidelines of tradition that the inclusion or non-inclusion of children within a family ritual is set.

The influence of culture may play a role within the formation of tradition, but the family system ultimately explicitly defines the constructs of their traditions. Through deciding who is involved, what will happen, and where and how the event will happen, families shape their traditions as they see fit. However, traditions are still closely related to culture. Similar to the cultural concept of self-asserted family identity within society, "family traditions seem to say, 'This is the way we are; this is our family'" (Wolin & Bennet, 1984, p.3). Thereafter, the level of significance that family members give to their traditions will influence their attachment to its practice, which will impact the potential creation of a ritual as a result. That potential creation may be affected by the involvement of younger generations as they would be the ones to maintain or break past (family of origin) traditions with their own nuclear families in the future.

Influences: Culture

As mentioned previously, a family's geographical location may affect their cultural expression due to a potential for adaptation, especially when considering migration. Family rituals may adapt or change depending on the family's comfort within their environment, whether newfound or original. That is, there are outside factors to be considered within society that will impact a family's ability to observe their cultural rituals. For example, a family's self-asserted and perceived identities within society may influence the way rituals are observed, as these factors affect their embeddedness within their community.

Through cultural influences, family celebrations take consistent form, such as holidays and special occasions. Wolin & Bennett (1984) categorize "rites of passage, such as weddings, funerals, baptisms, and bar mitzvahs; annual religious celebrations, such as Christmas, Easter, the Passover Seder; and secular holiday observances such as Thanksgiving, New Year's, or the Fourth of July," within culturally based rituals (p.2). That is, culture sculpts the events families will create rituals for throughout their development. Once again, these rituals may stem from family of origin and become adapted as individuals differentiate from the beliefs and practices they were raised with.

Lastly, as part of culturally influenced rituals, "patterned family interactions" should be included as Wolin & Bennett state they are the "least deliberate and most covert of family rituals," yet still influential to the daily function of families (1984). They further explain that these patterned family interactions are the ones "most frequently enacted but least consciously planned by the participants. In this category belong rituals such as a regular dinnertime, bedtime routines for children, the customary treatment of guests in the home, or leisure activities on weekends or evenings" (Wolin & Bennet, 1984, p.4). Even though the routines are part of a family's daily function, guided by societal norms, they can also be considered part of their rituals due to their impact on the roles and responsibilities of family members (Wolin & Bennett, 1984). These daily routines are attached to expectations that contribute to family function, which potentially become rituals through repetition.

Influences: Religion

In 1950, Bossard and Boll conducted "an extensive qualitative study of family rituals... they concluded that rituals were powerful organizers of family life, supporting its stability during times of stress and transition" (Fiese, et al., 2002, p.381). Inherently as "powerful organizers of family life," rituals can very well be influenced by family beliefs brought through the practice of religion. For example, from a Catholic religious background, rituals can be seen throughout their practice of celebrating sacraments, such as baptisms, communions, confirmations, and marriages as well. Religion may also contribute to the ritual practices surrounding marriage and its trajectory, more specifically considering whether divorces are accepted or not. However, this may also be dependent on the level of devotion for clients within their religious beliefs and how strictly they follow customs practices. An example of this is seen through the observance of religious holidays. When thinking about the holiday of Easter, Catholic communities observe rituals throughout 40 days of the Lenten season. Further, individuals may practice fasting behaviors (not consuming meat on Fridays during the season) or abstain from their indulgences to maintain their devotion. However, variation may be seen as religious traditions and rituals can be practiced differently and to various extents as families see best fit. Additionally, prayer customs within families can differ (e.g., between Muslim and Christian communities, etc.) as well, but would also be included within the rituals of a family. As individuals from diverse backgrounds join to form new families, it is important to consider differences across religions as influential factors within ritual formation as well.

Rituals Throughout the Life Cycle

It is evident that rituals are an important part of the human experience, coloring the lives of people, families, and communities all throughout the world. Take a moment to think about the rituals in your personal life or in the world around you. Are there some rituals that have withstood the test of time and have been passed down from generation to generation? Are there some rituals that have changed over time? Are there some rituals you realize have been lost or forgotten? In this section, we will explore the process in which rituals are maintained, broken, and transformed. We will start by taking a closer look at rituals throughout a typical family life cycle. According to cross-sectional data, there seems to be a cycle to family rituals across generations (Fiese et al., 2002).

Time and rhythm in relationships has a powerful, largely unrecognized, influence on quality and organization in couples lives (Papp, 2000). The timing and rhythm that couples develop together can often dictate what cycles and patterns they begin to develop within their relationship. As timing and rhythm consistently impact the outcome of every couples' interactions on some scale, this factor at times becomes difficult to break and can impact and create both healthy and unhealthy rituals. When couples become caught in the recursive nature of their unpleasant rituals, or their everydayness, the probability that the rituals lead to unpleasant interactions is more likely (Breunlin et. al., 2001). Breaking the recursive nature through reorganizing the timing and rhythm of rituals in a relationship can increase pleasant interactions throughout the life cycle.

Marriage: Negotiating Rituals

Marriage marks the beginning of a new family life cycle. New couples typically rely on their families of origin as a model for their own rituals (Wolin & Bennett, 1984). Spouses must negotiate to some level which rituals they would like to continue or not continue from their family-of-origin in their new family (Wolin & Bennett, 1984). There may be conflict throughout this process, especially if spouses have different religious and cultural backgrounds and attitudes towards roles and hierarchy in the family. The negotiations of the couple may lead to the commitment to continue, the decision to abandon, or the flexibility to adapt rituals from their families-of-origin. Furthermore, new couples are not only limited to rituals inherited from their families-of-origin. New couples can also create new rituals together. Decisions about rituals continue throughout the new couple's family life cycle, especially if the couple decides to have children. Rituals may be decided at first in one form to be later transformed to the changing needs of their partnership and family (Wolin & Bennett, 1984).

Child-Rearing: The Passing on of Rituals

If a couple decides to have children, they enter into the child-rearing portion of the family life cycle. When a couple first has children, they typically become increasingly ritual-centered in order to provide familiarity, cohesiveness, and continuity for their children (Wolin & Bennett, 1984). Rosenthal and Marshall (1988) found that 80% of the adults they interviewed continued rituals with their children from their family-of-origin practices (Fiese et al., 2002). Additionally, research shows that the meaning ascribed to family rituals becomes more central when individuals become parents themselves. Performing rituals that have been passed down from a previous generation gives a "familiar and right" feeling, offers comfort, and builds a sense of "home" within a family (Wolin et al., 1980). Rituals that are maintained through generations can act as a force against change within the family. Rituals offer reassurance that what is most important in the family remains the same and unbroken (Wolin & Bennett, 1984). The generational transmission of rituals ultimately strengthens the identity of a family.

Families often remain heavily involved with family rituals until children enter adolescence. As children grow and develop with age, they have a greater ability to be an active participant in rituals. Children are especially more involved in the practice of routines from elementary school through adolescence (Fiese et al., 2002). Children may be given increasing levels of responsibility in rituals by parents. This could be a son helping to set the table with his father for Sunday night dinner with the grandparents or siblings taking turns lighting the menorah for Hanukkah. Children may also build an increasing sense of ownership towards a ritual by adding their own "flavor" to it. This could be a daughter leading the decoration of the Christmas tree or choosing which Christmas carols to sing as a family.

Additionally, children also have an increasing capacity to understand the deeper meaning of family rituals. Rituals in a sense are a learning experience, whether through observance or participation (Wolin & Bennett, 1984). Research shows that the meaning ascribed to family rituals does not appear to be important until late adolescence (Fiese et al., 2002). Their natural curiosity may spark questions about why things are done the way they are done or why the family is doing what it is doing. Parents may see their children's engagement with rituals as a readiness to share the symbolic meaning and folklore behind the rituals. Through rituals, children are taught deeper messages that are important to the family. They may learn the family's spiritual or religious beliefs, cultural heritage, and attitudes towards roles and hierarchy.

Overall, children take more responsibility and ownership towards family rituals over time, gain a deeper understanding behind the family's rituals, and learn important values and beliefs to the family. All of this, along with the growing collection of warm memories associated with rituals, help children to maintain the rituals throughout their own life. Ultimately, parents passing rituals on to their children is how rituals are maintained and transcend the generations.

Launching Children and Later Life

As the aging couple witnesses the rise of a new generation, there is greater importance placed on ensuring an ongoing family heritage (Wolin & Bennett, 1984). The couple's legacy is seen as continuing through the rituals their children and their children's children carry on. Particularly in communities in which elders are revered, grandparents may play a significant role in passing on the practice and meaning behind important family rituals. During this time of the family life cycle, the aging couple has adult children who are focusing on their own emerging family and beginning their own family life cycle. Adult children, as mentioned earlier, are generally faced with decisions about abandoning or maintaining family-of-origin traditions, negotiating a blend between the unique family ritual systems with their spouse, and creating entirely new family traditions (Pett et al., 1992). It is possible that the aging couple's adult children may decide to abandon or transform the established family rituals. Aging parents may see this as a threat to family legacy, leading to strained, tense, and potentially disruptive interactions with their adult children (Pett et al., 1992). The pressures surrounding the maintenance of rituals will be discussed later in this section.

Disruptive Events in the Family Life Cycle

There are several disruptive events that may happen in the family life cycle that call into question whether a family ritual will be maintained, broken, or transformed. As a family gains or loses members through divorce, remarriage, and death, what will happen to the rituals in place? How will a family's rituals be impacted when a family migrates or is displaced into a different culture? What happens when family members have evolving views that challenge the beliefs and meanings behind established rituals? As we will discuss further in this section, families that are flexible and make appropriate changes to ritual performance over the family life cycle ensure rituals remain relevant and effective (Wolin & Bennett, 1984).

Separation, Divorce and Remarriage

A notable transition that threatens the practice of family routines is divorce (Fiese et al., 2002). Divorce is a disruptive process that starts in a malfunctioning marriage and continues for many years following the divorce (Pett et al., 1992). For years, the family will engage in the continued renegotiation and restructuring of roles, composition, and boundaries of previously valued family celebrations, traditions, ceremonies, and daily rituals (Pett et al., 1992). Naturally, some of the long-held family rituals will be maintained, lost, or changed with new rituals constructed from old ones (Pett et al., 1992). Post-divorce parenting and post-divorce living arrangements continue to be in a constant state of flux and thus the practice of family rituals continues to change over time (Bakker et al., 2015).

Pett et al. (1992) explored how late-life divorce impacts family rituals. For some families, divorce was a positive new beginning. Following divorce, these families experienced increased freedom to experiment with family celebrations and therefore built new traditions on previously established traditions (Pett et al., 1992). However, most respondents described a disruptive loss of family unity and traditions, holiday celebrations, birthdays, vacations, recreational activities, and everyday family interactions (Pett et al., 1992). Respondents reported that these traditions required extra planning and negotiation to accommodate both parents. In a Pett et al. (1992) study, some respondents reported problems with the spouses of remarried parents, which presented another barrier in continuing previously upheld family rituals (Pett et al., 1992). Along with the stress of complicated logistics, respondents reported discomfort, awkwardness, and increased tension surrounding family-get-togethers that resulted in fewer activities than before (Pett et al., 1992). Feelings surrounding the activity were different and many respondents reported that it was too emotionally painful to continue previously important family traditions.

Additionally, there is much diversity in how families restructure after separation and divorce, in turn affecting family rituals. Bakker et al. (2015) interviewed separated parents in the Netherlands and explored how rituals are affected in separated families. After separation, some families continued to practice pre-separation rituals with their children with both parents present. Efforts were made to maintain a ritual as it was practiced before the separation. Other separated families chose to "build a new life" in which children alternated living arrangements with each parent and practiced rituals separately. Children often celebrated birthdays, holidays, and major life events twice. Lastly, some families only had one parent involved in the children's lives post-separation and rituals were only practiced with that parent.

Following separation, some partners also chose to remarry. If a separated parent remarries and establishes another family system, children may have decreased daily contact with that parent (Pett et al., 1992). The lack of presence of the remarried separated parent will inevitably impact the previously established daily interactions and family gatherings of the family. If a parent remarries and a new parent enters the established family system, the new parental subsystem must negotiate new rituals. The family will have to restructure itself to include the new parent in existing rituals and to welcome any new rituals made by the new family unit.

It is evident that there is diversity and complexity among family's post-separation, post-divorce, and post-remarriage. Regardless of post-separation family structure, rituals continue to play a role in helping families identify as a coherent unit, whether "we are still family" or "this is my new family." Some rituals are maintained to create some semblance of familiarity and stability. Research has shown that maintaining regular routines and rituals in divorced and remarried families has been shown to promote better adaptation in children (Fiese et al., 2002). These routines and rituals ensure a sense of security and stability of family life during a time of profound change. Some rituals are lost with the decrease or loss of involvement of a parent. In other instances, with the absence of involvement of a parent, rituals can retain their original significance and importance while being modified in how they are performed. New rituals may also be created to adapt to the changing needs of the family. Clearly, the addition and loss of family members through separation, divorce, and remarriage forces families to restructure and calls into question the practice of previously upheld family rituals.

Physical/Mental Illness

Another disruptive event during the life cycle is the diagnosis of a family member with a mental or physical illness. Exploring family rituals and their disruptions can give insight into the state of the family's well-being. For instance, if a family's rituals are being disrupted by a pathological condition, it is proof that the physical or mental illness has had extensive repercussions in the family (Wolin et al., 1980). However, when the rituals are maintained, it is a sign that the family has retained some level of stability.

In the American population, 50% of men and 65% of women who have a diagnosed mental illness are also a parent (Power et al., 2016). Participants in a study by Power et al. (2016) reported that family life was unpredictable or chaotic due to a parent's mental illness. This includes unpredictable mood, availability, and care of the parent. In these families, the maintenance of everyday routines and family rituals are extremely important, allowing some predictability and relief from stress. This may be the continuation of previously upheld rituals or adapting rituals to better suit the capabilities and needs of the family. The consistent practice of rituals aided these families in fostering a sense of connectedness. Positive interactions with one another were a key ingredient for family resilience. The maintenance of everyday routines and family rituals were typically ensured by the parent who did not have a mental illness. However, in single-parent families or families with low access to resources, the diagnosis of a parent with a mental illness can disrupt previously active family rituals. This disruption may cause low stability and resilience for the family.

During the life cycle, family members may also be diagnosed with a physical illness. The financial, logistical, and emotional burdens on a family with a family member receiving treatment for a physical illness can be immense. The added burdens may cause family rituals to be disrupted, maintained, or adapted. The maintenance or adaptation of family rituals has been shown to promote better adaptation in families with a family member with a physical illness. It can foster stronger family ties by providing organization and increasing cohesion, all of which aid in disease management, treatment adherence, and roles adaptivity (Santos et al., 2015). A family with greater cohesion might share in illness-related responsibility, decision-making, and offer support. The maintenance or adaptation of family rituals can also increase feelings of hope through creating structure and support towards goal-directed actions. Increased feelings of hope from continuing family rituals can help adolescents diagnosed with a physical illness to adapt to their diagnosis and treatment. Increased feelings of hope from continuing family rituals can also help family members perceive an illness as a barrier to overcome rather than a threat or fatality. This in turn motivates family members to engage in more coping strategies that further aid adaptation.

Loss and Death

The loss of a family member is an inevitable but disruptive event in the family life cycle. When families attempt to "return to normal life" after the passing of a family member, they are faced with ongoing grief coupled with emotional, financial, and logistical stressors. Along with this enormous weight, families are also faced with the task of restructuring the roles of the family and adjusting to the change. Some families may continue previously upheld rituals to invite a sense of familiarity, warmth, and stability. The maintenance of these rituals can help bring the grieving family closer and increase resilience in coping with the loss. Since grief is unique to each person, some family members may see the practice of previously upheld family rituals as painful reminders of the loss. Other family members may struggle to accept that previously upheld family rituals will "never be the same." Some families who have a lack of support or resources and in turn struggle to deal with the loss may abandon important family rituals. Other families may choose to transform previous rituals to adapt to the changing needs of their family.

Migration

Another disruptive event in the family life cycle that calls into question the maintenance, disruption, or adaptation of family rituals is migration or displacement. Following migration or displacement, families must balance the importance of maintaining and honoring their cultural identity with the need to assimilate into the new culture. The task of assimilating into a new culture can deplete financial, emotional and time resources that make it challenging to continue rituals. Additionally, the absence of extended family members and larger community add an extra layer of difficulty in maintaining rituals from the country-of-origin (Migliorini et al., 2016). Rituals, however, can be a tool to reduce stress and cope with the ambiguous losses of migration (Migliorini et al., 2016). Some families may engage with re-creation rituals in which a collective cultural group recreates the meeting places of the past. Some families may also engage with memory rituals. Memory rituals consist of telling stories of the past or the migration experience to make meaning out of the present circumstances and develop hope for the future.

The rigid adherence to rituals from the country-of-origin can lead some members to view the rituals as a burden or chore. The rituals may become hollow and meaningless. Typically, first-generation immigrant children are navigating how to fit in and gain acceptance by adopting practices of the new culture. Parents may worry their children are losing their cultural heritage and become more forceful with continuing rituals of the past. In these cases, excessive reliance on the performance of the ritual may take on greater importance than adapting to the new culture. Also, adherence to the ritual may take on greater importance than its actual meaning. Children may rebel against the family ritual, symbolizing the rejection of the culture-of-origin, and resent ceremonial aspects of early life (Bossard & Boll, 1949).

The hollowing out of country-of-origin rituals may occur throughout the family life cycle as all family members change in how they uniquely relate to their cultural heritage. On the other hand, complete abandonment of country-of-origin rituals or inability to adapt these rituals to a new context may also be problematic. Family members may lose touch with an important part of their identity and the loss of rituals may also disrupt family unity and positivity. Hence, it is important that families who migrate or are displaced find a balance between maintaining cultural rituals and adapting to the new culture.

The Pressure to Continue Rituals

According to Wolin and Bennett (1984), rituals are passed on with the expectation or implicit assumption that the next generation will continue them, which may be interpreted as pressure as rituals are maintained. There may be fears that not maintaining a ritual may be met with disappointment, judgment, and rejection from the family or larger community. Since rituals reinforce a sense of belonging, not continuing a ritual threatens that sense of belonging. This is important because when children become adults, they form their own values, beliefs, and perspectives. Although this is guided by the family-of-origin, there may be some disparities between the child's beliefs and the family-of-origin's beliefs.

There are familial pressures in continuing rituals. Families naturally seek continuity and repetition over change and instability (Wolin & Bennett, 1984). Families with high-commitment rituals have been found to place importance on preserving family structure and clarity of roles across generations. Particularly, the hierarchy in the positions of parents and children is of utmost importance in maintaining rituals (Wolin & Bennett, 1984). Parents in these families may place great pressure on children to continue their legacy and to respect the hierarchy, learned roles, and upheld traditions of the family. Preservation of rituals can preserve the family's belonging to the wider group. However, some children may react to their parents' preoccupation with structure and roles by having minimal regard for the family's rituals (Wolin & Bennett, 1984).

There may also be cultural, religious, and societal pressures to maintain rituals. In cultural and religious communities, the continued performance of a ritual strengthens the identity of the group. The rituals pass down deeply important messages to individuals about their place in society and the cosmos (Wolin & Bennett, 1984). There may be fear of judgment, rejection, and loss of community when an individual decides to not practice a ritual and thus some may continue rituals for the sake of safety and belonging.

In conclusion, throughout the family life cycle and all the disruptive events that occur, it is crucial for families to consistently re-evaluate the current need for rituals. Rituals can become "hollow" when the commitment to the ritual prevails over the meaning of the ritual. Additionally, rituals can become "hollow" when the commitment to the ritual fails to adapt to the developmental needs and changes of their family. Flexibility to incorporate change in rituals that maintains the symbolic meaning and accommodates the needs of the family is vital.

Recognizing Rituals in a Culturally Sensitive Manner

In a world filled with people that have come from all walks of life, it is no surprise that there is a plethora of unique cultural norms. Everyone embodies distinct cultures with histories of rich tradition and rituals that have been passed down generation after generation. These rituals are often symbolic in nature, representing a significant aspect of the family's roots and values. Knowing this, it is paramount that clinicians recognize the importance of acknowledging all kinds of various rituals in a culturally sensitive manner. These rituals, in many cases, have not been shared outside the family and are foreign to people of different races, ethnicities, and cultural backgrounds.

A family's identity may be seen via its rituals as they are shaped by the family's tendency for certain emotional and behavioral patterns. Within the family system, members might embody certain roles and, in a way, develop components of their identity through their rituals as well. Roles are crucial for the health of the family unit and for its members to build a sense of belonging within their own system, at both a micro and macro level. Additionally, rituals help families preserve their homeostasis and stability. Establishing positive and healthy rituals can greatly impact the relationships of a system in the long term.

Most people would agree that when family members get together, opportunities for both positive and negative interactions arise over time. As family members unite, they develop emotional bonds with one another and form personal identities. Some family interactions may hold more weight than others, but this depends on the family itself. Moreover, the frequency of family interactions over time will also have an impact. Most family interactions can be divided into three categories: family celebrations, family customs, and structured family interactions (Wolin & Bennett, 1984).

While it may seem like all gatherings and events can be categorized as ritualistic, there are a few key differences worth pointing out. Holidays and other occasions that are commonly practiced across a culture and hold special meaning for a family are known as family celebrations. Family traditions are unique to each family and less culture specific. Even though they occur often in most households, they lack the yearly periodicity of holidays or the uniformity of rites of passage. In contrast to family festivities, family traditions are only mildly arranged. Patterned family interactions are the most unintentional and subtle of family rituals. These rituals are the most regularly performed, but the ones that the participants are least aware of planning. For example, some of these rituals include regular dinnertime, children's bedtime routines, how visitors are treated at home, and weekend or nighttime activities for fun fall under this category. These experiences hold emotional connections and value. When rituals are disrupted, family cohesion is threatened. Therefore, the meaning of belonging in the system can come into question. Thus, both routines and rituals have the potential to serve important roles in maintaining the structure and emotional climate of daily family life (Spagnola & Fiese, 2007).

Family Symptoms

In every family, both positive and negative family symptoms can appear. Symptoms of a family refers to the emotions and behaviors followed by a change that occurs in a family. These symptoms occur in order to keep equilibrium in the family system, and it can be both a positive and negative experience for those involved. For instance, a negative symptom can be of a family experiencing the effects of a divorce. Not all family members will be on board for a divorce, having an unwanted change taking place. Oftentimes, the original family splits apart and forms new family traditions with the new integrated family members (i.e., stepparents, step siblings, step-grandparents, etc.). "The stepfamily is not a variant form of the so-called normal nuclear family but is a distinct family form" (Gullotta & Blau, 2014). On the other hand, a positive family symptom can be the behavior and feelings followed by the experience of therapy itself. Going to therapy itself can promote positive family symptoms, such as increasing empathy, building connection, creating a safe space, and allowing for open communication between family members.

Family symptoms impact the emotions and behaviors of all family members involved. Major life events or transitions can push for unwanted change, challenging the family's norm. "Disruption of family rituals can have consequences well beyond the performance of the rituals" (Wolin et al., 1980), causing negative symptoms to appear more frequently. It should be emphasized that family symptoms take place in efforts to maintain stability in the system. With the help of a clinician, families can become aware and change their behavior to gain desired results.

Just as rituals are essential to the nuclear families' equilibrium, the integration of preexisting rituals and new rituals as well are essential to the overall wellbeing and success of the stepfamily. The ability to recognize the unique challenges that may arise during the development of this new family system will leave families in the best position for success.

While this is not a chapter dedicated to the challenges associated with stepfamilies and children, it's important that this population not be overlooked when discussing the significance of culture and rituals. Distinct cultures and rituals cross into all forms of unique family systems and while there is a wide range of varying opinions on how to successfully form and strengthen stepfamilies, most scholars will agree that at least some portion of the family's success will be determined by the establishment of rituals.

Resistance

Sometimes rituals are personal and specific to the person or people to whom they pertain. Due to the many differences in which families practice and perform their rituals, there are times when one or more members may resist the family's rituals . Children, for example, sometimes refuse to comply with rituals and try to deviate from the family norm. Examples of this may look like adolescents adopting more of a modern westernized set of rituals based on what they see and hear from their peers in school, or perhaps they have lost the connection to their family of origin and no longer wish to carry on traditional ways as they become adults. Another example of resistance can be seen when families invite new people, such as a friend, into their rituals. Resistance can be experienced by the friend, who may not know how to participate in the ritual, and by the family as well, who may not be accustomed to including newcomers into their ritual.

A popular example of the resistance of rituals can be seen widely throughout the history of religious confirmation and conformity. The significance of rituals is often seen, intergenerationally, because of the deeply rooted religious values that are essential to family development. However, there are times in which family members adopt variations of their religious backgrounds, potentially causing rifts amongst the family system that disrupt previously established rituals. For example, this can be seen through "The contemporary movement known as 'Spiritual but not religious,' in which one 'finds God in a sunset' and sees no need for any rituals or practices may also be an example of this sort of trivialization" (Chandler, 2019). To this end, sometimes, religion can be abandoned all together in lieu of a more fluid and spiritual belief system.

Cross-Cultural Rituals

In addition to the separation of families, rituals are also extremely relevant to the formation of two newly joined partners and their families as well. Whether it be the initial dating experience, marriage, or raising a family together, the rituals that each partner experiences from childbirth will impact how they build their relationships and often dictate how they pass on new rituals to their children. "It is increasingly common for individuals who are forming partnerships to come to their relationship from very different cultures in their families of origin; these cultures may vary by socio-economic status, religion and ethnicity, as well as family values and attitudes" (Pryor, 2006). While commonly shared rituals can become a bonding experience, it is important to note that partners coming from different cultural backgrounds may face challenges in integrating different rituals into their relationship.

Culturally Sensitive Strategies for Redesigning Rituals

Families can develop new rituals as their system grows and develops. Additionally, clinicians can gain insight that will let them guide families through forming and redesigning rituals, especially when rituals become harmful or negatively impactful. In order to redesign family rituals as part of treatment, clinicians can begin to take a culturally sensitive approach by using Wolin and Bennett's (1984) proposed framework. Wolin and Bennett highlight four key concepts surrounding decision-making in terms of forming new rituals: family units must be aware of the role and contribution of each family member, integrate heritage and values of all members involved in forming new family units, incorporate prior ritualistic behavior of each individual to blend with the demands of the family's current context and environment, and attend to developmental needs of family to accurately reflect present and past family essence and values (1984, p.12). The nature of rituals, though meaningful, may also generate a negative impact for family systems if they become harmful or disruptive to family function, which is further explored in the following, *Identifying Concerning Rituals*, section.

Identifying Concerning Rituals

According to Wolin and Bennett, in relation to alcoholism within families, "any chronic dysfunction tends to disrupt ongoing continuity of family rituals," (1984, p.11). This is considered a dysfunctional family symptom. Therefore, this begins to allude to the process of identifying how negative symptoms impact rituals for families. Clinicians can begin to assess the interactional cycles and patterns of families, specifically those that are harmful to family systems, through noticing a disruption of the "ongoing continuity of family rituals." A disruption can be seen when an unexpected interruption or change is made to a family ritual. Clinicians can then identify the symptoms caused by those unproductive rituals.

Disruption within family function due to rituals can be seen in many ways at all stages within family development. From the family's beginning stages to potential ends or modifications, as mentioned in other sections, rituals may need to be flexible and adaptable throughout family development. Noticing recent changes within a family system may be a starting point for clinicians to begin exploring the impact of rituals. Factors that clinicians can consider, which may require new ritual formation can include, change in religious beliefs, new and diverse marriages, differences between family identities (i.e., families of origin, nuclear families, stepfamilies), deaths within the family to address the need to create or understand rituals surrounding grief, funeral traditions, and assuming new family roles, among many others. Ultimately, considering the future impacts of ritual will allow families to work together with clinicians to understand the efficacy and longevity of their practices.

Clinical Intervention

While the importance and meaning of rituals may widely vary for all, one thing many share in common are the benefits that these traditions bring. Legare and Souza refute arguments from previous work that identifies rituals as "expressions of inner states of feeling and emotion, symbolize theological ideas or social relations, or represent psychophysical states," saying that "conceptualizing rituals exclusively in this way neglects the fact that the use of rituals for protective, restorative, and instrumental purposes is a pervasive feature of human culture" (2012, p.1). Clinicians must comprehend the full complexity of rituals in order to effectively treat patients in today's culture, from the concept that they are "inner states" to their exterior functions (being "protective, restorative, and instrumental") within human nature. It is crucial for clinicians to adopt a systemic perspective early on in treatment in order to comprehend how rituals affect all facets of family life in order to recognize the contributions of all family members to the unit. Facets of family life include, but are not limited to, daily activities, community building, interpersonal relationships, and individual factors of each family member, such as sex/intimacy, travel, art, music/dance, and health. Clinicians and families will have the chance to start coming up with solutions to address the impact of rituals, especially detrimental ones, when they understand the underlying family values that underlie them.

To move forward with treatment, it is essential to encourage client autonomy, allowing families to define how distress can be reduced through altering or dismissing certain family rituals. The intention to build new positive outcomes for families is the same, whether implementing ritual modification or dissolution. Spagnola & Fiese (2007) emphasize the positive outcome of family relationship satisfaction in terms of emotional investment in family rituals, while Wolin & Bennett (1984) note the importance of rituals addressing the families' current needs. These approaches, however, do not need to be separate. Through combining focuses between family needs and emotional investment for relationship satisfaction, clinicians can develop treatment in a manner that will be most efficient within the specific context for each family, which further promotes an acceptance for diversity within treatment and understanding of family rituals. Based on their applied theories of choice, clinicians will use interventions that fit their approach to treatment of families when redesigning rituals in a culturally sensitive manner.

Considering both options of treatment, if the family decides to dissolve the family ritual altogether, the family may need to adjust to no longer observing the ritual, which may impact their established practices thus far. This option of treatment could potentially challenge family member roles or senses of identity as they disconnect from rituals that have been consistent to them over longer periods of time. Additionally, clinicians can help families consider potential external consequences that may arise after ending a ritual. That is, families may need to consider what ending a ritual may mean in terms of generational impact (e.g., broken family ties due to differing values), in which case repair or coping may become a new goal for the family thereafter. Otherwise, if the family decides to modify their rituals, clinicians can help in that process of modification to create a new family ritual that will encompass the family's current needs, beliefs, and values.

In the beginning of treatment, if the family chooses to modify their existing rituals, clinicians should identify the origin and understand the meaning of the ritual for the family. Through discussing meaning-making with clients, clinicians can identify the importance and connection of a ritual to the family to help protect the symbolic meaning for the family. Clinicians can explore the history of the original rituals to understand the root of the problem brought by the ritual. By learning about the ritual meaning, behaviors, and actions, clinicians can then focus on identifying the negative emotions that rituals may create. To this end, they can address potential negative emotions and distress brought to the family system through the practice of the ritual within treatment. After gathering background information surrounding the original version of the ritual, when modifying the ritual, the clinician can assist the family to preserve the symbolic meaning within the ritual. In doing so, clinicians may find exceptions from the past, in which the ritual did not pose harm or problems to the families. Previous rituals can be further assessed through a form of mapping to identify all factors of the practice (i.e., who is involved, how, when, and where the ritual occurs, and so on).

The development of new rituals may be approached as an intervention of reframing from the clinician's perspective. However, the reframe may be a bit more interactive in the sense of creating a new practice rather than redefining the original meaning of previous rituals. An example of this intervention could look like having a family collaboratively define and create a personalized ritual during a session, if taking an Experiential approach. Although there are countless ways to take a creative approach to addressing the impact of rituals within family systems as couple and family therapists. To measure progress towards goals, clinicians may emphasize the importance of reducing negative interactions brought about by differing opinions surrounding rituals and instead encourage more awareness, open mindedness, and effective communication to help increase the frequency of the desired outcome (i.e., establishing new rituals). Throughout treatment of family symptoms brought by rituals, it is necessary for clinicians to maintain cultural sensitivity as practicing clinicians and respect client diversity.

Conclusion

The importance of broaching the topic of rituals with clients in a culturally sensitive manner is paramount to the joining process of a therapeutic relationship. Relationships and family systems are continually influenced by the development of rituals across generations, which are formed by traditions, religion, and culture. As time passes, demands and expected roles change, among other external elements within a family system that either preserve or break rituals. As clinicians, it is necessary to identify rituals in a culturally sensitive manner to show how they affect family systems. To help individuals, couples, and families through their therapeutic processes of recovery, clinicians are required to understand the significance of rituals for all family members. This chapter conceptualized the significance, development, impact, and progression of rituals to further generate a culturally sensitive approach for redesigning rituals internationally.

References

Bakker, W., Karsten, L., & Mulder, C. H. (2015). Family routines and rituals following separation: Continuity and change. *Families, Relationships and Societies, 4*(3), 365–382. https://doi.org/10.1332/204674314X13891971182856

Bossard, J. H. S., & Boll, E. S. (1949). Ritual in family living. *American Sociological Review, 14*(4), 463–469. https://doi.org/10.2307/2087208

Breunlin, D. C., Schwartz, R. C., & Kune-Karrer, B. M. (2001). *Metaframeworks: Transcending the Models of Family Therapy*. Jossey-Bass Publishers.

Chandler, M. (2019). Religion, ritual, and family. *Philosophy East and West*, 69(1), 20–29. https://doi.org/10.1353/pew.2019.0022

Fiese, B.H., Tomcho, T. J., Douglas, M., Josephs, K., Poltrock, S., & Baker, T. (2002). A review of 50 years of research on naturally occurring family routines and rituals. *Journal of Family Psychology*, 16(4), 381–390. https://doi.org/10.1037/0893-3200.16.4.381

Gullotta, T. P., & Blau, G. M. (2008). Family influences on childhood behavior and development. New York: Routledge.

Gullotta, T. P., & Blau, G. M. (2014). Stepfamilies and Children. In *Family influences on childhood behavior and development: Evidence-based prevention and treatment approaches* (pp. 161–161). Routledge.

Legare, & Souza, A. L. (2012). Evaluating ritual efficacy: Evidence from the supernatural. *Cognition*, 124(1), 1–15. https://doi.org/10.1016/j.cognition.2012.03.004

Li, M. (2018). Maintaining ties and reaffirming unity: Family rituals in the age of migration. *Journal of Family Communication*, 18(4), 286–301. https://doi.org/10.1080/15267431.2018.1475391

Migliorini, L., Rania, N., Tassara, T., & Cardinali, P. (2016). Family routine behaviors and meaningful rituals: A Comparison Between Italian and Migrant Couples. *Social Behavior and Personality*, 44(1), 9–18. https://doi.org/10.2224/sbp.2016.44.1.9

Papp, P. (2000). Couples on the fault line: New Directions for Therapists. Guilford Press.

Pett, M. A., Lang, N., & Gander, A. (1992). Late-life divorce: Its impact on family rituals. *Journal of Family Issues, 13*(4), 526–552. https://doi.org/10.1177/019251392013004008

Power, J., Goodyear, M., Maybery, D., Reupert, A., O'Hanlon, B., Cuff, R., & Perlesz, A. (2016). Family resilience in families where a parent has a mental illness. *Journal of Social Work, 16*(1), 66–92. https://doi.org/10.1177/1468017314568081

Pryor, J. (2006). *Beyond demography: History, ritual and families in the twenty-first century*. Families Commission.

Santos, S., Crespo, C., Canavarro, C. & Kazak, A. E. (2015). Family rituals and quality of life in children with cancer and their parents: The role of family cohesion and hope. *Journal of Pediatric Psychology, 40*(7), 664–671. *Journal of Pediatric Psychology, 40*(7), 664–671. https://doi.org/10.1093/jpepsy/jsv013

Smit, R. (2011). Maintaining family memories through symbolic action: Young adults' perceptions of family rituals in their families of origin. *Journal of Comparative Family Studies, 42*(3), 355–367. https://doi.org/10.3138/jcfs.42.3.355

Spagnola, M., & Fiese, B. H. (2007). Family routines and rituals. *Infants and Young Children, 20*(4), 284–299. https://doi.org/10.1097/01.IYC.0000290352.32170.5a

Ward, F., & Linn, R. (2020). The mother-in-law mystique: A tale of conflict, criticism and resistance. *Australian and New Zealand Journal of Family Therapy, 41*(4), 381–392. https://doi.org/10.1002/anzf.1430

Wolin, & Bennett, L. A. (1984). Family rituals. *Family Process*, 23(3), 401–420. https://doi.org/10.1111/j.1545-5300.1984.00401.x

Wolin, S. J., Bennett, L. A., Noonan, D. L., & Teitelbaum, M. A. (1980). Disrupted family rituals: A factor in the intergenerational transmission of alcoholism. *Journal of Studies on Alcohol, 41*(3), 199–214). https://doi.org/10.15288/jsa.1980.41.199

6

LIVED AND SUCCESSFUL SEXUALITY

A Challenge for Couple and Family Therapy

Ingo Zimmermann

Introduction

Sexuality is an important facet of human life. A soft porn with sadomasochistic overtones, the bestselling *Fifty Shades of Grey* trilogy by author E.L. James, sold 70 million copies in 2013 (Spiegel-Online, 2013). The great public interest in similar books and films can be explained not least by the tension between meaningful moral horror and an accompanying "horror" of relationships and sexual forms that may be considered strange or "deviant" and "perverted" and, at the same time, be perceived as identifiable experiences by many. While bestselling novels like the above have brought these things into focus in recent times, the phenomenon is not new. Among the classics of the genre of alternative and especially sadomasochistic sexual practices are the works of the Marquis de Sade (1740–1814) and Leopold von Sacher-Masoch (1836–1895), whose authors' names also established the terms sadism and masochism. Although their works were not among the most widely read writings during the authors' lifetimes – in the case of de Sade, they were even banned – they attracted such a great deal of social controversy that they still have a significance in the sadomaschostic scene and literature today. This also highlights a fundamental paradox of contemporary society: although the sexual seems to be omnipresent, the topic of lived sexuality in more intimate contexts, such as in private life, but also in psychotherapy and counseling, is communicated only marginally and with shame, and is limited to a morally legitimized normative range of lived sexuality (cf. Buddeberg, 2005; Ahrendt et al., 2011; Reinecke et al., 2006; Cedzich & Bosinski, 2010). Alternative sexual practices are pathologized not least by diagnostic manuals like the *Diagnostic and Statistical Manual of Mental Disorders-5th edition-TR* (APA, 2022) as well as the *International statistical classification of diseases and related health problems (11th ed.).* (World Health Organization, 2019), and excommunicated from prevailing medical and psychological discourses. Freud speaks here, following Krafft-Ebing's *Psychopathia Sexualis* (1894), of sexual aberrations or even perversions, which include sadomasochistic practices, fetishism, homosexuality, anal play, etc. (Freud, 2010, 42 ff). This social externalization may also be produced when the individual is precisely not suffering from nonconforming (i.e., seemingly deviant) impulses, as required by the ICD as a diagnostic criterion of sexual preference disorders.

DOI: 10.4324/9781003297871-7

In contrast, studies from recent years point to a broad acceptance of alternative ways of playing the sexual in private contexts (cf. Beier & Loewit, 2011, Joyal et al., 2014, Crepault & Coulture, 1980, Templeman & Stinnet, 1990). Publicly penalized, islands of the private obviously form where alternative practices are lived and loved.

State of Research

Sexual experience and behavior are characterized by biological, psychological, and social dimentions. The pleasure dimension characterizes the function of sexuality for experiencing positive feelings of sexual excitement, the reproduction dimension refers to the importance of sexual behavior for reproduction, and the relationship dimension has to do with the social aspects of sexual behavior in the sense of fulfilling basic needs for closeness, security, and safety. The respective modes of lived sexuality, the so-called preference patterns, are formed postpubertally and are largely irreversible over the lifespan (Beier & Loewit, 2004, 2011). Sexual fantasies and arousal-focused sexual practice correspond to the pleasure dimension of sexuality. Alternative sexual forms here refer to all practices and modes within the pleasure dimension that are distinct from "usual," traditional, and vaginal sexual intercourse between two people. Alternative or "deviant" sexual forms, although widespread, do not seem to gain the interest of researchers and thus the number of robust empirical findings is comparatively small. Sexuality cannot be considered independently of the social factors that norm and constitute it Sigusch (2005, 2013) Social relations affecting sexuality are historically linked to a series of drastic changes, which on the one hand release individuals from traditional role assignments, and on the other hand, not least due to economic motives and system imperatives (cf. Habermas, 1982), change relationship structures themselves and thus lead to a changed perception of partnership and sexuality. If in the 1960s the introduction of hormonal contraceptives led to a far-reaching decoupling of the reproductive sphere from the sexual sphere and thus to a dissolution of the traditional connection between sexuality, childbearing and family structure, in the period that followed quite different formations of the family as well as of sexual life were possible. A sexuality freed from the reproductive dimension was for the first time able to bring the pleasure dimension of sexual union to the fore and at the same time made it possible for women to decide more autonomously than before about children. Coupled with an increasing liberation of women from traditional role patterns and the accompanying decrease in the male role assignment as the breadwinner of the family, possibilities arose for completely new kinds of family constellations, which finally culminated in the movement of the 68ers (a West German student movement rejecting traditional ideologies), as well as numerous new communes. Seen from today's perspective, these movements did not lead to an "anything goes" promiscuous and norm-negating society, but they did loosen the traditional and Christian-based ideas of marital cohabitation.

The point here in this discussion is that of preference or sexual preference. This refers to an unique pattern of sexual responsiveness, which manifests itself on three different axes. The development of sexual preference is completed after puberty and is irreversible over the life course. Pedagogical and psychotherapeutic "re-education measures" prove to be ineffective and are merely attempts to persuade people to give up their sexual arousal patterns under the threat of discrimination. The resulting behavioral changes can at best be regarded as superficial adaptations, but not as genuine re-education. On the other hand, the fact that preference development can be considered to be completed after puberty does not now mean that the preference pattern of each person also becomes immediately conscious at this stage of life. Rather, it is the case that awareness of one's preference results from experience. In other words: Those who have a lot of sexual experience early on autoerotically or in connection with sexual partners become aware of their sexual preferences earlier. Practice makes perfect. The preference pattern proves to be uninfluenceable by therapeutic interventions and is not related to specific socialization experiences, traumatization, parental or family upbringing styles, religious orientation, or socioeconomic factors.

The preference pattern of a person (or one's modes of lived sexuality) includes three axes:

1. **Gender:** Every person has a preference for the gender of potential sexual partners upon completion of puberty. People are homosexual, bisexual, or heterosexual. The nearly equal distribution of homosexuality and bisexuality in different cultural and political contexts suggests an epigenetic or cell division-related causation, especially since purely genome-based factors can be largely excluded.
2. **The body scheme:** Each person has a preference for a specific body scheme. This does not denote a person's absolute age, but rather their physical appearance. A distinction can be made between pedophilic tendencies, a hebephiliac, prepubescent tendency, and a sexual responsiveness with respect to the body schema of younger, middle, and old adulthood. The latter can also be called gerontophilic.
3. **The mode:** The mode designates now (in contrast to the up-to-now) named factors of the way and manner sexuality is optimally lived. This includes all sadomasochistic practices, fetishism, and transvestitism, but also anal intercourse, exhibitionism, voyeurism, frotteurism, sexual cannibalism, necrophilia, and many others. The mode can be classified into three domains, each conceptualized as existing on a continuum, for each person:
   A) **Subject – object:** This refers to whether the sexual partner is understood as subject or object.
   B) **Activity – passivity:** Here it is decided whether the person in question behaves actively and proactively or passively.
   C) **Dominance – sub-dominance:** Here the power relations during the sexual act become clear. If it is primarily stimulating for a person to take command, they can be characterized as dominant. If it is more sexually arousing for someone else to take control, the person is more subdominant.

The preference patterns composed in this way are unchanging over the course of life. Accordingly, a successful partnership is one in which the partners' preference patterns are compatible with each other. An identical orientation is not advisable. Two dominant individuals or two subdominant ones are unlikely to experience satisfying sexuality. Thus, incompatibility of preference patterns is a key component of the quality of sexual experience. Research suggests that sexual satisfaction feeds back into overall satisfaction with the partnership. Incompatible preference patterns lead to earlier separations and to cheating. Cheating is often an attempt to satisfy the unsatisfied preferences within the relationship. In addition, the respective preference is not necessarily lived. Social taboos, religious norms, and values, or even personal reservations and negative, discriminatory, or devaluing experiences often prevent sexual fulfillment.

In the late 1960s, the emancipation movement led to an increasing awareness of the relevance of preference patterns within relationships. Sennett (1998) points out that it is modern societies that expect flexibility from individuals. This is not only true regarding spatial flexibility as a prerequisite for acquiring a new job after intermittent phases of unemployment and poverty, but also regarding loosening and reduced social relationships that require new psychological behavior patterns. Those who change jobs frequently are more often forced to establish new social contacts and abandon old ones. This lack of permanence generates anxiety and insecurity, which is perhaps another reason for the increasingly observable and clinical forms of sexuality disorders. In this way, contact becomes available less through personal presence and more virtually, mediated by corresponding Internet portals and social networks. Despite the prevailing normativity that still declares "marriage until the grave" as the social normal case, relationships are increasingly fragmented. As a result, serial monogamy tends to take the place of the monogamous life course relationship. Thus, mutual needs and the mode of satisfaction must be repeatedly negotiated. At the same time, new sexual forms develop that promise the thrill to those who are thus lonely, which the partnership cannot deliver due to its demanded flexibility and the uncertainties associated with it, so that fragmented sexual forms provide relief at least in the short term to compensate for the lost security – lust turns into pleasure (cf. Sigusch, 2005, 23). Against this background, the coordinates, not of relationship and partnership, but of sexuality, shift and let the reproduction and relationship dimensions recede into the background in favor of the pleasure dimension. Contemporary sexuality is characterized by (1) the dissociation of the old sexual sphere; (2) the dispersion of sexual fragments; and (3) the diversification of sexual relationships (cf. ibid., 29).

(1) Dissociation of the sexual sphere refers to the shattering of the perceived shared sexual experience. In this context, neo-sexualities consist "primarily of gender differences, self-love, thrills, and posterizations" (Sigusch, 2005, p. 30); sexuality, freed from its religious and historical contexts, is thrown back on the individual and demands its redemption from the individual, conceived as "pure sexuality" (ibid.); it is possible without a partner, with a partner, as masturbation in the sense of an independent form of sex, as well as with the use of countless purchasable aids. It becomes pure sexuality in that nothing can interfere achieving orgasm. This also applies to the partner. Sex is just sex and nothing more and is characterized by the "disembodiment of the Sexus and the genus" (ibid., p. 32).

(2) The dispersion of sexual fragments points to the fact that the thus individualized form of Sexus with all its practices is not only subject to a current push toward individualization, but also to a push toward commercialization. This goes hand in hand with the attempt "to press as many fragments and segments as possible into the form of a commodity, from media self-exposure to flirtation schools, dating agencies, the production of chastity belts or penis clothing (...) to the embryo trade" (Sigusch, 2005, p. 34). Every aspect is for sale, and all are available for purchase at any time. In this context, true to the principles of the market, new sexual forms and corresponding aids and prostheses emerge that make new experiences possible

(3) Finally, the diversification of intimate relationships is shaped by the very demands of the market for a self, freed from emotional and sexual needs, which is markedly willing to submit to the laws of supply and demand. This economically induced "compulsion to unconstraint" (Sigusch, 2005, p. 38), on the other hand, does not eliminate needs, but forces the individual into a different perspective on relationship; the emphasis on the emotionalization and itemization of social relations is reflected not only in the respective partnerships, but ultimately also in those who care for failed partnerships, including social workers, physicians, psychologists, and psychotherapists, who are primarily concerned with reducing the emotional misery in such a way that the individuals in question once

again function appropriately. Such over-emotional relationships, whose main point of reference is the relationship itself and whose main topic of conversation is the relationship itself, lead to the dissolution of the immediacy within the relationship, but also of the relationship itself. Or in the words of Sigusch: "Capitalism and love belong together" (ibid., p. 13). The retreat into individuality, the emphasis on the pleasure dimension at the expense of the relationship dimension, and the increasing prevalence of alternative sexual practices (Joyal et al., 2014) correspond exactly to the social framework of late capitalist, neoliberal societies. Contemporary sexuality is the result of a historically unique social individualization push.

The awareness of sexual preference and the spread of alternative sexual forms and sexual fantasies in capitalized Western societies is hardly empirically secured in a representative manner, and the collection of data is usually subject to considerable validity limitations. Especially in German-speaking countries, correspondingly differentiated studies are scarce. Crepault and Coulture (1980) interviewed 94 men regarding their sexual fantasies during masturbation and sexual intercourse. Among these, 61% reported fantasies of seducing young girls for sex, 33% reported fantasies of rape of adult women, 12% reported masochistic submission, and 5% reported zoophilic interests. Templeman & Stinnet (1990) studied 60 male college students in terms of sexual fantasies and sexual practices. In this study, 42% reported voyeuristic, 35% reported frotteuristic, and 5% reported sadistic practices. Moreover, 2% of the students studied practiced exhibitionistic behaviors and 8% reported making obscene phone calls. Overall, 65% of respondents reported at least one paraphilic tendency. Strassberg & Lockerd (1998) reported on a study of 137 female college students regarding their sexual fantasies. In this study, about half of the respondents reported fantasies with violent content, and such fantasies were found to be expressed predominantly by those with elevated levels of sexual experience. A connection with actual experienced sexual violence could not be proven biographically.

Renaud and Byers (1999) also found elevated scores for fantasies about group sex, involvement in orgies, sex with strangers, and sex with significantly younger individuals among males in a sample of 292 college students, and high scores for transvestite fetishism among females surveyed. Finally, in Robinson & Parks' (2003) study, 62.8% of the 128 women surveyed reported fantasies on the sadomasochistic spectrum. Khar (2007; 2008), in a study of 18,299 men and women in relationships, identified masochistic fantasies in approximately 30%. Another 30% fantasized about their partner engaging in masturbatory practices. No fantasies involving the relationship partner were reported by 42%. In a larger recent study of sexual fantasies from Canada, Joyal et al. (2014) identified fantasies involving oral stimulation in 78.5% of women and 87.6% of men using a 55-question inventory of different sexual fantasies. Sex with two women was fantasized by 36.9% of women and 84.5% of men. Fantasies of masochistic submission were reported by 64.6% of women and 53.3% of men, and dominance fantasies by 64.6% of women and 53.3% of men. Anal intercourse was fantasized by 32.5% of the women and 64.2% of the male respondents. Group sex was still imagined by 56.6% of women and 15.8% of men. Beatings and whippings were imagined by 36.3% of women and 28.5% of men, and rape fantasies were reported by 28.9% female and 30.7% male respondents. Fetishistic fantasies were reported by 26.3% of females and 27.8% of males. In the German-speaking world, Witte et al. (2007) examined individuals with sadomasochistic preference in relation to attachment behavior and found that individuals with sadomasochistic inclination had significantly higher educational attainment and showed highly significant differences in satisfaction with their sexuality, communication, and partner attachment: the sadomaso-chistic group tended to have higher satisfaction with partnership and sexuality (Witte et al., 2007). A chance finding on the prevalence of paraphilic arousal patterns occurred in a Berlin study (Ahlers et al., 2011; Beier & Loewit, 2011) in which 6,000 men were originally surveyed about erectile dysfunction.

In a subsequent survey with 373 selected participants (63 single, 310 in partnership) from the first study on sexual preferences, fantasies, accompanying fantasies during mas-turbation, and lived sexual behavior, structured interviews were again conducted. Among other things, the men were asked about their sexual fantasies in the areas of fetishism (ICD-10, F65.0), fetishistic transvestitism (F65.1), exhibitionism (65.2), voyeurism (F65.3), pedophilia (65.4), and sadomasochism (65.5). About 57.6% of the men had sexual fanta-sies from at least one of the domains presented, and 43.7% had acted out their fantasies. Particular practices, such as "secretly watching" (17.7%), arousal to objects (24.1%), but also "torturing" (15.3%) or "being tortured" (12.1%), were common in the studied group. Impressively most fantasies to a significant part also are experienced in real life. As many as 9.4% of the men surveyed reported pedophilic fantasies; 3.8% also lived out these – after all, criminally relevant – areas of sexual satisfaction. Overall, alternative forms of sexu-ality seem widespread. It is obvious that the above findings correspond to a development in society, which goes hand in hand with the decoupling of the sphere of reproduction and sexual pleasure as well as with the emancipation movement of women and current processes of flexibilization and economization in neoliberal societies.

In this context, two studies were conducted on the above-mentioned problem area, a smaller preliminary study and a very differentiated and, in terms of the participants surveyed, the world's largest study. The aim of the empirical surveys was, first, to obtain information about lived sexual forms and, second, to draw conclusions about family and sexual counseling processes. What is the significance of sexuality for couples and families?

Study

Methodical Approach

How common are alternative forms of sex in contemporary society? How satisfied with their relationship and sexuality are those people who practice alternative forms of sex compared to people who do not? To this end, a questionnaire with a total of 33 questions was developed and published as part of an online survey via www.soscisurvey.de for 30 days in the spring of 2014. In addition to socio-demographic data, the questionnaire collected a range of sexual fantasies and sexual practices, as well as information on satisfaction with the relationship and sexuality lived. The social network "Facebook" was primarily chosen to distribute the questionnaire. The link to the survey was promoted via Facebook from different (private) profiles. The link was shared several times, so that a broad distribution could be achieved (cf. Batinic et al., 1999). In addition, the URL was linked on different public profiles and forums in German-speaking countries. At the same time, the subjects were asked to share the link further online. The questionnaire consisted of two main parts. The first part collected sociodemographic data. The education and occupation items were equally related to the respondent's father to assess the milieu in which the respondent grew up. Questions on occupation and education were taken mostly from Sigusch and Schmidt's (1971) questionnaire on working-class sexuality, adapted and expanded. For the analysis, income and age were additionally divided into two groups: Income into "under 1000 € net/ month" and "over 1000 € net/month" and age into "under 30 years" and "over 30 years." The second part of the survey included questions about sexual fantasies and practices and frequency of occurrence. The practices were chosen so that the widest possible range of different preferences could be acquired. Finally, general questions about satisfaction in the relationship, with the relationship status, and with lived sexuality, were added to the questionnaire. Results A total of 434 questionnaires were recorded, of which 295 proved to be usable. The subsequent analysis of the data pool was carried out via SPSS 22. Descriptive statistics of the frequencies follow first, followed by an interference statistical analysis if this seemed necessary based on the data set of the descriptive statistics.

Sociodemographic Data

Of the total 295 records used, 152 were men and 140 were women (3 did not specify gender). Of these, the majority were heterosexually oriented (85.1%), 11.5% bisexual and 2.4% homosexual (3 o.A.). In the age distribution, the 20–30-year-olds dominated with a frequency of 155 (52.5%). There were 22 (7.5%) representatives of those under 20 years old, 65 31–40 years old (22%), forming the second largest group; 33 people were between 41 and 51 years old (11.2%). 18 participants (6.1%) were 51–60 years old and 2 even older (0.7%). When the age groups are divided, there is a relatively homogeneous distribution of 177 to 30-year-olds (60%) and 118 over 30-year-olds (40%). The sample included a total of 103 singles (34.9%), 58 married persons living in a household (19.7%), 67 persons were in a relationship and living together (22.7%), and 66 persons who were also in a relationship but not living together (22.4%) (1 o.A.). 72.5% of the sample were childless. In 74 participants, one to two children under the age of 18 lived in the household (25.1%) and only 1.7% (n=5) had more than two children living in the household (2 o.A.). Satisfaction with relationship status was reported as follows: 146 were satisfied with their relationship status as single, married, or in a relationship (49.5%). 87 (29.5%) individuals indicated they were "Somewhat Satisfied." "Somewhat dissatisfied" was indicated by 45 (15.3%) and "dissatisfied" was indicated by 16 (5.4%). The sample included an above-average number of participants with higher education. Higher professional positions such as managers (5.8%) or civil servants (3.4%) were also represented in the sample. After dividing "under €1000" and "over €1000," the income groups showed a distribution of 36.6% to 62.7%. Thus, there were significantly more people with incomes above the poverty line (about 60% of the average net income in German-speaking countries) in the sample. In the first group, there were 108 (36.6%) with the lowest income of up to €1000. In the second group, 21.4% earned up to 2000 € gross; 19.7% had gross earnings of 2001–3000 €; 3001–4000 € were earned by 24 people (8.1%) and 4001–5000 € by 17 (5.8%). The top earners with more than 5000 € monthly gross earnings were represented here by 7.8% (n= 23). Regarding the educational qualification and occupation of the father, the following values emerged: 7 of the fathers did not have a degree (2.4%). Most of the fathers of the respondents had completed a type of vocational training (33.2%) or a completed degree (21.7%). On the other hand, 14 people did not know which degree the father had (4.7%). The largest group of respondents came from social backgrounds in which the father earned a living through employment (28.1%). This was followed by executives with 16.9%. Forty-five fathers each were self-employed (15.3%) or skilled workers (15.3%), 11.5% were employed as civil servants, and 5.1% worked as semi-skilled or unskilled laborers. Only

3.1% received mostly social benefits and 1.7% lived from a mini/midi-job. 9 respondents (3.1%) could not provide information about the father's employment relationship

Data on sexuality, regarding the question on general satisfaction with sexual life, 27.5% claimed to be "very satisfied" and 33.6% "somewhat satisfied." 86 participants claimed to be "rather dissatisfied" (29.2%) and 25 were "very dissatisfied" (8.6%). 150 people reported not having enough sex (45.3%) or not having a suitable partner (30%) as the most important reason for sexual dissatisfaction. In each case, 9.3% reported that they could not satisfy their sexual desires or that their partner's preferences and desires did not match their own. Six percent cited other reasons. The average frequency of sexual activity in the past six months was more than twice a week, with a high of 25.4%, followed by 24.4% who claimed to be sexually active one to two times a week. 21.7% had sex one to three times a month and 15.6% less than once a month. 12.9% reported not having sex at all due to lack of partnership. Regarding the uptake of autoerotic stimulation and masturbation in the last six months, 38% claimed to have self-satisfied more than twice a week, 25.1% of respondents took up masturbation about once or twice a week, 15.3% satisfied themselves one to three times a month and 12.2% less than once a month. 9.5% claimed not to have taken up masturbation at all.

Fantasies

Only 4.4% of the respondents had none of the listed fantasies, 85.4% of all respondents stated that they had had fantasies about oral stimulation of the genitals with themselves or their partner. Of those who had fantasies about this, 90.9% also practiced it regularly or irregularly, and 9.1% had fantasies about it but did not live them out. Using sex toys or other objects to insert into the vagina was reported as a fantasy by 61.4%. Of these, 38.7% practiced it regularly and 40.3% did so irregularly. 21% did not live out their fantasies. 61% of respondents claimed to have fantasies of anal insertion of a member or object into themselves or another person occasionally or regularly. 27.8% practiced this regularly and 48.3% irregularly. In contrast, 43 (23.9%) respondents reported not practicing their fantasies. Role-playing games aroused keen interest among 49.1% of the respondents. 41% of these lived out their fantasy irregularly and 18.8% regularly. 40.3% did not put their fantasies into practice. A total of 51.9% of the sample reported having fantasies of power and/or submission in terms of sadomasochistic practices, practiced by a total of 101 respondents. Regularly practiced 26.1% of the respondents and irregularly 39.9% sadomasochistic practices. 34% reported not turning these fantasies into reality. Fantasies of tying up one's partner or being tied up were exhibited by a total of 59.5% of the total sample. Of those who described these fantasies, 69.7% acted out their fantasies regularly (19.4%) or irregularly (50.3%); 30.3% had the fantasies but did not act them out. A total of 63.9% were interested in partner swapping, group sex, attending erotic parties or swingers' clubs. 15.4% lived out their fantasies about this on a regular basis, 32.4% on an irregular basis; 52.1% said they had fantasies about this but did not act on them. Voyeuristic fantasies (watching or being watched during a sexual act) were affirmed as fantasies by 53.1% of the selectees; 14.7% acted out their fantasies regularly and 34.6% irregularly; 50.6% did not act out their fantasies. Using urine, feces, or vomit (urophilia, coprophilia, vomophilia) occurred in the fantasy of 16.9% of respondents. 12% of respondents used excreta regularly for sexual stimulation and 34% irregularly. 54% of respondents reported having the fantasies but not performing them. Sexual pleasure derived from engaging with a particular object or body part (fetishism) in fantasy was experienced by 25.3% of respondents. Of these, 20.3% also reported acting out the fantasy regularly and 41.9% did so irregularly. 37.8% did not live out their fantasies. Across the entire sample, 35.4% of respondents act out their fantasies regularly to irregularly. Only 8.9% did not practice any of their fantasies. Regarding the evaluation of successful sexuality, 61.7% of the participants shared that they considered a well-successful sexuality to be important in life. 28.5% said that there were more important things in life and only 2% answered that they were not interested in sex. 23 people did not give any information about this. 63.4% of respondents, on the other hand, would like to be able to live out their fantasies more often, and another 69.9% said they would still like to try out many things regarding their sexual practice that they had not yet practiced.

Descriptive Statistics in Group Comparison – Gender Comparison

Men are slightly more likely to be single (38.8%) than women in this sample, but also twice as likely to be married (25%). 31.4% of women were single; 12.9% married. Overall, 68.8% of women and 60.5% of men were in some form of stable relationship. Women tended to be more satisfied with their relationship status and sex life than men. On the other hand, it was striking that women had significantly lower incomes, which is largely consistent with the official data. 52.9% of women had incomes below €1000 compared to men at 21.7%. Since childlessness was extremely high in both groups (72.5%), this correlation could hardly be explained using parental leave or child-rearing periods. However, it is striking at this point that 37.9% of the women stated that they had a high school diploma and 55.7% were currently pursuing another degree. Thus, many women could have been studying or in training, which explains the lower income and the income from social and transfer benefits (BAföG) (w=22.1%; m=13.2%), as well as from mini/midi-jobs (w=18.6%; m=5.9%). Men, on the other hand, more often had completed vocational training or a degree and thus had a correspondingly higher income. Women had sex more often than men. 32.1% of women had sex more often than twice a week. For men, on the other hand, the figure was only 19.1%. Men showed a significantly higher frequency of masturbation. For a better representation of sexual frequency and masturbatory frequency.

The distribution of preferences is similar where only marginal differences were found, including: Women fantasized most about oral stimulation methods (77.9%), about being tied up or tied up (60%), about using sex toys or other objects (56.4). Oral stimulation (92.7%), anal stimulation (84.1%), and using sex toys or other objects (82.3%) were also most frequently implemented. However, all other practices were also frequently detectable in fantasy as well as in implementation in about 50% of the women. In men, oral stimulation in fantasy (92.2%) as well as its realization (89.3%) were also the most common, followed by anal stimulation in fantasy (75.7%) and group sex and/or partner exchange fantasies (74.3%). In realization, oral sex was followed by the use of sex toys and the like (76.8%) and anal penetration (71.3%). Successful sexuality was especially important to both sexes (m=63.8%; w= 59.3%). However, men (71.7%) tended to want to act out their fantasies more often than women (54.3%), with women generally describing a higher level of satisfaction with their sex lives than men. Men, on the other hand (78.9%), liked to try more things they had not yet done regarding sex than women (59.3%) and were thus possibly more willing to experiment.

Again, it remains to be assumed that the difference can be explained by differences in sexual frequency and satisfaction with sex life. If we divide the data sets into two age groups, we first notice that there are more singles in the younger group (39.5%) than in the older group (28%). In addition, 4.5% of the younger group were married, compared to 42.4% of the older group. Regarding the satisfaction with the relationship status, it is noticeable that with increasing age, the satisfaction with the partnership decreases successively. 18.7% of the group under 30 claimed to be dissatisfied or rather dissatisfied. 23,9% were it with the older ones. The age group between 40 and 50 years was most dissatisfied, whereby in this group also about one third singles were, and the existing dissatisfactions can be explained with this connection. Regarding having their own children, 43.2% of the group over 30 said they had children, compared with only 15.9% of the group of younger respondents. In the present sample, a significant predictor of satisfaction with sex life seems to be age itself: as age increases, satisfaction with sex life decreases significantly. Respondents indicated that the most common reason for dissatisfaction was "not having enough sex" (younger = 19.8%; older = 28%). It is well known that sexual frequency decreases with age anyway, and the present sample confirms similar findings: among younger people, 31.1% had sexual intercourse more than 2x/week, among older people 16.9%.

The group of the over 30-year-olds, however, shows all the higher frequencies in masturbation (43.2% satisfied themselves more than 2x/week; the younger 34.5%), so that here one can speak of sexual compensation. This may also be related to other variables shown by the interference statistics. Regarding the different fantasies and their realization, there are only marginal, hardly noteworthy differences in connection with age. Conspicuous, however, are the fantasies about group sex, partner swapping, and the like. 57.1% of the younger group fantasized about it and 73.7% of the older group. There was a tendency for the younger group to live it out slightly more (by 3.5%). Anal intercourse and watching or being watched was also more prevalent in the older group's fantasies by 15–20%, although there was minor difference in the percentage of implementation.

Overall, successful sexuality was about equally important to both groups. The older group, however, wished to be able to act out their fantasies more often by 13% more. The younger group tended more to try new things (71.2% to 66.9%). If one divides the sample regarding the degree of education, it is noticeable that persons with a low degree of education were most dissatisfied with their relationship status. The higher the level of education, the higher the satisfaction with the sex life and the relationship. The reason for the dissatisfaction described was "too little sex" in about 40% and across all educational levels. With increasing education, however, it was also stated slightly more frequently in the freely available items that the sexual desires, i.e., the sexual preference pattern did not appear compatible with those of the partners. Regarding fantasies and lived practice, however, there were hardly any differences among the educational strata.

In the sample, however, it is noticeable: The higher the level of education, the more likely it was that fantasies tended not to be acted out at all. Academics also had less interest in acting out more fantasies or trying out new things. Successful sexuality in life, on the other hand, was equally important to all levels of education. However, since the academics tended to be in higher age groups, and the interest in trying out new things decreases with increasing age, the existing differences can be explained by this. The frequency of sexual intercourse decreases significantly with the level of education and the frequency of masturbation increases slightly in the opposite direction (but only with a frequency of more than 2x per week). Regarding the educational degree of the father, it is noticeable that 85.7% of those whose father did not acquire a degree were dissatisfied with their sex life. Moreover, satisfaction in sexual life (and sexual frequency) increases with higher educational qualification of the father. When divided by income, there are few abnormalities. The higher income group was marginally more satisfied with their relationship status (by 6.7%), but not with their sex life. It is noticeable that the higher income group had fantasies more often and acted them out more often (by about 10% on average for each practice), which may be related to the more economically favorable living conditions. Regarding relationship status, it is noticeable that singles were more likely to be dissatisfied with their relationship status and sex life, primarily as a result of lack of experience. Their sexual frequency was also significantly lower. Overall, it can be demonstrated that satisfaction in relationships is strongly related to satisfaction with sex life. There is a statistically significant correlation here. Acting out sexual practices is also statistically significantly related to satisfaction with relationship status. Of those who were satisfied, 40.3% lived out their fantasies one hundred percent; 95.7% practiced at least one of their fantasies.

Of those who were satisfied, 32.1% realized their fantasies completely; 9.5% did not realize any of their fantasies at all. Among those who indicated they were dissatisfied, 32.6% lived out all their fantasies, and the percentage of those who practiced none of their fantasies increased to 16.3%. Among the very dissatisfied, only 15.4% still performed their fantasies completely; 30.8% did not perform any of their fantasies. Again, however, it can be demonstrated that the majority of those who indicated being very dissatisfied with their relationship status were single and thus had a lower frequency of sex. Dividing the group according to satisfaction with sex life reveals a statistically significant correlation between sex life and satisfaction with relationship status: the more dissatisfied respondents were with sex life, the more dissatisfied they were with relationship status. Here, too, as before, it was observed that satisfaction with sex life decreases significantly with increasing age.

In the group of those who said they were very dissatisfied with their sex life, 64% were over thirty years old and 60% were single. As dissatisfaction increased, sexual frequency also decreased significantly and the frequency of use of autoerotic self-stimulation increased, while the frequency of fantasies acted out decreased. 52.3% of dissatisfied couples did not act out their fantasies at all but had a desire to act out fantasies more often and try new things. Interestingly, couples who lived in separate households reported being least dissatisfied with their relationship and sex life.

Pearson Chi-Square Interference Statistics

The Pearson chi-square test was used in this study to test the hypotheses and other relationships between the variables. With decreasing size of the determined p-values, the claimed relationship is significant. Age: As already noted, satisfaction with sexual life decreases with increasing age. This result shows a statistical significance of $p=0.001$ and thus represents a highly significant correlation of the item satisfaction with sexual life and age. With a statistical significance of $p=0.033$, the desire to act out fantasies more often also increases with age. When divided into two age groups (under 30 and over 30), the result becomes even clearer ($p=0.027$) – cf. Tab. 8. Overall, the result is confirmed by the fact that with increasing age, sexual frequency also decreases significantly. Especially at the age of 31–40 years and 51–60 years the frequency decreases significantly and is most often 1–3 times a month. Here, a statistical significance value of $p=0.015$ is shown. Gender: Regarding autoerotic acts, men had a significantly increased frequency of masturbation: 80.3% of men masturbated at least once a week and more frequently. Only 43.6% of women masturbated as frequently and 21.4% had not masturbated at all in the past six months. Among men, on the other hand, only 4.6% did not masturbate themselves. Here, there is a highly significant correlation of p=0.000. Men also had the desire to act out their fantasies more often, by 17% more than women. The p-value here is p=0.003 and shows a highly significant correlation – see Tab. 9. Men were more interested in trying out new things: 78.9% of the men answered yes to this question; for the women, however, it was 59.3%. This correlation is significant (p=0.000). Crossing satisfaction with relationship status and satisfaction with sex life shows a significant correlation between both variables (p=0.000):

The more satisfied someone was with relationship status, the more satisfied they were with their sex life and vice versa. Thus, sexual frequency is also related to satisfaction with relationship status and satisfaction with sexual life: The more dissatisfied someone was with their relationship status or with their sex life the lower their sex frequency became. Here, a p-value of p=0.000 results for both intersections. An equally significant correlation results from the correlation of masturbation and relationship status. The higher the dissatisfaction in the relationship status was indicated, the more frequent was the frequency of masturbation (p=0.002) – cf. Tab. 10. Those who were more dissatisfied with their sexual life had the desire to live out their fantasies more often (p=0.000) and to try out new things (p=0.038, cf. Tab.12). However, only 35.8% of those who said they were very satisfied with their sex life expressed the desire to act their fantasies more often. Thus, the desire to realize fantasies more often already increased to 66.7% among those who reported being satisfied. The highest value (88%) was reached by those who were very dissatisfied – cf. tables 11 and 12. The respective relationship status is related to selected sexual practices: In particular, regular practice of oral sex is related to satisfaction with relationship status. The more satisfied the group, the more likely they were to practice oral sex (p=0.000).

Using sex toys or other objects was also statistically significantly related to relationship status satisfaction (p=0.044); the same was true for role-playing (p=0.008) and being tied up or restrained (p=0.015). The crosses with the other sexual practices did not reveal any other significances. As far as satisfaction with sexual life is concerned, only slightly different significances emerge concerning the sexual practices. Oral intercourse is also related to satisfaction in sexual life with the maximum value of p=0.000. The more dissatisfied someone was, the more likely they were to say they did not have such fantasies, but this tendency only applies to oral sex and using sex toys. Using sex toys (p=0.044) and performing role-playing games (p=0.008) are also related to sex life here. However, instead of bondage, practicing sado/masochistic practices is added here, which is statistically highly significantly related to satisfaction in sex life (p=0.005). Thus, some practices are dependent on satisfaction in relationships and/or on satisfaction with sexual life, while others are lived independently of it.

Interpretation

The present study finds that there is a great interest in alternative sexual practices among the German-speaking population, and likewise a high degree of willingness to live them out. Compared to other studies, the values and frequencies found are higher, but these discrepancies can be well explained. The studies described above show partly divergent definitions and perceptions of specific sexual practices. In the present study, pathology-related designations were avoided, and the corresponding behaviors were broadly defined, but at the same time the study allows for the possibility of assigning several items if specific fantasies are present. Those who have S&M fantasies may also have indicated the item being tied up or being tied up at the same time, since submission fantasies are often accompanied by fixations or the use of objects. Thus, the variety and number of fantasies increases, resulting in a summarily higher score. In the context of the Durex study, the results were collected internationally; results for Germany are available but are not accessible due to private-sector conditions of use. At this point, it may become clear that the lower figures determined how alternative sexual practices are not only related to the extremely broad formulation of the items there, but also to culture-specific peculiarities and political-normative conditions in other countries. According to Sigusch (2005), the processes of dissociation of the sexual sphere, the dispersion of sexual fragments and the diversification of sexual relationships described in the context of neo-sexuality primarily concern capitalist societies in Western industrialized countries: "Capitalism and love belong together" (Sigusch, 2005, p. 13). Since the other studies have been limited in terms of item selection of alternative sexual practices and have only formulated them in an unspecific way, the lower result of the spread of certain fantasies may be strongly influenced by the reductionist selection of practices. In addition, there are issues of differing study design. As far as the Durex study operated with a survey mix of online survey, door-to-door interviews and questionnaires and thus must be judged as uncertain regarding quality criteria, especially reliability and objectivity, its representativeness is additionally questioned. The Berlin study (Ahlers et al., 2011; Beier & Loewit, 2011), on the other hand, conducted its survey using personal interviews. An anonymous questionnaire on the Internet significantly lowers the inhibition threshold to provide information about certain intimate fantasies or practices.

In a concrete comparison of the Berlin men's study with the results listed in the present study, similar tendencies can be identified with various sexual fantasies and the implementation – cf. tab. 13. The values for "at least one responsiveness" can certainly be explained by the more diverse selection of practices in the present study and are therefore hardly comparable. For the implementation of at least one fantasy, a percentage deviation of 12% is shown. If one compares the percentage average values of the question to what extent the sexual practices mentioned in the table are lived out, percentage values of 67.6% (Berlin study) and 56.5% are shown, resulting in a deviation of just 11.1%. Since the values here appear remarkably similar, it must be assumed that the response bias in the present study can be described as minimal. A correlation between class affiliation and sexual forms could not be proven in the present study. A significant correlation existed only between higher income and higher fantasy occurrence (p=0.015). Although significant, this correlation must be viewed with skepticism. Since men overall had a higher fantasy occurrence (p=0.007) and significantly more often had a higher income than women (p=0.000), one must assume that the higher fantasy activity of the higher income group was influenced by gender.

Sigusch (2005) points out that the aspects of pluralization of sexual forms described by him claim validity across all educational stratification. Neither economic endowment nor educational attainment influenced sexuality or relationships in the present sample. Rather, general satisfaction factors are relevant predictors: Satisfaction with relationship status and satisfaction with sexual life are highly significantly related (p=0.000). Likewise, significant associations can be observed regarding satisfaction with sexual life as well as relationship status in relation to sexual frequency (p=0.000 and p=0.000, respectively).

Dissatisfaction with relationship status or sexual life is associated with lower sexual frequency (p=0.000), the need for more sex, and the desire to act out fantasies more often (p= 0.000). Dissatisfaction with sexuality increases the desire to try more (p=0.038), which is equally true for singles and couples. The fact that sexual life satisfaction decreased with increasing age (p=0.001) and that 42% of those over thirty reported being married (the percentage increases with increasing age) makes it clear that relationship length is the most significant predictor in terms of successful sexuality. The willingness to act out fantasies was significantly higher, even if the sexual frequency was high and the respondents were satisfied. Desire to try new things and willingness to experiment were significantly related to sexual dissatisfaction and reduced coitus frequency (p=0.038). According to Amendt et al.'s (2011) study, sexuality still takes place in committed partnerships and relationships for about 95% of all coital experiences, which was confirmed by the significant dissatisfaction and significantly lower sexual frequency of singles in this study (p=0.000). The desire to act out fantasies more often was also characterized by a deficient sexual life (0.000), dissatisfaction in relationship (p=0.000) and low sexual frequency (0.004). At this point, even if they were satisfied, men generally had an increased need to realize more fantasies (p=0.003) and try more practices (p=0.000). They exhibited higher fantasy activity (p=0.007) and thus seemed to be more sexually responsive overall than women.

Study: Sexuality and Sexual Preferences among Adolescents and Young Adults First Results of the German Sex Survey

In another study with a much larger number of participants, the "German Sex Survey," 2323 subjects from German-speaking countries were interviewed using a standardized questionnaire as part of an online-based, highly differentiated study on sexual fantasies and sexual practices. With a total age range between 11 and 68 years and a homogeneous gender profile, the group of 18- to 30-year-old adolescents and young adults predominated. 44 different sexual preferences were surveyed, intended to reflect the entire range of possible-preference patterns.

Results

Most respondents (> 96.6%) reported having at least one of the specified fantasies, with the majority reporting an average of 11.0 fantasies (median: 10.0). The situation is quite similar to the sexual practices experienced. Here, only 13.3% report not living any of the practices mentioned. On average, 6.7 fantasies were lived (median: 5). Overall, however, the proportion of over-30s in terms of the number of fantasies classified as arousing was highly significant (p = 0.00) above that of under-30s. The same applies to the lived practices (p = 0.00). In the sense that it must be assumed that the group of U-30-year-olds has less experience in the sexual field than the older ones, it must be assumed that this difference is explained by the higher age. Those who have more experience in the sexual sphere can perceive their preference pattern more consciously and align their sexual behavior to it. Sexually stimulating aids, pornographic material and sex toys are used by a broad majority to increase the feeling of pleasure, but here too, despite the considerable frequency of the under-30 group, the proportion of people over the age of 30 is higher. Pornographic material is not used at all by only 16.5% of the under-30 group (compared to 13.4% of the over-30 group); 46.6% of the under-30 group use pornographic material several times a month (compared to 50.8% of the over-30 group). It must be assumed, however, that the use of pornographic material by adolescents in particular is more likely to compensate for unfulfilled sexual desires and, within relationships, to aggregate consensual sexual creativity within the partnership.

The interviewed adolescents and young adults also emphasize the relevance of a successful partnership: 93 % (91.8 % Ü-30) of them stress the importance of talking to their partner about sexual desires, but 42.4 % (36.2 % Ü-30) do not dare to do so. 33.8% (44.1% Ü-30) would cheat on their partner or leave them if sexual desires remain unfulfilled, and 59.9% (65.5% Ü-30) wish to live out their sexual fantasies more often; 16.9% of the U-30 group (23.4% Ü-30) have a challenging time finding an adequate partner at all because of their sexual preference. There is hardly any difference between the two age groups in terms of satisfaction with their sex lives: on a six-point scale, 34.7% of U-30s are dissatisfied to very dissatisfied, compared with 37.2% of Ü-30s.

Discussion

Sexuality and relationships do not just belong together in a fragmentary way, but together form the basis of successful relationships. A good, stable relationship requires satisfying sexuality, and vice versa. Socioeconomic factors and social origin load above the significance level and are of little significance. If, on the other hand, sexual life loses quality and quantity and its subjectively experienced intensity declines, then there is a risk of imbalance, and the partnership becomes unstable. Different preference patterns, different distributions of sexual mode, body schema, and preferred sex reduce the likelihood of fully satisfying sexuality. While partnerships are characterized by an elevated level of sexual activity and mutual attraction at the beginning of the relationship, different routines develop over time, which can also take the form of decreasing sexual frequency and increasing uniformity in sexual life. According to the sex report of a German television station (with 55,992 participants), 61% of men and 50% of women would like to have more frequent sexual intercourse. If we assume that the desire for more frequent sexual intercourse corresponds to increasing dissatisfaction in sexual and relationship life (more than 50%3), it is easy to explain why the number of divorces and remarriages is so high.

Especially in times of economically necessary flexibilization processes in the life course (cf. Sennett, 1998, Sigusch, 2013), the social norm of lifelong relationships is increasingly undermined by socio-political "constraints" and economic necessities. The "marriage to the grave" is turning into life-stage relationships that are not only more short-term in nature, but also change the classic role patterns of men and women. In particular, the decoupling from economic dependence formulated during the women's rights movement is changing male supremacy and increasingly turning relationships into encounters at eye level. What was taken for granted a few generations before must be negotiated consensually (cf. Schmidt, 1998). This applies not only to questions of how to organize everyday life, but also to questions of successful sexuality. A relationship with sexual difficulties or different preference patterns between the partners thus lacks an essential stability factor.

The available studies can make it clear that sexuality is not a marginal phenomenon of relationships, but an integral part of partnership. If the sexual frequency becomes lower and thus the sexual diversity is reduced, this has an influence on the subjectively perceived quality of the relationship. The higher the dissatisfaction in relationships, the more likely partner conflicts occur, which in turn are considered a high stressor for the individual and the couple (cf. Fiedler, 2010), but can hardly be compensated sexually. The fact that this also results in demands for people in medical, psychological, and psychosocial fields of work is obvious, although hardly received (cf. Buddeberg, 2005). The fundamental openness to bring up sexuality, theoretical knowledge of sexual science, the examination of one's own and other people's varieties of sexuality should be the basis of medical, psychological, and psychosocial training courses.

A look at the curricula of universities and professional societies shows that this is not the case for the most part: sexuality is, if at all, predominantly discussed in a negative way, i.e., in terms of abuse, bullying, sexual violence and coercion. Sexuality thus becomes a mere appendage of the respective form of relationship and is thus excluded from prevailing therapeutic and counseling discourses. In this way, professionals also contribute to the tabooing of sexuality. Briefly: psychosocial counseling without consideration of the sexual dimension is like a bicycle without a saddle: it rides, but not well.

Implications for the Practice of Couple and Family Therapy

The studies described and the general data situation suggest that the topic of sexuality, in lived sexual practice, mutual desires and expectations as well as one's own sexual preference and that of the respective partner(s), is still a mostly taboo subject. Only about half of all couples can address these topics within their partnership. All other couples, on the other hand, seem to be more likely to speculate about what pleases and satisfies their respective counterparts sexually. However, this also makes it clear that a sizable proportion of couples obviously fall far short of their sexual potential. In public, on the other hand, lived and successful sexuality is also hardly an issue. Prudishness, sexual defensiveness, and sexually hostile milieus are more in the foreground here. If the topic is nevertheless addressed, it is usually with negative connotations, such as sexual abuse, coercion, or experiences of discrimination. Against this background, the still existing restrictive legislation of some states of the United States in connection with certain sexual practices as well as the current jurisprudence of the Supreme Court regarding the legality of abortion must be understood as additional current obstacles in dealing with sexual topics, which in view of highly taboo sexual topics and sexual preferences, additionally burden couple relationships and individuals.

This burden is also felt by couple and family therapists, who in practice often must deal with persons and couples who often conceal differences in sexual desire and in the desired sexual practice behind communication difficulties and conflicts in everyday cohabitation, because they lack the possibilities and the ability to openly address the corresponding topics within the partnership. If then – and studies from the European area suggest this – the family therapist is also subject to similar taboos, he will also have doubts about addressing and naming sexual topics and will thus contribute to the perpetuation of the problem. Couple and family therapy, on the other hand, is at best a co-evolutionary process that can facilitate learning on both sides. This requires the freedom to connote sexual issues positively and to bring them up appropriately. Clients often sense the therapist's intuitive rejection of the topic and then shy away from articulating the issue of sexuality and stating their own needs. In this context, the topic of successful sexuality, sexual preferences, arousal patterns and preferences belong in the curriculum of all psychotherapeutic trainings. If there is one topic that affects all people of this world equally, it is the topic of sexuality. No one would be present on this planet without sexuality.

Three Key Takeaways

From what has been said, there are some important implications for family therapy practice, which will be summarized here:

1. In the background of many, if not most, couple conflicts are issues of sexual dissatisfaction, usually related to incompatible preference patterns. This is also especially true in cases where the conception's reason relates to communicative misunderstandings or other everyday conflicts. Usually, the concrete experience of incompatibility of a couple's arousal patterns lies a long time, often many years, behind the presented problem. The task of therapy is then first to address the issue of sexuality and then to advance to the point in the couple's biography where the awareness of incompatibility arose.

2. The goal at this point of therapy is to make the different desires and needs present and discussable. The exercise of the "optimal sexual scenario" is recommended here. Both partners are asked to write out at home and each for themselves the best possible sexual intercourse from their point of view. The current partner does not have to be in the story. In the following session, possibilities can be worked out to approach the scenario of the other partner.

3. In the case of preference differences, there are only three viable solutions to the difficulties. This is essentially because preferences must be understood as largely stable sexual needs whose behavioral change is always accompanied by a loss of sexual excitability. The solutions are in detail:

   A) **The "lowest common denominator"**: Both partners decide by mutual consent to revalue the relationship. This means that less importance is attached to sexual satisfaction and instead the essential accent is placed on loving togetherness, a shared future, or other joint projects. Sexuality can then take place in a more relaxed way, even if sexual satisfaction may not reach the level that both partners' desire.

   B) **The opening of the relationship**: Both partners decide consensually, honestly, and openly, while living sexually with each other the lowest common denominator. The then unfulfilled preferences are lived with other sexual partners outside the relationship. This is where the issue of jealousy quickly arises. However, jealousy never refers to the sexual level of a relationship but is a consequence of the assumption that the partner could fall in love with the other person. Therefore, if it would be ensured that in case of existing sexual external contacts the partner does not fall in love, the acceptance of this solution strategy increases. In this context, it is the therapist's task to initiate a negotiation process, at the end of which a contract is made between the partners in which they commit themselves to certain behaviors that are suitable to minimize the jealousy of the other partner.

Example: In couples therapy there is a couple who have been married for over ten years. Both partners love each other and declare that they want to stay together in the future. They both run a horse farm together, he takes care of the financial matters of the farm, she gives riding lessons and looks after the welfare of the horses. The partners do not have children and do not wish to have any. During therapy, both partners learn to openly address the otherwise taboo subject of sexuality. The woman particularly has difficulties with this since she was bullied in her school days because of her figure and her other appearance. Both partners show a dominant preference, which together can be considered incompatible. If the man behaves dominantly during the sexual act, her desire dwindles; if the woman behaves dominantly, the man shows erectile dysfunction. During the following conversations, the woman broaches the subject of her jealousy at the idea that her husband might look for a submissive woman to have sex with. All the husband's protestations that he loves his wife do not initially change the jealousy. In a negotiated settlement, it becomes clear that the woman's jealousy is tied to the idea that her husband could fall in love elsewhere if they had repeated sexual contact. The two conclude a contract by mutual agreement: Both agree to look for other sexual partners outside the relationship. This is done openly and comprehensibly, which means that, for example, Internet contacts are openly communicated, and the wife has access to the husband's Internet account and vice versa. To minimize jealousy, both also agree to meet with any outside contacts only once each, so that mutual love cannot develop in the first place.

After four sessions, couples therapy is terminated, and a follow-up appointment is scheduled in six months. After this time, both partners have occasionally met with other sexual partners and have also had sexual experiences. Jealousy has not occurred, and contacts have been comprehensibly consummated, one contact also in threesomes. Erectile dysfunction no longer exists. Both spouses describe an emotional deepening of their relationship and a considerable increase in quality of life and mutual trust.

C) **Separation:** If the lowest common denominator is deemed insufficient by the partners and opening the relationship is not an alternative, the only remaining solution is separation. This lack of an alternative becomes even more apparent the more the partners adhere to rigid norms and values, such as those of a religious nature. If a separation does not occur because the corresponding norms and values also prohibit it, severe psychological disorders of the least resilient partner are usually the long-term consequence.

The aspects described here for couple and family therapy suggest the urgency of addressing the sexual. Those who are unwilling or unable to deal with the topic of sexuality, even in their own lives, and who devalue or are unable to accept their own preference and that of their counterpart, cannot conduct profitable couple and family therapy.

References

Ahlers, C. J., Schaefer, G. A., Mundt, I. A., Roll, S., Englert, H., Willich, & S., Beier, K. M. (2011). How unusual are the contents of paraphilia? Paraphilia-associated sexual arousal patterns in a community-based sample of men. *Journal of Sexual Medicine, 8*, 1362–1370.

Amendt, G., Schmidt, G., & Sigusch, V. (2011). *Sex tells: Sexualforschung als Gesellschaftskritik.* Konkret, Hamburg.

American Psychiatric Association. (2022). *Diagnostic and statistical manual of mental disorders* (5th ed., text rev.). https://doi.org/10.1176/appi.books.9780890425787

Arendt, H. J., Adolf, D., & Friedrich, C. (2011). Inzidenz sexueller Probleme in der gynäkologischen Praxis. *Sexuologie,18*(1/2), 25–29.

Batinic, B., Puhle, B., & Moser, K. (1999). Der WWW-FragebogenGenerator. In: Batinic, B., Werner, A., Gräf, L., Bandilla, W. (Hg.). *Online research: Methoden, Anwendungen und Ergebnisse.* Hofgrefe Verlag für Psychologie, Göttingen, 93–102.

Beier, K. M., & Loewit, K. (2004). *Lust in Beziehungen. Einführung in die syndyastische Sexualtherapie.* Springer, Berlin.

Beier, K. M., & Loewit, K. (2011). *Praxisleitfaden Sexualmedizin. Von der Theorie zur Therapie.* Springer: Berlin.

Buddeberg, C. (2005). *Sexualberatung. Eine Einführung für Ärzte, Psychotherapeuten und Familienberater.* Thieme, Stuttgart.

Cedric, D. A., & Bosinski, H. A. G. (2010). Sexualmedizin in der hausärztlichen Praxis: Gewachsenes Problembewusstsein bei nach wie vor unzureichenden Kenntnissen. *Sexuologie, 17*(1/2), 5–13.

Crepault, E., & Couture, M. (1980). Men's erotic fantasies. *Archives of Sexual Behavior, 9,* 565–581.

De Sade, M. (2010). *Gesammelte Werke.* Akzente, Neu-Isenburg.

Dilling, H., Mombour, W., Schmidt, M. H., & Schulte-Markwort, E. (2011). *Internationale Klassifikation psychischer Störungen.* ICD-10 Kapitel V (F). Diagnostische Kriterien für Forschung und Praxis. Huber, Bern.

Durex (2008). *Sexual Wellbeing. Global Survey.* www.durex.com/en-sg/sexualwellbeingsurvey/documents/swgs pptv2.pdf (7.5.14).

Fiedler, P. (2010). *Sexualität.* Reclam, Stuttgart.

Freud, S. (2010). *Drei Abhandlungen zur Sexualtheorie.* Reclam, Stuttgart

Habermas, J. (1982). *Theorie des kommunikativen Handelns.* Suhrkamp, Frankfurt a.M.

James, E. L. (2012). *Fifty Shades of Grey.* Geheimes Verlangen. Goldmann, München.

Joyal, C. C., Cossette, A., Lapierre, V., 2014. What exactly is an unusual sexual fantasy? *Journal of Sexual Medicine.* doi: 10.1111/jsm.12734

Khar, B. (2007). *Sex and the Psyche.* Basic Books, New York.

Khar, B. (2008). *Who´s been sleeping in your head? The secret world of sexual fantasies.* Basic Books, New York.

Krafft-Ebing, R. (1894). *Psychopathia Sexualis.* Ferdinand Enke, Stuttgart.

Prosieben, Sex Report (2008). www.myvideo.de/channel/ *sex_report* (Zugriff 6/2015).

Reinecke, A., Schöps, D., Hoyer, J., 2006. Sexuelle Dysfunktionen bei Patienten einer verhaltenstherapeutischen Hochschulambulanz: Häufigkeit, Erkennen, Behandlung. *Verhaltenstherapie, 16,* 166–172.

Renaud, C. A., Byers, E. S., (1999). Exploring the frequency, diversity and content of university students' positive and negative sexual cognitions. *Canadian Journal of Human Sexuality, 8,*17–33.

Robinson, J.D., & Parks, C.W. (2004). Lesbian and bisexual woman´s sexual fantasies, psychological adjustment and close relationship functioning. *Journal of Psychology & Human Sexuality, 15,*185–203.

Schmidt, G. (1998). *Sexuelle Verhältnisse. Über das Verschwinden der Sexualmoral.* Rowohlt, Reinbek.

Schmidt, G., & Sigusch, V. (1971). *Arbeiter-Sexualität. Eine empirische Untersuchung an jungen Industriearbeitern.* Luchterhand, Neuwied.

Sennett, R. (2010). *Der flexible Mensch. Die Kultur des neuen Kapitalismus.* Berlin Verlag, Berlin.

Sigusch, V. (2013). *Sexualitäten. Eine Kritische Theorie in 99 Fragmenten.* Campus, Frankfurt am Main.

Sigusch, V. (2005). *Neosexualitäten: Über den kulturellen Wandel von Liebe und Perversion.* Campus, Frankfurt am Main.

Sigusch, V., & Schmidt, G. (1973). *Jugendsexualität. Dokumentation einer Untersuchung.* Ferdinand Enke, Stuttgart.

Spiegel-Online (2013). Shades of Grey: Softporno rettet Bertelsmann-Bilanz. www.spiegel.de/wir tschaft/unternehmen/fifty-shades-trilogie-rettet-bertelsmann-das-geschaeftsjahr-a-888203.html (20.2.14).

Strassberg, D. S., & Lockerd, L. K. (1998). Force in women´s sexual fantasies. *Archives of Sexual Behavior, 27,* 403–14.

Templeman, T. L., & Stinnett, R. D. (1991). Patterns of sexual arousal and history in a "normal" sample of young men. *Archives of Sexual Behavior, 20,* 137–150.

Witte, E. H., Poser, B., Strohmeier, C. (2007). Konsensueller Sadomasochismus. Eine empirische Prüfung von Bindungsstil und Sozialisationseinfluss. (Hamburger Forschungsbericht zur Sozialpsychologie Nr. 76). Universität Hamburg, Arbeitsbereich Sozialpsychologie. http://psydok. sulb.unisaarland.de/volltexte/2008/2339/pdf/HAFOS_76.pdf

World Health Organization. (2019). *International statistical classification of diseases and related health problems* (11th ed.). https://icd.who.int/

SECTION II

Theories and Models in an International Context

7

SOCIOCULTURAL ATTUNEMENT IN FAMILY THERAPY

Socioculturally Attuned Family Therapy: Third-order Thinking

J. Maria Bermudez, Teresa McDowell, and
Carmen Knudson-Martin

Context

Socioculturally attuned family therapy is a transtheoretical framework that can be applied to existing couple and family therapy models in ways that encourage equity-based practice. We define sociocultural attunement as awareness of the impact of the relationship between societal systems, culture, and power along with the willingness to be attentive and respond to what is unjust. The approach relies on interdisciplinary concepts for recognizing the impact of culture, power, and societal systems on individuals, couples, families, and communities. It goes beyond analyzing between-group dynamics within a single society to understanding the politics of difference across local, national, and international contexts and the impact of these on relationship processes.

Socioculturally attuned family therapists support cultural democracy while promoting just relationships. They consider how each person's needs, interests, and wellbeing are reflected in how relationships are organized, decisions are made, and communication occurs. There is an emphasis on respecting and integrating a family's cultural values and idiosyncratic perspectives, while simultaneously confronting relational inequities and oppression. This is especially challenging. For example, unjust relationships that harm one or more family members may be common within a culture without being just. In other words, being culturally aware does not mean accepting commonly occurring practices that place some family members at greater disadvantage or risk than others. Consider intimate partner violence (IPV) as a case in point. IPV is ubiquitous across cultural contexts, yet few would argue that it is a preferred cultural arrangement for all involved. Socioculturally attuned couple and family therapists build on resilience by helping members consider how they can help each other navigate unjust societal systems, as well as how their relationships can buffer the impact of social inequity.

DOI: 10.4324/9781003297871-9

Third-order Thinking and Third-order Change

Family therapy has a history of differentiating between first and second-order change. This differentiation, we suggest, reflects first and second-order thinking. First-order thinking refers to conceptualizing problems in "common sense" terms. First-order change, therefore, leads to obvious solutions that may be helpful but fail to fundamentally change relationship rules, processes, or shared meaning. For example, encouraging a couple who are arguing over getting up with a newborn to take turns every other night might help ensure both parents get some rest and relief, but doesn't address relational dynamics that contribute to the problem. Family therapists more often use second-order thinking to target second-order change to help clients solve problems by shifting patterns in their relationships, as well as how they punctuate, or story, their experience. From a second-order perspective, the same couple might be invited to consider how it is that they have not been able to solve the problem; why a commonsense solution has not worked. This approach highlights relational dynamics that create and maintain the problem.

What we have termed third-order thinking and third-order change (McDowell, 2015; McDowell, et al., 2018; McDowell, et al., 2019) enables therapists to be socioculturally attuned. Third-order differs from first-order, which targets change within a set of alternatives, and second-order, which changes the set of alternatives itself. Rather, third-order thinking and third-order change involve sets of alternatives within systems of systems. This perspective expands choices in meta narratives and meta processes within which relationships are organized. Targeting third-order change might include asking the couple mentioned above to consider the relative social value of work-for-pay and parenting, societal expectations of gender roles related to infant care, and the impact of their identities on their ability to influence the relationship.

Third-order thinking requires therapists to connect the dots between clients' personal and relational problems and the broader social world and environmental context in which they are embedded. To do this, therapists must be aware of how they are organizing and making sense of vast amounts of information, including how their perspectives delimit their work with couples and families. Third-order thinking helps therapists attune to the experience of each client within the complexities of interconnected identities and relationships within social, economic, political, and environmental contexts. This requires keeping a keen eye on the impact of uneven distribution of resources and inequitable societal structures. In other words, third-order thinking provides a conceptual map by which therapists can integrate awareness of societal context and power processes into everyday practice.

Thinking About Thinking and Third-order Ethics

Third-order thinking invites us to take a meta perspective. It invites us to think about how we think, including the positioning of Western ethnocentric theories within globally diverse ontological and epistemological frameworks. This is particularly salient when considering what and how couple and family therapy knowledge claims become reified and shared across borders. Diverse ontologies – how we view the very nature of being – are rarely considered when producing professional knowledge. Our ontological imaginations (Norwalk, 2013) are constrained by what we consider true and possible within the framework of our accepted reality. For example, it is not common for Western family therapists to talk about the impact of a spirit world on relational problems, while they readily gravitate toward advancements in neuroscience. Awareness of ontological frameworks allows us to contextualize therapy, to recognize the potential harm of unintended colonization via sharing of professional "truth" across the uneven terrain of global resources and influence.

Epistemology is deeply tied to ontology. Epistemology refers to knowledge itself; what is considered to be knowledge and how knowledge is created or acquired. Consider the tension between evidence-based practices and use of clinical experience. Most relationship therapists who practice for an extended period are informed by research, theories, and models, but also have a sense of knowing that goes beyond formal learning to create a gestalt that guides them in what to do in each situation. Western, scientific epistemologies often value this knowledge less than that which is produced using random control trials (Harding, 1998; 2008). The dismissal and marginalization of non-dominant knowledge reflects a type of epistemological injustice (Fricker, 2007) in which many ways of looking at the world are not only devalued and rendered silent but are internally experienced without a language in which they can be described and developed.

Third-order ethics within diverse global contexts starts with recognizing and being accountable for the impact of how we think – what we consider to be true and right – on our everyday practice (McDowell, et al, in press). Ontological and epistemological diversity and flexibility allow us to move within, while thinking beyond, single systems of thought and limiting dichotomies. This metaview invites us to consider the impact of systems of thought on social discourse, societal systems, communities, and everyday life at the most local and intimate levels. Thinking about thinking includes acknowledging the value we, as authors, place on social and relational justice as not only a practical concern for mental and relational wellbeing, but an outcropping of our shared epistemology. Additionally, acknowledging and challenging our values is necessary to position ourselves to do this work.

Third-order thinking is connected to third-order ethics. Third-order ethics (McDowell, et al., in press) relies on family therapists considering their own worldviews and biases (first-order thinking), placing family and therapeutic systems in cultural and societal context (second-order thinking), and interrupting unjust power dynamics by shedding light on systems of systems that create inequities that promote and maintain mental health and relational problems (third-order thinking). This stance is necessary across and within cultural groups, in the United States and abroad. We have an ethical responsibility to critically examine the impact of inequity and abuse of power on therapeutic processes. From a third-order perspective, the therapist's awareness of societal context and power dynamics is a foundational and integrated part of their professional knowledge across all cultural contexts.

Third-order Positioning: Supporting While Disrupting

Working within and across borders requires us to repeatedly situate ourselves. Our social location, intersectional identities, and cultural experiences strongly affect how we see the world, including our perspectives of clients and their presenting problems (Collins & Bilge, 2016). We must engage in ongoing critical-contextual self-reflexivity to be able to be intentional in our work. This includes not only being accountable for the power and privilege associated with our professional role, but also being aware of how our own social locations or markers of identity afford additional privilege, while marginalizing and/or oppressing others. Although we all hold both dominant and subordinate aspects of identity (Tatum, 1997), regardless of our individual social locations, it is necessary for us to consistently examine and correct our biases that contribute to unjust relationships and social inequity. We must be able to attune to all clients within their cultural and social context (D'Aniello, et al., 2016; Knudson-Martin, et al., 2020). Taking a broad meta view of systems of systems helps us respect clients' values and beliefs without feeling the need to give up our own (McGoldrick & Hardy, 2019). As mentioned, cultural democracy is an important framework for socioculturally attuned family therapists (Kosutic & McDowell, 2008). This stance helps us actively value all cultures, while simultaneously taking steps to interrupt the dominance of one culture or group over another. We contend that this stance is ethical on various levels.

This critical self-awareness is vital and must be ongoing. When we fail to inspect our own epistemological frameworks, we run the risk of inadvertently marginalizing the experience and lifeworlds of others and judging/labeling them pathologically. As Fricker (2007, p. 91) stated, "epistemological responsibility requires a distinctly reflexive critical social awareness." The need to navigate tensions inherent to socioculturally attuned practice and third-order challenges is never-ending. Although this work is uncomfortable, hard, and tiring, not doing this critical self-work may unintentionally lead to further subjugation of those who hold less societal power, such as with benevolent racism, sexism, classism, homophobia, and ableism, among others.

Third-order positioning requires family therapists to honor the cultural values and personal perspectives of clients, while simultaneously challenging oppression. Questions we often consider include: How do we honor beliefs, goals, and values that we believe may inadvertently oppress another or contribute to a client's own subjugation? How do we navigate the potential consequences of raising social awareness among family members when doing so may disrupt relationships? How do we differentiate between what is common in a culture and what may be common but is also oppressive? How do we help clients to explore the implications of taken-for-granted cultural practices and assumptions that are not just? And finally, how do we maintain a meta-view that allows us to identify when symptoms are a result of and/or forms of resistance to unjust exertions of power? In essence, we contend that third-order positioning is necessary for challenging the practice and the field of family therapy as an agent of colonization and subjugation.

Colonizing and Decolonizing in Family Therapy Practice

Family therapy has grown and developed worldwide, in part, by importing U.S.-based models of family therapy into other societies. Simultaneously, practitioners continue to use family therapy models without consideration of the biases, values, and beliefs embedded in these ways of researching, assessing, and intervening with diverse families within all societies, including within the United States. When therapists/researchers have a sense of superiority or lack of consideration for sociopolitical and cultural context, we can unknowingly impose the dominant schema of the Standard North American Family (SNAF) (Smith, 1993) and the mythical norm (Lorde, 2007). As socioculturally attuned therapists, we must reflect on the ramifications of imposing our worldviews when exporting family therapy to other countries (e.g., clinical training, research, and practice). We must be vigilant about what informs the creation, interpretation, and application of the guidelines of our profession, especially within and across cultural and societal contexts.

Although movements are in place to decolonize family science and family therapy (Bermudez et al., 2018; McDowell & Hernandez, 2010), colonialism is prevalent worldwide and must continue to be challenged. The consequence of colonialism is the creation of unequal relationships and an establishment of hierarchical power structures that benefits people from the dominant group over others. On every continent there is evidence of colonialism, which has created imbalances of power, privilege, resources, and wealth that continue to have intergenerational effects on families and communities (Miller & Garran, 2008; Uttal, 2009). In this process, the ideologies and practices of persons from a dominant group are given precedence, and the cultural voices, beliefs, and practices of others are subjugated (McDowell & Hernández, 2010; Tatum, 1998). Colonization occurs when the cultural values, beliefs, and practices of the dominant group are centered as preferable, normal, best and right (Denzin et al., 2008; Harding, 1998; McCall, 2005; Mohanty, 2003; Swadener & Mutua, 2008; Tatum, 1998). This is not simply a matter of "different" beliefs. Dominant cultural practices determine cultural capital (e.g., language, traditions, religion), social capital (e.g., who you know, social influence), and even symbolic capital (e.g., skin tone, immigration status, education) (McDowell & Hernandez, 2010), creating life-long cumulative advantage as methods and systems of inequality (DiPrete & Eirich, 2006; Zrenchik & McDowell, 2012). All of these are connected to economic capital (Bourdieu, 1986) and power to dominate and control groups of people. Consequently, colonizing processes at an international level reflect attitudes that determine what is good, right, and true based on a country's level of power, such as technological advancement, material wealth, and military power. A similar dynamic occurs within societal systems (e.g., education, government, business) and families.

Re-Thinking Best Practices

Being a socioculturally attuned family therapist in cross-cultural and international contexts includes recognizing and being responsible for how family therapists potentially serve as a colonizing force, especially when we export our ways of thinking and working as "best practice." As family therapists, we are at risk of colonizing on a broad societal level when we export family therapy theory and practice across national and cultural contexts. This is particularly concerning when "best practices" are imported from powerful, high resource countries in the West. For example, our unexamined use of empirically supported treatments and theoretically based family therapy models often privilege Western-based science and values such as individuality, emotions, independence, personal achievement, and self-focus, often undermining the values of those who embrace collectivistic and communal worldviews. As mentioned, worldwide, Western-based ideologies and practices are often thought of as "best," which is often privileged, prioritized, and held in high esteem by professionals in countries who often have a history of colonization.

Scholars in other fields are challenging and critiquing the Eurocentric biases embedded and imposed by neoliberal global one-size-fits-all "best practices." For example, Keating (2012) examined the effects of importing these standards in higher education in sub-Saharan Africa and Southeast Asia. Murray et al. (2007) contend that systemic power is reproduced and guarded by gatekeepers of what is deemed "good science," and that the regime of evidence, along with corporate standards of accountability, best practices, and methodological fundamentalism, has led to decreases in innovation, scholarship, and care in the health sciences in Canada. Petr and Walters (2005) offer a multidimensional framework that broadens current approaches to "best practices" inquiry to include perspectives of consumers and practitioners by making it more inclusive of the experiences, preferences, and wisdom of consumers and professionals in any given field.

Colonizing Effects of Professional Standards and Diagnostics

Broadly defined, psychotherapy is considered a Western professional practice. Diagnostic criteria (i.e., DSM 5 from the American Psychiatric Association) and professional standards are grounded in empirically supported clinical models and theories primarily developed in the United States. These practices are often assumed to be the gold standard for psychiatric and psychotherapy training and practice worldwide. Likewise, professional expectations and standards are deeply embedded in values developed and enforced by the most dominant groups of a society. Elsewhere, we discussed the implications of the potential ethnocentric and colonizing effects of the professional codes of ethics, specifically for the field of Marriage and Family Therapy (McDowell, et al., in press).

We contend that in general, all standards and ethical guidelines are steeped in cultural values, most of which are covert and unexamined. For example, the AAMFT code of ethics is a set of standards situated within the field of family therapy in the United States. As licensed practitioners, we value the structure, order, and principles of this code, primarily because it reflects important sets of expectations founded on our unified commitment to ethically and professionally serve the public. However, these standards and the clinical actions that follow are rarely critically examined to assess the taken-for-granted values and cultural biases underlying what we make explicit. Dominant beliefs and values can lead practitioners to assume our professional standards are universal, benevolent, and neutral; however, sociocultural attunement requires us to consider the effects of dominant cultural biases and how persons in central positions of power influence what is deemed as competent, professional, and best practice. Family therapists are critically evaluating the effects of Western-based practices and superiority across cultural contexts (Jordan, et al., 2021; Seponski et al., 2020).

Decentering Western-Based Family Therapy

Decolonizing processes have begun to loosen the grip of dominant discourses and practices that assume one culture's superiority over another (Laenui, 2006). According to Tourse and colleagues (2018) "postcolonial theory provides a lens through which to understand identity, gender, race, racism, 'color,' and ethnicity... and underscores how knowledge of the world is generated under specific relations between those who have power and those subjugated by it" (p. 111). Engagement with this critical stance heightens our awareness of biases embedded in context, culture, knowledge, and dominant discourses of influence. A decolonizing approach highlights and privileges ways of knowing that are often ignored, disregarded, and/or marginalized and attempts to honor subjugated, marginalized people and their local knowledge.

Third-order thinking helps us engage in family therapy to critically examine systems of systems that operate to maintain or dismantle what is deemed legitimate, normative, or empirically supported practice. In the United States, we continue to suffer the ripple effects of colonization, slavery, immigration policies, and heteronormative oppression through policies and practices that keep those with less power in subjugated positions. The legacy of colonization is evident in systems and structures worldwide and third-order international family therapy requires us to consider all systems as involving systems of oppression and privilege. Our commitment to help transform these systems is reflected in our stances and action toward third-order change.

Third-order Thinking in Clinical Practice

Socioculturally attuned therapists know that what they see and do – how they think about cases and respond – is not neutral. They strive to recognize the impact of their clinical decisions so as to interrupt and transform societal-based power inequities and colonization rather than perpetuate them. They know good practice must be equitable and use a third-order lens to integrate an analysis of power and societal context with their clinical model (McDowell et al., 2018).

Tracking the Flow of Power

Power dynamics impact all aspects of wellbeing, including relational processes such as communication, intimacy, and conflict resolution (Knudson-Martin, 2013). Power, as we use it here, is a social process that focuses attention and legitimacy on the needs and interests of some persons or groups rather than others. Power processes are constructed as people interact with each other and create and reinforce inequitable social structures. Social power is reflected in who feels worthy and valued, expectations about what one has a right to expect in a relationship, whose experiences are part of shared language and knowledge, who is deemed credible, and who influences or accommodates the other (Bava, 2023; Fricker, 2007). The more powerful tend not to notice the less powerful or be aware of their needs and interests. People with less power tend to be attentive and responsive to those with more power, which can be necessary for survival. It typically falls to those in less powerful positions to "keep the peace" and avoid disappointing, disturbing, or upsetting powerful persons in their families, workspaces, or communities. Those in more powerful positions may be unaware of the accommodations people are making and do not necessarily feel powerful (Kimmel, 2016; Tatum, 1997).

Tracking the flow of societal power processes within relationships enables therapists to develop interventions that take their impact on power into account. For example, if a female client from a low-income family of origin tells you that "low self-esteem" keeps her from being assertive enough at work, an intervention that helps her identify societal messages that her perspective is not worthy would interrupt the societal flow of power that diminishes credibility of her voice (Fricker, 2007). In contrast, a clinical intervention that moves directly to assertiveness training would replicate the dominant power system that says she is the problem without taking into account how willing and open the system is to hearing and valuing her voice. Similarly, with a cisgender heterosexual relationship in which the male partner says he does not know what his partner wants because she doesn't tell him, interventions that put the burden on her to express herself, without first exploring *how* their relational power processes limit her voice and his attunement, would replicate patriarchal power patterns (Knudson-Martin, 2013).

Attending to Context

It is important to understand each client within their sociocultural niche (Falicov, 2014). Individual identities are intricately connected to a wider set of intersecting power differentials depending on one's gender, socioeconomic status, sexual orientation, age, ability/disability, religion, ethnicity, Indigenous heritage, and national origin, among other social locations. The unique impact of these also depend on ecological context, migration/acculturation, family life cycle, and family organization (Falicov, 2014). Wherever one lives, all of these intersecting factors influence experience with social justice and cultural diversity.

Socioculturally attuned therapists seek to apprehend each person's felt sociocultural experience, recognizing that people may be privileged in some aspects of their social location and oppressed or marginalized in others (Tatum, 1997). Therapists need to also consider concepts such as hierarchy and individuality within cultural context. In Western cultures, norms of individualism tend to mask power differences and make them covert; people are expected to be responsible for their own well-being and the effects of implicit social hierarchies are minimized (Silverstein et al., 2006). In contrast, individual well-being in collectivist cultures is experienced in the context of interdependence, shared relational responsibility, and overt hierarchies and people are expected to communicate indirectly to preserve harmony (Bermudez, 2011; Hofstead, 2001). Equity and mutual care may be enacted while respecting hierarchy and tradition (Knudson-Martin & Kim, 2023; Moghadam & Knudson-Martin, 2009). The guidelines described below are presented in the spirit of offering a framework for being a socioculturally attuned family therapist whose aim is to respect and respond to these cultural differences – rather than colonizing – while also centering equity and third-order ethics.

Guidelines for Socioculturally Attuned Practice

We use the acronym ANVIET to identify six guiding principles that socioculturally attuned therapists can use to maintain ethical, socially responsible practice regardless of community or nation. They include (1) **A**ttune to context and power; (2) **N**ame injustice; (3) **V**alue what is minimized; (4) **I**ntervene in power dynamics; (5) **E**nvision just alternatives; and (6) **T**ransform to make the imagined a reality. These principles apply across cultural contexts and theoretical models. To illustrate them, we use the case of the Robertson family. The Robertsons live in a working-class neighborhood in a small city in a Southwestern U.S. state. This case, which represents a composite of several, demonstrates the ANVIET approach and issues relevant across sociocultural contexts.

The nuclear family is composed of Mia (34) a cisgender multicultural woman of Latinx, Euro-American, and Indigenous heritage, James (39) a cisgender male of Northern European heritage, and their three sons Liam (13), Elijah (12), and Noah (9). Mia called to make an appointment based on a referral from the school counselor because Elijah is engaging in physical fights in school and at risk of failing several classes. The therapist, Angela (35), identifies as a cisgender Mexican-American female and is a single mother of a 14-year-old daughter. She tells Mia her usual practice is to begin by meeting with the entire family. After some struggle to find a time in which James can participate, all attend. The therapist observes that based on their attire, hair, etc., each of the boys presents as cisgender. The boys fight among themselves as they enter the room, and James glares at them and admonishes them to "be quiet and sit down."

From the intake form, Angela learns that James is a foreman of a roofing crew and Mia works as a home healthcare aide. During the COVID-19 pandemic, Mia cut back significantly on her work hours to oversee the boys' online school but has since returned to full-time work. They report no current religious involvement and no problems with substance use. Liam and Noah are actively involved in multiple sports teams, which James helps coach. The parents indicate that their marriage is stable but also report high stress levels. They say their concern is with Elijah, who seems irritable and disengaged and is having trouble at school. Angela begins the first session interested in learning more about the family and the sociocultural context in which the concerns regarding Elijah have arisen. She is mindful that while she shares some identities with Mia, her experiences may be very different, and that though her heritage is Mexican-American, most of the theories she learned in graduate school developed within Western, Global North contexts.

Attune to Context and Power

As the family describes the concerns that brought them to therapy, the therapist seeks to understand, resonate with, and respond to their experience within societal contexts. She wants to append – to "get" – each family member's unique sociocultural experience. She brings both a knowing and not-knowing perspective (Knudson-Martin et al., 2020), in which she uses what she knows about social discourses, norms, and societal power processes to inform her curiosity and areas to explore, while also avoiding stereotypes and being responsive to what is salient to clients. For example, when Mia says she "just wants Elijah to be happy and stop getting in trouble," Angela begins to expand the lens outward to get a sense of the social context around parenting for her:

Therapist: (to Mother) You want Elijah to be happy – to not get in trouble. As his mother, what does that mean to you?

Mia: That I don't have to worry; that he's going to be OK. (pause) That he can get along with people.

Taking in Mia's statement raises a number of contextual curiosities for the therapist. She knows many cultural messages tell mothers they are responsible for child outcomes, so Angela wonders if/how Mia experiences this role. The therapist also wonders how Mia pictures the world in which Elijah's well-being will be determined and how that shapes what getting along with others means.

Therapist: (to Mia) what is your sense about what it takes to get along in the world, what do you think people expect of someone like Elijah?

Mia: To follow the rules. To do what is expected; to not question everything and everyone!

The therapist continues to socioculturally attune to the contextual meaning of parenting and Elijah's behavior. She asks James similar questions. Angela learns that both parents are trying to prepare their children for life as they've experienced it in their work environments, where willingness to conform to expectations is necessary and acts of independence and defiance get people in trouble (Lareau, 2011; Tuttle et al., 2012). Neither can feel successful as parents when Elijah does not comply with school standards or get along with his peers. James worries that people see Elijah as too soft, not man enough, easy to bully. For this reason, he is somewhat encouraged when Elijah defends himself by getting in fights. The therapist now has an initial sense of how patriarchy, gender, and class may intersect in this family. As she explores these in the emerging identities of the boys, she finds that Elim and

Noah are learning to follow these contextualized gender messages. Elijah is not. The therapist begins to gently explore their responses to the idea of more flexibility around gender expressions and identity.

Therapist (to Elim): It sounds like you enjoy being an athlete and get a lot of recognition for that. Are there other parts of being a person or being you that you think people don't notice as much or give as much credit to?

Attuning to societal contexts and power from the beginning of therapy helps set a larger frame for the clinical work. The therapist will continue this kind of attunement throughout the sessions, paying attention to how social power processes contribute to each person's experience and relational processes.

Name Injustice

Socioculturally attuned therapists identify what is unjust or has been overlooked and amplify silent voices. For example, in this case the therapist gives voice to some of the injustices created by patriarchal social structures and engages family members in considering the consequences. Note that she does this by helping to draw connections between their experience and larger societal contexts:

Therapist: Elim said he thinks qualities like being kind or being artistic don't get much acknowledgement or credit – not just in this family, but in the larger society. Who do you think that hurts?

Mia: Well, it hurts girls and women. We try to be kind, but we get walked on, don't necessarily get kindness back.

It's not surprising that when the therapist created an opportunity, Mia raised inequities that she otherwise would likely not have voiced. After following up on what this means to Mia and her place in the family, Angela brings the conversation back to the effect on boys and men:

Therapist: Mia, you described hurts you've experienced by how women are minimized or put down. James, you expressed some surprise that she felt this way and this sounds like an important conversation to continue. (pause) I'm wondering too about the effect of putting down more [makes air quotes] feminine qualities has on boys? On men? On relationships. How do you think it has affected you, James?

James: What do you mean?

Therapist: What parts of you have been affected or hurt by having to tow the line – to being the strong, tough guy?

James: I don't know. (slowly) Well. My dad was always really hard on me. Still is. I never seemed to be good enough for him. He was always telling me to be tough and to "suck it up!" I came out OK...

Therapist: You came out OK (pause), but it seems like it's been at a cost. Is that right?

Angela continues to develop the conversation of the cost to men and boys of such rigid societal ideas about masculinity, and makes a mental note to come back to the price of patriarchy in the relationship between James and his father at another time. She invites the family to consider Elijah's fights and struggles through a more inclusive value frame.

Value What is Minimized

An important way socioculturally attuned therapists center equity is through the values they represent and clinical responses that acknowledge the worth of that which has been minimized or devalued. In this case, the therapist intentionally values "soft" qualities that are frequently overlooked. She is curious about what has not been valued in Elijah's experience and highlights those that tend to be overlooked in the dominant U.S. culture.

Therapist: Noah, I know there is a lot of fighting and rough and tumble in this house. But I'm curious – How are your brothers kind to you? How do they show they care for you?

Noah: (giggles and looks around).

Therapist: You're not used to talking about being kind...about caring. I'm guessing that your brothers are kind sometimes. How do they show that?

This question challenges the dominant patriarchal ideological structure within which the family is living. As Angela persists in raising kindness as an important value, Noah begins to describe a variety of ways that Elijah, in particular, is kind to his younger brother. He especially highlights that Elijah plays silly games with him and lets him win. Then on a somber note Noah says, "some guys say he's a sissy, (pause) a fag." The therapist names this as hurtful and unjust:

Therapist: Sounds like those guys are trying to hurt Elijah, to be intentionally mean. That sounds very unfair to me.

Intervene in Power Dynamics

Socioculturally attuned therapists develop interventions that disrupt oppressive power dynamics and support equitable relationships. Angela recognizes signs of many oppressive power processes as the Roberston family engages with each other and tells their story. She is mindful that all family members appear to accommodate and placate James, that Mia tends not to openly disagree with James, but had a lot to say when invited to share her experience. Though Elijah does not verbally confront his father, his nonconforming behavior can be viewed as a form of resistance. As a working-class family "playing by the rules," Angela also sees them as potentially limited by the work/economic structures they inhabit and the gender ideology that supports it. She develops interventions that interrupt these power dynamics as they are enacted in the Robertson family, as in this example with James:

Therapist: Elijah, Noah says some guys call you a "fag." What does that word mean to you? What message do you take from it?

Elijah: (looking down). They're just stupid...just dumb guys.

James: (to Elijah) I don't know what you expect! Guys will pick on you if you don't man-up.

Therapist: (to James) You don't like to see your son hurt. (pause) Where do you think you got the idea there is only one way to be a man? Or that being a woman or gay is bad?

James: Not bad, but...different, lower. It's how things are.

Angela continues this conversation, which interrupts the father's enforcement of hegemonic masculinity (Pascoe, 2007). She intervenes again when James discredits Mia's perspective and Mia seems to agree:

Mia: Sometimes I think Elijah isn't sure we love him, that we could support him more...

James: (interrupting). That's silly! Elijah knows we love him. He's lucky to have two parents who take him wherever he needs to go, puts food on the table, and pays the bills.

Mia: I know. We both work hard. We take parenting seriously.

It would be easy for the session to move forward based on James' perspective, which Mia seems to endorse. Instead, Angela notices how quickly Mia accommodated and intervenes in this power process by highlighting the importance of Mia's earlier contribution:

Therapist: Yes. you take parenting seriously. And, Mia, what you said, that Elijah may not be sure you love him, sounds important. Could you say a little more about that?

Mia: (slowly) Elijah has always seemed sort of vulnerable to me...like he wants to please us.

Angela helps Mia develop her thoughts on this topic and then encourages James to attune to her perspective, which also intervenes in the usual flow of power. When the couple repeats the pattern of Mia accommodating James' view, the therapist responds by inviting James to notice and reflect upon his part in this pattern and the relational consequences:

Therapist: James, did you notice just now that when you spoke with such certainty about what the boys need, Mia shut down on the subject? I'm guessing you'd like to know her thoughts [James agrees]. How do you think your adamant style affects Mia's response?

James: She should speak up! I get tired of her not saying what she really thinks.

Therapist: You want to know what she thinks. How do you think it happens that there is little space for her thoughts or to speak her mind? How could you invite them in?

This intervention opened space for additional conversation about how the patterns in their family are connected to larger societal systems and values, which sets the stage for envisioning something different. Angela will also encourage Mia to speak up, but not before making it likely that she will be heard.

Envision Just Alternatives

Socioculturally attuned therapists know identifying problems is not sufficient. They provide space to imagine just relational alternatives beyond those prescribed by the dominant systems within which they are embedded, to see possibilities within larger systems of systems. In this case, Angela draws on awareness of the history of colonization in the United States, which systematically wiped out Indigenous cultures and imposed patriarchal colonialism and binary gender structures on the Diné people (Jaimes-Guerrero, 2003). This brings the previously silenced part of Mia's native legacy (which valued multiple gender expressions, feminine skills and roles, and egalitarianism) into the family's relational process:

Therapist: Mia, you indicated that part of your heritage is Indigenous. [Mia nods]. I know that many Indigenous people have a tradition of more than two genders. Has this been part of your legacy?

Mia: My grandmother – on my mother's side – is Diné. But I don't know her very well. She lives a long ways away. We hardly ever see that side of the family. She married a White man, but he was mean I guess, and she left him and went back to the Rez. When my mom married my dad, she hardly ever went back there. She doesn't talk about it much. My father is a 5th generation Mexican-American. His family is very big and until I married James, that was the family I knew.

Therapist: You come from a lot of different people, with very different experiences in this country. It will be helpful to learn more about all of them. At this moment, I'm curious about your Diné heritage. What have you heard or learned about gender among the ancients?

Mia describes hearing about two-spirited people who went back and forth between genders or embodied both masculine and feminine characteristics and roles. She said she had been interested in learning more about that when she was a girl – about the ages of her boys now – but as she got older she got busy and let it go. The therapist uses this as an opportunity to engage the family in envisioning a wider, more fluid range of perspectives on gender:

Therapist: (to everyone) Have any of the rest of you heard about two-spirit people?

Elijah: I have actually. I read about it online. It sounded kinda cool.

Therapist: What do you think it would be like if people acknowledged more different ways to express gender?

Elijah: I think people would get along better. There'd be less pressure.

Therapist: What would it look like in this family if there was less pressure to express gender in a certain way?

This opens a lively conversation in which all the boys readily engage. It is a kind of talk they have never had before. James does not say much, but he listens. Angela uses this as an opportunity to open possibilities regarding father-son relationships as well:

Therapist: James, you said your father was hard on you; that's it's always been hard to seem like you were good enough. How do you think your relationship with him would be different if what it meant to be a man was less rigid?

James: (long pause). I think we might talk more – maybe get to know each other better.

After expanding on what James and his father could come to know about each other, Angela invites the family to envision other possible ways to engage. She and Mia also discuss how she can connect with her Diné grandmother and learn more about the Diné People and their history and traditions, which is a step in transforming the effects of colonization.

Transform to Make the Imagined a Reality

Socioculturally attuned therapists collaborate with their clients to make what is imagined real. Therapists apply their systems models and practices through an expanded lens to help couples and families create third-order change. This means facilitating clients' ability to enact the just ideals and relational patterns they envision, continuing to interrupt unjust power dynamics when they reappear, and helping clients develop strategies to transform and overcome them. In the case of the Robertson family, this means helping the parents become more aware of the social world within which they are raising their children so they can make more intentional and informed parenting decisions. It means moving beyond Elijah's presenting behavioral problems to seeing them related to larger systems of class, gender, sexuality, and race, so he – and all members of the Robertson family – have the opportunity to learn and know more about themselves and how they wish to express their genders and sexualities and relate to each other. For example, in one of the closing sessions, the family reports an argument about a forthcoming trip to a baseball game with James' father. The therapist uses her role to help the family clarify how to respond more equitably to the patriarchal legacy inherent in this event. Notably, Elijah is now more able to openly express his position.

Elijah: We're having this fight about the baseball game we're supposed to go to with grandpa [James' father] next week. I think baseball games are boring. I'll go to respect grandpa, but I'm not going to pretend that I want to be a jock.

Liam: Me either. I like baseball and I'm good at it. But I sometimes want grandpa to do different things with me, not only sports.

Therapist: Elim and Elijah, when you say you want your grandpa to do different things with you. What ideas do you have? How could it change your relationship with him? What would you say? Where would you go? What would you do? [the boys detail these]. James, how can you support your sons? What will it mean for you to help them expand their definition of what it means to be a man, especially with such a rich cultural heritage? How could this be helpful to them now and in the future?

As the therapist applied the ANVIET principles when working with the Robertson family, they were able to acknowledge and explore the personal consequences of societal power patterns, including migration and colonization, and to see and embody options within larger systems of systems. This enabled them to relate outside the demands of heteropatriarchy that had previously limited their relationships and caused Elijah significant distress.

As this example illustrates, socioculturally attuned family therapy can occur within and across borders. Couple and family therapists can use the ANVIET principles to connect any presenting issues and family processes to larger societal patterns across sociocultural contexts. In order to resist culturally endorsed inequity and injustice, therapists must intentionally take stances that actively interrupt societal-based power processes and resist reifying colonizing ideologies and practices.

Conclusion

By attending to power and context, therapists can engage in third-order thinking by critically examining our worldviews and biases and the inequities they create and endorse. We have a responsibility to scrutinize our professional standards, best practices, and codes of ethics that privilege dominant discourses and maintain hegemonic processes and power structures. As family therapists, we are increasingly working in multifaceted, complex, cross-cultural, and international contexts. This work requires that we attune, name, value, intervene, envision, and transform in ways that support just and equitable relationships and communities. At the end of this chapter, we offer reflexive questions to engage in this process. Our hope is that these questions create space for new questions to emerge and continue the evolution of third-order thinking and equitable practice.

Reflexive Questions

- What happens when ethical and practice standards are created in one culture and country and imported to another culture and country, especially those that have a history of colonization?
- What challenges do we face or overlook when we assume that clinical models made for the dominant group of a particular society will be appropriate for members of non-dominant groups?
- What are the intentions and ethics involved in decolonizing practices that support just relationships?
- How do we honor all perspectives and demonstrate cultural relevance and respect, while challenging oppression?
- In what ways are we accountable to recognize and support resistance to oppression?
- In what ways do we corroborate with oppressive forces when we fail to use our power to name and interrupt what is unjust? What are the costs?
- What relational values do you want your work to support? In what ways do they align or interrupt the dominant discourses in your cultural context?
- What does it mean to do international family therapy within and across borders in ways that expands possibilities for more equitable and just relationships and societies?

References

Bava, S. (2023). A relationally responsive world: The politics of collaborative dialogic Practices. In H. Anderson & D. Gehart (Eds). *Collaborative-dialogic practice: Generative relationships and conversations across contexts and cultures.* (pp. 37–53). Routledge.

Bermúdez, J. M., & Stinson, M. A. (2011). Redefining conflict resolution styles for Latino couples: Examining the role of gender and culture. *Journal of Feminist Family Therapy 23*(2), 1–87.

Bermudez, J. M., Muruthi, B., & Jordan, L. (equal authorship) (2016). Decolonizing Research Methods for Family Science: Creating space at the center. *Journal of Family Theory & Review, 8,* 192–206.

Bourdieu, P. (1986). The forms of capital. In J.G. Richardson (Ed.), *Handbook of theory and research for the sociology of education* (pp. 241–258). Greenwood Press.

Collins, P. H., & Bilge, S. (2016). *Intersectionality*. John Wiley & Sons.

Curtis, M. G., Ellis, E., Ann, S., Dai, Y., & Bermudez, J. M. (online, Dec. 2020). A Decade in Review: Intersectionality within family studies and family therapy journals from 2010–2020. *Journal of Family Theory & Review*. https://doi.org/10.1111/jftr.12399

D'Aniello, C., Nguyen, H. N., & Piercy, F. P. (2016). Cultural sensitivity as an MFT common factor. *American Journal of Family Therapy, 44*(5), 234–244.

Dannefer, D. (2003). Cumulative advantage/disadvantage and the life course: Cross-fertilizing age and social science theory. *The Journals of Gerontology Series B: Psychological Sciences and Social Sciences, 58*(6), S327-S337.

DiPrete, T. A., & Eirich, G. M. (2006). Cumulative advantage as a mechanism for inequality: A review of theoretical and empirical developments. *Annual Review of Sociology, 32*, 271–297.

Falicov, C. J. (2014). Psychotherapy and supervision as cultural encounters: The multidimensional ecological comparative approach framework. In C. A. Falender, E. P. Shafranske, & C. J. Falicov (Eds.). *Multiculturalism and diversity in clinical supervision* (pp. 29–58). American Psychological Association.

Fricker, M. (2007). Epistemic injustice: Power and the ethics of knowing. Oxford University Press.

Harding, S. (2008). Sciences from below: Feminisms, postcolonialities, and modernities. Duke University Press.

Harding, S. G. (1998). Is science multicultural? Postcolonialisms, feminisms, and epistemologies. Indiana University Press.

Hofstede, G. (2001). *Culture's consequences*. Sage

Jaimes-Guerrero, M. A. (2003). Patriarchal colonialism and indigenism: Implications for native feminist spirituality and native womanism. *Hypatia, 18*, 58–69.

Jordan, L. S., Seponski, D. M., Hall, J. N., & Bermudez, J. M. (2021 online). "Hopefully you've landed the Waka on the shore": Negotiated spaces in Aotearoa/New Zealand's bicultural mental health system. *Transcultural Psychiatry*. https://doi.org/10.1177%2F13634615211014347

Keating, M. F. (2012). Global best practices, national innovation systems, and tertiary education: A critique of the World Bank's accelerating catch-up (2009). *International Journal of Public Policy, 8*(4–6), 251–265

Kimmel, M. (2016). *The gendered society* (6th ed.). Oxford University Press.

Knudson-Martin, C. (2013). Why power matters: Creating a foundation of mutual support in couple relationships. *Family Process, 52*, 5–18.

Knudson-Martin, C., & Kim, L. (2023). Socioculturally attuned couple therapy. In J. L. Lebow and D. K. Snyder (Eds.), *Clinical handbook of couple therapy*, (6th ed., pp. 267–297). Guilford.

Knudson-Martin, C., McDowell, T., & Bermudez, J. M. (2019). From knowing to doing: Guidelines for socioculturally attuned family therapy. *Journal of Marital and Family Therapy, 45*(1), 47–60.

Knudson-Martin, C., McDowell, T., & Bermudez, M. (2020). Sociocultural attunement in systemic family therapy. In K. Wampler & R. Miller (Eds.). *Handbook of Systemic Therapies, Vol 1*. p. 619–637. Wiley.

Kosutic, I., & McDowell, T. (2008). Diversity and social justice issues in family therapy literature: A decade review. *Journal of Feminist Family Therapy, 20*, 142–165.

Laenui, P. (2006). Processes of decolonization. www.sjsu.edu/people/marcos.pizarro/maestros/Laenui.pdf

Lareau, A. (2011). *Unequal childhoods: Class, race, and family life*. University of California Press.

Lorde, A. (2007). Sister outsider: Essays & speeches by Audre Lorde. Crossing Press.

McDowell, T. Knudson-Martin, C., & Bermudez, J. M. (in press). Socioculturally Attuned Ethical Practice in Family Therapy. In AAMFT Ethics.

McDowell, T. Knudson-Martin, C., & Bermudez, J. M. (in press). Socioculturally Attuned Family Therapy. In J. L. Lebow, A. L. Chambers, and D. C. Breunlin (Eds.) *Encyclopedia of Couple and Family Therapy*. New York: Springer. https://doiorg/10.1007/978-3-319-49425-8_1093

McDowell, T., & Hernández, P. (2010). Decolonizing Academia: Intersectionality, Participation, and Accountability in Family Therapy and Counseling. *Journal of Feminist Family Therapy, 22*, 111–93.

McDowell, T., Knudson-Martin, C, & Bermudez, J. M. (2019). Third order thinking in family therapy: Addressing social justice across family therapy practice. *Family Process, 58*(1), 9–22.

McGoldrick, M., & Hardy, K. V. (3rd. Ed.) (Eds.). (2019). *Re-visioning family therapy.* Guilford Publications.

McNeill, T. (2010). Family as a social determinant of health: Implications for governments and institutions to promote the health and well-being of families. *Healthcare Quarterly, 14,* 60–67.

Moghadam, S., & Knudson-Martin, C. (2009). Keeping the peace: Couple relationships in Iran. In C. Knudson-Martin & A. Mahoney (Eds.,), *Couples, gender, and power: Creating change in intimate relationships* (pp. 255–274). Springer Publishing Co.

Murray, S. J., Holmes, D., Perron, A., & Rail, G. (2007). No exit? Intellectual integrity under the regime of "evidence" and "best-practices." *Journal of evaluation in clinical practice, 13*(4), 512–516.

Nowak, A. W. (2013). Ontological imagination: Transcending methodological solipsism and the promise of interdisciplinary studies. *AVANT. The Journal of the Philosophical-Interdisciplinary Vanguard, IV*(2), 169–193.

Petr, C. G., & Walter, U. M. (2005). Best practices inquiry: A multi-dimensional value-critcal framework. *Journal of Social Work Education, 41*(2), 251–267.

Seponski, D. M., Lewis, D., Bermudez, J. M., & Sotelo, J. M. (2020). Cambodian therapists' perspectives of Western-based psychotherapy models: Addressing the challenges for service providers. *Journal of Family Psychotherapy, 31*(1–2), 36–55.

Smith, D. E. (1993). The Standard North American Family: SNAF as an Ideological Code. *Journal of Family Issues.* 14(1), 50–65.

Tatum, Beverly Daniel. (1997). *"Why are all the Black kids sitting together in the cafeteria?" and other conversations about race.* New York: Basic Books.

Tourse, R., Hamilton-Mason, J., & Wewiorski, N. (2018). Systemic Racism in America: Scaffolding as Social Construction. Springer Publisher.

Tuttle, A., Kim, L., & Knudson-Martin, C. (2012). Parenting as relationship: A framework for assessment and practice. *Family Process, 51,* 73–89

Zrenchik, K. & McDowell, T. (2012) Class and Classism in Family Therapy Praxis: A Feminist, Neo-Marxist Approach, *Journal of Feminist Family Therapy, 24*(2) 101–120.

8

SOCIO-RELATIONALLY RESPONSIVE SUPERVISION FOR INCLUSIVE LEARNING

A Discursive Anti-Dominance Perspective

Saliha Bava

Introduction

In the closing episode of the third season of a popular US science fiction dystopian HBO series Westworld, Delores, our robotic protagonist, explains to, Caleb, a human she deeply cares for, that long before the privacy laws of 2039 kicked in there were data companies that tracked each of their lives, collecting data and in this process making profiles about how people would act and what directions their life would go, ultimately programming them into that existence [Spoiler alert].

Previously, in Caleb's story, we see him talking to his army pal, Francis, who keeps checking in on Caleb, reminding him to keep progressing and to keep his eye on the ball. Initially, we are left wondering what Francis's story is. As the story continues, we learn that Francis died on the battlefield and is now a programmed voice, part of Caleb's computerized programmed psychological treatment. The treatment both keeps him alive while also conditioning him to be a candidate for suicide. Unaware that he is programmed into this contradiction, Caleb stays hopeful until Delores reveals his contradictory storylines. This prompts him onto an alternate path, ultimately confronting the rigid control-based structure that programmed him into these contradictions.

As the camera pans out, we see the two characters—Caleb and Delores—leaning against the pier's railing gazing into the turbulent yet beautiful waters of the ocean. A metaphor no doubt.

I'm drawn into the implications of what the series Westworld is offering us for today's world. It sheds light on identity, human–nonhuman interactions, and how we are being profiled and programmed by social media even as we deny its capacity to shape our self-concept (Englemenn et al., 2022). A commentary on a neoliberal world (Bhatia & Priya, 2018; Sugarman, 2015) driven by greed-based capitalist politics, where our fluid, emergent, and plural identities are reduced to zeros and ones to profile us and simultaneously feed us insecurities and remedies as part of the global psy-complex that shapes well-being and treatments (Hardy & Ness, 2015; Sullum, 2020). It is within such a context that our

DOI: 10.4324/9781003297871-10

process of supervision becomes a rudder that steers us either into becoming gatekeepers for the psy-complex or responsive radicals who ride the wave, or better still, become the emergent swells of responsiveness and change.

As is explored in this chapter, Westworld reveals that the choice of how we engage in relationships and conversations is a political one. The politics of us acting back in response to our social world, as it acts on us, presents itself every day in our supervision, inviting us to step up with our responsiveness. How, in our everyday supervision interactions, are we creating the world around us? As there is no escaping politics, how might we politically engage in supervision instead of maintaining the illusion that we remain apolitical?

In this chapter, I illustrate how our training conversations are sites of knowledge construction that are identity- and world-making. How might we create conditions for learning *with* people-in-training to reflect on the political nature of dialogic practice? Adopting a socio-relational pedagogical perspective drawn from collaborative-dialogic practice (Anderson, 2007b, 2012), I illustrate how to engage with people-in-training to think and act critically from both an anti-oppression *and* discursive perspectives. By unpacking the frame of participation, I offer how I position myself to engage the critical, creative voices of emerging therapists in orienting to the politics of socio-relationality within the emerging context. I locate teaching and learning, and thereby supervision, within the interplay of the interactional and social discourses. I offer the *Relational ADEI* and the *Relational Discursive Loop* as conversational resources for a polyphonic anti-dominance orientation in supervision talk. I illustrate this as a socio-relationally responsive orientation toward the current call for engaging racial and social justice within supervision across global contexts by interweaving reflexive examples.

A Political Call and the Activity of Knowledge Construction

The political nature of our lives is being delineated in ever starker terms by the pandemic, calls for anti-racism and anti-oppression, the media, and the increasing divisiveness as evidenced by the culture wars. There is increased contextual awareness. Calls are increasing to address social justice in therapeutic practices, calling for the decolonization of therapy (McDowell & Hernández, 2010; McDowell, 2015; polanco, 2022), socio-cultural attunement in therapy (Knudson-Martin, McDowell, & Bermudez, 2020), addressing structural racism (Kelly, Jérémie-Brink, Chambers, & Smith-Bynum, 2020) and racial trauma in therapy (Menakem, 2017). Systemically oriented therapy theorists are forerunners in this work. They contextualized therapy as an initial response to the call for social justice, which was foundational for the field's evolution. The pursuit of social justice in the form of emphasis on social and larger systems (Imber-Black, 1992), working with marginalized families (Minuchin, Colapinto, & Minuchin, 2007), contextual awareness, power dynamics (Hare-Mustin, 1978), and unpacking our knowledge and language practices by the questioning our grand narratives and social discourses (Anderson & Goolishian, 1988) have shaped the evolution of couples and family therapy (Lebow, 2019, p. 3).

Despite our impressive evolution, reflecting our society's struggle, couple and family therapy (CFT) educators and trainers have "struggled with how to teach and implement what we call socioculturally attuned practice; a practice that is aware and responsive to the intersections of societal context, culture, and power in client experience and positioned to promote equity" (Knudson-Martin, McDowell, & Bermudez, 2019, p. 47). One could read this struggle as not reflective but constituted by the very nature of the social challenges we seek to address. The willingness to use dominance and hegemonic practices, to define who matters by defining what matters and how, lies at the heart of our social challenges, leaving our field of practice similarly impacted.

These matters of definition and whose voice matters are knowledge-making matters. And, as a field, we have failed to look at our knowledge-making practices as contributing to dominance-based structures within our practice. "Knowledge is socially constructed…all knowledge and knowing are embedded within history, context, culture, language, experience, and understanding" (Anderson, 2007a, p. 8). Supervision and training are interactional spaces where knowledge of systemic and relational expertise is the currency of practice. The supervisory space is not limited to knowledge transmission, rather, it is a space of critically engaging knowledge and knowing to co-create new understandings since knowing is a social process (Anderson, 2007a, 2012). More importantly, supervision is a space for a "third kind of knowledge"—one that arises "from within a social situation, a group, an institution, or a society, and which exists only in that situation. We might call it a 'knowing-from-within'" (Shotter, 2010, p. 26). Thus, *how might we engage in the practice of knowing-from-within the training and educational relationship and context to honor its sociality?*

Dominance seeks hegemony, a reliance on a singular top-down voice, rather than a polyphony that contextually generates diversity and belonging in the construction of knowledge, system creation and evolution, empowering the diversity that is reflected in families, organizations, and society. In supervision a polyphonic approach also requires an orientation to the marginalization of voices due to the historical, social-cultural, and local institutional contexts in order to fully embrace an anti-dominance stance. So, how might we create conditions for learning where people engage in the entanglements of what matters and how? How might we decolonize training practices when inherent in the training and supervisory relationships is a built-in hierarchy? Not all hierarchy has to be dominance-based, but hierarchy lends itself to dominance when we fail to foreground reflexive process-oriented conversations that foster and engage equity and inclusion. So, how might we do so? The answer lies in acknowledging the political nature of CFT or systemic therapy supervision. "Political is *what people do together*" (Bava, 2022, p. 37).

Supervisory (Relational) Interactions: Sites of Meaning Making

I teach at Mercy College in the marriage and family therapy program that is located in the New York City metropolitan area, a microcosm of the global context. Our students are ethnically, culturally, and linguistically diverse, representing traditions from Argentina, Bangladesh, Caribbean Islands, China, Columbia, Dominican Republic, India, Ireland, Italy, Jordon, Mexico, Russia, South Korea, Sudan, Ukraine, U.K, U.S., etc. This rich international context offers a diversity of nationalities and immigration statuses that intersect with race, ethnicity, gender, sexual orientation, class, etc. In a number of these countries, racism takes the form of colorism and structural inequities, making it both visible and invisible depending on one's gaze. We have students who identify as cis and genderqueer (Gender and gender identity at a glance, n.d.; Stockton, 2021) of varying sexual orientations. A majority of our students are first-generation college and graduate students. Given this diverse mix of social identities, our supervisory conversations afford us a rich training array of politics, positionalities, and intersectionality that shapes and is shaped by our trainees' participation. Our supervisory conversations are relational interactions that become sites of meaning and understanding as we learn from each other. Often, we have to go slow to unpack the nuances that might otherwise be lost or rushed by the time barrier of our meetings.

Some conversations have ease, while others are experienced as difficult. Difficult conversations feel risky, can make us uncomfortable or confused, and can create tension, anger, silence, or the sensation of being silenced. Difficult conversations can also feel unfamiliar; even though the topic of conversation is part of one's lived experiences, the conversation itself is not part of one's professional or educational context, thus leaving us uncertain about how might we speak and engage. Such self-reflective difficult conversations often are those about race, class, sexuality, shame, our family of origin or culture, etc. Difficult conversations might evoke an emotional response from us that we might view as negative or avoid feeling vulnerable in a public space. Such conversations can be focused on our work product, our styles of engaging, professionalism, or how others are engaging us, etc., all carrying identity-shaping potentials. These identity-informing conversations can also be about differences in perspectives underpinned by the power differentials in our society based on gender, race, religion, politics, money, ability, etc. These power differentials are very much present in our classrooms (Curtis-Boles, Chupina, & Okubo, 2020) and organize all conversations, including supervision. How we lean into such difficult conversations is an action that can either constrict or open the space for feeling seen and heard. So, how might we host everyday conversations within the training context, where people feel seen and heard, especially within the conversations that shape our identities?

Relational ADEI

Hosting conversations where people feel seen and heard is about dignity and equity. While the diversity of voices is inherently present in the makeup of our student body (at Mercy), equity refers to *how* one is included (Hardy, 2016). I offer the Relational Anti-Racist/ oppression, Diversity, Equity, and Inclusion (ADEI) Buckets as an anti-dominance process guide for engagement within any dialogic context as described below. Each of the three buckets are in relationship to other (see Figure 8.1), informing and being informed by the other two buckets and contextually shaping our supervisory and teaching/learning interactions.

1. **Diversity and Plurality of Views/Voices:** *How do we honor and dignify?* There are many knowledge-making perspectives and practices from the voices of dominant discourses to global majority voices, from Global South to Global North voices, what might be called the multiverse. Acknowledging that there are many ways of knowing, being, and doing is at the heart of plurality. At times these might conflict with one another, within communities, organizations, and families. Even within the same person, there may be divergent viewpoints; for instance, several of my trainees reflect on their uncertainty with how to relate psychological ideas to their Spiritism belief where the dead communicate with the living. It is in connecting and understanding each other and these divergent voices we avoid being divided and polarized. The Public Conversations project (called Essential Partners today) founded in 1989 by family therapists is an excellent example of this work in communities (Gergen, 2009; History, 2022).

2. **Anti-racist, Anti-oppression Stance:** *How do we orient?* Honoring our differences without acknowledging the differentials is harm-inducing and maintains our social-structural

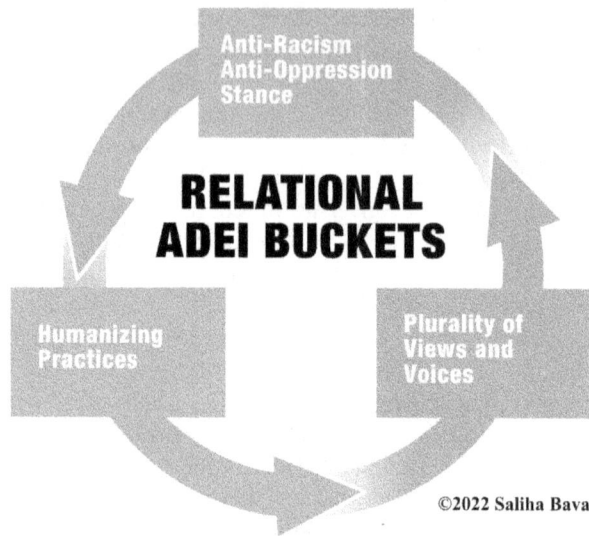

Figure 8.1   Relational ADEI buckets.

arrangements as a natural order of things. The differential refers to how we are socially organized, by the collective circulation and location of power (Reed, 2013). Simultaneously, invisiblizing the power of resistance, liberation, and collaboration—what we do collectively—in the way power and power analysis is constructed (Bava, 2022; Escobar, 1991). In this way, power differentials are maintained while furthering dominance-based social and structural systems that block marginalized groups of people from realizing their potential by creating avenues of potential for privileged groups of people serving as the norm. For instance, privileging the Global North as power centers compared to Global South, norming whiteness as pure or epitomizing it as beauty, gender norming leadership on male dominance, heteronormativity of sexual attraction or making of families, and so on. These systems of dominance get institutionalized and create insidious social and relational dynamics that impact peoples, communities, and organizations, creating dehumanizing conditions. Dominance-based systems aim to be hegemonic and divisive to create an us-against-them system built on a scarcity mindset. The goal is to favor one group's way of being as superior to another, creating a system of elitism rather than egalitarianism. An anti-oppression stance aims at egalitarianism with a shared-resource mindset. It seeks to make visible the dynamics of oppression and resistance while organizing a culture of equity that builds on our sensibility of inter-connectedness and interdependencies between all humans and non-humans (our pets, environment, AI, or for that matter Caleb and Delores). Rather than put any one group down to create a sense of security, well-being or specialness, we organize to lift everyone ensuring access and processes to bring all to the circle. The valuing of connectedness and interdependencies is core to systemic, relational therapy making an anti-racist, anti-oppression stance a logical progression of our evolving field.

3. **Humanizing Practices:** *How do we engage?* Connecting, collaborating and co-creating (Anderson, 2007b, p. 54) are the processes by which we not only undo dehumanization but also transform and grow systems that dignify people and create a sense of belonging.

These relational processes (Anderson, 2012; Bava, 2022; Gergen, 2009; McNamee, 2008) include orienting towards relationality, inclusion, and sustainability. We orient to people and their stories rather than the social labels that typify them. Labels are limiters. Instead, by participating *with* others, drawing on an abundance mindset, we engage in curiosity, dialogue, collaboration, reflexivity, witnessing, systemic thinking, awe, play, circle practices, and many other relationality-oriented practices to enhance a sense of belonging and possibilities.

"Dialogue is a responsive situated activity" (McNamee, 2008, p. 9). And, these ADEI buckets offer us the frames by which to engage in such a situated activity. We reflexively engage our language and interactions to create understanding, thereby constructing meanings and stories, setting the context for inclusive responsiveness and what arrives next. The meaning of that which arrives and that which will arrive next is shaped and shapes our conversations and relationships (Anderson, 2007b). What we attend to within this organic flow is situated (McNamee, 2008) and is a "spontaneous responsive, living bodily inter-activity" (Shotter, 2003, p. 436) rather than an intellectual activity. What we notice and act on as spontaneous bodily responses have been shaped and often grown from within the frames we have cultivated over time via our relational coordinations (Gergen, 2009; McNamee, 2008). Thus, giving our spontaneous embodied responsiveness its situated texture.

How might we perform our supervisory interactions to be relationally ethical within the moment of an interaction while also being responsive to how the larger socio-cultural context is invoked and constructed from within our interactions (Bava & McNamee, 2019)? How are we shaping this world even as it shapes our everyday encounters? For me, the answer lies in one's reflexive relational responsiveness (Shotter, 2004).

Reflexive Relational Responsivity

Relational responsiveness is a way of orienting to the process of making meaning **together**, locally in our utterances and interactions. *Reflexivity* refers to the situated and constitutive nature of such responsivity. As per McNamee (2008), such responsiveness is situated or contextualized by our histories, social, cultural, relational, and local expectations and repertoires. Relational responsiveness is a way of engaging what is between people and not as something that belongs or is limited to one person's action. Rather than focus on the individual actors we focus on the relational coordination (Anderson, 2012; Gergen, 2009; McNamee, 2008). For instance, within a teaching and learning context, when we view a student's participation as a relationally responsive (interwoven) activity, it shifts our frame from "is the student participating or not" to "*how are we relating with each other*?" How are we listening, understanding, and responding to each other's frames and positionalities? How do we engage in mutual inquiry to construct our meanings? How do we engage together to move the conversation forward? These questions are not limited to teaching and learning, they apply to any context where two people are in conversation.

These questions of reflexivity are an invitation to attend to the discursive process that is co-created by the participants. Discursive refers to the social actions rising from within the daily interactions, talk, or text (Tseliou & Borcsa, 2018), consequentially constructing and constructed from within our materialized lives and realities. *The discursive process is one that is an interplay of language, interaction, and meaning-making, which continues to emerge and get reshaped as the conversation flows. To understand and engage this discursive process as a situated activity, I offer the relational discursive loop as a conversational guide* in the following section.

Drawing on John Shotter (2003, 2004), communicative action theorist and philosopher of living moments, I view participation as a relationally responsive activity; the intertwining of our spontaneous responsiveness with each other. Shotter states that participation occurs only in the intertwining of people's spontaneous responses to each other and to their surroundings, it cannot be explained by giving any person's reasons or justifications for his or her individual actions. What is produced in such responsively interwoven, dialogically structured activity is a strange third realm of always ongoing and always unfinished activity of its own unique kind (2003, pp. 456–457).

Thus, for Shotter engagement between people is not something that belongs or is located within one person's action. Participation is crafted from within our engagements rather than it being located in any one person, a.k.a. therapist-in-training. Thus, it raises the question: how are we speaking, listening, hearing, and understanding each other's frames and positionalities even as we engage to move the conversation forward? The answer lies in the discursive flow that is co-created by the participants. Within this flow, there is a constant interplay between our social discourses and somatic selves, which invokes our positionality. Positionality is not devoid of our social and relational processes (Bava, 2020; Davies and Harré, 1990; Shotter, 1993). To teach and learn this complex interplay is a creative challenge since it is the water we are always swimming in that which we seek to gaze upon. Thus, to facilitate this understanding, I created the relational discursive loop as a conversational guide.

Relational Discursive Loop

In conversations, daily utterances, and interactions, we create our relationships, social stories, and the world around us. Anderson and Goolishian (1988) in their classic paper, *Human Systems as Linguistic Systems* state, "meaning and social systems are created in and through dialogue" (p. 375). Drawing on the communicative action perspective, they draw our attention to the dynamic, constructive nature of communication by which structural and systemic processes come into being and get reified.

As I pondered how to create a context for learners to notice the interplay of their embodied sense, utterances, frames of meaning, and the social, I arrived at the illustration of this discursive understanding (as shown in Figure 8.2). I illustrated the process of making our social systems and structures in and through dialogue, thereby drawing our attention to the recursive interplay of the structural and processual.

It is the constitutive power of communication that I sought to bring forth in my training. Communication's constitutive power affords us one of the resources by which we can respond to the call of action for just lives. In supervision conversations as I sketched this interplay, an early draft of the figure (Bava, 2019) arrived as an invitation for the trainees to notice where they were speaking or listening from as they engaged with each other.

Reflexive relational responsiveness, a political activity, positions us to see how our somatic experiences, utterances, and interactions are deeply intertwined discursive processes resulting in and resulting from the structural and systemic processes that in turn shape and are shaped by our storied realities (Figure 8.2).

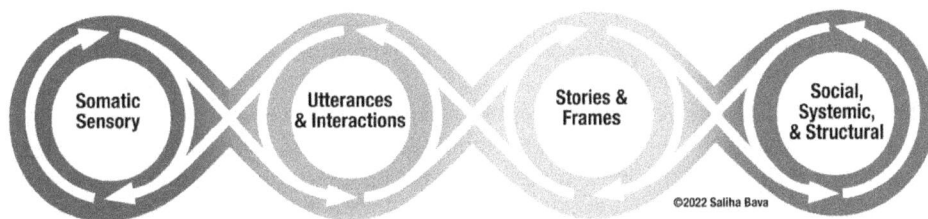

Figure 8.2 Relational Discursive Loop.

A. **Somatic Sensory:** Beginning at the physical level, our bodies somatically respond to how we interpret our everyday experiences. These somatic experiences in turn shape our words, actions, and interpretations.
B. **Interactional Utterances:** At the interactional level, utterances and exchanges are the ingredients for making meaning with others. Our words and inter-actions simultaneously shape and are shaped by our understandings. Words, gestures, and utterances, while giving meaning to somatic experiences, are understood/interpreted from within social and relational frames of meanings that we draw upon to negotiate and coordinate within the relational moment. We calibrate to each other's expression as we speak by spontaneously making micro-adjustments with our words and gestures to coordinate and create shared meanings. There is a tremendous amount of play here.
C. **Stories/Frames:** The frames and stories are interpretations that occur *in relationship*. Our interpretations and meanings emerge from within the relationally, socially, culturally, and historically situated narratives that become the invisible frames for sense-making. In relationships, we negotiate and navigate these situated meanings thus creating local shared meanings.
D. **Social, Systemic, Structural:** From within the engaged dialogic process, the social, systemic, and structural dynamics emerge and become sedimented. Thus, over time they both influence and are influenced by our frames, stories, and meanings. For instance, the making of a constitutional process emerges from the founders' engaged dialogue. And, over time, the interpretation of the written constitution continues to shape and get amended.

I seek to visualize this invisible interlinked discursive process as a double infinity loop affording us a resource for engaging and tracking conversations. The Relational Discursive Loop represents the water we swim in, influencing us even as we collectively influence our worlds. Thus, how might we position ourselves if we came to understand our supervision conversations (and organizations, families, social systems, structures, and discourses) as emergent byproducts of our utterances and interactions? How might we understand our tensions when we view the current relational moment as a discursive interplay of the present relational context and the social, cultural, and historical contexts?

The two "ends" of the double infinity loop—the somatic and the social—are two resources that are present with us, but often ignored when we engage with each other. While the social is always present in our stories and frames of meanings, the somatic is a felt embodied experience. And, though the somatic and social are navigated and mediated by our utterances and interactions, they are also access points by which to enter into a conversation that is engaged and situated. The meaning of all of these experiences is created and sustained through dialogic interactions. Any conversation can be mapped to one, two, three, or all of the four spaces.

The Relational Discursive Loop is one way to visualize the complex process of communicative action and is as such applicable to supervision conversations. The Loop along with the Relational ADEI buckets offers supervisors and supervisees reflexive resources to stay present and curious about our ways of knowing, including knowing-from-within, thereby transforming supervision as a site of meaning-making by engaging in meaningful identity-forming conversations. So, how might we use these conversational resources? The ways to use them are only limited by our imagination. I offer two possibilities in how I use them in my practicum course when CFT therapists-in-training are at their internship sites seeing clients.

Socio-Relationally Responsive Supervision in Practice

I offer a couple of ways to be responsive to our larger social context from within our relational moments within the supervisory context. Noticing how the social is connected to the relational and how from within the relational interactions, we shape the social is the goal of these offerings. There are many ways to operationalize and materialize these ideas in practice. Since improvisation and spontaneous responsiveness is key to humanizing, what I describe below will have additional moving parts depending on the context and the interactional moment. These offerings are not meant to be prescriptive but offered as food for thought with the invitation to adapt, build, and make anew what is offered here.

Locating Self: A Reflective Exercise and Presentation

At the start of the internship, in the practicum course, our therapists-in-training begin by reading about four interrelated concepts regarding the construction of our social identities: social location, intersectionality, positionality, and hyperlinked identities.

Social Location: This is the way social and political contexts position our identities based on group identification. These group identities are socially categorized and organized based on power differentials creating a hierarchical system with those on the top valued more than those on the lower rungs. The material impacts of such a socially organized system are evidenced by the research on the social determinants of health (World Health Organization, n.d.).

Intersectionality: Legal scholar and Black feminist Kimberle Crenshaw (1989; 1991) coined the term intersectionality to challenge single-issue analysis. She challenges single identity categorizations and invites us to notice and engage in the unpacking of the confluence of multiple social influences that define our identities such as gender, race, class, ability, sexual orientation, etc. She calls us to notice the various ways these identity threads intersect to shape our lives politically and structurally "because the intersectional experience is greater than the sum of" any two threads that any analysis does not take up intersectionally (Crenshaw, 1989, p. 140).

Positionality: This is the way we uniquely perform ourselves based on our lived experiences as we navigate and negotiate our intersectional social identities in everyday interactions within a social and relational context. In language and interaction, our positionality is invoked and performed.

Hyperlinked Identities and Conversations: Hyperlinking refers to the unique ways we surf the web in search of an understanding of a term. Similarly, we weave conversations and identities as we negotiate meanings, seeking a coordinated, coherent understanding in the process of interacting with each other. The metaphor of hyperlinking offers a way to attend to the intersection of our intertextual, flexible, emergent, and plural identities as we engage in such identity-shaping conversations (Bava, 2019).

Drawing on these concepts and more, trainees are required to do a presentation titled "Locating Yourself." It is a reflective exercise on their social location that leads to a class presentation. I introduce the exercise with the following words:

> Oppression is a big concept, and it acts on people in many ways, especially by dehumanizing us. It is also enacted in many ways in everyday interactions and daily conversations. It is related to mental health. It affects not only how we feel about ourselves (personal/micro), but also how we relate with each other (interpersonal/meso) and how society gets organized and the institutions that govern our lives (social/macro). To humanize is an anti-racist, anti-dominance practice. Socio-cultural, relational- and emotional attunements are ways to humanize that which is distancing and splitting.
>
> (Bava, 2021, p. 1)

The purpose of the exercise is to unpack the concept of social identities and learn how it is organized from within their own life while understanding to not stereotype clients based on it (Knudson-Martin, McDowell, & Bermudez, 2020). Clinically, to develop a contextual curiosity of how the socio-political context mediated by the person's relational context organizes the person as understood from the person's perspective. A hard task to do without making interpretations from within the conversations. Thus, noticing our process of making interpretations while understanding each other's stories is a pathway to notice our biases. The exercise is designed to invite each student to self-reflect on their lives by drawing upon their cultural, familial, and temporal narratives, thus locating themselves contextually.

As the course proceeds, students prepare their presentations on how they are socio-relationally and temporally located. Based on their ethnicity, the learners do a critical reading of a chapter from the book *Ethnicity and Family Therapy* (McGoldrick, Giordano, & Garcia-Preto, 2005) reflecting on what fits or doesn't fit in the chapter(s) based on their reading and lived experiences. Thus, inviting them to reflect on ethnicity while going beyond an ethnicity-based understanding to an intersectional understanding of socio-cultural-political processes. Additionally, they construct their cultural genogram (Hardy & Laszloffy, 1995). In addition to the questions offered by Hardy and Laszloffy, I ask them to reflect on what their group identity affords them or not, that is, the ways in which it opens and closes doors in the world for them. I invite them to identify one or two themes of shame and pride for their 20–25-minute presentation, which is followed by a 20-minute discussion.

On the day of the presentation, I invite us to notice how our "understanding is relational and dialogic" (Anderson, 2007a, p. 14). To notice how we participate and engage in conversations, setting the stage for us to self-reflect on our process of relating—listening, hearing, speaking, and understanding (Anderson, 2012). Drawing on Anderson, I emphasize that they all go hand-in-hand. I invite them to notice their positionality and relational intersectionality (Addison & Coolhart, 2015) as they interact. Drawing on the Relational

Discursive Loop, I may say, "notice how your language might be evoking a frame or a story. Be curious about your own story as you are curious about the presenter's story." I ask, "What social and/or familial frames are being evoked by such stories" drawing their attention to the right two loops—stories/frames and social/systemic/structural. This allows us to reflect on what each of us offers (me included,) to invite questions of curiosity, and to notice our interactions and exchanges rather than keeping the focus solely on the presenter. This fosters a reflexive relational responsiveness in the form of curious questions to learn more, statements of appreciation for the presenters' vulnerabilities, and style of presentation, including the way they weave their family and cultural stories to shed light on their positionality as a therapist.

At other times, there are comments of support and giving of advice as presenters talk about their vulnerability, loss, and/or painful stories. With permission, I engage the responders to inquire where they are speaking from or what compels them to give advice to the presenter, inviting them to notice the relational intersectionality and/or the meaning they are making. For instance,

> Jay (in a reassuring tone to Eli, who had just presented): One day, your family will accept you.
> Me (to Jay): That is a beautiful offering. If I may, I'm curious, where are you drawing your hope from?
> Jay: I'm realizing I have a lot in common with Eli's family story. So, in offering comfort to Eli, I'm expressing my hope for what I might receive from my family.

The conversation shifts from the presenter to the responders, spontaneously interweaving multiple voices and creating learning conditions that invite us all into reflection. In the above example, we reflected on the performance of acceptance, how it is showed or not, our feelings about our family's acceptance or not, cultural differences in the performance of acceptance, and its relationship to love. As conversations go, we discursively unpacked meaning, language, and our curiosity about our interactions with each other. For instance, I inquired of Jay how they felt about me asking about their offering to Eli.

As the supervisor instructor, I see myself as the host of the conversation. I ground myself in the Relational ADEI buckets by tracking for the plurality of voices, actively adopting an anti-oppression stance by being curious about the social contexts based on how the conversation turns as a way to humanize what might be made invisible within our conversations.

And driven by time, I'll draw the conversation to a pause acknowledging the unfinished nature of our conversation and the arbitrary pause produced by time. In closing, by drawing upon the Relational Discursive Loop, I invite us to collectively notice the conversational threads and how we shifted back and forth from our felt experiences (sensations) to the interactions to the frames and social stories we evoked. Thus, inviting them back to notice the entanglements of how or where we are speaking from, with what intent, and what was being created by our conversations.

Reflections on (Not) Norming of Identity and Practices

One of the challenges of holding and opening space for divergent views is the relational intersectionality among the learners and between the learners and faculty. This impacts what we collectively create as the classroom culture. As the facilitator, the supervisor instructor is responsible for creating conditions for learning while tending to the classroom culture. My intent is to create a context for humanizing conversations and interactions while creating space for a plurality of voices by adopting the anti-oppression stance (the Relational ADEI touchstones). In this way, I remain mindful of the local interactive moment while verbalizing (or inquiring) how we are invoking the social scripts and dynamics from within our interactions. How might we do this, given the intersectional flow of conversations and identities? Are we disrupting the dominant discourses? Or are we reproducing them? How might we be curious about what's emerging? How do we hold space for plurality while also noticing which discourses drive the supervisory conversations? And who decides how to name the discourse? Is it the supervisor? Or do we invite the learners to name the multiplicity of discourses present? These questions are touchstones and offer us an organizing compass in the midst of the complexity of everyday supervisory conversations.

I aim for us to notice the plurality of the interweaving discourses while acknowledging that my role as a teacher has an impact on how my words and ideas are received in comparison to the others in the room. Even the telling of this story is from my point of view. We cannot escape the privileged position I participate, speak, and write from when positioned as a supervisor instructor. While acknowledging my other voices I bring into the mix, I'm first received as an instructor, an expert, and as an evaluator (who grades their assignments). To reduce the hierarchy of my role, I attend to my stance and presence by being conversational rather than instructive. Also, I set up the room as a semi-circle for our meeting and sit among the students as they present. I acknowledge the institutional power granted to me in the position of instructor and open it up for conversation.

Additionally, I offer multiple invitations to work together to co-design our space in terms of our agenda, how to organize our time together, what the students would like to prioritize, etc., to reduce the level of hierarchy in the room. I'm also aware that I enter with my other intersecting social locations as a cis-gendered, able-bodied, immigrant Indian woman with a number of invisible, but organizing, identities such as religion, health, age, etc. While, at one level, there is no separating of the intertwined voices, at another level, I'm reflexively present to the multiple voices that speak through me (Bakhtin, 1981). According to Bakhtin, this joining and disjoining of different voices within a spoken moment or text is known as heteroglossia. Thus, I seek to invite all to reflexively notice ourselves as intertextual beings in how we weave our intersectional stories and relational intersectionalities.

As we seek to understand concepts of social location, intersectionality, positionality, etc., students sometimes report feeling overwhelmed and confused. Also, "in dialogue, we are steeped in uncertainty, incompleteness, and multiplicity" (McNamee, 2008, p. 9). Thus, I acknowledge the complexity of such conversations by stating, "this is a challenging conversation with many tangled threads, so let's continue to make meaning together! Let's ask questions, make sense, and be lost, confused, delighted, mad, sad, hopeful, and/or curious...all voices are welcome!" I continue to invite creativity and ask them to present their stories in ways that reflect their uniqueness. It takes a few conversational turns to shift from approaching the "Locating Self" exercise as a traditional assignment to seeing it as food for thought. I frame their presentations as creative offerings by which we will be exploring these concepts through our lived experiences. For instance, exploring how our social locations are not labels or demographics but are our lived stories (Bava, 2019).

And while doing so, I also invite them to notice how our social scripts *perform us*. I refer to social script as norms. "How are we being normed? How are we being organized?" In the box below, I offer an example of an email I might send out to the students inviting them to notice how our identities and practices are both interconnected and shaped by the larger social stories. It is in these ongoing, interwoven dialogues that we grow our capacity to notice how the parts of the Relational Discursive Loop show up, inform, and impact our norms and stories.

As we reflect on all the wonderful presentations on locating ourselves. I want to invite us all to reflect on *how social norms perform us*, especially if we belong to a group whose ways of being and moving through the world are considered the norm. How do these norms organize us?

A norm is never having to ask ourselves, "how else should it be?" because the water we swim in is so familiar that it is comfortable. Or the water flows in our favor. At times, we don't ask these questions because we have been socialized to not notice "the thing" as a norm or if we do notice, schooled into not questioning it but living with the tension or discomfort of it.

But the water we swim in is our environment and it shapes not only what we do or don't, how we show up or don't but also our sense of well-being. And our well-being (or lack of) can show up as health issues—physical, mental, relational, behavioral, and emotional health.

What is Saliha talking about?

Let's take a look at this 13-min video where a leading voice in Narrative Therapy, David Nylan, reflects on a day from his life: www.youtube.com/watch?v=HD6ojWB05Gg as a way to reflect on norming.

And, more as we continue to reflect and share our stories to make sense of how to position ourselves as therapist.

While on this topic of norming, check out the attached article (Lannamann & McNamee, 2020) that invites us to *reflect on how trauma norming happens within our field.*

One takeaway is norming is not limited to our personal identities, it also shapes how we practice ideas from within our professions; how we move through the world. *Norming informs all forms of practice and thus the performance of our "roles"*—as therapists, teachers, interns, clients, partners, humans, etc.

Most presentations are very moving and inspirational as they talk about their family stories and stories of shame and pride. I have been honored to see interpersonal tension shift as students get to glance behind the curtain of each other's lives, creating community, support, and admiration for each other while critically orienting to the other's context, which helped co-create our collective learning context. The dialogue continues with the presenters sharing a written reflection after the presentation.

Implications for Therapist Training: Takeaways

Research shows how creating a collaborative way of talking with others depends on the participants´ skillfulness to attend and react to the most minute of details. When people are in conversation the (sic) do not passively register messages, rather they are responsive; they react to the content, the packaging and timing of such utterances.

(Martínez, 2014, p. 98)

Martinez (2014) drawing on his research echoes Shotter's notion that responsiveness to the other's utterances allows for a collaborative way of talking. He speaks to the participants' skillfulness and attention to details as key for collaborative participation. By creating a learning condition where participants reflect on their social location and engage each other with curiosity while enhancing their reflexivity of where they are speaking from, people become increasingly responsive. They become their stories, and the stories become them, propelling them further into becoming and curiosity. Pires and Sobral (2013), drawing on Bakhtin, remind us "we are always changing according to the relationships we enter into." And, so it is with supervisory conversations, we engage in creating space for knowing-from-within our relationships and conversations even as we explore theoretical and skill-based knowledge.

The power of these self-reflective presentation-based conversations lies in what the therapists-in-training are sharing about what they are learning. I ask them, "Based on these presentations, readings, and discussions, what is your takeaway? What are the implications for our clinical work?" The student responses are categorized below:

1. **Engage with clients to seek understanding and make new meanings**
   - Understanding the client's identity by letting them express themselves and asking questions of curiosity
   - Get more curious about cultural values and how it ties into their own beliefs
   - Seeing the client as their stories and their values, and not as their labels
   - Dig deeper into family stories
   - Breaking the textbook barriers that describe client's ethnicity and instead learning about their culture in how clients tell their story
2. **Learn to engage complexity with curiosity**
   - Contextually unpacking their social location
   - How culture in the family is internalized
   - How it can become stories of shame and pride
   - Listening for what is missing
   - Listening for people's priority
   - Get comfortable asking uncomfortable questions
   - Don't be afraid to go there: "We didn't talk about X. Can I ask you about it?"
3. **Problematizing one's role as a therapist or helper**
   - It is more important for clients to understand the situation rather than for me to define it to them
   - Asking clients open-ended questions about the process, that is asking how questions rather than seeking explanations by asking why questions
   - Noticing how I'm asking questions
   - Being curious about where my questions are coming from
   - Becoming aware of my implicit biases by reflecting and self-reflexivity
   - Seeking to be self-compassionate

We make the path as we walk together. The power of socio-relationally responsive supervision lies in its experiential sensibility of how we co-create knowledge from within our interactions. It creates public reflection around how systems of dominance privilege some voices above others. By employing the Relational ADEI buckets and the Relational Discursive Loop, we invite the full range of personal, interactional, social, and systemic influences into the therapeutic process and supervisory conversations ensuring an inclusive context for ongoing exploration by all—learners and facilitators. It reframes participation as an activity of engagement and interaction between people where "knowledge and the knower are interdependent" (Anderson, 2007a, p. 8).

These are unfinished conversations. Shotter (2003) reminds us participation is an ongoing, unfinished activity. The politics of participation (Bava, 2022) lies in how we view participation as an intertwined activity and in how we hold space for not-knowing; staying curious for what emerges as we learn with our fellow learners. To lean in and learn how they are learning (even as we keep our eye on what they need to be learning) is what creates participation. Without the focus on how we are engaging our intersecting positionalities, we fail our students in developing a context for critical thought about what they are learning. Because it is in *how* we engage along with *what* we teach (e.g., structural analysis) that systemic/structural shifts occur. The form needs to match the content or else it lacks the dynamic relational resonance of what we are teaching.

Our social, systemic structures operate like Westworld character Caleb's computerized psychological treatment, unknown to us, programming us into our profiled identities of compliance and complacency. Mindlessly, maybe with some discomfort and resignation, we reproduce the programming through our talk, language, and interactions, unknowingly becoming each other's Francis (Caleb's army buddy)—relationally echoing, and even becoming foot soldiers for, our harmful social arrangements of dominance. However, a discursive mindset, embodied by Dolores and Caleb's relationship, is a reminder of the importance of how in talk and interactions we are also shaping the very systemic structures that are otherwise invisibly shaping us. In talk and interactions, we make them visible through our curiosity giving form to the formless. Thus, making our local knowledge-making processes a reflective socio-relational process. In the process, noticing our own agency, interdependencies, and choice points by which to engage our interconnectedness to actively dismantle a dominance-based system. Such humanizing includes adopting an anti-racist, anti-oppression stance as a crucial ethical position within supervision by which we interact to dignify each other. Such is the positionality that actively shifts us towards equity and inclusivity within and outside supervision.

References

Addison, S. M., & Coolhart, D. (2015). Expanding the therapy paradigm with queer couples: A relational intersectional lens. *Family Process, 54*(3), 435–453.

Anderson, H. (2007a). A postmodern umbrella: Language and knowledge as relational and generative, and inherently transforming. In H. Anderson & D. Gehart (Eds), *Collaborative therapy: Relationships and conversations that make a difference* (pp. 7–19). Routledge.

Anderson, H. (2007b). The heart and spirit of collaborative therapy: The philosophical stance— "A way of being" in relationship and conversation. In H. Anderson, & D. Gehart, *Collaborative therapy: Relationships and conversations that make a difference* (pp. 43–59). Routledge.

Anderson, H. (2012). Collaborative practice: A way of being "with." *Psychotherapy and Politics*, 130–145.

Anderson, H., & Goolishian, H. (1988). Human systems as linguistic systems: Preliminary and evolving ideas about the implications for clinical theory. *Family Process, 27*, 157–163.

Bakhtin, M. M. (1981). *The dialogic imagination: Four* essays (M. Holquist, Ed.; C. Emerson & M. Holquist, Trans.). [Kindle version]. University of Texas Press.

Bava, S. & McNamee, S. (2019). Imagining relationally crafted justice: A pluralist stance. *Contemporary Justice Review, 22*(3), 290–306. DOI: 10.1080/10282580.2019.1644174

Bava, S. (2019). Hyperlinked identity: A generative resource in a divisive world. In M. McGoldrick & K. Hardy (Eds), *Re-visioning family therapy* (pp. 318–335). The Guilford Press.

Bava, S. (2020). Play creates well-being: The contingency and the creativity of human interaction. In S. McNamee, M. M. Gergen, C. Camargo-Borges, & E. F. Rasera (pp. 516–527). *The Sage Handbook of Social Constructionist Practice.* Sage

Bava, S. (2021). *Humanizing: Unpacking oppression and its impact within therapeutic spaces. Unpublished.*

Bava, S. (2022). A relationally responsive world: The politics of collaborative-dialogic practices. In H. Anderson, & D. Gehart, *Collaborative dialogic practice: Relationships and conversations that make a difference across contexts and cultures* (pp. 37–53). Routledge.

Bhatia, S., & Priya, K. R. (2018). Decolonizing culture: Euro-American psychology and the shaping of neoliberal selves in India. *Theory & Psychology, 28*(5), 645–668. https://doi.org/10.1177/09593 54318791315

Crenshaw, K. (1989). Demarginalizing the intersection of race and sex: A black feminist critique of antidiscrimination doctrine, feminist theory and antiracist politics. *University of Chicago Legal Forum:, 1989*(1), 139–167. Retrieved from http://chicagounbound.uchicago.edu/uclf/vol1989/iss1/8

Crenshaw, K. (1991). Mapping the margins of intersectionality, identity politics and violence against women of color. *Stanford Law Review, 43*, 1241–1299.

Curtis-Boles, H., Chupina, A. G., & Okubo, Y. (2020). Social justice challenges: Students of color and critical incidents in the graduate classroom. *Training and Education in Professional Psychology,* 14(2), 100–108. https://doi.org/10.1037/tep0000293

Davies, B., & Harré, R. (1990). Positioning: The discursive production of selves. *Journal for the Theory of Social Behaviour, 20*(1), 43–63.

Engelmann, S., Scheibe, V., Battaglia, F., & Grossklags, J. (2022). Social Media Profiling Continues to Partake in the Development of Formalistic Self-Concepts. Social Media Users Think So, Too.. In Proceedings of the 2022 AAAI/ACM Conference on AI, Ethics, and Society (AIES'22), August 1–3, 2022, Oxford, United Kingdom. ACM, New York, NY, USA, 15 pages. https://doi.org/10.1145/3514094.3534192

Escobar, E. (1991). Language, identity and liberation: A critique of the term and concept "people of color." *Yale Journal of Law and Liberation*: Vol. 2:1, Article 10: 93–98

Gender and gender identity at a glance. (n.d.). Retrieved 10 31, 2022, from Planned Parenthood Federation of America Inc. www.plannedparenthood.org/health-topics/sexual-orientation-gender/gender-gender-identity-26530.htm

Gergen, K. (2009). *Relational being: Beyond self and community.* Oxford University Press.

Hardy, B., & Ness, O. (2015). Beyond the therapeutic state. *European Journal of Psychotherapy & Counselling, 17*(4), 322–325. doi:10.1080/13642537.2015.1096813

Hardy, K. (2016). Toward development of a multicultural relational perspective. In K. Hardy, & T. Bobes, *Culturally sensitive supervision and training: Diverse perspectives and practical applications* (pp. 3–10). Routledge.

Hardy, K., & Laszloffy, T. (1995). The cultural genogram: Key to training culturally competent family therapists. *Journal of Marital and Family Therapy, 21*(3), 227–237.

Hare-Mustin, R. T. (1978). A feminist approach to family therapy. *Family Process, 17*, 181–194.

History. (2022, July 17). *A brief history of essential partners.* Retrieved from Essential Partners: https://whatisessential.org/history

Imber-Black, E. (1992). *Families and larger systems: A family therapist's guide through the labyrinth.* Guilford Press.

Kelly, S., Jérémie-Brink, G., Chambers, A. L., & Smith-Bynum, M. A. (2020). The black lives matter movement: A call to action for couple and family therapists. *Family Process, 59*(4), 1374–1388. https://doi.org/10.1111/famp.12614

Knudson-Martin, C., McDowell, T., & Bermudez, J. M. (2019). From knowing to doing: Guidelines for socioculturally attuned family therapy. *Journal of Marital & Family Therapy, 45*(1), 47–60. https://doi.org/10.1111/jmft.12299

Knudson-Martin, C., McDowell, T., & Bermudez, J. M. (2020). Sociocultural attunement in systemic family therapy. In R. B. Karen S. Wampler, *The Handbook of Systemic Family Therapy: Volume 1, First Edition* (pp. 619–637). John Wiley & Sons Ltd.

Lannamann, J. & McNamee, S. (2020). Unsettling trauma: From individual pathology to social pathology. *Journal of Family Therapy, 42*: 328–346. doi: 10.1111/1467-6427.12288

Lebow, J.L. (2019). Editorial: Social justice in family therapy. *Family Process, 58*, 3–8. https://doi.org/10.1111/famp.12430

Martínez, A. I. (2014). Collaborative forms of talk in supervision: A View from discursive psychology. *International Journal of Collaborative Practice, 5*, 98–116.

McDowell, T. (2015). *Practicing critical decolonizing family therapy*. Retrieved 10 29, 2022, from https://link.springer.com/chapter/10.1007/978-3-319-15633-0_7

McDowell, T., & Hernández, P. (2010). Decolonizing academia: Intersectionality, participation, and accountability in family therapy and counseling. *Journal of Feminist Family Therapy, 22*(2), 93–111. Retrieved 10 29, 2022, from https://tandfonline.com/doi/full/10.1080/08952831003787834

McGoldrick, M., Giordano, J., & Garcia-Preto, N. (2005). *Ethnicity and family therapy*. Guilford Press.

McNamee, S. (2008). Transformative dialogue: Coordinating conflicting moralities. *The Lindberg Lecture 2008*. Retrieved July 17, 2022, from https://mypages.unh.edu/sheilamcnamee/publications/transformative-dialogue-coordinating-conflicting-moralities

Menakem, R. (2017). *My grandmother's hands*. Central Recovery Press.

Minuchin, P., Colapinto, J., & Minuchin, S. (2007). *Working with families of the poor*. Guilford Publication.

Pires, V., & Sobral, A. (2013). Implications of the subject's ontological statute in the Bakhtin, Medvedev, Vološinov circle's discursive theory. *Bakhtiniana, 8*(1), 207–220.

polanco, m. (2022). Why Am I A Woman? Or, Am I? Decolonizing White Feminism and the Latinx Woman Therapist in Academia. *Women & Therapy, 45*(2–3), 248–268. doi:10.1080/02703149.2022.2097597

Reed, I. A. (2013). Power: Relational, discursive, and performative dimensions. *Sociological Theory, 31*(3), 193–218.

Shotter, J. (1993). Becoming someone: Identity and belonging. In N. Coupland & J. Nussbaum (Eds.), *Discourse and lifespan development* (pp. 5–27). Sage.

Shotter, J. (2003). "Real presence": Meaning as living moment in a participatory world. *Theory and Psychology, 13*(4), 435–468.

Shotter, J. (2004). Expressing and legitimating "actionable knowledge" from within "the moment of acting." *Concepts and Transformation, 9*, 205–229.

Shotter, J. (2010). *Social construction on the edge: "Withness"-thinking and embodiment*. Taos Institute Publications.

Stockton, K. B. (2021). *Generder(s)*. The MIT Press.

Sugarman, J. (2015). Neoliberalism and Psychological Ethics. *Journal of Theoretical and Philosophical Psychology, 35*(2), 103–116. Retrieved 10 29, 2022, from https://apa.org/pubs/journals/features/teo-a0038960.pdf

Sullum, J. (2020, July n.d.). Curing the Therapeutic State: Thomas Szasz interviewed by Jacob Sullum. *Reason*, p. 28 "et seq.". Retrieved October 29, 2022, from http://reason.com/archives/2000/07/01/curing-the-therapeutic-state-t/

Tselious, E. and Borcsa, M. (2018) Discursive methodologies for couple and family therapy research: Editorial to special section. *Journal of Marital & Family Therapy, 44*(3): 375–385.

World Health Organization. (n.d.). Social determinants of health. Retrieved October 20, 2022 https://www.who.int/health-topics/social-determinants-of-health#tab=tab_1

9

EMOTIONAL DIVORCE AND COUPLES THERAPY IN IRAN

Afarin Rajaei and Parmida Safavi

Introduction

Divorce rates in Iran have increased over the past 10 years with an estimate of 183,193 couples getting divorced in 2020 (National Organization of Health Center in Iran, 2020). Besides the official figures on divorce rates, there exists another form of divorce called emotional divorce, which is often overlooked. In an emotional divorce, couples continue living together, but they lead separate lives and maintain a distant, aloof relationship without necessarily contemplating an actual divorce (Matthews, 1998). Iran is an Islamic country, and although a recent study shows that only one-third of the population claims to observe Islam, some of the Islamic policies and rules are entrenched in society. There are people who live together without an official marriage in Iran, and also there are LGBTQ communities in Iran, but because of the mentioned reason above, we don't have official data on those matters and populations.

The rate of emotional divorce is two to three times higher than legal divorce (Mashregh NEWS, 2016). This implies that the prevalence of emotional divorce in Iran may be linked to the societal shame and negative perception associated with seeking a legal divorce, particularly within the country's collectivist cultural framework. There is a famous Farsi/Persian proverb, which says that women enter the marital relationship dressed in a white gown and exit wrapped in a white shroud after they die, which means women leave marriage only after they die. In addition, Islam also promotes a negative view of divorce. There is a narration (hadith) from Prophet Mohammad saying: "Of all things permissible, divorce is the most reprehensible" (Haeri, 2014). Therefore, the taboo attached to divorce in Islam has deeply permeated Iranian culture (Sheikhi et al., 2012). While the intensity of the taboo surrounding divorce has significantly reduced with the passage of time and people have become more willing to end unsatisfactory relationships sooner, divorce is still perceived as an act that carries shame and social stigma, leading to unfavorable judgments from both the family and the wider community (Sheikhi et al., 2012).

Another factor to consider is gender biases in the policies and rules of Iran against women. Women usually don't have the right to have custody of children after the divorce, and based on Islamic rules that exist in Iran, custody goes to men most of the time. Therefore, a likely

DOI: 10.4324/9781003297871-11

solution for women to keep children can be an emotional divorce, which leads couples to have less positive affection, connection, and expectations.

Furthermore, research suggests a growing trend in the incidence of conflicts among Iranian couples due to changes in global factors that impact personal choices, cultural norms, and marital satisfaction (Askari et al., 2012; Najafi et al., 2015). Despite these developments, there is a shortage of research studies that investigate marital conflicts and appropriate interventions for Iranian couples. Although the Gottman method is a well-known approach to couples therapy with some evidence-based studies on its effectiveness (Cornelius & Alessi, 2007; Cornelius, Shorey, & Beebe, 2010; Denton et al., 2001; Hawkins et al., 2012), few studies have explored the relational challenges faced by Iranian couples while taking into account their collectivist cultural context, as opposed to the individualistic cultural context typical of western couples (Rajaei et al., 2019).

Clinical Application

It is important to see the role of couple therapy based on the Gottman method on the improvement of Iranian couples' relationships (Gottman et al., 1977). While this may seem obvious on the surface, few studies have been done on Iranians' culture from a collectivistic perspective. Based on these few studies, marriage and family therapists (MFTs) working with Iranian couples can focus on the Gottman method and its specific concepts (friendship system, meta-emotion, emotional divorce, conflict management, and shared meaning; Gottman, 2000; Gottman & Levenson, 2000) that can lead to satisfactory changes for couples (Rajaei et al., 2019). Family therapists should remind couples that marriage is not a box full of joy and Hollywood stories. A high-quality relationship is something that partners build together. Marriage is akin to an empty container, which can either be filled with unresolved conflicts, struggles, negative attributions, and violence, or it can be infused with positive emotions such as love, intimacy, companionship, friendship, and effective communication (referred to as the "emotional bank account" by Gottman and Silver, 1999; Gurman, 2008). The latter approach empowers couples to flourish in their relationship and achieve a successful marriage.

As a reminder, marriage therapists need to be mindful of cultural humility when they work with Iranian couples. For example, sex has been a taboo subject in Iran and conversations surrounding the sex lives of Iranian couples may not be as direct as in some western cultures. As a result, therapists need to modify questions and some of the interventions in Gottman method such as dreams within the conflicts (e.g., in the event that a persistent sexual disagreement is causing distress for an Iranian couple, and the therapist recognizes that the couple may feel uneasy discussing the matter, the therapist may choose to introduce "dreams within conflict intervention." The modification may involve suggesting a physical sensation (and not sexual) in the session, and then asking the couple to practice the main tool in private at home (and not in the therapy session in front of the therapist), Gottman & Silver, 2015). In addition, in Gottman's method, accepting influences from your partner is another important concept. Despite the fact that patriarchy affects all marital relationships worldwide, its impact is more apparent in certain cultures. The MFT needs to share studies and data on egalitarian relationships and how couples have more satisfaction and fewer health-related issues in those relationships (Gottman, 1989; 1994; 1999; 2004; Grey, 1999). Accepting the influence of one's partner, as observed in the Gottman Method's conflict management approach, poses challenges within Iranian culture. In this context, there exists a delicate balance. On one side, women are encouraged to actively listen to their partners, but this can result in reduced relationship satisfaction as their own agency and independence may be disregarded. Conversely, men are discouraged from being influenced by their partners due to the presence of toxic masculinity. However, according to the Gottman Method, maintaining high-quality relationships often necessitates being influenced by one's partner, making it extremely difficult to avoid. (Rajaei et al., 2019)In summary, cross-cultural studies provide valuable insights into the aspects of human relationships that are universally applicable and those that are shaped by specific cultural contexts. It is crucial to distinguish these factors from Western-centric methods and perspectives and examine them through a diverse cultural lens, particularly when exploring Eastern societies and cultures. This approach proves to be effective in promoting cosmopolitanism and fostering a sense of shared humanity, encouraging progress based on compassion and interconnectedness rather than animosity and alienation.

Considerations for Iranian Couples

To serve better work and create a stronger bond while working with couples, no matter their nationality, the clinician needs to know about their client's culture. The therapeutic relationship in therapy plays a significant role, so therapists should be aware of and familiar with their biases. In addition, it is essential to remember that not all individuals, families, and couples are the same. Therefore, instead of generalizing and making assumptions, therapists should stay informed and curious. The following are some considerations to keep in mind when working with Iranian couples and immigrants:

1. MFTs should play a role in addressing and bringing awareness to the phenomenon of the invisibility syndrome among Iranian couples.. The *invisibility syndrome* describes a pattern of racial discrimination that a person repeatedly experiences, leading to feelings of low self-esteem and self-worth (Franklin & Boyd-Franklin, 2000). This lived experience creates the "paradox of invisibility" such that, on the one hand, Iranian women and people experience being incredibly visible as stereotypic characters (e.g., Iranian men as violent, aggressive, and Iranian women as victims and helpless individuals), but on the other hand, they may feel equally invisible for not being noticed for their talents or strengths (e.g., bravery, wisdom, and resourcefulness; Franklin & Boyd-Franklin, 2000). MFTs should avoid stereotyping Iranian couples and making comments such as "you feel helpless 'because' you are from Iran and it is a theme there, right?." In C/MFT training settings, we always give students vignettes for role-plays and practice. It is shocking how many times professors have seen supervisees or trainees say "I am going to ask safety questions since the husband is from the Middle East." MFTs should be mindful of their biases, and ask informed questions, instead of going with their own assumptions.
2. In Iranian couples, sometimes in-laws' families are involved in stories and complaints. It is important for MFTs to use the Gottman method to challenge their definition of health/unhealthy boundaries and relationships. Sometimes, what seems unhealthy in western society is very common and functional in eastern societies.
3. Focusing on communication is a significant aspect for Iranian couples. Developing effective communication skills, which are essential for conflict management according to

the Gottman method (Gottman, 2000), involves acquiring learned abilities. Mos of the time, these skills are not taught in schools or families in Iranian culture.

4. In Iranian culture, there is a tendency for individuals to engage in indirect communication and maintain a practice known as "Taarof." Taarof is a form of polite behavior that promotes equality within a hierarchical society. For instance, when a group of Iranian friends approach a doorway, they will often insist that others go through first. Understanding this cultural aspect is crucial in the context of couples therapy, particularly when it comes to expressing one's needs and communicating them effectively, which is an important aspect of the Gottman method (Gottman, 2015). Iranian couples may require additional support in recognizing their needs and overcoming the potential barrier posed by the concept of "taarof" to express themselves openly.

5. The Iranian government does not recognize the LGBTQ+ community in Iran, which brings up a lot of social injustice issues. This is important to know because Iranian couples from LGBT+ communities depending on where they are living might not a ge`t chance to explore their romantic relationship enough due to the norms and rules of Iran society. It is crucial that couple therapists be mindful of their own biases and stay present and curious with their LGBTQ+ Iranian couples. There might be some traumas in the past (or present) that need to be addressed while working on the relationship.

6. Iranian women face various social injustice issues in Iran (Rajaei et al., 2020). They grew up/live in a culture that took away their voice and silenced them. This is a global issue that varies country to country. MFTs should be mindful of intersectionality and the power dynamic in their sessions. They should keep asking themselves "does my couple especially the female partner/s feel heard and understood?" to avoid retraumatizing couples and deconstructing power dynamics in their sessions.

7. Therapy is not as common in Iran as it is in western countries. Therefore, MFTs may use more psychoeducation for Iranian immigrant couples. In the context of couples, psychoeducation involves providing couples with information and education about various aspects of relationships, communication, conflict resolution, and intimacy. The goal is to enhance their understanding of each other, improve their relationship dynamics, and equip them with skills and strategies for building a healthy and fulfilling partnership.They may also need to expand the therapeutic conversation in working with Iranian immigrant couples. Iran has a unique relationship with western countries and because of that, there are many stereotypes about Iranians, which usually leads to the experience of discrimination against Iranian immigrants. Therefore, the MFTusing the Gottman method can help couples by using stress-reducing conversations (a tool/technique in Gottman method; Gottman, 2000) about the impact of society on the daily lives of couples.

8. Language barriers might be another complication in couples therapy with Iranian and/or Iranian immigrants. One solution is promoting telebehavioral health (TBH) for Iranian immigrant couples. Studies highlight the significant role of language between clients and providers via TBH and in-person (Hilty et al., 2015; 2017). TBH provides more flexibility and options for Iranian immigrant couples to have a MFTwho speaks their native language and/or has an interpreter (Rajaei & Sahebi, 2021).

9. Cultural humility is a lifelong journey and is about constant self-reflection (Tervalon & Murray-Garcia, 1998). Regarding Iranian couples' culture, MFTs should try to be humble, flexible, and have a client-oriented approach (Hook et al., 2013). In addition, recognizing and addressing power imbalances in working with Iranian couples is another

aspect of cultural humility (Rajaei & Jensen, 2020). Power imbalances and concerns regarding injustice can arise due to the intersecting differences between the couple therapist, Iranian couples' social position, cultural and contextual factors, and the influence of the dominant culture. These factors contribute to significant challenges in maintaining an equitable therapeutic relationship. Therefore, MFTs are encouraged to be mindful of their own social location factors, implicit biases, the position of privilege, and the intersectionality of the parts of the identities that intersect with Iranian couples' social locations.

10. Regarding cultural humility, McDowell et al. (2018) proposed a framework that MFTs can apply in their clinical practice when working with Iranian couples. This framework recommends the incorporation of socioculturally sensitive family therapy as a guideline for treatment in clinical settings. McDowell et al. (2018) pointed out a movement to the third-order change. This change involves couples understanding of how social forces shape and shift their life narratives and impact intimate partner relationships as well as material/relationship realities. Therefore, MFTs are encouraged to explore how dominant discourses are tied to vehicles of marginalization, systemic oppression, and interactions with privilege for Iranian couples. MFTs are also encouraged to invite Iranian couples to explore the ways in which sociocultural dynamics intersect with their presenting problems as constraints. MFTs join in the effort by listening attentively and deeply in the search for the couple's experiences, shared values, and meanings while navigating Iranian couples' attempts to cocreate their preferred narratives/lived experiences (McDowell et al., 2018; Rajaei & Hodgson, 2019). This manifests itself in various interventions in the Gottman method such as dreams within the conflict, stress-reducing conversations, shared fondness and admiration, etc. (Gottman, 2000). It is noteworthy that the attention on third-order change increases the likelihood of increasing the Iranian couple's awareness. MFTs can help Iranian couples view dominant narratives from a multisystemic lens, which includes a sociopolitical framework and facilitates the deconstruction of power-embedded relational injustices and empowered resistance (McDowell et al., 2018).

Future Clinical Directions

MFTs who use the Gottman method have the opportunity to incorporate recent research findings into their work with Iranian couples. To achieve optimal health outcomes for these couples, therapists can employ the biopsychosocial-spiritual (BPSS; (Engel, 1977, 1980; Wright et al., 1996) framework and systems thinking (von Bertalanffy, 1968). It is important for therapists to utilize a systemic BPSS lens when assessing and treating Iranian couples, and to collaborate with healthcare providers to consider both individual and dyadic influences on relationship quality and stability (Rajaei et al., 2021). Additionally, therapists should have knowledge of complex BPSS factors that affect Iranian couples and provide support and education to help these couples develop a systemic understanding of their relationship quality and stability. It is important to address potential barriers such as lower health literacy, lack of social support, and high anxiety that may affect understanding of Iranian couples and their day-to-day lives (Hodgson et al., 2018).

Iranian couples may experience the impacts of their stories differently due to gender differences, power, and other BPSS factors (Burwell et al., 2008; Rajaei & Jense, 2020).

For example, Iranian women may report more perpetual problems(i.e., a concept in Gottman method) than men. We need more clinical and research work on these differences, so MFTs can embrace a culturally sensitive approach when exploring contextual factors (e.g., age, gender, race, and reproductive stages; Galanti, 2015). The Four Cs of culture may be helpful for MFTs using the Gottman method, which includes asking questions about what the couples call their experiences (i.e., Call), what they think caused it to happen (i.e., Cause), how they cope with it (i.e., Cope), and what concerns they have about it (i.e., Concern). It is important for therapists to practice cultural humility, which means continually self-evaluating their biases, attitudes, and beliefs in order to reduce and ultimately eliminate health disparities (Tervalon & Murray–Garcia, 1998).

Furthermore, MFTs may also consider how cultural discourses regarding relationships in the country in which they are seeing Iranian couples (i.e., where the therapist lives and where the clients are living) affect how Iranian couples interact with their MFTand the Gottman method in the course of treatment. Couples may feel voiceless when attempting to fully express their concerns about their relationship because they are concerned about a therapist's dismissiveness or discomfort surrounding their shared experience of the relationship or their own lived experience in the context of their relationship. Using the Gottman method therapists can help Iranian couples and the healthcare system see the pervasiveness of societal systems of power and facilitate the deconstruction of power-embedded relational injustices and resistance (McDowell et al., 2013; Rajaei & Jensen, 2020).

Finally, MFTs should increase collaboration between providers, couples, and the healthcare system (Rajaei & Jensen, 2020). MFTs who utilize the Gottman method in integrated healthcare settings should collaborate with other healthcare providers such as primary care providers, oncologists, and social workers to provide evidence-based, culturally appropriate, and systemic BPSS care for Iranian couples. This collaboration can lead to better care for Iranian couples by strengthening the relationships between providers (McDaniel et al., 1992, 2013).

Future Research Directions

To enhance our understanding of the impact of biological, psychosocial, spiritual, and interpersonal processes on the quality and stability of romantic relationships in Iranian couples, it is crucial for therapists and researchers to use the Gottman method. Future research should adopt mixed methods to obtain a comprehensive understanding of the experiences of Iranian couples. In addition, studies with larger sample sizes and objective observational measures should be conducted to ensure the validity and generalizability of results (Bruce & Desmond, 1997). Research on LGBTQ+ Iranian couples and their similarities and differences in processes that affect relationship quality and stability is also necessary. The actor-partner interdependence model (APIM) should be used to investigate systemic challenges affecting Iranian couples, considering both relational and micro- and macro-level health domains. Longitudinal dyadic data techniques, such as the longitudinal actor-partner interdependence model (L-APIM), could be employed to analyze changes in both partners' relationship quality and stability based on the Gottman method over time.

Three Key Takeaways

1. Couple therapists using the Gottman method should pay close attention to their own social location factors, implicit biases, position of privilege, and the intersectionality of the various aspects of their own identities that intersect with the social locations of Iranian couples.
2. MFTs should contribute to demystifying the invisibility syndrome in Iranian couples. The *invisibility syndrome* describes a pattern of perceived racial discrimination that occurs repeatedly and leads to a sense of low self-esteem in the person affected (Franklin & Boyd-Franklin, 2000).
3. Cross-cultural studies provide insights into the universal and culturally specific aspects of human relationships. It is important to distinguish these issues from Western perspectives and examine them through a diverse cultural lens, particularly when considering Eastern societies and cultures. This approach serves as an effective means of embracing a cosmopolitan perspective and advancing as human beings on this planet. By prioritizing humanity and connection over hatred and disconnection, we can move forward in a more harmonious and inclusive manner..

References

Askari, M., Noah, S. B. M., Hassan, S. A. B., & Baba, M. B. (2012). Comparison the effects of communication and conflict resolution skills training on marital satisfaction. *International Journal of Psychological Studies, 4*(1), 10. doi:10.5539/ijps.v4n1p182

Cornelius, T. L., & Alessi, G. (2007). Behavioral and physiological components of communication training: does the topic affect outcome? *Journal of Marriage and Family, 69*, 608–620. https://doi.org/10.1111/j.1741-3737.2007.00395.x

Cornelius, T. L., Alessi, G., & Shorey, R. C. (2007). The effectiveness of communication skills training with married couples: does the issue discussed matter? *The Family Journal, 15*, 124–132. doi:10.1177/1066480706297971

Cornelius, T., Shorey, R., & Beebe, S. (2010). Self-reported communication variables and dating violence: Using Gottman's marital communication conceptualization. *Journal of Family Violence, 25*(4), 439–448. https://doi.org/10.1177/1066480706297971

Denton, W. H., Burleson, B. R., Hobbs, B. V., Von Stein, M., & Rodriguez, C. P. (2001). Cardiovascular reactivity and initiate/avoid patterns of marital communication: A test of Gottman's psychophysiologic model of marital interaction. *Journal of Behavioral Medicine, 24*(5), 401–421. https://doi.org/10.1023/A:1012278209577

Engel, G. L. (1977). The need for a new medical model: A challenge for biomedicine. *Science, 196*, 129–136. https://doi.org/10.1126/ science.847460

Gottman, J. M. (1994). *What predicts divorce? The relationship between marital processes and marital outcomes.* Hillsdale, NJ: Lawrence Erlbaum Associates.

Gottman, J. M. (1999). *The marriage clinic: A scientifically-based marital therapy.* New York, NY: W. W. Norton.

Gottman, J. S. (2004). *The marriage clinic casebook.* New York, NY: W. W. Norton.

Gottman, J. S., & Gottman, J. M. (2015). *Book Review: 10 principles for doing couples therapy.* New york, NY: W.W. Norton & Company.

Gottman, J. M., & Krokoff, L. J. (1989). Marital interaction and satisfaction: A longitudinal view. *Journal of Consulting and Clinical Psychology, 57*(1), 47–53. https://doi.org/10.1037/0022-006X.57.1.47

Gottman, J. M., & Levenson, R. W. (2000). The timing of divorce: Predicting when a couplewill divorce over a 14-year period. *Journal of Marriage and Family, 62*(3), 737–745. https://doi.org/10.1111/j.1741-3737.2000.00737.x

Gottman, J. M., Markman, H., & Notarius, C. (1977). The topography of marital conflict: A sequential analysis of verbal and nonverbal behavior. *Journal of Marriage and theFamily, 39*, 461–477. https://doi.org/10.2307/350902

Gottman, J. M., & Silver, N. (1999). *The seven principles for making marriage work (1st ed.).* New York: Crown.

Gottman, J. M., & Silver, N. (2015). *The seven principles for making marriage work (2nd ed.).* New York, NY: Harmony Books.

Gray, W. R. (1999). Tuning in to the conversation: Twenty-five years later. *The Journal of Popular Culture, 33*(2), 123–130. https://doi.org/10.1111/j.0022-3840.1999.3302_123.x

Gurman, A. S. (2008). *Gottman Couple Therapy. Clinical handbook of couple therapy* (pp. 129–161). (4th ed.). New York, NY: Guilford Press.

Haeri, S. (2014). *Law of desire: Temporary marriage in shii iran, revised edition.* Syracuse: Syracuse University Press.

Hawkins, A. J., Stanley, S. M., Blanchard, V. L., & Albright, M. (2012). Exploring programmatic moderators of the effectiveness of marriage and relationship education programs: A meta-analytic study. *Behavior Therapy, 43*(1), 77–87. https://doi.org/10.1016/j.beth.2010.12.006

Hilty, D. M., Crawford, A., Teshima, J., Chan, S., Sunderji, N., Yellowlees, P. M., Kramer, G., O'Neill, P., Fore, C., Luo, J. S., & Li, S. T. (2015). A framework for telepsychiatric training and ehealth: Competency-based education, evaluation and implications. *International Review of Psychiatry, 27*(6), 569–592. https://doi.org/10.3109/09540261.2015.1091292

Hilty, D. M., Maheu, M. M., Drude, K., Hertlein, K., Wall, K., Long, R., Luoma, T., & Ford, D. (2017). Telebehavioral health, telemental health, e-therapy and e-health competencies: The need for an interdisciplinary framework. *Journal for Technology In Behavioral Science, 2*(4), 1–19.

Hook, J. N., Davis, D. E., Owen, J., Worthington, E. L. Jr., & Utsey, S. O. (2013). Cultural humility: Measuring openness to culturally diverse clients. *Journal of Counseling Psychology, 60*, 353–366.

Mashregh NEWS. (2016). Retrieved July/August, 2018, from www.mashreghnews.ir/

Matthews, W. (1998). Long-term effects of divorce on children. North Carolina Cooperative Extension Service. North Carolina A&T State University, U.S. Department of Agriculture, and local governments cooperating.

McDaniel, S. H., Doherty, W. J., & Hepworth, J. (2013). *Medical family therapy: A biopsychosocial approach to families with health problems.* Basic Books.

McDaniel, S. H., Hepworth, J., & Doherty, W. (Eds.). (1992). *The shared experience of illness: Stories of patients, families, and their therapists.* Basic Books.

McDowell, T., Knudson-Martin, C., & Bermudez, J. M. (2018). *Socioculturally attuned family therapy.* New York, NY: Routledge.

Najafi, M., Soleimani, A. A., Ahmadi, K., Javidi, N., & Kamkar, E. H. (2015). The effectiveness of emotionally focused therapy on enhancing marital adjustment and quality of life among infertile couples with marital conflicts. *International Journal of Fertility & Sterility, 9*(2), 238.

National Organization of Health Center in Iran. (2013). *Iran: Health – Pars Times.* www.parstimes.com/cr?IG¼893FB47B044141B9AE540F70EC24681B&CID¼16D4DBBB1D316 A0919F4D0241C9E6BC2&rd¼1&h¼3qAINvWHMbO7KUvWlnRMkeOOHAuIr9tkV4o-C1G5CQ0&v¼1&r¼http%3a%2f%2f w.parstimes.com%2fhealth%2f&p¼DevEx,5087.1

Rajaei, A., Daneshpour, M., & Robertson, J. (2019). The effectiveness of couples therapy based on the Gottman method among Iranian couples with conflicts: A quasi-experimental study. *Journal of Couple & Relationship Therapy, 18*(3), 223–240.

Rajaei, A., & Jensen, J. F. (2020). Empowering patients in integrated behavioral health-care settings: A narrative approach to medical family therap. *The Family Journal, 28*(1): 48–55. https://doi.org/10.1080/15332691.2019.1567174

Rajaei, A., Nasrollahi Shahri, M. N., & Jensen, J. (2020). The lived experience of recent Iranian graduate student immigrants in the United States. *New Diversities, 22*(2). ISSN-Print 2199-8108; ISSN-Internet 2199-8116.

Rajaei, A., Jensen, J. F., Brimhall, A. S., Torres, E. T., & Schwartz, A. J. (2021). Dyadic Function of Couples with Cancer: A Review. *Journal of Couple & Relationship Therapy, 20*(3), 279–302. https://doi.org/10.1080/15332691.2020.1841055

Rajaei, A., & Sahebi, B. (2021). Re-Visioning immigrant couple therapy: Immigrant couples in the United States and telebehavioral health. *The Family Journal*, 29(4), 442–448. https://doi.org/10.1177/10664807211000070

Sheikhi, K., Khosravi, J., Gharibi, H., Gholizadeh, Z., & Hassanzadeh M. (2012). Understanding of divorce and its positive consequences (A qualitative research). *Journal of Family Counseling & Psychotherapy*, 1(4), 64–77 (Persian).

Tervalon, M., & Murray-Garcia, J. (1998). Cultural humility versus cultural competence: A critical distinction in defining physician training outcomes in multicultural education. *Journal of Health Care for the Poor and Underserved*, 9, 117–125.

Von Bertalanffy, L. (1968). *System theory: Foundations, development, applications*. George Braziller.

Wright, L. M., Watson, W. L., & Bell, J. M. (1996). *Beliefs: The heart of healing in families and illness*. Basic Books.

10

'IT'S MORE THAN I CAN MANAGE'

Psychosocial Counselling and Family Therapy for Refugees in Mecklenburg–Vorpommern

Barbara Bräutigam, A. H. Lohrasbi Nejad, and Lisa Werle

Introduction

This passage was taken from a novel, and it illustrates clearly how fugitive people suffer. It presents not so much an objective description as a subjective report on what it means to be a refugee or one of the 'boat people'. The motivation behind our concern with transcultural psychotherapy for refugees, immigrants and their families is mainly based on the hospitation of one of the authors in the Immigrant and Refugee Children's Mental Health Research Unit. This unit is part of the Department of Social and Transcultural Psychiatry, which was founded by Lawrence Kirmayer and is probably one of the most famous departments in this field. Both the unit and the department belong to McGill University in Montreal, which also offers summer schools, workshops and training courses in the field of transcultural psychotherapy. Its family-related approach entails a special focus on the narratives and subjective understandings of the client's disorder, with an ongoing emphasis on strength-based interventions. Emphasis is placed on the possible transgenerational aspects of the symptomatology presented. Overall, studies show that multicultural skills and cultural sensitivity lead to lower discontinuation rates in therapy, and enable the regular termination of therapy (Gries et al., 2020, pp. 425–443).

'It's more than I can manage' – the title of our chapter – was a statement by one of our clients. It well describes the situation of many refugees in Germany, who often face much bureaucracy, many insecurities and daily racism. The chapter describes our attempt to support refugees and their families through counselling and therapy that takes a culturally sensitive approach. First, we point out the main principles of counselling and therapy with refugees and their families who have suffered and survived different types of trauma, focusing on female refugees. Second, we explain the concept behind our counselling center in Western Pomerania, and some of the challenges and barriers caused by external conditions. Third, we concretize our experience on the basis of three case studies, and highlight some ideas which seem important to us in the context of our work with couples and families. Finally, we summarize our considerations regarding a therapeutic approach that

DOI: 10.4324/9781003297871-12

emphasizes the elaboration of clients' highly individual perspectives on their own problems and solutions.

Culturally Sensitive Counselling and Psychotherapy

The combination of multiple complex fields into one presents a challenge for both counsellors and therapists in culturally sensitive counselling. Basic counselling principles are extended by trauma-specific counselling methods and sensitivity towards cultural features, and this all needs to be held in mind while one deals with traumatic experiences and clients' culturally specific mechanisms for coping with those experiences. This complexity reveals how urgently more research in this field is needed. At the same time, the complexity also entails a need to proceed by small individual steps. Refugees come from different places and cultural backgrounds, and they have different ways of understanding what traumatisation has done and can do to their mental health. In this context more than any other, counselling needs to be understood first and foremost as a process of communication in small steps that offers a safe environment to the client and gives them a strong, mindful and trustful partner with whom to speak about the unspeakable. The process will develop over time, and informed, reflexive counsellors will encounter needs for intervention along the way. Some of these possible interventions are specified in this chapter.

The expression 'traumatic experience' is understood in terms of one's having had to live through or watch situations that triggered emotional and somatic responses of fear for one's life. Successful trauma therapy helps clients to reintegrate these experiences of traumatisation into their biography and personality (Hantke & Görges, 2012, p. 53).

The prevalence rate of mental trauma among refugees is significantly higher than in the general population, at about 30% (Liedl, 2018). It must be mentioned that some people also develop resilience or 'post-traumatic growth' (Kleefeldt, 2018). However, there are clear indications of a connection between psychological stress, traumatisation and flight (Gavranidou et al., 2008). There were some diagnostic advances regarding the definition and concretisation of traumatic stressors in DSM-5 – for example, it was expanded to include sexual violence (Schellong et al., 2019), which also affects many refugees. Importantly, it is not so much the immediate traumatic experiences before flight but rather the social and family burdens of exile that are linked to psychological problems among refugees and their families (Measham et al., 2014). On the other hand, we wish to stress the political meaning of refugees' suffering. Most of these people have psychological problems because of external conditions; they are not mentally ill. It is very important to discuss this aspect again and again with clients – which means telling them that they are not crazy, but that they do not feel well because they have had a lot of difficult experiences. 'With the current diagnosis of entire population groups as "traumatised" and the boom in trauma projects and therapy offers... the political dimension of trauma and trauma work is in danger of being lost' (Mlodoch, 2017, p. 22, our translation). Nevertheless, psychosocial interventions have positive effects for refugees both with and without diagnoses (Turrini et al., 2019).

It must be emphasised that counselling sessions with refugees usually occur at a stage of life when people have experienced nothing but instability and uncertainty on all levels: emotional, social, financial, and environmental. Not only have they fled from violence, war or oppression, but they are now living in a transitional place and have to battle with the authorities for their safety. This uncertainty affects not only clients themselves but also their families. Therefore, creating a safe space amid all this uncertainty, where clients can open up and speak about unresolved trauma, is the key to successful trauma therapy.

The topic of family life can be highly sensitive. Most refugees become separated from their families enroute and are unable to stay in touch with people at home. During counselling sessions, it is important to understand that some refugees are uncertain whether their close relatives, parents and siblings are even still alive. Some interviews conducted as part of a study on the lives of young women who had escaped from Somalia (Werle, 2020) showed what an impact the uncertain whereabouts of family and friends can have on asylum seekers' mental well-being. In that study, the interviewees' traumatic experiences were directly connected to family structures. Sometimes family members had been the initiators of trauma. One of the women had survived an abduction; she had been beaten and made watch her father being tortured, before being taken away for forced marriage. The man to whom she was to be married was supposedly a militia member; he had previously been married to her sister, who had died during pregnancy a few months into the marriage. All of these traumatizing experiences had led her to initiate her escape and were related to the topic of family. Another woman reported having lived with and been oppressed by her uncle, and she still feared for her family. Some of the female adolescents that flee to northern Europe have a constellation of role responsibilities similar to those of adult women, and these responsibilities are another reason why they are trying to find a safe new place to live – not only for themselves, but often also for their children. Thus there are educational aspects that can be helpful for work with asylum-seeking families, adolescents, and/or minors, including the children of adolescent women. Three principles have been identified as the main elements of this work, again all revolving around the element of safety: first, the inpatient facility/institution as a safe space for the client; second, emotion oriented dialogue between counsellor and client, and a sheltered setting that establishes a safe space during counselling sessions (Quindeau & Rauwald, 2017); third, the building of the client's trust and feeling of safety. There are multiple helpful tools and manuals to adequately meet the needs of individual clients within this safe space, according to the client's gender, age and biographical background.

In our counselling and psychotherapeutic work in an intercultural context, we follow the model presented in Table 1, which gives a good overview of the multidimensionality of this type of work.

Table 10.1 The three-pillar model

Post-migration process	*Stressful everyday life*	*Mental aspects*
Concepts of migration	Stressful housing conditions	Clinical psychology
Search for identity between two cultures	Uncertain future	Trauma therapy
Mourning/homesickness	Structural discrimination	Culturally specific concepts of aetiology
Loss of social references	Experience of racism	Culturally specific expectations of help
Loss of resources	Little access to provision of help	Value orientation

Source: Liedl & Abdallah-Steinkopff, 2017, as cited in Liedl, 2018, p. 17.

Cultural biases can be another difficult obstacle. Depending on their cultural heritage or religion, some people may not have formed a scientific understanding of mental health; if they believe that mental health issues derive from the existence of bad spirits or even witchcraft, they may consider it a very dangerous and shameful topic (Gutmann, 2019). In such cases there is an especially strong need to proceed in small educational steps and to refer to the client's specific symptoms and their consequences and origins. Liedl et al.'s (2013) 'psychoeducation on post-traumatic stress disorder' (PTSD) is exemplary here. These authors present multiple individual step-by-step approaches, structured in chapters on the development of traumatisation, with tools for coping with emotional consequences such as anger and fear. These manuals can be worked through at any pace and in any order, depending on the client's individual needs.

In resource-oriented counselling, culture can help to provide a framework and everyday structure for clients' lives. Refugees and their families can learn to practise important elements of their own culture, religion, and everyday rituals so as to regain their confidence and trust in their own actions. This can support the counselling process, as it can be utilised in a resourceful manner. Positive reinforcement and the use of supporting structural elements can empower clients and improve their well-being. Using culture as a framework and channel for motivation can help to re-establish much-needed structure and stability (Altenthan et al., 2008).

Basic knowledge of the client's former home country, its possible cultural features, and its current political situation lays the groundwork for one's trustworthiness as a counsellor. Not only may one be able understand the client's experiences more easily, but the client will also not need to provide detailed descriptions of their intrinsic attitudes towards groups of people, behaviours, or institutions. The focus of sessions can be placed on the topics that are most important to the individual client, which are usually how to regain a feeling of safety (Völter & Reichmann, 2017). A study conducted in Mecklenburg-Vorpommern also found that the resetting of clients' individual boundaries after losses of control and experiences of physical and mental violence may be enhanced through sports and physically strengthening activities such as self-defence classes (Preitler, 2016).

Not all basic counselling principles need to be applied in a culturally sensitive manner. Client-centred counselling that closely follows the principles developed by Carl R. Rogers shapes counselling sessions in a manner that is independent of culture. The three principles in question are congruency of the counsellor with the client and their emotions, unconditional positive regard towards the client, and an empathetic understanding of the client (Rogers, 1983). These are universal, and can be dealt withoutside of one's cultural background or understanding. If the counsellor opens themselves up to fully and sympathetically comprehend the physical and emotional world of the client, there will be complete mutual understanding regarding feelings and circumstances. Clients must be treated as experts on their own individual biographies, and should be met without prejudice (Völter & Reichmann, 2017).

It is important to constantly explain throughout the counselling process that even if the counsellor engages intensively with the client's emotions and listens to intense details of trauma, they can manage what is said. Thus, the counsellor becomes a strong but empathetic counterpart to help and guide the client through this difficult and painful process in the best way possible.

Psychosocial and Family Counselling for Refugees

In this section we give a brief overview of the state of research on low-threshold psychosocial interventions for refugees in Germany, and describe the barriers that refugees have to overcome in order to receive psychosocial support. The aim is to better identify the special situation of refugees and clients, and to gain better insight into their real needs and difficulties. Our counselling center wants to be a place where refugees can speak about their personal and flight-related experiences. It is important for us to support clients in their everyday lives and focus on their strengths and resources.

According to the Federal Ministry of the Interior, around 1.7 million refugees are living in Germany as of 30 June 2020 (Media Service Integration, 2020). These refugees are of different ages and have come to Germany from many different parts of the world (Bundestag, 2020). They can be divided into three groups according to their residency status: refugees who are entitled to asylum, refugees who are going through the asylum procedure, and refugees whose asylum applications have been denied (Federal Office of Statistics, 2021). One's residency status plays a significant role in one's well-being and quality of life (Gahleitner et al., 2017, p. 25).

Refugee problems cover a wide range of issues, such as residential, legal, social, psychological, and family problems. Problems related to family can be divided into three categories: family problems that occur in the refugee's country of origin, family problems that occur during their escape, and family problems that occur in the host country.

Family problems in the refugee's country of origin can be seen both as a cause of flight and as problems in their own right with which the refugee is still dealing. These problems are usually due to pressure from refugees' families to do things that the refugees do not want to do: for example, sexual abuse by a family member; forced marriage or the prevention of divorce by threats from one's own family; the risk of female genital mutilation to oneself or one's children, threats of murder in a dispute over inheritance, or because of a failure to perform one's religious duties. In addition, some refugees' desire for a lifestyle that differs from common practice in their own societies – such as a preference for same-sex relationships, which is still taboo in many societies and families – causes family problems. Ethnic and tribal affiliations can also be mentioned as a cause of family problems: individuals or even whole families may face death threats to avenge a family member because of problems between different tribes. These are problems refugees will face again if their asylum application is rejected.

Problems related to the family that occur during flight may include the death or disappearance of a fugitive family member, as well as the sexual abuse or rape of a family member by human traffickers or other strangers – all traumatic experiences for refugees and their families. These experiences manifest themselves in the form of flashbacks, nightmares, and feeling of guilt.

Family problems that occur in the host country are the focus of our work. These problems are due to the lack of facilities, or to the restrictions imposed by asylum laws and regulations. For example, in the state of Mecklenburg-Vorpommern, the obligation to reside in refugee community shelters is a major problems for two groups of refugees: those who are going through the asylum procedure, and those whose asylum applications have been denied. The issues about which refugees complain during counselling sessions with regard to community shelters include the witnessing of violence, frequent police presence in some dormitories, lack of privacy, poor hygiene in bathrooms and public lavatories, loud noises from neighbouring units, and the sale and consumption of drugs. These problems affect not only parents but also children. The obligation to reside in community shelters worsens the well-being of traumatised people and reduces the effectiveness of counselling. A large proportion of refugees request a change of their place of residence. Rrefugees also face numerous barriers to labour market access. For example, refugees in both groups who arrived in Germany after 31 August 2015 from 'safe' countries of origin – that is, European Union member states, Albania, Bosnia and Herzegovina, Ghana, Kosovo, Northern Macedonia, Montenegro, Senegal, and Serbia – are not allowed to work. Refugees with unclear identities may also not be granted work permits (Asylum and Migration Information Network, 2019a, 2019b).

Moreover, the consequences of trauma significant within our clients. Such consequences may include substance abuse, PTSD, anxiety disorders, depressive disorders, etc. Among refugees who visit our counselling centre, more than half show symptoms of depression and about a third show symptoms of severe depression. Homesickness and the experience of discrimination and daily racism contribute to these problems. Problems that manifest as intense worries about the future are very common.

To deal with such a variety of problems, we have created a concept of counselling that combines several approaches and counselling techniques to find proper and practical solutions for the physical, psychological, and social problems of refugees who seek counselling.

Refugees find themselves in a critical circumstances for reasons such as war, political, or religious persecution, natural disasters etc., they are forced to leave their hometowns immediately. They are forced to leave behind not only their physical possessions but also their family and social ties, and enter a new and unfamiliar environment – the host country – without knowing much about its culture, customs, or social and legal structures. This means that refugees lose their most important protective factor, i.e., the stable bond that most people have with other people. The absence of trusted people such as family members or friends, and the lack of information, leads to insecurity and mistrust. Therefore, the first step in providing a proper consultation is to build a relationship with refugees and gain their trust (Gahleitner et al., 2017, pp. 20–26). This requires our unconditional acceptance and understanding of our clients as well as honesty to provide the best care (Weinberger, 2011). This professional relationship based on trust creates a safe external place for refugees (Kühn, 2013, p. 33) where they can talk about and work on experiences related to their escape as well as interpersnal problems such as marital infidelity, domestic violence, etc. Next, we determine the needs of the refugee through the use of various methods such as diagnostic interviews and tests, as well as through collaboration with organisations in the field of medicine and psychiatry, and then we concretise the problems and classify them into three categories: physical, psychological, or social problems. In addition, and with the help of resource-oriented techniques, during counselling sessions we analyse the client's strengths and weaknesses in individual categories (such as education) and social categories (such as interpersonal relationships, friends, family, etc.). In the third step, we develop an assistance programme, based on the information collected and the need to address the problems and the extent to which the refugee has access to social services. We provide counselling according to this assistance programme so that the client can solve their problems step by step (Gahleitner et al., 2017). In addition, through our established networks, we refer refugees to other organisations in the field for medical, psychiatric, therapeutic, and social services. As mentioned before, since the client's residency status is crucial to their well-being and quality of life, we pay special attention to the asylum procedure and residency status during counselling sessions, so that legal and litigation counselling can be accessed if necessary through the relevant organisations in order to increase the chances of success.

The following describes three vignettes where, in addition to counselling regarding everyday problems, the complexity of couple- and family-related dynamics also becomes clear. We treat these three cases therapeutically.

Dealing with Guilt and Shame: Three Case Studies

Ms A: *the primacy of family*

Ms A is in her early 30s and comes from Chechnya. She has six children, of whom the two youngest were born in Germany. Her residency status is not secure: she has a tolerated stay permit, and she and her family have feared deportation for several years. She receives psychosocial counselling sessions because she suffers from depression and severe concentration problems.

At our first meeting she was dressed completely in black, wore a headscarf, and answered questions very monosyllabically. She made almost no eye contact with me, and fixed her gaze on the interpreter; my impression was that she was very careful with what she said. She reported that since the birth of her youngest child she had not been able to rest. There had been a mix-up at the hospital, her child had been given a wristband with the wrong name, and since then she had been afraid that this was not her child.

In the course of our conversations it became clear that as a child she had always had doubts as to whether she was her own mother's child, because she had looked different from her sisters. Her siblings had also teased her with the idea that she might be a 'cuckoo child'. Furthermore, the client suffered from a strong sense of guilt towards her husband and family: she had supposedly 'betrayed' her husband to the Chechen militia, and he had subsequently been captured and tortured. A large part of the therapy concentrated on our finding out together what possibilities for action and decision-making she had had in the past, and what possibilities she had available in the present. The client experienced relief when we established that in all her decisions she had always had the well-being of her family in mind and considered her own well-being to be secondary.

It became very clear in this case that Western therapeutic ideas about stronger self-development or the strengthening of emancipatory thoughts would have been rather counterproductive for the client at first. Interestingly, it later became possible for her to consider things such as taking a language course, after she had internalised the primacy of her family for herself.

Ms H: *Cut off from everyone*

Ms H and her two sons (aged 8 and 12 years) came from a Central American country. Her ex-husband had been persecuted by organised criminal gangs and seriously injured several times and had died in a German hospital. Ms H was afraid for her parents, who still lived in her homeland, because they were being constantly threatened by the same criminals. Ms H now lived with her sons in a small German village where no one spoke their language, and she suffered primarily from social isolation. The therapeutic sessions were held alternately with her alone and together with her sons. During one session, it emerged from the younger son that his mother sometimes became angry to the point of beating him – for example, when he did not clean his room. In the subsequent conversation it became clear that the mother was under considerable pressure to establish herself as an authority in front of her children because no male authority figure was present. Together we worked out other ways for her to show her assertiveness, such as by establishing clear rules about who had to do what and when, but also by establishing shared family time (e.g.,when all three of them cuddled up together to watch a film). Furthermore, the family's situation improved abruptly when another Spanish-speaking family moved into the village, alleviating the social loneliness.

Culturally varied evaluated methods of upbringing became recognisable in this case, and were communicated as such. Nevertheless, we could still discuss how violent upbringings had been proven to be harmful, and how it was necessary to apply alternatives without undermining the mother's parental authority.

Couple B: What cannot be expressed

This was an Iranian couple who had been living in Germany for some time. The woman suffered from depression and several psychosomatic symptoms; there was an unfulfilled desire for children, which was one of the reasons for the consultation. She seemed extremely tense, and her husband seemed exhausted. At the beginning of one session, the woman asked to be allowed to speak with me alone. Her husband then left the room, and she began to cry violently and could hardly speak. She said that she loved her husband but could hardly bear it if he approached her physically; if they had sex, she had to think about something else. She was always forced to recall that she had been abused as a child and teenager, first by her cousin and then by her father. She had kept silent about it for a long time, and had said nothing about it during her last stay in a psychiatric hospital, but she could not go on like this any longer. Her husband was not allowed to know about it; I had to promise not to tell him. While speaking she threatened to lose her ability to regulate several times, and it was constantly necessary to ground her in the here and now. The following sessions focused on how to deal with sexuality. The man suffered from his wife's distant behaviour, while the woman was constantly afraid of losing him because of it. In one-to-one conversations with the woman, it became clear that she was afraid that her husband would hold her responsible for the sexual abuse she had experienced, because she had been a teenager at the time. Initial relief was offered by the introduction of a complete temporary suspension of sexual activity, and also by addressing and reducing the woman's feelings of guilt during one-to-one sessions.

Conclusion

What are the central elements of family therapy and counselling work with refugees? One significant element is the permanent confrontation with powerlessness and loss of control, which also has a significant impact on therapists' and counsellors' experience of self-efficacy. These feelings must be contained, and require continuous clinical supervision. However, there are also methods and techniques that are helpful for working with this target group.

Manuals can be used to communicate information about traumatisation during the first period of counselling sessions (i.e., psychoeducation). Psychoeducation can be a resourced-based tool, but it can also be independent of clients' backgrounds. It is one of the first steps in any process concerning work with traumatisation, and it lays the foundation for successful therapy (Preitler, 2016, p. 78). It is not only clients who must be educated and thus prepared for the physical and psychological aftermath of their experiences, but also all staff working with traumatised people. The United Nations Inter-Agency Standing Committee has published the 'do no harm' guidelines. These state that all work with refugees needs to focus on the benchmark of not worsening their situation in any way, and on how staff can manage to achieve this (Inter-Agency Standing Committee, 2008, p. 7). Unfortunately, we also should not forget the significance and negative effects of everyday racism. Another important aspect of psychoeducation is offering information in the clients' first languages, or facilitating interpreters to do so (Machleidt et al., 2005).

Intercultural exploration, following Liedl and Abdallah-Steinkopff (2017, as cited in Liedl, 2018, p. 81), can be very helpful. This process involves six steps with respect to clients' cultural backgrounds:

- Exploring clients' views on their traumatisation, its origins, and possible help and interventions based on experiences in their home country
- Reviewing their biographical background, such as their culture and religion
- Identifying their individual 'taboos' regarding mental health
- Explaining possible scientific steps during the counselling process
- Conveying the origin of the disease, based on a scientific background
- Finding intercultural commonalities that may be helpful during counselling

In conclusion, we would like to point out some central principles in our work. First, family therapists and counsellors have to reflect on their own cultural stereotypes and face their own inner tensions in cases where values diverge (Rober & De Haene, 2014) – for example, regarding children's upbringing. Further, we have to focus on the detection of possible post-migration stressors (Liedl, 2018) and pay special attention to the quality of language mediators (Mucker et al., 2018). One of the most important aspects is the significance of resource-activating interventions and the search for resources (Schweitzer et al., 2019). We also have to consider the clients' disturbances and ideas about healing, and the significance of transgenerational aspects. Ultimately, the primary goal has to be helping clients mend their broken trust in other people and to counterbalance those feelings.

References

Altenthan, S., Betscher-Ott, S., Gotthardt, W., Hobmair, H. Höhlein, R., Ott, W., Pöll, R., & Schneider, K.-H. (2008). *Pädagogik*. Bildungsverlag EINS.

Asylum and Migration Information Network. (2019a). Asylsuchende. www.asyl.net/themen/bildung-und-arbeit/zugang-zu-arbeit/asylsuchende/

Asylum and Migration Information Network. (2019b). Geduldete. www.asyl.net/themen/bildung-und-arbeit/zugang-zu-arbeit/geduldete/

Bundestag. (2020). *Zahlen in der Bundesrepublik Deutschland lebender Flüchtlinge zum Stand 30. Juni 2020* (Bundestag Printed Document 19/22547). https://dip21.bundestag.de/dip21/btd/19/224/1922457.pdf

Federal Office of Statistics. (2021). *Migration und Integration: Schutzsuchende*. www.destatis.de/DE/Themen/Gesellschaft-Umwelt/Bevoelkerung/Migration-Integration/Glossar/schutzsuchende.html

Gahleitner, S. B., Zimmermann, D., & Zito, D. (2017). *Psychosoziale und traumapädagogische Arbeit mit geflüchteten Menschen.* Vandenhoeck & Ruprecht

Gavranidou, M., Niemiec, B., Magg, B. & Rosner, R. (2008). Traumatische Erfahrungen, aktuelle Lebensbedingungen im Exil und psychische Belastung junger Flüchtlinge. *Kindheit und Entwicklung, 17*(4), 224–231.

Gries, S., Longley, M., Kästner, D., & Gumz, A. (2020) Therapeutenmerkmale und Therapieabbruch. *Psychotherapeut, 65*, 425–443.

Gutmann, J. (2019). *Humane Psychiatrie: Psychosoziale Versorgung zwischen Anspruch und Wirklichkeit.* Kohlhammer Verlag.

Hantke, L., & Görges, H.-J. (2012). *Handbuch Traumakompetenz: Basiswissen für Therapie, Beratung und Pädagogik.* Junfermann Verlag.

Inter-Agency Standing Committee. (2008). *Guidelines on mental health and psychosocial support in emergency settings.* https://interagencystandingcommittee.org/system/files/legacy_files/Checkl ist%20for%20field%20use%20IASC%20MHPSS.pdf

Kleefeldt, E. (2018). *Resilienz, Empowerment und Selbstorganisation geflüchteter Menschen.* Vandenhoeck & Ruprecht

Kühn, M. (2013). Macht Eure Welt endlich wieder mit zu meiner. In J. Bausum., L. U. Besser, M. Kühn, W. Wilma. (Eds), *Tramapädagogik: Grundlagen, Arbeitsfelder und Methoden für die pädagogische Praxis* (3rd ed., pp. 24–35). Juventa & Beltz Juventa.

Liedl, A. (2018). *Psychotherapeutische Versorgung von geflüchteten Menschen: Konzepte und Methoden im interkulturellen Setting.* Vandenhoek & Ruprecht.

Liedl, A., Schäfer, U., & Knaevelsrud, C. (2013). *Psychoedukation bei posttraumatischen Belastungsstörungen.* Klett-Cotta.

Machleidt, W., Garlipp, P., & Calliess, I. T. (2005). Die 12 Sonnenberger Leitlinien -Handlungsimpulse fur die psychiatrisch-psychotherapeutische Versorgung von Migranten. In H. Assion (Ed.), *Migration und seelische Gesundheit* (p. 215–216). Springer Verlag.

Measham, T., Guzder, J., Rousseau, C., Pacione, L., Blais-McPherson, M. & Nadeau, L. (2014). Refugee children and their families: Supporting psychological well-being and positive adaption following migration. *Current Problems in Pediatric and Adolescent Health Care, 44 (7)*, 208–215.

Media Service Integration. (2020). Zahl der Flüchtlinge: Wie viele Flüchtlinge leben in Deutschland? https://mediendienst-integration.de/migration/flucht-asyl/zahl-der-fluechtlinge.html

Mlodoch, K. (2017). *Gewalt, Flucht – Trauma?* Vandenhoeck & Ruprecht.

Mucker, J. Bautz, W. u., & Hadzic, E. (2018). Rahmenbedingungen für Psychotherapie und Beratung unter Einsatz von Sprachmittlern und Sprachmittlerinnen. In S. Schriefers & S. u. E. Hadzic (Eds), *Sprachmittlung in Psychotherapie und Beratung mit geflüchteten Menschen* (pp. 25–39). Vandenhoeck & Ruprecht.

Preitler, B. (2016). *An ihrer Seite sein: Psychosoziale Betreuung von traumatisierten Flüchtlingen.* Studienverlag.

Quindeau, I., & Rauwald, M. (Eds). (2017). *Soziale Arbeit mit unbegleiteten minderjährigen Flüchtlingen: Traumapädagogische Konzepte für die Praxis.* Beltz Juventa.

Rober, P. u. L., & De Haene, L. (2014). Intercultural therapy and the limitations of a cultural competency framework. *Journal of Family Therapy, 36*(Supp. 1), 3–20.

Rogers, C. R. (1983). *Therapeut und Klient: Grundlagen der Gesprächspsychotherapie.* Fischer Verlag.

Schellong, J., Hansschmidt, F., Ehring, T. Knaevelsrud, C., Schäfer, I., Rau, H., Dyer, A. & Krüger-Gottschalk, A. (2019). Diagnostik der PTBS im Spannungsfeld von DSM-V und ICD-11. *Nervenarzt, 90*. https://doi.org/10.1007/s00115-018-0668-0

Schweitzer, J., Schliessler, C., Kohl, R. M., Nikendei, C., & Ditzen, B. (2019). Systemische Notfallberatung mit geflüchteten Menschen in einer Erstregistrierungsstelle. *Familiendynamik, 44*, 144–154.

Turrini, G. et al. (2019). Efficacy and acceptability of psychosocial interventions in asylum seekers and refugees: Systematic review and meta-analysis. *Epidemiology and Psychiatric Sciences, 28(4)*, 376–388.

Völter, B., & Reichmann, U. (Eds). (2017). *Rekonstruktiv Denken und Handeln: Rekonstruktive Soziale Arbeit als professionelle Praxis.* Verlag Barbara Budrich.

Weinberger, S. (2011). *Klientenzentrierte Gesprächsführung: Lern- und Praxisanleitung für psychosoziale Berufe.* (13 ed., pp. 37–65). Beltz & Juventa.

Werle, L. (2020). *Kultursensible Beratung von jungen Frauen mit Traumaerfahrungen: Perspektiven für die psychosoziale Gesprächsführung* [Unpublished master's dissertation]. Hochschule Neubrandenburg.

11
BI-NATIONAL AND MULTICULTURAL EXPAT COUPLES IN MEXICO CITY

Exploring Covert Cultural Contracts

Jason James Platt and Elizabeth Ann Willems

Introduction

Clinical Vignette

Salome was born in Barranquilla, Colombia and moved to Bogota to study accounting. After she finished her degree, she was hired at an international Non-Governmental Organization (NGO). Two years later she was promoted and given additional responsibilities. This led to the opportunity to be a part of a team that worked closely with the emergency financial services program of the United States embassy. It was in this role that she first met Cory, who was completing a twelve-month assignment at the embassy. Cory was born in the United States in Sherwood, Oregon and after earning a degree in economics he was hired as an economic Foreign Service officer. He was very excited about his emerging international life, both professionally and personally.

Cory had invited Salome out for drinks a few times, but she had always declined because she was still self-conscious about her English. One night though she was at a karaoke bar with a few friends and ran into Cory. After the group shared a few aguardientes, Cory began flirting the best he could in his broken Spanish. They ended up drinking and dancing until near daybreak and after that evening, they began dating. Three months later, Cory learned about a position available in Mexico City, Mexico and applied. Once he knew he had been hired, he decided he could not go without Salome, so he asked her to marry him. Salome agreed and two months later they were married and living in Mexico.

It was an exciting whirlwind romance, but soon the profound changes they had experienced, as well as the challenges of being from two different national contexts and differing cultures, began to weigh on their relationship. Salome identifies as Afro-Colombian, but it should be understood that the notion and terms regarding ethnic and racial groups have distinctive meanings linked to Colombia's unique history, cultural groups, politics, linguistic, and territorialized communal and traditional life forms (Restrepo, 2018). Cory views himself as a White U.S.-American but has not given significant thought to his own

DOI: 10.4324/9781003297871-13

race or culture. He prefers to think that "we are all just humans." In recent months, it has become a challenge for them to discuss the ways their differences influence their relationship. They were also dealing with the challenges of being in a third national and cultural context that neither of them knew well. A significant portion of daily tasks fell on Salome to handle because she spoke Spanish. Also, while both of them had improved their ability to speak in a second language, Salome was frustrated that they primarily spoke in English. This was particularly difficult in arguments because she struggled to put her feelings adequately into words and felt disadvantaged. She also could not begin seeking employment because of a limitation with her current visa. Her career was important to her and she did not like feeling dependent on Cory for financial support. Cory was gone most of the day and she was left alone in the apartment and felt isolated. Cory on the other hand was excited about this new stage of his career and the connections and friends he was making at work. Cory felt blindsided when Salome told him one night that she was considering going back to Colombia. They began to try and work on their relationship, but things escalated again several weeks later when they discovered that Salome was pregnant. It was at this point that they reached out to set up an appointment for couple therapy.

Clinical Work with Global Citizens

Dr. Willems and I have been providing therapy to bi-national and multicultural expatriate (used interchangeably with "expat") mixed-sex and same-sex couples in Mexico City, Mexico for over 15 years. This fictional story of Salome and Cory's history highlights many common challenges and themes to consider when providing clinical services to expatriate and bi-national couples. A central factor in the struggles of couples like Salome and Cory is that there are often many unexamined cultural assumptions that can result in misunderstandings and feelings of both resentment or even betrayal. Additionally, the quid pro quo or unconscious "something for something" reciprocal behaviors that develop in all couples (Lederer and Jackson, 1968) often need to be renegotiated following a change of national context.

For many reasons, as we will explain in the chapter, a new country can cause an upheaval in previous relational agreements. In this chapter we discuss how clinicians can assist expats in negotiating changes and evolutions in their individual identities and relationships and to gain increased consciousness of the covert cultural contracts influencing their relationships. We share thoughts about why it is beneficial for expat couples to explore the many different layers of cultural adjustment. This may involve gaining insights about each of their own cultural backgrounds as well as how their current national context might have an influence on their relationship. There are also a number of common challenges that expats may face, including shifts in their identities, cross-cultural adjustments, adaptation to a new host culture, complex and competing conceptualizations about race, class, and other social issues, balancing cultural traditions, language issues, logistics fatigue, isolation, complex work and career issues, and raising third culture children. In our experience, for many couples from different nationalities, these issues tend to go unexplored until conflicts and misunderstandings develop.

There is no single story about expatriate and bi-national couples. We (Drs. Platt and Willems) would like to recognize that intimate partner relationships can come in varied forms, including but not limited to distance and in-person relationships, short- and long-term, consensual non-monogamous, and polyamorous relationships. In this chapter, we primarily focus on long-term intimate partnerships between mixed and same-sex monog-amous couples who live locally and who are residing in Mexico by choice rather than due to forced displacement. All names and biological-sociological data in this chapter have been altered to protect client confidentiality. Also, as can be observed in our introduction, in some instances we have also created fictional case examples that illustrate common themes we have observed in our clinical work.

Covert Cultural Contracts

As we think about the common difficulties faced by expatriate and bi-national couples, perhaps the most common theme is frustration about their partners not living up to expectations. These expectations are often based on differences in assumptions linked to their nationality. We think of these in terms of covert cultural contracts, where each partner has expectations that they may not have voiced overtly, but still result in a sense of betrayal, confusion, and resentment when the unspoken contract is broken. For example, a common covert cultural contract among expat couples in Mexico City that often results in tensions is about how each partner expects to spend their weekends. Halverson, Hancock, and Platt (2016) found that many partners from the United States hold the expectation that weekends will be spent engaging in individual- or child-focused leisure activities (e.g., resting at home, group activities, etc.) while many Mexican partners hold the expectation that weekends are to be spent with extended family, particularly the parents of the partners. These types of differences in expectations may lay dormant for many years and only emerge years later, perhaps if the couple returns to one of their home nations or after children are born.

This phenomenon of covert cultural contracts is particularly likely when the relationship had its origins in an event (e.g., the couple met during a study abroad program or on a tem-porary assignment or other whirlwind beginnings) versus when it was a relationship-driven courtship that developed over time. Event-driven courtships are more likely to result in a divorce or termination given that couples may not have had sufficient time to get to know one another at a deep level (Rahmati and Bahrami Nejad, 2019). A beginning step we find useful is to ask about their courtship and to determine if there is a need for expat couples to engage in more relationship development work. Research has shown that couples who do not develop some shared perceptions of reality during courtships are likely to have less sta-bility in their relationships (Wilson & Huston, 2013). Below we share a few of the common topics in which bi-national couples may have different perceptions of realities, linked to their nationalities and cultures.

Expat and Identity: What Is in a Name?

It is estimated that 258 million people (or one out of every 30 people) currently live abroad and it is predicted that number will continue to rapidly increase in the coming years (Stroud, Jones, & Brien, 2018). With the highest number of people in the earth's history currently living outside their nation of origin, therapists will increasingly be called on to support individuals and couples in navigating expat life and challenges. A central component of this work will likely be linked to changes in one's identity and how those changes may influence their relationships.

Most U.S.-trained therapists have limited exposure to healing and change practices around the world and are primarily only educated in U.S.-originating psychological concepts and theories of mental health (Arnett, 2008; Platt, 2022). This includes the majority of identity models, which are generally from an individualistic perspective. These models tend to suggest that identity and personality are inherent traits or that they tend to be consistent across the lifespan. That is not our experience. Young, Natrajan-Tyagi and Platt (2014) have noted, "Most models that explore the concept of identity were developed in a context that predates modern globalization. Psychologists have yet to understand the consequences that globalization will have on self-identity" (p. 177). Given systems theorists' recognition of how much a person's sense of self is influenced by (and can change) based on the interactional patterns in which their lives are embedded (Watzlawick, Beavin, & Jackson, 1967), family therapists may be able to utilize a different and useful perspective of identity for bi-national expat couples. We suggest that a systems framework may be particularly useful when considering the unique challenges faced by expatriate couples. One could argue that from this lens, human Iidentity is far more fluid and changeable. In our experience, most of the people we work with have found moving to a new national context to be profoundly transformative and often involves a period of identity crisis. A person's personality and identity are often linked to the expectation of consistency of behavior by important others in their lives. When a person moves abroad, where both relational and cultural expectations are not the same, this often creates a re-evaluation of one's identity. This reconsideration of one's identity can be occurring for both members of a couple and can lead to a need to re-evaluate their relationship. For some, this can be freeing and lead to growth and change and increased intimacy. For others, the experience can be disorienting and can lead to significant relational difficulties.

A relevant piece of the expat puzzle is how a person comes to think of and label themselves. An expatriate is someone who lives outside their nation of origin. We use this umbrella term in this chapter, but therapists working with this community should be aware that individuals may consider the term as pejorative. Many expats feel the term is limited in its ability to capture their experience or at least a desire to clarify which meaning the term holds for them. The unique aspects of their life abroad may get lost when they are lumped in with such a vast and diverse group. The term is sometimes linked with the idea that a person has rejected their nation of birth, or on the other extreme, the term may imply that people only intend to stay in the new nation temporarily. Others may feel the term implies that they are superficially immersed within the new nation and culture and reside within a bubble among fellow expatriates. However, on the other hand, many people embrace the term expat and being part of the expatriate community might be very central to their identity. Diversely, the term may be considered biased, based on country of origin, socioeconomic status (SES), and/or racialized ethnicity. In general, terminology becomes an important point of reflection when it is used as a political tool or to dehumanize. For example, often individuals with roots in a North Atlantic country are described as expats, whereas individuals with home countries in Africa, Asia, the Middle East, South America, and parts of Oceana may have other intercultural terms applied to them. One's socioeconomic status can also be a factor in how one identifies (e.g., working abroad versus immigrating).

There are many reasons someone may live outside the country in which they were born and the way they label themselves signals how they have incorporated the experience into their identity. Individuals might identify as immigrants, refugees, engaging in a study abroad, global nomads, having relocated due to work, missionaries, on international assignment, retirees, or as the partner of a local. We recommend that therapists ask and learn how their patients have come to live in the current nation in which they are residing and create a space to discuss how the process has influenced their views of themselves. While the stories may overlap, we have found that providing an opportunity for couples to discuss both their history moving across national boundaries and their courtship history (sometimes these are stories that overlap and sometimes they occurred at different times) is therapeutic both as an assessment and intervention.

CROSS-CULTURAL ADJUSTMENT

Intercultural Model

Milton Bennett's Developmental Model of Intercultural Sensitivity (DMIS; 1986, 1993, 2004, 2013) was created as a framework to explain people's responses to cultural differences. Bennett observed how people confront cultural unlikeness as they learned to become more competent intercultural communicators. He placed these observations into positions along a continuum of sensitivity to cultural heterogeneity. Bennett's model posits a positive correlation between complexity of experience of cultural difference and competence in intercultural relations. The DMIS continuum stretches from ethnocentrism, the experience of one's own culture as fundamental to existence, to *ethnorelativism*, the experience of culture (both one's own and others) as contextually based. Intercultural sensitivity may not come naturally and can contribute to conflict and misunderstanding within the context of multicultural couple dialogue.

Benette's DMIS can be observed in Arabella's cultural conceptualizations. Born in the Netherlands, a self-identified introvert, Arabella preferred to "safely" remain in her small hometown. However, after having met and wed her Mexican-born partner, Antonio, Arabella moved with him to Mexico City. Arabella began to resent residing abroad making negative generalizations about her host culture. Given that one's nationality is linked to one's identity, the disdain she felt toward Mexico felt very personal to her partner. The couple began to experience conflict and this ultimately led to their separation.

Throughout our work together, I (Dr. Willems) both validated Arabella's emotional response to personal experiences and provided counterexamples for her negative cultural generalizations of Mexico. We built rapport in our work together while she also forged strong social networks with Mexicans and non-Mexicans alike. Following an eventual divorce from Antonio and an understandably lengthy deliberation about where she would live next, Arabella began preparing to return to her home country with their children. Given that she would still have a relationship with Antonio as a co-parent and that she would be raising bi-national children, her work on intercultural communication remained important. Having lived away from her home country and experiencing meaningful interactions with members of other cultures she began to develop greater ethnorelativism. She also developed a more complex view of her own national context of origin and was better able to contextualize both positive and negative experiences in her host country, rather than make wholly negative generalizations.

As therapists, an important part of the work needed to assist couples to find a more balanced perspective regarding their different national contexts involves engaging in our own self-of-the-therapist work around nationality. This helps us limit the problematic forms of nationalism that can creep into clinical practice. In particular, we seek to demonstrate in our work the idea of critical patriotism, or "the ability to honestly and fairly reflect and assess the values, history, culture, and traditions of one's country. Inherent in this process is the ability to consider the nation's virtues and vices in a balanced way" (Platt & Laszloffy, 2013, p. 442). While we do not directly teach this concept in our work, we have witnessed the relational implications of clients holding nationalistic views. We believe it is helpful to facilitate dialogues that can help couples to gain more nuanced views about both their nations of origin and their host nations.

Psychological Comfort with Host Country Culture

Like Arabella, an individual's comfort in their host country can vary over time. For example, Zainol, Tambi, Ali, and Azami (2020) found that among a sample of Malaysian professionals living in a host country, four components were found to influence psychological distress including interaction, adjustment, reward, social life, and living environment. Unmet needs for psychological comfort were projected to negatively affect the working environment. This can be exemplified in my work with Angela and Jonas, a Portugal-born, married mixed-sex couple who lived in two host nations before beginning their three-year assignment in Mexico City. The capitol city was a mutually agreed upon location for Angela and Jonas. After arriving and beginning her new position Angela began to adjust with relatively low distress.

While Angela's career trajectory was improved by the move, Jonas had a very different experience. Limited by visa restrictions, Jonas, a mid-40s professional, found himself expending increasing time on a dwindling number of professional tasks. Jonas' interactions were limited to those with his wife and brief conversations with the contractors working in their building. His limited and superficial exposure to the inhabitants of this megalopolis contributed to increasing acculturation stress.

While together in their apartment Jonas' increasingly disclosed his frustrations with their host culture. Angela experienced internal conflict between her need for independence and pressure to *provide* an enjoyable acculturation experience. Jonas, while socially isolated, began to focus intensely on Angela's behaviors, which she found intrusive. The two entered into couple therapy when they reached the brink of separation. Over time, and with the support of couple therapy, Jonas found a rewarding job and built rapport with peers. The two met others and engaged in subjectively meaningful activities, participating in group day-tours of the towns outlying Mexico City. As they began to explore the nature of their problems in couple therapy, their psychological comfort increased, and they decided to remain in their marriage. Their story illustrates what Zainol, Tambi, Ali, and Azami (2020) found within their research regarding the vital importance of a person's social life on the success of the individuals living in a host culture.

Cultural Conceptualization of Social Justice

Just as Angela and Jonas observed different responses to Mexico and different degrees of psychological comfort, many couples experience challenges in managing their different approaches to a novel culture. Specifically, when living in a host cultural differences in decisions related to social justice may contribute to relational discord. Leung and Stephan's (2001) model of justice posits that morality and justice are simultaneously culture-specific and universal. The authors elaborate that rules and abstract constructs combine with distinct, context-relevant information to yield morality and justice-related decisions (2001).

The complexities of social issues being both culture-specific and universal can be partially exhibited in the dynamic between Andrea, a White U.S. American-born cisgender woman and her multiethnic Mexican-born cisgender husband, Manuel. They welcomed children into their family during the length of her four-year post. As the domestic and professional workload increased for both parents the family increasingly relied on the support of their domestic employee Isabel, a Hispanic childcare professional with Nahua ancestry. As Isabel began to work enough hours to be considered a full-time employee, Andrea and Manuel experienced conflict as they discussed Isabel's employment package.

Andrea was less conscious of the historical events and current political realities of Mexico and filtered her experience through her U.S.-formed lens of social justice. She expressed concern about her potential bias while reviewing Isabel's employment benefits. In her discussions with Manuel, Andrea communicated a desire to mirror aspects of the worker's rights she observed in U.S. employment (e.g., authoritative managerial communication style, access to insurance plans, paid leave, etc.). She had been reared in a middle-income home and had little exposure to domestic employment management. Manuel, raised in an upper-income household, had been exposed to at least two generations of family members who continually hired domestic employees. He was hesitant to include benefits and pay above the average daily wage for the role ($300MXN; $15USD). He experienced the aforementioned wage as a common-practice rate and went on to consult with his mother for recommendations. Ultimately, with independent reflections and mutual exploration regarding the contributing factors for their different viewpoints, the two were able to mutually agree upon an approach to their employment practices with the support of couple therapy. As Leung and Stephan's model (2001) posits, in this case we observed that providing a space for a dialogue about rules and abstract constructs combined with assisting the couple to gain more contextual information helped them in making decisions that worked for both of them.

Multilingual Couples

Facilitating Language Agreements

As individuals living in host-cultures are often living and using multiple languages, we suggest that couples should be encouraged to consider the ways that language can influence their relationship. Language is not just words and grammar; it is central to how we make meaning of and experience the world. Many words in one's language have no exact translation into another language. Language is personal and tied to our cultures and identities. When partnering with a person who does not share the same native or first language, it is often a recipe for miscommunication and misunderstanding. Klerk (2001) has suggested that "When two languages coexist within one family, on a micro-level, spouses, either consciously or unconsciously, work out their own 'language policy', and the patterns of language maintenance or language shift are set in motion" (p. 1). In our experience with couples in crisis, the language policy that develops is rarely an overt agreement and often one partner is left feeling a loss of self and possibly a degree of resentment.

Patterns linked to power that occur at the macro level are often isomorphically recreated in a couple's relationship. Dominant or major languages, based on economic, social, or nationality prestige, tend to be privileged over minority languages (Wolff, 2000; Igboanusi & Peter, 2005; Wolff, 2000). There may also be an intersection between language and gender politics that can play out in couples. Research has found that women are "more likely to adapt their language use than men in cross-language partnerships" (Lyon, 1996, p. 188). Given the importance of language, as well as John Gottman's extensive research into the importance of men being able to accept the influence of their partners, we suggest that there is value in expat couples being encouraged to dialogue about decisions about language use.

Beyond the issue about which language is spoken by couples, sociolinguistic research points to other surprising challenges that multilingual couples may face. For example, Lev-Ari, Ho and Keysar (2018) found that "merely expecting nonnative speakers to have lower linguistic competence can lead people to remember their interaction with them in less detail and in a manner that is more in line with their expectation" (p. 845). In a couple, this may be happening in two directions. Couples may not be accurately remembering their conversations with their partner. Rather than relating to them, they are interacting with an internalized and storied version of their partner. Lev-Ari and Keysar (2010) also found that because of the extra mental effort it might take to understand someone speaking in a second language, people tend to give less credibility to what is being said by the second language speaker. Trust is a core component of successful relationships, thus this finding may be important for a therapist to explore.

We have found it useful to ask bi-national and bilingual couples, "How do the two of you decide when to speak which language?" Aimed at making the covert process that has occurred overt, the question usually strikes couples as funny. Fairly quickly though, the question can spark conversations that reveal meaningful couple dynamics. A follow-up question might be "When the two of you argue, what language do you typically argue in?" When the emotional stakes are higher, it can be particularly frustrating to be required to speak in a second language.

Logistics Fatigue

Rodrygo (52) met Henrick (31) while in Copenhagen, Denmark, for several months providing consultation for a shipbuilding company interested in partnering with a firm in Brazil. Born in Brazil and educated in the United States, Rodrygo speaks Portuguese, English, Spanish, and rudimentary Arabic. His work has allowed him to live as a global citizen for several decades. Henrick was born in Sønderho, a village with a population of about 300 people and he had moved to Copenhagen just a few years earlier where he worked for a landscaping company. He speaks Danish and English and has an interest in going to college to study business. They met at a smoky jazz concert at a popular gay club and felt an instant connection. They began seeing each other regularly and Henrick became an invaluable informal cultural ambassador for Rodrygo, who confidently was able to help him navigate many of the complexities of Danish life. Henrick also felt as if Rodrygo was an emissary for him as he was exposed to international and affluent communities in Copenhagen. As the time drew closer for Rodrygo to leave Copenhagen, both desired to have more time to see how their relationship might develop. Rodrygo ultimately invited Henrick to join him for his next assignment in Mexico City. Henrick, having never been abroad, was excited and accepted.

The first month in Mexico was exciting and fun for both of them. Soon though, it became evident that the quid quo pro of their early relationship had changed. Henrick's inability to speak Spanish and limited experience navigating new cultures hampered his ability to assist Rodrygo as he did in Denmark. Rodrygo began to manage the majority of the logistics of their new life, such as often complex processes such as renting a place locating and arranging housing, setting up banking accounts, completing important forms in Spanish such as those related to their visas, etc. as well as the majority of endless mundane tasks such as figuring out how to get rid of garbage, where to get dry cleaning done, how to get potable water delivered, and other household-related issues. Fairly quickly Henrick began to experience an uncomfortable dependence and loss of personal power. Rodrygo began to feel overburdened and resentful from the logistics fatigue and one result was that he began to find it easier to go places alone. The unaddressed shift in the prior quid pro quo of their relationship completely altered their relationship satisfaction and threatened the still developing romantic connection.

Research on expatriates has suggested that most people who move to a new nation experience a stage of disintegration, which is characterized by a loss of sense of competence in the handling of daily tasks (Furnham & Bochner, 1989). Oddou (2005) describes this challenge stating that, "In the general environment, the expatriate knows how and where to purchase items, find locations, use public transportation, register vehicles, and all the other things associated with general living. In the foreign environment, the expatriate must learn all of these things – and often in a foreign language" (p. 759). We have found that this stage can last for many years and that people can feel fatigued due to constantly having to accomplish tasks that would be simpler for them in their nation of origin. It can also result in relationship strains when an imbalance develops between partners, due to factors such as language. It also can lead to a partner feeling a loss of independence and unhealthy dependence on their partner.

Personal Reflections

As expatriates ourselves, logistics fatigue can also become a self-of-the-therapist issue to address. The deadline for this chapter has come and gone. The last section to be written is on logistics fatigue. I (Dr. Platt) message Dr. Willems promising to finish the section soon, but first I need to prove to a U.S. university in the Midwest that I am a U.S. citizen. The power grid in Mexico is overburdened and my building's wiring system is old and I currently do not have electricity. I have taken the day off to wait for an electrician who was scheduled to come at 10:00am. It is now 4:00pm and the electrician has messaged me to say that he will be arriving "ahorita," which loosely culturally translates to "later," "tomorrow," "never," or "please stop bothering me." I am hesitant to leave the house in case he arrives, but I need to find a place to print and scan the forms for the university. In the meantime, I have spent hours on the phone trying to find a way to get a replacement social security card. I could do it online if I had a U.S. driver's license, but I only have my Mexican one. One Social Security staff member tells me the only way to get a replacement card is by mailing my passport to them (making it impossible for me to leave Mexico if any family emergency occurred). I am also informed that they would return my passport and replacement card through the highly unreliable national mail system that few people use in Mexico. Ultimately, I discover that I can get a replacement card through the United States embassy, but the semester would likely be over by the time I can get an appointment.

Dr. Willems and I commiserate. She shares the frustration that U.S. banks often wrongly identify transactions in Mexico as fraudulent, which can lead to card cancelations. Working internationally means working in different currencies and needing to figure out ways to transfer from one currency in one country to another currency in another country. That also has tax implications in the different national contexts we work. Dr. Willems shared how her U.S. bank will not allow her to add the Mexican bank for wire transfers and how often she cannot verify her identity easily because she does not have a U.S. cell phone number. Both of us have needed to rely on friends and family members to receive confirmation text messages. We both feel a little burdensome and dependent on other people to help us manage U.S.-based online platforms and mail while in Mexico. We also discuss the ways language influences our day-to-day lives. While we may both feel confident in our Spanish language abilities, in Mexico City one also needs familiarity with Nahuatl words and we each find ourselves often asking, "What is that again?" Also, there is not just one Spanish language to learn. For example, the name of food products in Spanish is country-dependent, so if we are at a Spanish, Mexican, Argentinian, or Uruguayan restaurant, the words used change. We have both noticed how easy it is to fall into the habit of handing the phone over to a native Spanish-speaker when there are administrative tasks to accomplish by phone and the language barriers feel too strong.

It could be easy for Dr. Willems and I to fall into an expat habit of simply ranting about the challenges we face, but we attempt to shift our dialogue into a form of peer supervision and engage in self-of-the-therapist work. We recognize that many of our frustrations are rooted in privilege (nationality, economic, racial, language, etc.). It is important to work through these issues in order to be able to model for clients productive ways of managing logistics fatigue. While for us it could be easy to fall into ineffective gripe sessions with our expat clients, domestic therapists may have different self-of-the-therapist work to do. For example, there may be either the tendency to underestimate the level of complexity that their expat clients may be navigating or perhaps the other extreme of conveying a message that living abroad is not a viable life choice given challenges being a global nomad can create.

There is something empowering for clients as they learn they are not alone in their struggle and that there are stages beyond disintegration. It was also helpful to become conscious and therefore able to dialogue and brainstorm about ways to share the tasks of daily living. Both had not considered the way logistics fatigue was having an influence on their relationship. As with other common themes, they did not have a conscious awareness of how the shift to living in a new nation had changed their previous way of being in relationship with each other. Not only does overt discussions about the shift in previous agreements normalize their experience, it makes it possible to create new agreements.

Isolation and Building Community

A 2020 study (Jobbatical, 2020) found that 43% of international hires and 48% of relocating spouses find making local friends challenging. This was the case for Noah, a cisgender man in his mid-twenties who had built positive relationships with his family of origin, an active lifelong membership in his religious community, and several strong friendships all in his U.S. hometown. He felt content in his recent marriage to Caleb, a cisgender male who was raised in Mexico City. The two decided to begin their married lives together in the bustling Mexican metropolis. Despite Noah's natural social agility, the fledgling networks he built in his host-culture left him devoid of kindred connections.

In Mexico City, it is customary for couples to spend significant periods of time together with extended family members on weekends. Noah initially enjoyed sharing traditional meals with his in-laws. However, the expectations of reuniting every weekend became challenging. He was conflicted with managing family expectations, work demands, and the crescive void, which his hometown religious community once filled. He attempted to connect with local coreligionists but found the cultural differences difficult to overcome. This attests to what Hobson et. al. (1998) asserted, that change in home or career path is an important life stressor.

Noah provides an example of common challenges to expat adjustment. Despite having a secure attachment with his partner, he has struggled to develop a sense of community apart from her. He has not experienced a loss of network, difficulty to finding or connecting significantly will develop either friendships or professional connections. local community members and he negatively compares his present social situation against his prior social life before moving to Mexico. unsatisfactorily contrasting novel social relationships with friendships built from childhood over decades. Similarly, Shen and Kram's (2011) study, which examined developmental networks among individuals living in host countries, highlighted the importance of psychosocial and cross-cultural transition support in these individual's intercultural adaptation. Moreover, Filipič Sterle, M., et al. (2018) found that increased subjective availability of socioemotional support was related to expatriates' increased work adjustment and interaction. Correspondingly, after discussing cultural differences in therapy, Noah's positive acculturation process eventually included scheduled calls to his childhood confidants, increased visits to his hometown, alternating weekend schedules of schoolwork and in-law gatherings, as well as mindful engagements with other community members in his host culture. Like in the case of Noah and Caleb, many expat couples (either one or both individuals) are initially far removed from previously-built support system – family, friends or community – that might have bolstered a struggling marriage

Working Internationally

Millions of people work abroad in host countries and 90% of them are accompanied by a relationship partner (Slobodin, 2019). Adjusting to a host culture can trigger *acculturative stress* (Berry, 1970), or a reduction in health status, which may relate to an individual's experiences of acculturation. Mental health symptoms associated with moving internationally and the resulting high acculturative stress include depression, anxiety, somatization, suicidal thoughts, identity confusion, and subjective alienation (Castro, 2003; Hovey & King, 1997). The experiences of acculturative stress may differ within a couple. For example, one partner may be experiencing the stresses related to working within a new national context and culture. McNulty (2015) noted the extraordinary levels of stress that can overwhelm an expat's coping mechanisms and "frequently results in polarizing behaviors such as infidelity, excessive drinking, abuse, and workaholism as a means of coping" (p. 127). Whether their partner may be experiencing Trailing Spouse Syndrome (TSS), the isolation, depression, dependency, and identity crisis that can result from making sacrifices related to their careers and other goals to support one's partner's success (McNulty, 2012) can be difficult to navigate. These experiences can be happening simultaneously and can lead to partners feeling alone.

Cross-cultural employees need not confront these challenges alone, however. Intercultural researcher Sally J. Walton (1990) asserted that intercultural training programs should ideally incorporate the concepts of hardiness, thoughtfulness, and coping, self-efficacy, and social support to decrease acculturative stress and build growth and learning for employees working cross-culturally. With these interventions available we are able to expand our clinical approach with couples and individuals in Mexico to consider the unique experience of having a bi-cultural employee within the family system. Recent statistics have shown that 44% of relocating spouses were not fully employed outside of domestic/parenting capacities, though 17% were looking for work (Jobbatical, 2020). Throughout my (Dr. Willems) work in Mexico I have come across various combinations of legal work permission within expat couples. While the primary visa holder (i.e., the partner who initiated a relocation through first receiving work permission in a host country) may have administrative support through the sponsoring employer in the host country, intimate partners may be expected to independently procure legal working status in the host nation. If unable to work outside the home (in a domestic capacity) in the host country, the non-visa procuring partner may experience difficulty in adjusting to a novel identity. I have observed that failure to psychologically process this change in advance of a relocation can contribute to resentment within couples. Additionally, unmarried couples may face pressure to form a legal union in order to obtain a visa for the non-primary visa-holder. This can confuse the way the intimate relationship is conceptualized and experienced.

While living in a host culture the members of a couple may experience adjustments in their careers. For example, several of my clients began working remotely (pre-dating the structures of remote work established during the COVID-19 pandemic lockdown) while transitioning to life in Mexico. For employees whose companies were based in a different time zone, work-day schedules adjusted in response. The change in schedule (e.g., sleep/wake schedules that differed greatly from their partners) in some cases contributed to insomnia, conflict, and unmet needs for togetherness with one's partner. Furthermore, couples living in a host culture who lose community support, such as childcare during working hours, may have to divide these responsibilities among themselves. I have observed among my clients that this restructuring of domestic work within the couple can contribute to conflict.

Parenting Third Culture Kids

Parenting practices vary significantly around the world and cultural norms influence parenting behaviors (Johnson, Radesky, & Zuckerman, 2013). Parenting is a thematic point of contention in most marriages (Crippen & Brew, 2007), and understandably, perhaps more so among couples with different cultural foundations. Accordingly, intercultural couples may experience conflict or confluence regarding parenting expectations. In my (Dr. Willems) work in Mexico, I have observed bi-national parent conflict related to parenting style (e.g., authoritarian, permissive, uninvolved, authoritative; Maccoby & Martin, 1983), rites of passage, spiritual practices, meal choices, and sleep schedules. Likewise, I have observed culturally similar couples raising their children in this host country while confronting parenting expectation asymmetry between themselves and their community.

Ruth Hill Useem conceived the term Third Culture Kids (TCKs) to describe children who may have complex identities based on their experiences as global citizens. The term now includes a person of mixed culture, of mixed ethnicity, children of individuals who have immigrated, children of those with refugee status, children of racialized-ethnic minorities, international adoptees, and those who live in a minority culture within their passport nation (Van Reken & Pollock, 2017; Wells, 2020). Within my clinical work in Mexico City, I have observed TCKs contemplating the benefits and drawbacks of living interculturally. Some have struggled to feel rooted in long-term friendships while others thrived by developing strong social skills applicable in novel circumstances. TCKs have reported feeling like cultural Others (Said, 1978). Clients of mixed ethnicity felt disallowed from claiming their ancestry. This cultural imposter syndrome (Harrison & Lane, 2000), likened to racial imposter syndrome (Demby & Meraji, 2017, 00:04), can leave individuals feeling self-doubt if their internal self does not match others' perception of their identity.

The question then arises as to how parents of TCKs can work together to support the unique needs of their children. Wells (2020) recommended recognizing and validating TCK's unique needs by 1) processing grief following a relocation, 2) offering a transitional object, 3) discussing what a child can anticipate in their new environment, 4) maintaining stable attachment figures across changing circumstances, 5) transmitting family traditions, and 6) seeking out small communities of TCKs with similar heritage for example. Differences in parenting styles may be subjectively insurmountable to some multicultural couples. Nevertheless, clinicians can also assist parents in identifying the ways their children may also benefit from their varied parenting practices. Regardless of the circumstances, couples raising TCKs will undoubtedly benefit from discussing their unique circumstances and values around parenting and to develop strategies for finding common ground.

We would also like to briefly mention that when expat or bi-national couples with children divorce or separate, issues of custody can become extremely complicated. The laws regarding custody vary in each nation and there may also be power differences between the couple based on their visa status, gender, or nationality. Couples may disagree on which country has jurisdiction and where the divorce should occur; a decision that can have profound financial and custody implications. It is not uncommon for an expat parent to feel trapped in a nation or limited in their ability to cross boarders as freely as they might have historically. A parent may feel it is within their right to take a child to their home nation, yet such actions can be treated as child abduction and have significant consequences. In our experience, we have found it useful to assume more of a mediator role and to encourage the parents to base decisions on their shared concern for the well-being of their children.

Race and Seeking Intimate Relationships Internationally

Gillain is a cisgender woman of African ancestry. She exhibits attachment-style dimensions (Bowlby, 1969/1982), which in various studies (Noftle & Shaver, 2006; Mikulincer, Florian, Cowan, & Cowan, 2002; Noftle & Shaver, 2006; Simpson, 1990) have related to higher relationship quality. She envisioned herself one day marrying and having children. However, while living in Mexico City and actively seeking an intimate partner she felt unseen and unappreciated as contrasted with her local White cisgender female friends. Gillain questioned if her romantic interests in Mexico viewed her as a fetish rather than a potential long-term intimate partner.

Given Gillain's dating history, she felt uniquely validated and intellectually aligned with Adriel, a Diné Native American cisgender male, who was able to discuss the nuances of racialized racism microaggressions and ethnocentrism in Mexico. The two formed an intimate relationship and welcomed a child into their lives. Adriel later experienced significant difficulty decreasing the intensity and frequency of his mental health-related problems. Ultimately their romantic relationship ended. Gillain was left questioning if she might have avoided these relationship challenges if she were not living in Mexico and had a greater breath of choice in potential romantic partners elsewhere.

Gillain is not alone. In fact, sociologist Sarah Adeyinka-Skold (2020) argued that women of color, especially women with African ancestry, face significant challenges in their search for intimate partners, which in turn may reduce the likelihood of marriage compared to Asian, Latina, and White college-educated women. Adeyinka-Skol further concluded that dating technology reifies and sustains racial and gender inequality (2020).

Three Key Takeaways

We hope readers of this chapter take away three main points. The first point is that there will be an increasing need for therapists prepared to work as global citizens; those who may be shifting between varied national contexts and who might also partner with someone who is from a different national origin. A second main point we have hoped to convey is that bi-national couples often hold expectations of their partners, linked to their nations of origin, that may have never been overtly expressed. Therapists can assist these couples in improving their relationships by assisting them in making these expectations overt. The final takeaway and challenge is that most therapists are not likely trained to work from a global perspective, particularly those trained in the United States. To address this challenge, we hope this chapter encourages therapists to engage in self-of-the-therapist work around nationality.

Concluding Thoughts

It is challenging for the field of couple's therapy to keep pace with the speed in which changes linked to globalization are occurring. Much of the research that forms the basis of our approaches with couples does not consider the influence that shifting national contexts has on relationships. We believe that future research must focus on better understanding the ways in which nationality is relevant both for couple relationships and as a self-of-the-therapist issue for therapists. Future research also needs to find ways to address U.S.-centric discourse, content, and attitudes, as well as overt nationalism, limits the effectiveness of our approaches with global citizens and couples. This will require us to reconsider many of the core concepts that many may assume to reflect reality, such as attachment, identity, personality and the deeply-rooted U.S. values (and blind spots) found in DSM diagnostic labels. Future research may also need to explore how U.S. values inform what is considered ethical and professional. Capitalism and the litigious culture of the United States has a significant influence on what U.S. practitioners consider to be ethical practice. For example, is it really in the best interest of couples to be required to begin with a new therapist each time they change locations around the globe? The work of couple's therapists must also find a way to access and incorporate increased international research on couples and research that is conducted in languages other than in English. Thus, we suggest that the existing research on which we base our mental health practices has only begun to scratch the surface in regard internationalizing our conceptualizations of mental health and clinical practices.

The writing of this chapter has served as a useful process of critical reflective practice. It has allowed us to become more conscious of clinical themes occurring among expats, the theories and ideas that guide our work, as well as an opportunity to see where we can improve our methods as mental health providers and healers. While we seek to draw on the best practice, empirically supported treatments available to couple therapists, we also recognize the need for ongoing efforts to internationalize our approaches and to draw on mental health practices beyond those privileged within the United States. One of the most evident aspects about this community is that there is no single story about bi-national and multicultural expat couples. In this spirit, rather than offering a prescriptive checklist, we would like to end by offering a Covert Cultural Contract Questionnaire (Table 11.1). This is not intended to be given to the couple to fill out, rather as a possible framework that therapists can use to facilitate dialogues with bi-national and multicultural expat couples.

Table 11.1 Covert Cultural Contract Questionnaire

Identity
- How has living in different national contexts influenced how you see yourself and your partner?
- Are there parts of yourself that you feel have been lost or changed in different national contexts?
- What is one of your personal traits that is difficult for your partner to understand given the cultural differences between the two of you?
- Are there ways you have seen your partner differently since moving to a new nation?

Language
- What is the primary language spoken at home and how did this eventuate?
- How well do you speak each other's language?
- In what ways do the languages you speak influence your identity?
- Are there times when communicating in another language triggers anxiety?
- Does your personality differ when you are communicating in the different languages you speak?
- What subjects are difficult to express in a second or third language?
- Between the two of you, what misunderstandings were based on your different languages?
- How might language be linked to the problems we are addressing in therapy?
- Do you correct each other's language? If so, how does that feel to each of you?
- In which language do you think you are the funniest?
- In what language are you able to flirt or feel sexiest speaking?
- When you are with your extended families, what happens, linguistically?
- Do you have a community of local friends with whom you speak a common language?
- What are the positive aspects of being in a bilingual or multilingual relationship?

Career
- As an expatriate, what do you see as the challenges in your career?
- As a couple, what aspect of your careers/work balance do you both find most difficult?
- What sacrifices related to your career did you make in moving to this country?
- What are the unique employment-related challenges in this country?
- What do you need from your partner in order to bolster success in your career?
- What are the restrictions/allowances of each of your visas in this country?

Parenting Third Culture Kids
- What differences in your parenting styles do you think may be related to where you raised?
- Are there particular challenges you have noticed your children experiencing since moving to a new national context?
- As parents with different cultural backgrounds from your child(ren), what are the unique child care challenges in this national context?
- What hopes do you have regarding your child(ren)'s religion/ spiritual education or practices?

(Continued)

Table 11.1 (Continued)

- When there are parenting responsibilities or child care emergencies, how will you decide who makes adjustments at work?
- What are your thoughts about which primary language your child(ren) will speak?
- Are there differences in parenting styles you are noticing in this national context?

Logistics Fatigue
- How have household tasks been divided up between you and how what the division decided?
- What tasks do you find more difficult to accomplish in this new national context?
- How is your level of comfort with the local language a factor in how daily life tasks have been divided?
- How might imbalances in all the tasks that must be handled influence your relationship?

Isolation and Building Community
- Do you have any local friends here?
- By what means do you meet new people here?
- Do you two feel that there is an equity of opportunity for each of you to spend time with friends?
- How connected are each of you with your non-local support network?
- What differences have you noticed in how people date here compared to how they date in your nation of origin?

Resources and Further Reading

Arnett, J. J. (2008). The neglected 95%: Why American psychology needs to become less American. *American Psychologist, 63*, 602–614.

Martín-Baró, I. (1994). *Writings for a liberation psychology*. Cambridge, MA: Harvard University Press.

Platt, J. J., & Laszloffy, T. A. (2013). Critical patriotism: Incorporating nationality into MFT education and training. *Journal of Marital and Family Therapy, 39*, 441–456. https://doi.org/10.1111/j.1752-0606.2012.00325.x.

Watters, E. (2010). Crazy like us: The globalization of the American psyche. Free Press.

References

Adeyinka-Skold, S. (2020). *Dating in the digital age: Race, gender, and inequality* (3816).[University of Pennsylvania]. Publicly Accessible Penn Dissertations. https://repository.upenn.edu/edissertations/3816

Arnett, J. J. (2008). The neglected 95%: Why American psychology needs to become less American. *American Psychologist, 63*, 602–614.

Bennett, M. (2013). *Basic concepts of intercultural communication: Paradigms, principles, & practices*. Boston: Intercultural Press.

Bennett, M. J. (1986). A developmental approach to training for intercultural sensitivity. *International Journal of Intercultural Relations 10* (2), 179–95.

Berry, J. W. (1970). Marginality, Stress and ethnic identification in an acculturated aboriginal community. *Journal of Cross-Cultural Psychology, 1*(3), 239–252. https://doi.org/10.1177/135910457000100303

Bowlby, J. (1969/1982). *Attachment and loss, Vol. 1. Attachment* (2nd ed.). New York: Basic Books (1st ed. pub. 1969; 2nd ed. pub. 1982).

Castro V.S. (2003). Acculturation and psychological adaptation. Westport, CT: Greenwood Press.

Crippen, C., Brew, L. (2007). Intercultural parenting and the transcultural family: A literature review. *The Family Journal, 15*(2),:107–115. https://doi.org/DOI: 10.1177/1066480706297783

Demby, G., Meraji, M.S. (Hosts). (2017, June 6). A Prescription For "Racial Imposter Syndrome" [Audio podcast episode]. In Code Switch. NPR. www.npr.org/podcasts/510312/codeswitch. Ogilvie, K. (Listener)

Filipič Sterle, M., et al. (2018). Social Support, Adjustment, and Psychological Distress of Help-Seeking Expatriates. *Psychologica Belgica, 58*(1), pp. 297–317., DOI: https://doi.org/10.5334/pb.464

Halverson, E., Hancock, C., & Platt, J. J. (2016). Sexpectations and Globalization. Paper presented at the 2016 Annual the International Family Therapy World Congress in Kona, Hawaii, U.S.A.

Harrison, S., & Lane, M. (2000). The Cambridge History of Greek and Roman Political Thought (The Cambridge History of Political Thought) (C. Rowe & M. Schofield, Eds.). Cambridge: Cambridge University Press. https://doi.org/doi:10.1017/CHOL9780521481366

Hobson, C. J., Kamen, J., Szostek, J. et al. (1998). Stressful Life Events: A revision and update of the social readjustment rating scale. *International Journal of Stress Management, 5*, 1–23. (1998). https://doi.org/10.1023/A:1022978019315

Hovey, J. D., & King, C. A. (1997) Suicidality among acculturating Mexican-Americans: Current knowledge and directions for research. *Suicide and Life-Threatening Behavior, 27*(1), 92–103. https://doi.org/10.1111/j.1943-278X.1997.tb00506.x

Igboanusi, H., & Peter, L. (2005) Languages in Competition: The struggle for supremacy among Nigeria's major languages, English and Pidgin. Frankfurt am Main: Peter Lang.

Jobbatical (2020). Relocations and Global Mobility Trends and Data, Jobbatical, Tallinn, Estonia. DOI: https://jobbatical.com/resources/global-mobility-trends

Johnson, L., Radesky, J., & Zuckerman, B. (2013). Cross-cultural parenting: reflections on autonomy and interdependence. *Pediatrics, .131* (4), 631–633.; DOI: https://doi.org/10.1542/peds.2012-3451

Klerk, Vivian. (2001). The cross-marriage language dilemma: His language or hers?. *International Journal of Bilingual Education and Bilingualism, 4*, 197–216. https://doi.org/10.1080/13670050108667728

Lederer, W. J. & Jackson, D. D. (1968). *The mirages of marriage.* W. W. Norton & Company: New York.

Leung, K., & Stephan, W. G. (2001). Social justice from a cultural perspective. In D. Matsumoto (Ed.), *The handbook of culture and psychology* (p. 375–410). Oxford University Press.

Lev-Ari, S., & Keysar, B. (2010). Why don't we believe non-native speakers? The influence of accent on credibility. *Journal of Experimental Social Psychology, 46*(6), 1093–1096. https://doi-org.ezproxy.uvu.edu/10.1016/j.jesp.2010.05.025

Lyon, J. (1996). *Becoming Bilingual.* Multilingual Matters: Clevedon.

Maccoby, E. E., & Martin, J. A. (1983). Socialization in the Context of the Family: Parent-Child Interaction. In P. H. Mussen, & E. M. Hetherington (Eds.), *Handbook of Child Psychology: Vol. 4. Socialization, Personality, and Social Development* (pp. 1–101). New York: Wiley.

McNulty, Y. (2015). Till stress do us part: the causes and consequences of expatriate divorce. *Journal of Global Mobility, 3*(2), 106–136. https://doi-org.ezproxy.uvu.edu/10.1108/JGM-06-2014-0023

Mikulincer, M., Florian, V., Cowan, P.A. and Cowan, C.P. (2002), Attachment security in couple relationships: A systemic model and its implications for family dynamics. *Family Process, 41*, 405–434. https://doi.org/10.1111/j.1545-5300.2002.41309.x

Noftle, E. E., & Shaver, P. R. (2006). Attachment dimensions and the big five personality traits: Associations and comparative ability to predict relationship quality. *Journal of Research in Personality, 40*(2), 179–208. https://doi.org/10.1016/j.jrp.2004.11.003

Platt, J. J. (2022). What shall I teach my blond blue-eyed son?: Thoughts on love, interbeing and accountability. In M. E. Gallardo (Ed.), *Developing cultural humility: Embracing race, privilege and power* (199–221). Thousand Oaks, CA: Sage.

Platt, J. J., & Laszloffy, T. A. (2013). Critical patriotism: Incorporating nationality into MFT education and training. *Journal of Marital and Family Therapy, 39*, 441–456. https://doi.org/doi: 10.1111/j.1752-0606.2012.00325.x.

Pollock, D. C., Van Reken, R. E., & Pollock, M. V. (2017). Third culture kids: Growing up among worlds. Boston, MA: Nicholas Brealey Publishing

Rahmati, A., & Bahrami Nejad, H. (2019). Signs of divorce before marriage: The role of premarital events in Iran. *Journal of Divorce & Remarriage, 60*(4), 301–315.

Restrepo, E. (2018). Talks and disputes of racism in Colombia after multiculturalism. *Journal of Cultural Studies, 32*(3), 460–476.

Said, E. W. (1978). *Orientalism.* New York: Pantheon Books.

Shen, Y., & Kram, K. E. (2011). Expatriates' developmental networks: Network diversity, base, and support functions. *The Career Development International, 16*(6), 528–552. https://doi.org/10.1108/13620431111178317

Simpson. (1990). Influence of attachment styles on romantic relationships. *Journal of Personality and Social Psychology, 59*(5), 971–980. https://doi.org/info:doi/

Slobodin, O. (2019). "Out of time": A temporal view on identity change in trailing spouses. *Time & Society, 28*(4), 1489–1508. https://doi-org.ezproxy.uvu.edu/10.1177/0961463X17752283

Stroud, P., Jones, R., & Brien, S. (2018). Global People Movements. London: Legatum Institute Foundation in partnership with Oxford Analytica.

Walton, S. J. (1990). Stress management training for overseas effectiveness. International *Journal of Intercultural Relations, 14*(4), 507–527. https://doi.org/10.1016/0147-1767(90)90033-S

Watzlawick, P., Beavin, J. & Jackson, D. (1967). *Pragmatics of human communication: A study of interactional patterns, pathologies, and paradoxes.* New York: Norton.

Wells, L. (2020). Raising Up a Generation of Healthy Third Culture Kids: A Practical Guide to Preventive Care. Canby, OR: Independently published

Wilson, A., & Huston, T. L. (2013). Shared Reality and Grounded Feelings During Courtship: Do They Matter for Marital Success? *Journal of Marriage and Family, 75*(3), 681–696. https://doi.org/10.1111/jomf.12031

Wolff, E. H. (2000) Language and society. In B. Heine and D. Nurse (eEds.) *African Languages: An introduction.* (pp. 298–347). Cambridge: Cambridge University Press

Young, J. T. L., Natrajan-Tyagi, R. & Platt, J. J. (2014). Identity in flux: Negotiating identity while studying abroad., *Journal of Experiential Education,* 1–14. https://doi.org/10.1177/1053825914531920

12

SYSTEMIC FAMILY THERAPY IN AFRICA

Past, Present, and Future Trends

Ronald Asiimwe, Michelle Karume, and Rosco Kasujja

Introduction

In recent years, the eminent disparities in accessing scalable mental health care for communities in lower-middle-income countries (LIMCS) has dominated the global mental health discussion (Bischoff et al., 2017; Patel et al., 2011). Although psychological and relational interventions in general have been perceived as effective treatments for a wide range of mental, emotional, behavioral, and relational problems, barriers such as limited skilled human resources and negative perceptions of Western mental health models have meant that majority beneficiaries of mental health interventions particularly in LMICS have limited access to services. As a result, multi-country research programs such as the Emerging Mental Health Systems in Low- and Middle-Income Countries (EMERALD; Semrau et al., 2019) and the Program for Improving Mental Health Care (PRIME; Breuer et al., 2014) have been established to try and create sustainable mental health solutions in LMICs, including those in Africa (Shah et al., 2017).

Consequently, the growing field of systemic family therapy (SFT) has not been left behind, and in fact, the past decade has seen several systemic family interventions being adapted and implemented across the African continent (Asiimwe et al., 2021). Because SFTs are trained to use systemic/relational approaches as core mechanisms for treating individual, couple, and family mental health problems (Bond, 2009; Sim & Sim, 2020), many mental health practitioners in Africa, the majority of whom were trained in individual psychotherapy approaches, have excitedly acquired extra training in systemic interventions to improve their clinical skillsets and outcomes with individuals, couples, and families in their unique contexts. Indeed, the emergence of family therapy as a new mental health profession on the African continent has led to the development of unique approaches to intervening with individual, marital, and family problems. Particularly, within the past 10 years, there has been increased widespread implementations of relational interventions aimed at improving parent-child relationships in traumatized families (e.g., Wieling et al., 2015), strengthening emotional connection in couple relationships (e.g., Lesch et al., 2018), interventions to reduce domestic violence and violence against children (e.g., Ashburn et al., 2017; Lachman et al., 2016), and interventions for treating relational trauma due to war

DOI: 10.4324/9781003297871-14

and violence (Morgan et al., 2018, 2020). The two most influencing factors for this shift have been: 1) the desire to shift from individual approaches to treatment by most African mental health professionals, and 2) the increased collaboration between African and systemic family therapists from the West (mostly the United States, Australia, and Europe).

In discussing family therapy trends on the African continent, it is important to first note that family therapy takes many forms and variations. These range from a therapist meeting with one individual, one therapist with a family, a therapist working with a couples or groups of couples, a therapist working with siblings, and families in groups. Additionally, larger systems involving multiple therapists and communities are all considered family therapy. Jithoo and Bakker (2011) note that all these modalities share a common phenomenon, that is, they treat individual behavior using a social and contextual lens. We will see these variations in systemic family therapy practice in the sections below.

Further, while it might be exciting to read a chapter on family therapy in Africa, combining African countries together might lead some readers to conclude that we imply that families from various African countries are homogeneous. This is far from the truth; Africa is a heterogeneous and multiethnic/racial continent comprising of 54 countries, more than 1,000 ethnic groups, each with people who practice different traditions, speak different languages, different dress styles, food, and many others. Thus, it is unrealistic to assume that what we cover in this chapter is a comprehensive picture of families and family therapy in this large multiethnic continent. However, recognizing African diversity does not mean we overlook the reality of some of the commonalities and homogeneity in African societies.[3] Therefore, we encourage the reader to approach the content with a sense of curiosity and appreciation for diversity that distinguish Africans from other cultures around the world. Our number one goal is to demonstrate the strength of African cultural values and how these have historically shaped and continue to shape different aspects of family life and the family therapy profession on the continent of Africa. Our second goal is to highlight past and current trends of Western models of family therapy in Africa. We end this chapter by offering reflections on where we think the research agenda in SFT is likely to advance in the future on the African continent.

Africa, a Multi-Ethnic Continent

Many people around the world tend to think of Africa as a homogenous continent comprising one language, culture, and traditional practices. However, Africa is a culturally, linguistically, and religiously diverse continent comprising 54 countries. There are roughly 6,700 languages in the world, and almost 30% (over 2000 languages) of these are spoken on the African continent (Bamgbose, 2011). Due to the history of colonialism and slave trade, most African countries' languages and cultural practices are largely influenced by Indigenous, Arabic, and European civilizations (Iliffe, 2017). Although European colonial regimes attempted to extinguish African languages in favor of their languages (e.g., French, English, and Portuguese), the majority Africans today are multilingual and can speak both their native language(s) as well as the language of their former colonial masters. In Senegal, for example, although French is the official language, most Senegalese people can speak Wolof, Pulaar, Mandika, and Sereer (Sall, 2009). Wolof is in fact the primary language spoken by the majority of people in the countries of Senegal, the Gambia, and Mauritania. Similarly, in Nigeria, most people primarily speak major native languages, including Igbo, Yoruba, and Hausa, in addition to English (the country's official language) (Nwadiora,

1996). Further, countries such as Cameroon and Rwanda combine two colonial languages (i.e., French and English) in addition to native languages (i.e., Duala and Kinyarwanda). Some countries approve more than two languages as their official languages. For example, besides English, South Africa has ten additional official languages, each representing a particular ethnic group in the country (Van Dyk & Nafale, 2005).

Africa's population is growing rapidly, and the United Nations (UN) projects that by 2050, the population of Africa may be close to 2.5 billion (about 26% of the world's total population), and nearly 4.5 billion by 2100 (about 40% of the world's total). As a result of increased migration, globalization, social media, and information technology, African countries have increasingly grown to be in close and constant intersection with each other, and as well between cultures in the East and West (Ojagbemi & Gujere, 2020). Thus, practicing systemic family therapy in such linguistically and culturally diverse settings in Africa carries several opportunities to advance the field as well as several challenges. For example, in many African societies, it is not uncommon for people to practice and engage in traditions from more than one ethnic group. When these individuals encounter mental, emotional, or relational problems and need the help of a psychotherapist, it is challenging to try and conceptualize the main presenting problem for both the client and the therapist because often the problem or conflict is influenced by practicing multiple cultural traditions.

It Takes a Village: Indigenous Knowledge, Distinct and Commonly Shared African Cultural Values

Despite immense cultural and linguistic diversity on the African continent, there are certain philosophies that are emblematic and values that distinguish Africans from the other cultures around the world (Idang, 2015). One such a philosophy is known as *Ubuntu* (pronounced as 'uu-Boon-too'). The word Ubuntu is derived from the Nguni-Bantu people of South Africa, and it means "humaneness" or "personhood" (Ewuoso & Hall, 2019; Nassbuam, 2003). Although the term has origins in South Africa, it is found in many African Bantu languages across the south of the Sahara (Mnyaka & Motlhab, 2005). For example, it is known as *Vumuntu* among the ShiTsonga of Mozambique, *Omuntu* among the Baganda and Banyankole of Uganda, *Umundu* among the Kikuyu of Kenya, and *bumuntu* among the Sukuma people of Tanzania. The philosophy of Ubuntu underscores the strong sense of interconnectedness, shared humanity, oneness of purpose, and collective unconsciousness that many Africans espouse (Ojagbemi & Gureje, 2020). Put differently, "One's humanity is made possible through the humanity of others."

The individual's sense of "self" in the African perspective is rooted in community with others and therefore cannot solely be described by one's physical or psychological attributes (Kamya, 2018). There are three communities an individual African represents; they include the community of one's origin, the community of locality, and the community of ancestors (Shambare, 2021). Shambare (2021) further emphasizes, *"No one is born outside Ubuntu because one is born in a community, exists within a community, and when one dies, they are committed to a community of ancestral lineage"* (p. 5). This sense of rootedness in one's community is often expressed as *"umuntu ngu muntu nga bantu"* (in Zulu language, South Africa), which literally translates as *"I am because we are"* (Van Dyk & Nafale, 2005; Mbiti, 1990). While values such as self-determination and respect for autonomy are espoused in most Western cultures (Metz, 2010), Africans under the Ubuntu philosophy value "processes geared towards seeking consensus, mutual understanding, and harmony of the community" (Nassbaum, 2003, p. 22). Living by the communal principles of Ubuntu does not mean that an individual's pursuit of happiness is prohibited or subordinated, but rather, it is strengthened through the individual's pursuit of good for others in the community.

Further, Van Dyk and Nafale (2005) discuss three fundamental dimensions of Ubuntu. The first dimension is that of *God* the "uncreated creator Who breathes life in all people, hence giving us the shared humanity" (p. 55). To many Africans, God-centered humanity through the Ubuntu spirit is foundational and gives purpose and meaning to life. Further, God and other supreme spiritual entities (e.g., divinities and ancestors) enable the person to live in community with others. The second dimension of Ubuntu is on an *intrapsychic level*. According to Van Dyk and Nafale (2005) Ubuntu does not mean merely possessing positive human qualities, but it is "the very human essence itself" (p. 55). Without Ubuntu, individuals can experience extreme intrapsychic problems, tension, and disconnection in their human relationships (Ewuoso & Hall, 2019). Third, Ubuntu is also experienced at an *interpersonal dimension* where the ideal person embraces values of living in harmony and a commitment to share with others (i.e., what is Yours is ours and What is ours is yours). A commitment to share with others is characterized by virtues such as kindness, generosity, discipline, honor, and respect upon which the person is judged (Van Dyk & Nafale, 2005). In summary, the Ubuntu philosophy carries deep meaning, purpose, and is a vehicle for healing for many Africans who have been historically oppressed, divided on religious, political, and cultural/ethnical grounds. In fact, Wilson and Williams (2013) contend that Ubuntu philosophy enables us as Africans to "understand and define mental health from an African Worldview which is missing from most Western psychological discourse" (p. 3).

Applications of Ubuntu in the African Societies

The philosophy of Ubuntu influences how Africans plan, organize, and celebrate several life and family events. Birth, marriage, funerals, and mourning rituals are some examples (Kamya, 2018). During these events, it is common for family members and friends to travel long distances to participate and/or celebrate these events. The ceremonies that mark these events are characterized by masses getting together to prepare and share traditional elaborate meals, traditional dances, and other various forms of entertainment (e.g., art, drama, and stories) (Ojagbemi & Gureje, 2020). These practices are deeply meaningful for many Africans because they "evoke the sacred in the life of the community" and "underscore the connection to the past, present, and the future" (Kamya, 2018, p. 6). In general, Africans believe that genuine and authentic humanity (ubuntu) is expressed mostly in nonverbal symbolic language of works, rituals, attitudes, and behaviors. Thus, to many Africans, "explicit actions (intentional and unintentional) speak louder than words" (Jithoo & Bakker, 2011, p. 162).

Ubuntu Parenting

Further, Shambare (2021) discusses how Ubuntu philosophy has expanded to influence parenting in many African communities. According to Shambare, parenting in the African context goes beyond one being a biological parent. Parenting has a spiritual and religious connection that involves caring, socializing, and grooming, not only of one's children but other children in the community, to grow into positive contributing members of the society.

Thus, *Ubuntu parents* ensure that children learn culturally appropriate expectations for behavior, and encourage skill development and accountability in their children. In doing so, children understand the importance of community and aligning their goals to conform with the overall expectations of the family and community at large. Further, Ubuntu parents in Africa teach children to be practical problem solvers. One example that is common in most farming and rural communities in Africa is the practice of children (usually between 9–18 years) being entrusted with the responsibility of taking care of the family's wealth in the form of domestic animals like cows, goats, and sheep. Shambare (2021) contends that such skills are not listed in the mainstream curriculum of education but they teach children to be trusted stewards of their family's wealth, heritage, and traditions. Lastly, Ubuntu parenting principles are also manifested through kinship networks and childrearing practices that emphasize multiple caregivers (e.g., siblings, aunts, uncles, and friends in the community) common in countries in sub-Saharan Africa (Roelen et al., 2017; Skelton, 2012). Although several crises (e.g., HIV/AIDS, wars, and most recently, the COVID-19 global pandemic) have weighed on many families in Africa, research shows that kinship networks and the extended family still play a significant role in parenting children across Africa (Abdullah et al., 2020; Roelen et al., 2017).

Ubuntu Therapy: An Integrative Approach to Mental Health Treatment

The undermining or subordination of indigenous African cultural practices in the psychotherapy profession is perhaps the number one critique of most Western theories of psychotherapy in Africa (Somni & Sandlana, 2014). This undermining is evident in the default Western graduate training in psychotherapy that tends to focus primarily on the nuclear family structures and often pathologize/label (e.g., as dysfunctional) families whose structures, values, and practices do not align with the Western notions of a 'normal family' (Jithoo & Bakker, 2011). As a result, many African psychotherapists who acquire Western-based training in psychotherapy often seem unprepared to work with clients in African settings. This is primarily because most theories of psychotherapy developed in the West tend to be individualistic in their approach to treatment, yet African clients live in environments that espouse collective and communal ways of living (Somni & Sandlana, 2014).

Thus, Afrocentric scholars have called for models of psychotherapy practice that are rooted in indigenous African philosophies. One major model that has been developed to work specifically with Black clients and families in Africa is *Ubuntu therapy* (Rautenbach, 2015; Van Dyk & Nafale, 2005; Wilson & Williams, 2013). Like Western family therapy, Ubuntu therapy considers African clients' unique contexts, and in its intervention, the approach integrates both Western psychotherapy theories with African traditional practices to intervene in client mental health problems. The main goal of Ubuntu therapy is to address clients' conflicts at the three core dimensions of Ubuntu philosophy: psychotheological, intrapsychic, and interpersonal dimensions (Van Dyk & Nafale, 2005). Thus, in treatment, the Ubuntu therapist assesses three aspects: 1) the nature of the relationship the client has with God; 2) the intrarelational feelings that the client might have towards self, family, and community, and 3) the client's interpersonal relational challenges to facilitate relationship building and increase human value, dignity, and trust, which all enhance social harmony and cohesion.

Regarding treatment techniques, storytelling is the most commonly used treatment technique in Ubuntu therapy. Traditionally, Africans are oral people who believe as White et al.

(1990) believed that "life is lived through stories." In Ubuntu therapy, the therapist guides the client to tell the story of the problem from their own perspective. The therapists listen to the client's perspective of the story to determine the level of symptoms and treatment. Another technique is *life script*. This includes anything from family of origin scripts to parental and communal messages that one has internalized. The Ubuntu therapist collaboratively works with the client to map his/her life script. This process helps the client to gain insight into their presenting problem and the subsequent symptoms. Similar to the technique of reauthoring in narrative therapy (White et al., 1990), treatment involves the therapist guiding the client to write a new script that reflects the client's preferred future. Other Ubuntu techniques include *burning platform* and *art*, in the form of drawings, paintings, acting, and dances that help clients manage and cope with emotional struggles. Clients are helped to draw and/or make visual representations of their problems as well as illustrate their past and present family or communal dynamics that may be influencing the problem. Through art, the client can identify certain destructive practices embedded in the context of which the client exists that do not reflect Ubuntu living.

Since the introduction of Western psychotherapy, many African clients (and some mental health practitioners) have often oscillated between Western psychotherapy and traditional African healing practices (Van Dyk & Nafale, 2005).

In psychology, Freud referred to this phenomenon as *"splitting of the ego,"* that is, the coexistence of the self between two opposing and unintegrated attitudes (Brook, 1992). Thus, the development of Ubuntu therapy is considered the most culturally appropriate theory for psychotherapy practice in Africa (Somni & Sandlana, 2014; Van Dyk & Nafale, 2005). Despite the seemingly cultural appropriateness of Ubuntu therapy in African contexts, research regarding the clinical utility of this approach is still limited. The few empirical studies (e.g., Somni & Sandlana, 2014) validating the clinical utility and effectiveness of Ubuntu therapy perhaps explains why the approach is not widely known by many Western-trained psychotherapists both in Africa and in Western countries. We discuss this later in the section on research agenda in family therapy.

Africans and Aesthetic Values

Aesthetics is a general term used to refer to a "discipline concerned with the perception, appreciation, and production of art" (Vessel, 2013, p. 2). Aesthetics goes beyond mere preference of an object, a person, or an experience and encompasses a deep appreciation or being in awe of beauty and art attached to an individual, object, or experience. For centuries, the African view of personhood has always combined aesthetics (i.e., beauty) e.g., in a person, art, music, poetry, and storytelling (Idang, 2015; Ikuenobe, 2016; Tuwe, 2016). Art in the African cultures is expressed in various forms including portraits, handmade crafts, clothes, songs/music, and paintings, and is meant to serve the community. The African perception of art is that it is "a social activity, a way of life, and a technique of living that cannot be simply shaped or created sorely by one individual's imagination" (Ikuenebo, 2016, p. 130). Rather, works and processes of art are meant to serve deep meaningful and practical purposes for the community. Thus, to the African, art has no relevance and is not art if it does not meet the needs of the community; it is just a 'thing,' 'an object,' or 'junk' (Ikuenebo, 2016). As a social activity, art is guided and shaped by social norms and standards. Thus, for the art and the artist to be appreciated, they must be sensitive to the interests and values of the community.

Further, aesthetic values in Africa are also manifested in Africa's oral tradition of folktales and storytelling (Achebe, 1987; Hart, 2009). Although writing traditions exist in Africa, Africans are primarily oral people; most of their art forms and stories are oral rather than written. In ancient Africa, families would gather around a central fire to listen to stories (Achebe, 1958). Storytellers were usually elders and respected community members who told captivating stories usually with a moral and educational ending. These folktales would not follow any order or sequence, and often, the storytelling would be accompanied by music, drums, clapping, and dancing by the locals. According to Ngugi wa Thiongo (1980), stories and folktales served to entertain people, transmit cultural knowledge and information across generations, and teach morals, values, expectations for culturally appropriate conduct. Tuwe (2016) further argues that although storytelling traditions vary across cultures, they tend to share similar traits such as oral narration, moral teaching, and the use of gestures and repetitions. In the words of Africa's greatest poet and storyteller Chinua Achebe, a story entertains, informs, and instructs. He further goes on to say, the story continues beyond the war and the warrior. He emphasizes that it is the story that outlives the sound of the war drums and exploits of the fighters, pointing to the importance of stories saving our offspring from stumbling blindly into the future. Ultimately, Chinua Achebe insightfully shares that it is the story that owns us and directs us, for without it we are blind.

Spirituality, Religion, and Mental Health in Africa

In Africa, religion and spirituality are central to life. As Mugisha et al. (2013) put it, the two are "strong social forces that permeate all aspects of community life and decision-making" (p. 344). A recent nationwide panel study from South Africa found that 92% of South Africans identified with a particular religious group, and 90% found religion to be important in their day-to-day lives (Tomita & Ramlall, 2018). These statistics were divisible across the multiple ethnicities in South Africa. To Africans, religion and spirituality are often used interchangeably and usually characterized by 1) a belief in, and a connection to a Supreme Being (s) who is sacred, invisible, and transcendental, and 2) a unified sense community (Bayers, 2010; Idang, 2015; Ojagbemi & Gureje, 2020). In traditional African religion (ATR), spirituality could mean connectedness to relevant spiritual entities (e.g., including divinities and ancestors). Many Africans believe in the existence of good and bad spirits. According to Idang (2015), the spirits are "what inspires an individual to communicate with the Supreme Being" (p. 104).

Prior to the introduction of Western religion, sorcerers, diviners, and soothsayers were the main mediators between God and man in the ATR. The three served as interpreters of God's wishes for the people and helped to streamline behavior in society (Idang, 2015). Although there are diverse religious practices and deities in Africa, Mbiti (1970) contends that, "God takes the highest possible position" over all others forms of deities. To the African, God is acknowledged as the supreme creator of the universe; He is omniscient (all knowing), Omnipresent (everywhere) and accessible to every human, Omnipotent (all-powerful), transcendental, and immanent (Mbiti, 1970). Further, He is acknowledged as the "consoler, helper, and comforter of those in pain for various reasons including mental health problems" (Mugisha et al., 2013, p. 349). In contemporary Africa, it is not uncommon to find many who integrate both the African traditional religious practices in addition to Christianity and/or Islam.

Religion and spirituality play a huge role in how contemporary Africans perceive mental health, family problems, and subsequent treatment (Ojagbemi & Gureje, 2020). For example, studies from Uganda and Ghana exploring perceptions of suicide among religious communities indicated that suicidal behavior was unacceptable and perceived as a breach of God's doctrine of 'life as sacred' and against God's rule of agape (e.g., Mugisha et al., 2013; Osafo et al., 2011). Because most Africans believe that God owns their lives, individuals have no right to take it away (e.g., by suicide). From a religious perspective, some Africans believe that a person who experiences suicidal thoughts, attempts, or commits suicide deserves to be punished by God and the Church. Although spiritual and faith-based mental health care has been an important aspect in most of Africa, it is still an invisible and informal component of the many mental health systems and policies of various African countries (Ojagbemi & Gureje, 2020).

Family Structure and Marital Relationships in Africa; Traditional and Contemporary Perspectives

Relational interconnectedness and social bonds are highly esteemed as meaningful experiences in Afrocentric paradigms (Wissing et al., 2020). In the African Traditional Society (ATS), the family structure was highly hierarchical with elders such as parents and grandparents, followed by aunties and uncles occupying and playing executive functions (Ajayi & Buhari, 2014). These included setting rules for culturally proper conduct, child discipline, offering advise/wise counsel, and intervening in family and marital conflicts. Additionally, roles regarding headship, boundaries, and other family obligations were clearly articulated based on gender. A deviation from these roles and boundaries was considered taboo and carried serious consequences for the offender. Old age in many African societies was associated with wisdom due to long life experiences. Thus, when people became old and could not help themselves, they would move in to live with their children's families, often the adult male child's family.

Further, parenting and childrearing in the ATS were a communal responsibility as espoused in a famous African proverb, *"it takes a village to raise a child"* (Shambare, 2021). For example, when two related families lived in the same area, it was common for parents to seek help with childcare giving responsibilities from the members of the extended family or community members. Children are socialized early on regarding culturally appropriate expected gender roles and behavior using oral traditions like folktales and proverbs (Pohoață, 2019). For example, in most sub-Saharan Bantu cultures, young boys are taught to take care of domestic animals like cows, sheep, and goats, while girls are taught motherly roles (e.g., cooking and cleaning the house). These roles are meant to eliminate confusion and prepare children for their future responsibilities as husbands and wives. Thus, many Africans reject the Western idea of the couple discussing and agreeing upon responsibilities before marriage since these are already culturally prescribed.

To render respect to their parents and other elders in the community, children in the ATS were not expected to overtly show anger, frustration, or resentment when disciplined. Thus, when disciplined, many children tried to hide their feelings, and instead, many used indirect techniques (e.g., faking a sickness, refusing to eat food, and going at a sluggish pace when assigned house chores) to communicate their anger or annoyance to the parent(s) (Nwoye, 2004). Although the increased migration, urbanization, and globalization has increasingly fragmented these traditions, many contemporary African families still practice them. For example, to date, it is still a common practice for family members to visit their extended family members or send their children to the villages during school holidays and annual holidays such as Christmas, Easter, and Eid al-Fitr.

Further, because collective values are highly esteemed in many African societies, marriage in both the ATS and contemporary African societies was/is considered a permanent social and community event (Mafumbate, 2019). Thus, divorce and separation of two married people was unheard of and culturally unacceptable in the ATS. Marriage to the African is not only perceived as a coming together of two people (a man and a woman) but a coming together of two families sometimes. Traditionally, the communities in the ATS had law enforcement officers, traditional police, courts, and extended families as arms that regulated and ensured that marriage was preserved by resolving the marital disputes and reconciling both disputing parties (Umubyeyi & Mtapuri, 2019). Moreover, marital conflict, divorce, and other external threats were and continue to be viewed as a threat to the stability and sustainability of the institution of marriage (Amadi &Amadi, 2014). As a result, several mechanisms, such as involving elders, traditional healers, and seeking professional therapyhave been developed to try and mitigate marital conflicts in families (Theresa, 2014). For example, when women are unable to bear children, the majority of them tend to seek help from the traditional healers as a way to strengthen their marriages with their husbands and to prevent the husbands from marrying other women (Duijl & Nijenhuis, 2010). Traditional healers were revered for their capacity to manipulate natural forces and communicate with the spiritual realm to help local people solve their problems. And in the ATS, visiting traditional healers was a part of everyday life, with rituals and offerings to ensure that the gods support well-being, safety, and preserve marital relationships (Van Duijl et al., 2010).

Finally, because Africans are extremely religious, marriage was, and still is, considered a religious obligation that requires and as well bring blessings from the ancestors and God. To date, many people aspire for and do all that is necessary to make their marriages durable in order to retain a good relationship with God and their ancestors. Religious or spiritual components mark the African man's relationship with their wife, the divine God, and/or the ancestors (Hosegood et al., 2009). This religious sensibility is believed to promote moral excellence in the African community. In conclusion, although marriage is still highly esteemed in the African culture, the institution has and continues to face significant changes because of westernization, urbanization, modernization, and globalization (Sodi et al., 2010). These changes call for changes in the approaches used to solve these problems. Presently, there are families that seek professional services from western-oriented psychotherapists (e.g., counselors, couple and family therapy, psychologists, religious marital therapists) in addition to indigenous African marital treatment.

Family and Marital Problems in Africa; Historical and Current Perspectives

Globally and in Africa it is well documented that the family constitutes the most important component and basic unit of a community's or society's survival (Brian et al. 2019). Despite this recognition, marital and family conflicts have continued to threaten the existence of marriages and families, both in developed and developing countries (Ali et al., 2020; Umubyeyi & Mtapuri, 2019). Marital and family conflict takes several forms including verbal, physical, sexual, financial, and psychological. Conflicts usually involve application of manipulative, aggressive, and violent approaches to subdue or control a partner, child, or relative. In many African contexts, increases in family and marital conflicts have been directly or indirectly attributed to 1) increases in labor migration (e.g., Umubyeyi & Mtapuri, 2019) and 2) to oppressive social and political structures and processes created during colonial dispensations (Hosegood et al., 2009). In migration cases, tension arises in families as they attempt to acculturate and adapt to the cultures and lifestyle of the host cities or countries while attempting to maintain their own culture and traditions (Olaoba et al., 2010). In countries such as South Africa, unfair apartheid policies separated couples and families; partners who acquired paid employment in urban areas were prohibited from traveling back to their rural homes where their spouses resided. As a result, these individuals found new people to marry and started a second family in the urban towns.

Due to increased socioeconomic challenges, it is still a common trend in most of Africa for individuals (mostly men) to migrate to urban areas and leave their families in rural areas in search for better employment opportunities. This pattern has affected family functioning and shifted roles within the family. For example, in many African countries today, women are increasingly participating in the labor market to sustain their families (e.g., children and grandparents) in rural areas. In general, several studies from Africa (e.g., Mtika, 2007; Smit, 2001; Umubyeyi & Mtapuri, 2019; Yabiku et al., 2012) and systematic reviews from around the world (e.g., Antia et al., 2020) have documented the negative effects of labor migration on the mental health and well-being of families. Specifically, studies have reported cases of increased marital instability, separation and divorce, child depression, anxiety, and mortality in worst cases.

Further, customary and cultural practices embedded in most African societies have also been highlighted as potential influencers of marital and family problems. Two practices including early marriages (i.e., marriage before the age of 18 years) and bride price are worth noting. Although there several African states have adopted laws to attempt to curb the custom of early marriages (Walker, 2012), most countries still have provisions within those laws that accept early marriages in certain circumstances, such as under customary law or if the girl becomes pregnant (Yaya et al, 2019). Regarding bride price, this ancient African marriage tradition involves the exchange of girls/women for material and financial gains by the groom's family. This custom has raised some contentious debates among contemporary scholars including those from Africa. While some (e.g., Bonye et al, 2020; Kaye et al., 2005; Princewill et al, 2019) argue that bride price perpetuates unequal gender power relations and restricts women's independence, others (e.g., Mbaye & Wagner, 2017) argue that the practice has less power over economically independent women. Nonetheless, many Africans including women still take pride in this ancient traditional practice.

Historically, men/husbands in Africa were absolute "heads, protectors and providers" of the family for centuries with the responsibility of shouldering all the financially inclined duties on their heads; on the other hand, women/wives were viewed as helpers of their husbands with their main role to prepare food, maintaining the cleanliness of the home, making their husbands happy, and rearing the children (Best & Puzio, 2019; Bassey & Bubu, 2019). This patriarchal setup that systematically placed women in underprivileged and oppressed positions has greatly contributed to the increased marital and family conflicts. The World Health Organization (WHO) in 2013 released a report on aggregated global and regional prevalence of interpersonal violence (IPV) with findings showing that almost 30% of women globally who had been in a relationship had experienced physical and/or sexual violence by their male partner with figures going up to 37% in African regions (WHO, 2013). In Rwanda, a recent Demographic and Health Survey (DHS) report showed that 40% of women and 18% of men that had ever been married reported to have experienced emotional, sexual, or physical violence from their current or most recent partner; 36% of women reported spousal physical violence while men reported only 9%. Further, 35% of women and 17% of men reported to have experienced spousal emotional violence, and 16% of women and 1% of men reported to have experienced sexual violence (Rwanda DHS, 2021). In Nigeria 36% of women who had ever been married reported to have experienced emotional, sexual, or physical violence from their current or most recent husband, and 30% reported that they had experienced it the previous year (Nigeria DHS, 2018).

Research shows that on average, women living with HIV/AIDS experience more incidences of physical, sexual, and emotional violence by their partners, which is considered as one of the key risk factors for the increased IPV cases (Tenkorang et al, 2021). It also shows a high prevalence rate of IPV among women in sub-Saharan Africa with 44% of them reporting to have experienced emotional, physical, and sexual violence (Muluneh, 2020). Although most studies in Africa have historically focused on male perpetrated IPV, recent studies have focused on incidences of IPV perpetrated by women (Tenkorang, 2021; Zacarias et al., 2012). In general, these studies indicate that women who experienced violence as children were more likely to perpetrate IPV against men as adults. These women used violence as a form of self-defense against male dominance and control. Most women reported using emotional violence and a few have used sexual and physical violence against men (Tenkorang, 2021). Studies from Africa have concluded that contrary to popular opinion (i.e., that IPV is only perpetrated by men), IPV seems to be a mutual and bidirectional phenomenon, and that IPV interventions should consider these complexities.

In addition to sociocultural and economic factors, marital and family problems in Africa also stem from intergenerational family and war-related trauma. Studies indicate that experiencing early trauma predisposes an individual to long-term attachment problems, irrational expectations of interpersonal relationships, reduced ability to learn, and inability to self-regulate (Baryshnikov et al., 2017; Ford & Blaustein, 2013). Many families in Africa have endured long periods of political instability, notably the Rwandan genocide (1994), Lord's Resistance Army (LRA) war in Uganda, Wars in Liberia, Mali, South Sudan, and other central African countries. A recent United Nations High Commissioner for Refugees (UNHCR) report indicated that almost one-third of the world's refugee population (over 30 million) internally displaced people (i.e., refugees & asylum-seekers) living in Africa (UNHCR, 2020). Wars and conflicts have increased relational trauma (Morgan et al., 2018), disorganized family structure and values, and increased the number of child-headed families and gendered-based violence (GBV) and IPV.

Perceptions of Marital and Relationship Problems; African Indigenous Approaches to Treatment

Despite research highlighting the prevalence of mental, emotional, and relational problems among families in Africa, many Africans to date are still skeptical about Western forms of professional psychotherapy. Preexisting cultural and spiritual perceptions about mental health and seeking psychotherapy and a general lack of appropriate/accurate information regarding mental health and relational problems are perhaps the top two reasons for this skepticism (Knizek et al., 2021). Because the life of an African is lived through a community of relationships with others (i.e., Ubuntu), many traditional Africans believe that mental illness or family problems are an indication that society order, equilibrium, and harmony have been disrupted (Jithoo & bakker, 2011). Thus, to these Africans, illnesses and problems are a sociological phenomenon that affect not only the individual but the entire family, clan, and community.

Further, in African cultures, mental illness and family problems are believed to be religious concepts caused by malevolent intervention of evil spirits and witchcraft (Amadi & Amadi, 2014; Atindanbila & Thompson, 2011). Witchcraft and witchdoctors (*isangomas*) were and are still believed to possess mystical powers transmitted through charms, medical portions, and rags and are used to protect families, cattle, and other properties (Nandutu, 2017). For example, among the Baganda people, the largest and historically dominant tribe in Uganda, most people still believe that the failure of a woman to conceive is related to her ancestors not being happy about the couple's marriage. This scares people, and, in most cases, the woman is likely to be chased from her marital home (Kabagenyi et al., 2016).

Given this context, many individuals and couples when faced with family and marital problems consult traditional healers (e.g., Herbalists, Faith healers, Diviners/Spiritualists) as their first line of treatment (Maluleka & Ngulube, 2018). In fact, Jithoo and Bakker (2011) contend that traditional healers are at the "forefront of spirituality and health in many African communities" (p. 156). They are easily accessible to the masses especially those who reside in remote areas where there are no adequate mental health facilities (Atindanbila & Thompson, 2011). A majority operate in sites that are easy to access, where the cost of treatment is cheaper, and one could also call them to attend to clients in crisis situations. Finally, traditional healers are often members of the community who are familiar with the local cultural traditions (e.g., medicinal plants). As a result, they are easily trusted by the masses because they provide more culturally acceptable explanations regarding the causes of their clients' problems than clinicians trained in Western psychotherapy approaches.

According to the World Health Organization (WHO; 2003), 80% of Africans use traditional medicine as the first line of treatment for their basic healthcare requirements including marital and family problems before exploring other treatment options. Many report that traditional approaches to treatment are holistic in that they consider the spiritual, physical, and psychosocial aspects of health and wellness (Atindanbila & Thompson, 2011; Mathibela et al., 2015). Traditional pharmacopoeia (i.e., the use of plant and animal elements) and music and drama therapy are some of the common approaches traditional healers use to combat their clients' symptoms (Atindanbila & Thompson, 2011). Treatment success is also impacted by the highly symbolic physical aspects of plant and animal parts, as well as the sort of symptoms addressed, with pain reduction and depression being the most typically improved (Boakye et al., 2014). Individual variations in attention, compassion, anxiety, heredity, learning mechanisms, and personality qualities can all impact treatment success, and a favorable relationship between a competent healer and a believing patient increases the likelihood of a successful outcome (Boakye et al., 2015).

Some monotheistic religions, particularly Christianity, Islam, and Judaism have historically dismissed traditional healing throughout the years (Esan et al., 2019). For example, although certain Christian churches have parallels with indigenous religious traditions and some Christian churches tolerate traditional African practices, most Christians consider what African traditionalists do to be traditional witchcraft (Gureje et al., 2020; Paul, 2019). Some churches actively prohibit their members from contacting traditional healers, claiming that traditional healers worship the ancestors and evil spirits rather than God, which is considered sin in the Christian worldview (Peprah et al., 2018). The stigma and negativity associated with traditional healing practices has led to most consultations taking place in private, late at night (Rummun et al., 2018). Despite these forces of resistance, many Africans still consult traditional healers when faced with problems including marital ones.

Religious and Faith-Based Mental Health Providers

In addition to traditional healers, faith/religious healers (e.g., Christian clergy, Muslim clerics, and traditional priests) are frequently consulted for many mental, marital, and family problems in Africa (Jithoo & Bakker, 2011). Because religious beliefs influence and shape perceptions of mental health among many Africans, religious and faith leaders are thus considered important complementary and alternative mental health service providers (CAPS) in most African cultures. Faith and religious healers are sought after in Africa because the proportion of trained mental health professionals is very low, and the few that are available practice only in urban areas and their services are costly. Conversely, faith leaders often live in the community and are available to offer reliable and consistent emotional and spiritual support to their masses sometimes at no cost. Second, like traditional medicine men, many practices, values, beliefs, and worldviews of faith healers are believed to be congruent with those of their service users (Baum et al., 2006). For example, many Africans who subscribe to the Christian tradition believe in soul care, which is understood from a perspective of salvation that comes through Jesus Christ and is manifested in the hearts and bodies of people through God's Holy Spirit. This is the idea of the Trinity in the Christian worldview. According to Jithoo and Bakker (2011), Christian faith leaders (e.g., reverends, pastors, prophets, and church elders) support the masses with psychospiritual help when faced with existential struggles. Further, their intervention approaches tend to emphasize relational spirituality that is evidenced by followers getting together in small groups to recite Bible scriptures, listening, and praying for their loved one who is facing a mental health and/or family crisis. This kind of care nurtures, liberates, and instills hope in the person or family facing difficulties. It is important to note that although several are made to fit the cultures in Africa, the notion of 'pastoral care' originates from the Christian traditions that are predominantly rooted in Western societies' conceptual understanding of life and humanity (Jithoo & Bakker, 2011).

To gain a wider perspective regarding the role of faith leaders in supporting people with various mental health and family problems in Africa, we reviewed and summarized a few recent studies from various countries on the continent. The first study combined multiple studies highlighting research about how local spiritual beliefs and norms can facilitate and meet the mental health needs of clients in Africa (Ojagbemi & Gureje, 2020). This review included studies from Nigeria, Kenya, South Africa, and Uganda. The scholars reported that across the four African countries, pastoral, or spiritual care (not biomedical mental health care) was a predominant form of mental health care for many people. A second study we found was a survey of traditional and faith healers providing mental health care in three sub-Saharan African countries (Ghana, Kenya, and Nigeria) (Esan et al., 2019). Participants in this study were 205 CAPS from Ghana, 406 from Kenya, and 82 from Nigeria. The authors reported that over 70% of CAPS (traditional and religious healers combined) treated both physical and mental health problems in families. Alcohol and drug use, psychosis (insanity), depression, epilepsy, and others were among the mental illnesses commonly treated by CAPS in the three countries. In these countries, the scholars reported that CAPS received training through many years of apprenticeship (Esan et al., 2019). A third and final study we present is a recent qualitative study examining the role of religious leaders (n= 28) in suicide prevention in Ghana (Osafo et al., 2021). The religious leaders interviewed in this study described their role as 'frontliners' with "an obligation towards any individual in crisis, but more importantly prioritized suicide because it led to death" (p. 529). Authors reported that religious leaders were reliable sources of healing for the community; they provided lay counseling, offered prayer and deliverance, induced hope, and, in some cases, provided referrals to mental health professionals for the people suffering. Osafo et al. (2021) concluded that gatekeeper training and interprofessional collaborations were needed between trained mental health professionals and local religious leaders because they played key roles in intervening in mental health crises for their communities.

In conclusion, mental health services offered by faith and religious leaders are believed to be effective because they reflect the cultural and spiritual practices, beliefs, and worldviews of the African people. Although differences exist between the training and services offered by faith leaders and those of trained mental health professionals, there are overlaps in that both seek to improve the mental and family well-being of families in the community. Because of these overlaps, there are calls in Africa for more open collaborations between mental health professionals and religious leaders in many African countries (Ojagbemi & Gureje, 2020).

How Do Africans View Going to a Professional Psychotherapist?

If I (Michelle Karume) speak to my grandparents and their age groups and ask about how they resolved conflict or issues, they would confidently lean on their tribal ways and traditional dictates. First, they would explain that family problems were not to be discussed outside of the home. Second, they would speak of respected family members, elders, and religious leaders as those whose duties were to resolve marital and family disputes if the immediate family were unable. These elders were considered 'family' because they were part of the community. Going to a 'stranger' (i.e., the psychotherapist) was unheard of. However, the emergence of more psychosocial problems outweighed the traditional healing methods, and was thus a gateway to the emergence of professional therapy (Koinange, 2004). Nonetheless, many Africans are still skeptical about going to therapy. When they gather the energy to go, their affect during sessions is often hostile and one of discomfort. Like in some Western therapy contexts, initial therapy sessions with clients in Africa are used to build trust and gain buy-in from clients.

Common barriers to seeking psychotherapy are largely sociocultural, religious, and economic, and include a fear of being stigmatized, or perceived as weak by society, financial strain, and limited understanding of the difference between 'counseling' and 'therapy' (Muhorakeye & Biracyaza, 2021). In many African countries, the words 'counseling' and 'therapy' are used inter-changeably and are often confused to mean 'advise giving.' In Kenya, for example, the professional counselor was recognized by three emerging events: 1) the rise of HIV/AIDS in the country, which led to the development of Voluntary Counseling and Testing (VCT); 2) the 1998 American Embassy terrorist attacks; and 3) guidance and counseling as needed for the Kenya National Youth policy. Other factors such as post-election violence and unrest in schools increased the need for more professional counselors to provide psychological services to the masses. Thus, as psychotherapy made its way to the African shores, the age-old utilization of counseling techniques is seen to be synonymous given that both deal with the mental health issues.

However, I (Michelle Karuma) have noticed a significant change in better understanding of what therapy is, and more importantly, more people seeking therapy today. Specifically, in my cultural setting (Kenya), I have noticed that people are more openly talking about going to therapy and giving psychotherapy as a referral source when marital and familial challenges arise. Social media platforms have been another place where I have seen Africans talking about psychotherapy and how it has been meaningful to them. Most health insurance companies in Kenya now include mental health as a service they cover. This has truly helped with the reuptake of the services. Employers are more readily discussing and providing mental health services to their employees. In 2017, an article released by the Ministry of Health Kenya discussed the importance of mental health in the workplace as well as the financial implications when mental health is not catered to. It is movements such as these from African governments that have lessened the stigma and slowly shifted the perceptions of people towards mental health and recognizing seeking psychotherapy as treatment.

The History of Western Systemic Family Therapy in Africa

In attempting to trace the history of SFT in Africa, one cannot neglect the social-psychological influences of oppressive colonial regimes on the African continent. When colonialists came to Africa (mostly from Europe), they introduced Western science and cultural practices. These permeated the lives of individuals in many African societies; Western ways of knowing were considered supreme and were therefore forced onto Africans at the expense of existent African indigenous knowledge and practices, the majority of which were considered primitive, barbaric, and unscientific. Eventually, this psychological subjugation faced by Africans resulted in a deep sense of inferiority in who they were as a people, a culture, and a continent (Nwoye, 2004). This inferiority complex was further compounded by many years of countless prejudiced writings by Western historians and anthropologists that portrayed Africa as a 'dark continent' (Bassil, 2011).

With a history such as this, post-colonial Africa needed time to rehabilitate, heal, and restore a sense of self-belief in their culture, traditions, and practices. Thus, between the 1940s and the 1970s, the pioneers of family therapy in Africa, most of whom were religious leaders, artists, psychiatrists, and social/political thought leaders and writers (e.g., Wole Soyinke, Achebe; 1958; Namdi Azikiwe, Ngugi, wa Thiong'o; 1972; Nkrumah; 1970, etc.), thought to utilize psychotherapy as a weapon to "liberate, restore, and integrate the culture of the African people" (Nwoye (2001), p. 65). These pioneers, although not trained as family therapists, conceptualized the entire African society as one large family that suffered from collective psychological trauma due to negative aspects of colonialism (Nwoye, 2001). Thus, they saw psychotherapy as a vehicle to educate and inspire Africans towards a new sense of self and cultural togetherness that was lost during colonialism. A second goal of FT pioneers was to mentally prepare Africans with a 'solid structure inside themselves' that would enable them to persevere amidst new cultural dilemmas they would face post-colonialism.

The second phase of family therapy pioneering in Africa began in the early 1980s and 1990s (Nwoye, 2001). During this time, it was believed that some form of restoration of

African culture had been achieved but new challenges had arisen that complicated the psychology and mental health of the continent. These challenges were due to modern forces of globalization and urbanization, poor economic and political structures, ethnic wars and violence, and the HIV/AIDS epidemic that swept across Africa in the early 1980s. With these challenges, many individuals and families lost their jobs, loved ones, lost hope, and were demoralized about the purpose of living. This meant that the focus of family therapy again had to shift to focus on spirituality and restoring hope. As a result, many hope-healing communities were created in various African countries to try and help people defeat self-doubt, regain hope, and persevere amidst these new structural challenges (Nwoye, 2001).

In the years following the 1980s, mental health professionals around Africa began to embrace the idea of Western family therapy and hence some African countries started regulatory bodies to unite all psychotherapists doing family therapy work. For example, in South Africa, the First International Conference of Marital and Family Therapy was held in Durban (Mason and Shuda, 1999). It was at this conference that the South African Institute of Marital and Family Therapy (later called the South African Association of Marital and Family Therapy; SAAMFT) was started. The vibrant membership of the SAAMFT worked closely with the International Family Therapy Association (IFTA) to plan and organize trainings and conferences on family therapy in South Africa, and in other African countries. Unfortunately, the vibrant SAAMFT dissolved in the 2000s and has not been reestablished since then (Asiimwe et al., 2021). In Nigeria, the Association of Marriage and Family Counselors was established in the 2000s to support counselors in Nigeria who were involved in providing marital counseling services (Okocha & Alika, 2012).

Today, many family therapists such as two of the authors of this chapter are of the view that many of the systemic family therapy theories and techniques fit well with the collectivistic cultural values espoused in mostly sub-Saharan African countries (e.g., Uganda, Kenya, South Africa, Ghana, Zimbabwe, etc.). The systemic lens is already a part of the African way of being where community is greatly important and social support is valued. The cultural sensitivity embedded in many of the SFT theories creates safety for African clients and hopefully from what we see diminishes the threat of the Western techniques pushing out their traditional ways of being. As systemic family therapy training programs continue to expand in Africa, such as Kenya having master's and Doctorate level MFT programs (Asiimwe, 2021), the hope is that family therapy will increasingly become a legitimized mental health profession on the African continent. Our desire is that in the coming years, SFT will become the first line of treatment when individuals, couples, and families in Africa face mental health or relational challenges.

Recent Trends in the Application of Systemic Family Therapy in Africa

Perhaps the most recent exciting and innovative trend in the development of systemic family therapy on the African continent has been the establishment of two graduate training programs (a masters and a doctoral program) that provide exclusive specialty training in marital and family therapy for students in Africa (Asiimwe et al., 2021). Both programs are in Nairobi, Kenya, and in fact, one of these programs is focused on training systemic therapists with skills to intervene in trauma, family violence, and mindfulness. Besides established SFT graduate training programs, other available evidence shows that there have been other efforts to equip Africans in family therapy skills, concepts, and techniques. For example, McDowell et al. (2011) conducted a 7-day family therapy workshop in Uganda. Participants in this training were students in training and alumni of Bishop Magambo Counselor Training Institute (BMCTI) located in Fort portal, Western Uganda. The content of the training included general systems theory as well as concepts primarily from structural family therapy, Bowenian family therapy, and narrative therapy. They included concepts, intergenerational family dynamics, family assessment skills, narrative, and the use of stories in family work, genograms/ecomaps, multiple embedded systems, rituals in families and communities, and many others (McDowell et al., 2011).

During the training, trainees were allowed time to practice, through role plays, the skills they had learned. Post-training, trainees were asked to discuss (in focus groups) what ideas and concepts seemed most and least applicable in Uganda. Overall, trainees reported that structural family therapy would be most applicable to most families in Uganda given its emphasis on subsystems, roles, and rules, which are also emphasized in Ugandan families. Because Ugandans love to tell stories and re-tell life experiences, narrative therapy was also seen as useful in Uganda. Particularly, participants reported that storytelling helped people in Uganda overcome build resilience and strengths to overcome family and community challenges. Lastly, most participants also reported that ecomaps and genograms were other applicable family therapy techniques that could work well in Uganda.

Similarly in neighboring Kenya, Puffer and colleagues (2021) adapted concepts from solution-focused therapy, systems-based therapies, cognitive behavioral therapy, and concepts from parent training programs to develop and implement a family therapy intervention for eight lay counselors. This program was named "Tuko Pamoja" (TP; Kiswahili), which literally translates to "We are together" (English). Post-training, the counselors delivered between 12–15 sessions of the intervention to 10 families over a period of 30 weeks to test its initial feasibility and acceptability. Results from the qualitative interviews indicated that the program and its concepts were feasible in the Kenyan setting. Particularly, both counselors and families reported that they liked the program because it was in the community and sessions were delivered by local counselors who the families already knew. Families highlighted the usefulness of TP techniques (e.g., the tree metaphor) to explore family functioning and goals. Some reported that thetree represented the various parts of their family such as parents (middle) and roots (clan) (Puffer et al., 2021).

Besides the above highlighted trends in training, it is difficult to track what other countries are doing in terms of training family therapists. In most universities across Africa, graduate training in psychotherapy that is available follows an inclusive model that involves clinical and counseling psychologists, social workers, psychiatrists, and religious ministers (Nwoye, 2001). In these programs, systemic family therapy is often offered as a one-time lecture. The idea behind this model of training is to produce clinicians who are diversely competent in working with individuals, couples, families, and groups (Nwoye, 2001). Thus, although several mental health practitioners from Africa have acquired and continue to acquire SFT from Western countries (e.g., the United States, Europe, and Australia) (Sim & Sim, 2020), it is still difficult to estimate and track the number of trained SFTs in Africa.

Systemic Family Therapy Research in Africa

In line with the broader tenets of systemic family therapy, existing research shows that many African family therapists in general collaborate with international scholars (mostly from Europe and the United States) to implement various evidence-based systemic interventions.

Research in these interventions can be grouped into three broad categories. The first and largest category are parenting and family strengthening interventions for treating various family problems. Through Parenting for Lifelong Health (PLH), an initiative established by the World Health Organization (WHO), the United Nations International Children's Emergency Fund (UNICEF), three universities (Oxford, Cape Town, and Stellenbosch) (Ward et al., 2020), several evidence-based parenting interventions have been developed and widely implemented across Africa to prevent harsh parenting (e.g., child maltreatment) and improve overall wellbeing of children ages 2 to 18 years. For example, in South Africa, the two prominent programs under the PLH initiative are the PLH for children from ages 2 to 9 years, and PLH for parents and teens (10 to 18 years). Both programs are implemented mostly in groups (clusters of families) and are usually supplemented by home visits (Ward et al., 2020). Although both programs were initially tested in randomized controlled trials in South Africa (e.g., Lachman et al., 2016; Cluver et al., 2018; Ward et al., 2020), the programs have been tested and implemented in over 25 counties in sub-Saharan Africa including Uganda, Tanzania, Zimbabwe, Botswana, the Democratic Republic of Congo, and many others (Shenderovich et al., 2020). Outside of programs under the PLH initiative, other examples of parenting interventions implemented across Africa in the last 10 years include adaptation of the Parent Management Training Oregon (PMTO; Forgtach & Patterson, 2010) for families affected by war and trauma in Northern Uganda (Wieling et al., 2015), programs for treating families of children with disruptive behavioral problems (e.g., Sensoy et al., 2020), and programs for preventing violence against children (e.g., Ashburn et al., 2017). For an extensive review of these and other parenting programs in Africa, we recommended Asiimwe et al. (2022)'s article, "*Training of Interventionists and Cultural Adaptation Procedures: A Systematic Review of Culturally Adapted Evidence-Based Parenting Programs in Africa*" published in the *Family Process* journal.

The second category of systemic/relational research in Africa are interventions for treating couple's relational trauma, intimate partner violence, and overall strengthening of the couple's relationships. In this category, we want to highlight a study that pilot-tested the Hold Me Tight (HMT) relationship psychoeducation program among 10 Black South African couples (Lesch et al., 2018). The HMT program is founded on the core tenets and processes of Emotionally Focused Couple Therapy (EFT; Johnson, 2019). The main goal of this psychoeducational program is to sensitize partners in a committed relationship of the critical importance of emotional awareness, closeness, and responsiveness in strengthening the couple relationship. This program is designed to be conducted over eight sessions, with each session lasting two hours long. In the South African initial HMT study, all 10 couples reported relating very well with the principles of the program and that it helped them to deepen their emotional understanding and connection with their partners. Consequently, a larger study testing the feasibility of the HMT program is currently ongoing in several low-income communities in South Africa (Asiimwe et al., 2021).

Further in the Democratic Republic of Congo (DRC), Morgan et al. (2018) implemented a Torture-Surviving Group Couple intervention among 13 couples (26 participants) who were survivors of the war in the DRC between 1998–2004. Couples who experienced the intervention were interviewed about its impact on their relationships. All couples reported significant improvements in their relationship distress because of participating in intervention groups. Most importantly, couples highlighted the concept of being able to discuss their experiences related to war in a group with other couples as the most powerful in terms of healing their relational trauma (Morgan et al., 2018). These are just a few selected examples of couple's interventions on the continent. Other studies have aimed at combating intimate partner violence (e.g., Hossain et al., 2014).

A third and final category are interventions for supporting families affected by HIV/AIDS. Because most Africans understand the impact of HIV/AIDS to be collective rather than individual, recent efforts to combat the impact of the epidemic on families have been devoted to both preventing individual transmission of HIV as well as supporting couples and families living with HIV (Doherty et al., 2013; Rosenberg et al., 2015). Thus, in most African countries today, couple counseling includes HIV testing and encouraging the open sharing of results with each other. Although it is challenging for most couples to openly discuss their HIV results (especially if they are positive) with their spouses (Morton et al., 2021), studies show that openly discussing HIV results with one's partner improves relationship functioning. In conclusion, as relationships in families continue to be impacted by the increasing forces of globalization, urbanization, and problems such as intimate partner violence, substance use, and increased mental health challenges due to pandemics like COVID-19, there is increased need for well-trained psychotherapists to respond to the needs of the people of Africa.

The Clinical Fit of Western Family Therapy Models in African Cultures

African family therapy researchers such as Nwoye (2006) and proponents of culturally responsive therapeutic practices such as Seponski et al. (2013) have called for the implementation of therapeutic approaches that are respectful, sensitive, and responsive to the context-specific needs of a certain culture. Based on research and our clinical experience as African family therapists, certain approaches to family therapy, although have origins in Western societies fit well with African clientele. One such approach is narrative therapy (Denborough, 2014; White & Epston, 1990). The narrative therapy emphasis on exploring individual, family, and cultural narratives is one that transcends across cultures. Because most African traditions are oral, Africans love to tell stories about themselves, their families, their ancestry, animals, and even stories about nature. Further, the collectivistic and social nature of African cultures makes narrative a unique fit (Williamson & Williamson, 2020). Further, narrative therapists can use the stories that already exist in many African tribes to draw inspiration and help individuals and families re-author their life stories. The power of the narrative therapist to help families tell and co-create a shared story can unite the family and cause them to be resilient amidst adversity. As White and Epston (1990) stated, "in a therapy of oral tradition, the reauthoring of lives and relationships is achieved primarily, although not exclusively, through a process of questions" (p. 17). We agree with White and Epston in that family therapists in Africa can take the advantage of oral traditions in many African cultures and use narrative therapy techniques to help clients in Africa overcome mental and family problems.

One narrative intervention that can be helpful to clients is externalizing the problem. Like in other cultures, when individuals in Africa have problems, it is common for them to feel like they are the problem rather than victims of the problem. Through externalization, family therapists help clients to "separate from the problem which makes its destructive effects more apparent to both the client and the therapist" (Nichols, 2013, p. 276). Instead of asking the client "why are you ashamed or angry?" narrative therapists use *relative influence questions* such as "how does shame or anger affect you?" Asking such questions frees clients from the problems and enables them to discover their ability to find solutions to the problem. Further, externalizing conversations can help individuals and families to 1) minimize or eliminate unproductive family conflicts, 2) undermine a sense of failure, and 3) create new possibilities for individuals in a family or a community to relate to one another (Williamson & Williamson, 2020). Studies from Africa have discussed the clinical utility of narrative therapy treating various family and community problems in Africa. One example is a community-based approach model known as 'Narrative Theater' that was created by community workers in Northern Uganda to address domestic violence and improve outcomes at family and community levels in this cultural setting (Sliep et al., 2004). Because families and communities in Africa have endured decades of trauma due to various socioeconomic, political, and health challenges, approaches like narrative theatre could create new avenues for families to process painful memories and re-author their life stories. Other applications of family therapy models in Africa are also available (e.g., McDowell et al., 2011; Nwoye, 2006; Puffer et al., 2019).

To further gain understanding of the clinical utility of particular family therapy models in African contexts, we share a case example.

Case Application

The following clinical case is an example from a client family of Dr. Michelle Karume's that she worked with in Nairobi, Kenya. We have used pseudo-names to protect the confidentiality of the family. As you will see, Dr. Karume's case conceptualization and interventions integrate three family therapy approaches: Narrative therapy, Bowenian family therapy (Kim-Appel & Appel, 2015), and Structural family therapy (Minuchin, 1978). Using her cultural knowledge of the Kenyan family structure, Dr. Karume adapts the three models to help the family resolve their problem of a child with behavioral problems.

Mr. and Mrs. Mutua and their three children came to family therapy to work on 'behavior issues' from Makau the eldest son; he was 17, his sister Mueni was 13 years old. Makau as described by his mother was a smart boy and did well in school, however, she found that his behaviors had changed for the worse. He "is rude to us, does not follow through with instructions and is not abiding by the rules of our house," his father added. Both children sat quietly as their parents described the challenges they were facing as a family. As the therapist, I could not help but notice Makau's affect change upon hearing the negative reports that were given about him by his family members. His sister on the other hand kept trying to interrupt their parents and speak up for Makau. Every attempt was met with a stern look and instruction to not interrupt when "the grownups are talking." His father explained "Ever since his mother and myself divorced he has truly changed." So you are divorced? I asked, yes, yes Mr. Mutua stated. We are only here because "the mother seems to be having it really rough with him." I made some hypotheses. The dominance by which Mr. Mutua spoke in was probably influenced by the gender values prominent in Kenya. Mrs. Makau may also subscribe to the same gender roles-but I needed to observe more of their interaction to arrive at this conclusion. The children did not have a say, which is a typical African expectation where children are to be heard and not seen as is often stated by elders in the community.

To get a better picture of their family dynamics I asked them if I could draw their genogram. I specifically wanted to hear from the children in terms of their perspectives of the family relationships. What did those relationships mean to them? Mueni and her father appeared to be very close so much so that he often asked her to take on responsibilities that would oftentimes pull her apart from her brother. One example of this was when he got upset with Makau, he asked Mueni to check on what time he came back from the party, to determine if he did his chores, or to check on how he was doing in school. This I could tell really hurt Makau.

I opted to use Narrative and Structural family therapy with this case. I wanted to know the meaning attached to how things were for each of them. I wanted to readjust the subsystems and have the parents be parents and hopefully restore the sibling subsystem. Cultural sensitivity was a key element I needed to factor in. I asked the parents about the roles in the family and my hypotheses were correct. The father was not just the head of the house;his voice dominated in family decisions. I needed to remain sensitive to the 'divorce narrative,' so I adjusted some of my intervention techniques to fit the family context. For example, I used narrative therapy questions to understand Mr. Mutua's childhood and to determine if he ever had opportunities to share his opinions with his parents. He answered no, so I was curious as to how that made him feel. Exploring childhood narratives, particularly the silence in his family as a child, opened an opportunity for the father to see his son and understand his pain when his voice is silenced. We slowly progressed to the parental subsystem and how a healthy dynamic between the parents would translate to the children. This appeared to resonate well with all of them.

From my clinical observations, this family innately wanted harmony, but the cultural influences were getting in the way of what they experienced versus what they 'had to do' based on those gender roles. Throughout the sessions I made sure to give Makau the opportunity to speak his mind and share his views. The sullen affect from the initial sessions changed to that of confidence and joy. In the subsequent sessions, his parents noted that they had not seen him laughing and smiling like they had seen in sessions. Him and his sister were back to being playful with each other and the parents had a much better co-parenting relationship.

Family Therapy and the Years Ahead in Africa; Reflections on Research and Practice Agenda

Although systemic family therapy practices have gained increased prominence in the global context (Roberts et al., 2014), research on families in Africa is still underdeveloped. As we conclude this chapter, we want to offer the reader some of our reflections on where we envision future research and practice agenda in family therapy is likely to advance in the future on the African continent. We offer these reflections as starting points believing that to understand the application and usefulness of Western models of family therapy in Africa one must first understand the lived experiences that shape family relationships in Africa, as well as the global challenges facing the field of psychotherapy in various African countries. Because SFT is practiced differently and distinctly across and within various cultures/nations (Muruthi et al., 2015), family therapists in Africa have faced several changes related to training, practice, research, and supervision, as well political/structural challenges as they attempt to establish family therapy as a respectable and independent profession in their respective countries. Challenges such as the unfavorable socioeconomic climates, general negative perception of mental illness and western psychotherapy, limited educational and training opportunities, and general low priority of mental health at national levels in many African countries are all potential barriers to the widespread application of family therapy in Africa (Asiimwe et al., 2021; Bird et al., 2011). These challenges are further compounded by a lack of an identity as a field of family therapy in many African countries. The confusion surrounding what family therapy is (e.g., form of advice), and what family therapists do (e.g., give advice), is a huge barrier that family therapists in Africa must work to overcome to create a cohesion in our profession. In general, confusion and limited or differing understanding of mental health and psychotherapy has been identified as a common phenomenon contributing to the underutilization of mental health care in many African countries (Kyei et al., 2014; Shah et al., 2017). Thus, in our view, all SFT research, training, and practice, if it is going to be sustainable and useful to Africans, must be developed and conducted in full partnership with Africans, so that they are culturally responsive and matches the local and context-specific needs.

Thus, given the challenges above, traditional models of care (i.e., one-on-one in-person therapy sessions) and criteria (e.g., minimum of a master's degree) required to develop or implement evidence-based interventions in most developed countries might not be feasible in many African settings. Therefore, research in family therapy must focus first on sampling scalable and flexible interventions that have a large impact on the diverse communities of Africa. These interventions in Africa must have the capacity to 1) coordinate local resources; 2) encourage capacity for the community to generate local solutions; 3) have a diverse portfolio with both conventional and nonconventional strategies of treatment; and 4) have the capacity to deliver services in unconventional settings (Bischoff et al., 2017). Particularly, because Africans are communal people and problems are viewed as attacks on the entire community, it is our view that the availability of scalable and affordable parenting and couple interventions would help eliminate and/or control the mental and relational health impacts of diseases like malaria and HIV/AIDS, improve child outcomes and family functioning, and build community resilience.

Second, in line with the core tenets of sociocultural attuned family therapy (e.g., McDowell et al., 2017) and principles of culturally responsive therapy (e.g., Seponski et al., 2013), previous research (e.g., Kyei et al., 2014; Shah et al., 2017) has examined overall community perceptions of mental health in several African countries, but research examining perceptions of local experts (e.g., psychotherapists and spiritual/religious leaders) and whether they believe Western family therapy models should be implemented in African settings is needed. In agreement with Seponski et al. (2020) research with local experts should particularly examine if traditional ways of healing, which have been commonly used in many African settings for centuries, are more appropriate and effective for treating individual, marital, and family mental health problems in contemporary African societies. And if so, what empirical evidence is there to decide how this is determined.

Third, given that many psychotherapists including marriage and family therapists (MFTs) in Africa acquire (d) their advanced graduate training in Western countries (e.g., mostly the United States, Europe, and Australia) (Muruthi et al., 2015; Sim & Sim, 2020), and some end up returning to Africa or continue to work in Africa (in some fashion) while living in the host countries, future research should examine these therapists' perceptions regarding the clinical utility, applicability, and cultural appropriateness of prominent SFT theories. For example, the second author of this chapter (MK) received both her masters and PhD in MFT in the United States and is now practicing MFT in an African country. Similarly, the first author (RA) received his master's in MFT at a U.S, university and is currently completing his doctorate in MFT at another U.S. university. While the two of us believe that Western/American MFT theories and practices, if appropriately culturally adapted, are clinically relevant in our native African contexts, we cannot claim to speak for other

African psychotherapists about their perceptions of Western theories of family therapy. Thus, future research should explore this topic with African psychotherapists trained in the Western industrialized countries who are currently practicing in Africa.

Fourth, given the limited opportunities for therapists in Africa to acquire advanced training in systemic family therapy and the masses confusion about what family therapy is, research should examine how local/indigenous knowledge could be integrated into Western family therapy models to affect clinical processes and client outcomes. For example, we discussed *Ubuntu therapy,* an African approach to therapy that integrates western models of psychotherapy with indigenous African practices. Although this approach has been in existence for a long time, there is limited empirical evidence to validate its clinical utility in African communities. Thus, future research should examine the clinical utility of this approach with families and communities in Africa from a local experts' perspectives. In general, we know that due to the increased focus on survival in harsh socioeconomic and political circumstances, especially in urban settings in Africa, the Ubuntu principles are becoming increasingly less prominent among many youths and families living in urban settings (Asiimwe et al., 2021). It would advance family therapy practice if researchers could provide empirical evidence regarding how the integration of African practices (e.g., Ubuntu) would improve family therapy practice and overall clinical outcomes in Africa. These questions are particularly critical to explore given the emergence of several Western systemic interventions that have already shown promise in treating mental, emotional, and relational problems in various African communities (e.g., Morgan et al., 2020; Puffer et al., 2020; Wieling et al., 2018).

Fifth, research should focus on developing and empirically testing culturally responsive models of training family therapists as well as strength-based models of studying families in Africa. These models should build upon and incorporate relevant cultural values such as strong faith traditions, aesthetics values, and oral traditions (e.g., storytelling and songs) that characterize many families in Africa. Relatedly, research should focus on developing effective ways to train the future generation of family therapists in Africa to become critical thinkers about social justice issues (e.g., privilege, power, and oppression). This would give future African family therapists opportunities to "question, discuss, gain new insights, and collectively solve problems as members of a historically oppressed and marginalized continent" (Nwoye, 2018, p. 211). Second, it would help family therapists to develop conscious ways to "liberate themselves from the history of oppression" and empower them to make significant contributions to national and international issues pertaining to social justice and mental health disparities. Given the limited availability of empirical evidence on the use of family therapy theories and models in Africa, it is our view that the availability of well-trained SFTs in Africa will produce more empirical research on culturally responsive and strength-based models that work in African contexts. More training programs need to be developed, perhaps starting with one masters and doctorate level MFT program in every African country, in order to increase the legitimacy of family therapy on the continent and decrease the systemic challenges crippling individuals and families.

Final Reflections; Three Key Takeaways

In this chapter, the authors explored sociocultural values, traditions, and practices that have historically shaped and/or distinguished psychotherapy practice in Africa from the Eurocentric approaches. Western SFT approaches and theories were broadly commended for their valuable contribution to the development and professionalization of family therapy in various African countries. As we conclude this chapter, there are three key takeaways for the reader.

The first is that contrary to the mystical view that Western or "first-world" family therapy principles and theories are culturally inappropriate and/or oppressive to Africans, the evidence presented in this chapter shows that most Western SFT principles and practices (if culturally adapted) fit well with most African cultural values and practices. Drawing from existing literature (e.g., McDowell et al., 2011; Nwoye, 2001, 2006; Puffer et al., 2021), our research, and clinical experiences as African family therapists, we find that African value systems such as collective values espoused in the *Ubuntu philosophy* match well with the theoretical underpinnings of most models of western family therapy. The example shared by one of the authors (MK) a family therapist in Nairobi, Kenya further supports this takeaway. This is not meant to suggest in any way that African cultures and family values are homogeneous or similar to Western cultures. Rather, an acknowledgement that although family therapy was introduced to Africa through primarily oppressive regimes, over the years, African family therapists have found several ways to embrace that which was foreign (i.e., family therapy), adapted it, and made it useful for their clientele.

Second, in agreement with the tenets of culturally responsive therapy (Seponski et al., 2013, 2020), Western-trained family therapists planning to conduct research or implement a family therapy intervention must carefully reflect through aspects of Western family therapy theory and practice that can be usable and transferable into the African community (McDowell et al., 2011). Conversely, they must be willing and ready to abandon theories, concepts, ideas, and techniques that are not useful or transferable to Africa. Given the obvious ethnic and linguistic diversity in African countries, it is important that systemic family therapists (both African and non-African) learn to acknowledge that there are multiple ways to do family therapy in various African cultures (Nwoye, 2006). Thus, rather than trying to teach and do family therapy in the same way it is taught and conducted in developed countries, family therapists must be flexible and genuinely open to learning other ways of doing family therapy in Africa. Our view agrees with that of Nwoye (2001) that this will allow opportunities for self-correction, decolonizing family therapy, and improving the overall cross-cultural exchange of scientific knowledge particularly in the field of psychotherapy.

Most importantly, non-African therapists must "remain culturally humble and acknowledge their position of privileged as outsiders from mostly rich Western nations, bringing Western models of mental health" in Africa (Seponski et al., 2020, p. 52). This process requires a certain level of intentionality, critical consciousness, and active participation by researchers and clinicians in the local cultural settings before thinking to introduce, adapt, and implement a family therapy model. By recognizing the unique diversity between African and Western cultures, the process of actively engaging with the target African culture will help family therapists to determine what family therapy techniques and concepts could be applicable and useful in the target African setting. If non-African therapists fail to apply and uphold principles of culturally responsive therapy, they "risk operating from an ethnocentric and colonizing perspective" (Seponski et al., 2020, p. 52).

This takeaway also applies to African psychotherapists including psychologists, counselors, and family therapists (e.g., including the authors of this chapter) who are educated and trained in the Western approaches of mental health and family therapy. First, as educated African psychotherapists, it is our responsibility to defend the integrity of our cultures and take leadership in developing culturally responsive models of family therapy research and practice. In doing so, we must recognize that although we are Africans, our relevance to the African clientele when we acquire Western-based education has historically been questioned. In particular, we have often been accused of being elitist, Eurocentric, neo-colonial, and oppressive towards our own people whom we ought to be helping (Bakker & Snyders, 1999). Essentially, we have been criticized for arrogantly representing the values of the dominant Western cultures, which is seen as a continuation of the colonial mission. Thus, we need to be careful and culturally sensitive to how we apply Western family therapy models with African families. If we are not culturally attuned and sensitive, we run the risk of unintentionally oppressing and 're-colonizing' our own people.

Our final takeaway is inspired by the article *"Family Therapy and the Pedagogy of the Oppressed; Therapeutic Use of Songs in Apartheid South Africa"* by Professor Augustine Nwoye, one of Africa's celebrated advocates and scholars of family therapy. In this article (citation listed under 'Resources for Further Reading'), Nwoye (2018) articulates the "therapeutic value and psychological potency" of songs of struggle during the apartheid regime in South Africa. Inspired by ideas such as 1) the Black Consciousness Movement (BCM) by Steven Bantu Biko and others (Hook, 2012) and 2) *kuku-nku* psychology (the use of songs of provocation, for social correction, or social practice in oppressed majority Black South Africans used struggle songs to resist and fight against the apartheid regime. Zulu and Xhosa songs such "Sanzena na?" ('what have we done' in English), *"Pasopa Verwoerd"* ('here is a Black man'), *"Sarafina"* ('Freedom is coming tomorrow'), and English songs such as *"My Black president,"* were composed and produced by Black South African artists, poets, and musicians such as Mbogeni Ngema, Miriam Makeba, and Brenda Fassie.

According to Nwoye, the liberation/struggle songs have several psychological benefits including improving the mood of the people, decreasing depression and anxiety, and enhancing relaxation for individuals in desperate situations during apartheid South Africa. Further, songs 1) help people verbalize and make sense of their feelings related to apartheid; 2) nurture and enhance group morale; 3) promote resilience; and 4) serve as a coping mechanism for injured individuals and families, and "eased the boredom and alienation of apartheid imprisonment and helped prisoners to cope with tension, depression, and nausea while in jail" (Nwoye, 2018, p. 209).

Essentially, Nwoye (2018)'s idea of *family therapy as the pedagogy of the oppressed* stresses that family therapy can be used as 'a tool for social change' to help individuals (including therapists) to "recover the words and the agency they lost in their previous experiences" (Sluzki, 2017, p. 398). According to Nwoye, this can be achieved through our clinical work as therapists but can also be achieved using educational platforms (e.g., mass media, lectures, workshops, songs, and theatre), some of which are already embedded in the daily life experiences of many Africans. In staying with the tenets of culturally responsive therapy (Seponski et al., 2020), our final takeaway is therefore that family therapists (particularly those in Africa) must break away from the traditional one-on-one in-person approaches to psychotherapy and be involved in campaigns that promote social change. Because we as family therapists have "unique insights into how social policies and political discourses shape our client's lives and the lives of our profession" (Jordan & Seponski, 2018, p. 19), we must look beyond the four walls of our practice and participate in policy-making and in shaping political discourses in our respective countries. We can act as social change agents by using family therapy as a pedagogy to share creative ideas (e.g., songs) and inspire our clients and students to understand their past and work to advocate for their future. According to Nwoye (2018) using and seeing family therapy as a pedagogy entails two fundamental principles. First, it entails "teaching family therapy students to understand how the oppressed can pathologized and blamed in psychological literature," and second, it entails "seeing clinical work with families as a pedagogical practice" (p. 210). In doing this, family therapy can continue to shape not only the lives of individuals in Africa but also social and educational processes and institutions on the continent.

In conclusion, systemic family therapy is slowly gaining prominence and legitimacy in many mental health systems in Africa. With more family therapy training programs and models of culturally responsive practice developed, one can only hope that family therapy will continue to be widely acknowledged and accepted as the first line of treatment for mental and relational problems on the African continent. Nonetheless, researchers and family therapy practitioners in Africa should continuously and intentionally reflect on key themes related to specific sociocultural concepts, ideas, and theories embedded in Western notions of mental health and family therapy, that do not align with African cultural settings. Borrowing from critical questions posed by Seponski and colleagues (2020), family therapy practitioners in Africa should reflect on: 1) What influences their use of certain models of family therapy over others in Africa? 2) What are the secondary gains of systemic family therapy intervention implementers in Africa? And finally, 3) How are local ways of healing used, integrated, and honored in the designing of interventions for masses in Africa? (Seponski et al., 2020). These questions should not be viewed as an attack on specific systemic interventions that have already been implemented in Africa but rather, as reflection questions to keep our biases and cultural lens in check, as we develop interventions to help individuals and families in Africa. For long, Africans have endured periods of Western pathologizing and discrimination and thus we want to be sensitive that our clinical work and research is empowering rather than pathologizing to families in Africa.

Lastly, with the emergence of women's rights increasing globally and similarly in Africa, with more women in leadership positions, it is our view that systemic family therapy will become one of the forerunners in career choices and resources for all (Glebova et al., 2014). Our sincere hope is that in the coming years, SFT will be the first line of treatment when individuals, couples, and families in Africa face mental health or relational challenges. Second, that African governments, international, and local agencies will apportion more funding to family therapy training, research, and practice and that all Africans will finally have equal access to family therapy resources when needed. With the unfortunate heightened levels of family dysfunction the unique skillset that SFTs bring will be greatly sought after in the years to come.

Select Resources for Further Reading

Asiimwe, R., Dwanyen, L., Subramanian, S. M., Kasujja, R., & Blow, A. J. (2022). Therapist training and cultural adaptation procedures: A systematic review of culturally adapted evidence-based parenting programs in Africa. *Family Process Journal*

Asiimwe, R., Lesch, E., Karume, M., & Blow, A. J. (2021). Expanding our international reach: Trends in the development of systemic family therapy training and implementation in Africa. *Journal of Marital and Family Therapy.*

Bakker, T. M., & Snyders, F. J. A. (1999). The (hi) stories we live by: Power/knowledge and family therapy in Africa. *Contemporary Family Therapy, 21*(2), 133–154.

Idang, G. E. (2015). African culture and values. *Phronimon, 16*(2), 97–111.

Jithoo, V., & Bakker, T. (2011). Family therapy within the African Context. *Counseling people of African ancestry*, 142–154.

Jordan, L. S., & Seponski, D. M. (2018a). Public participation: Moving beyond the four walls of therapy. *Journal of marital and family therapy, 44*(1), 5–18.

Jordan, L. S., & Seponski, D. M. (2018b). "Being a Therapist Doesn't Exclude You From Real Life": Family Therapists' Beliefs and Barriers to Political Action. *Journal of marital and family therapy, 44*(1), 19–31.

Kamya, H. (2018). Harnessing spirituality within traditional healing systems: A personal journey. In Engaging with spirituality in family therapy (pp. 67–81). Springer, Cham.

Lesch, E., de Bruin, K., & Anderson, C. (2018). A pilot implementation of the emotionally focused couple therapy group psychoeducation program in a South African setting. *Journal of Couple & Relationship Therapy, 17*(4), 313–337.

Mason, J., & Shuda, S. (1999). The history of family therapy in South Africa. *Contemporary family therapy, 21*(2), 155–172.

McDowell, T., Brown, A. L., Kabura, P., Parker, E., & Alotaiby, A. (2011). Working with families in Uganda and the United States: Lessons in cross-cultural professional training. *Journal of Systemic Therapies, 30*(2), 65–80.

Nussbaum, B. (2003). Ubuntu: Reflections of a South African on our common humanity. *Reflections: The SoL Journal, 4*(4), 21–26.

Nwadiora, E. (1996). Therapy with African families. *The Western Journal of Black Studies, 20*(3), 117.

Nwoye, A. (2000). Building on the indigenous: Theory and method of marriage therapy in contemporary Eastern and Western Africa. *Journal of Family therapy, 22*(4), 347–359.

Nwoye, A. (2001). History of family therapy: The African perspective. *Journal of family psychotherapy, 12*(4), 61–77.

Nwoye, A. (2006). A narrative approach to child and family therapy in Africa. *Contemporary Family Therapy, 28*(1), 1–23.

Nwoye, A. (2018). Family therapy and the pedagogy of the oppressed: Therapeutic use of songs in apartheid South Africa. *Australian and New Zealand Journal of Family Therapy, 39*(2), 200–217.

Van Dyk, G. A. J., & Nefale, M. C. (2005). The Split-Ego Experience of Africans: Ubuntu Therapy as a Healing Alternative. *Journal of Psychotherapy Integration, 15*(1), 48.

References

Achebe, C. (1897). Anthills of the *Savannah*. New York, NY: Anchor.

Ajayi, A. T., & Buhari, L. O. (2014). Methods of conflict resolution in African traditional society. *African Research Review, 8*(2), 138–157.

Ali, P. A., McGarry, J., & Maqsood, A. (2020). Spousal role expectations and marital conflict: perspectives of men and women. *Journal of Interpersonal Violence*, 0886260520966667.

Amadi, U. P., & Amadi, F. N. (2014). Maritial Crisis in the Nigerian Society: Causes, Consequences and Management Strategies. *Mediterranean Journal of Social Sciences, 5*(26), 133–133.

Antia, K., Boucsein, J., Deckert, A., Dambach, P., Račaitė, J., Šurkienė, G., ... & Winkler, V. (2020). Effects of international labour migration on the mental health and well-being of left-behind children: a systematic literature review. *International Journal of Environmental Research and Public Health, 17*(12), 4335.

Asiimwe, R., Lesch, E., Karume, M., & Blow, A. J. (2021). Expanding our international reach: Trends in the development of systemic family therapy training and implementation in Africa. *Journal of Marital and Family Therapy 47*(4), 815–830. https://doi.org/ 10.1111/jmft.12514.

Ashburn, K. & Kerner, B., & Ojamuge, D., & Lundgren, R. (2016). Evaluation of the Responsible, Engaged, and Loving (REAL) Fathers Initiative on Physical Child Punishment and Intimate Partner Violence in Northern Uganda. *Prevention Science*, 18. 10.1007/s11121-016-0713-9

Atindanbila, S., & Thompson, C. E. (2011). The role of African traditional healers in the management of mental challenges in Africa. *Journal of Emerging Trends in Educational Research and Policy Studies, 2*(6), 457–464.

Bakker, T. M., & Snyders, F. J. A. (1999). The (hi) stories we live by: Power/knowledge and family therapy in Africa. *Contemporary Family Therapy, 21*(2), 133–154.

Bamgbose, A. (2011). African languages today: The challenge of and prospects for empowerment under globalization. In Selected proceedings of the 40th annual conference on African linguistics (pp. 1–14). Somerville: Cascadilla Proceedings Project.

Baryshnikov, I., Joffe, G., Koivisto, M., Melartin, T., Aaltonen, K., Suominen, K., ... & Isometsä, E. (2017). Relationships between self-reported childhood traumatic experiences, attachment style, neuroticism and features of borderline personality disorders in patients with mood disorders. *Journal of Affective Disorders, 210*, 82–89.

Bassey, S. A., & Bubu, N. G. (2019). Gender inequality in Africa: a re-examination of cultural values. *Cogito, 11*(3), 21–36.

Bassil, N. R. (2011). The roots of Afropessimism: the British invention of the 'dark continent.' *Critical Arts, 25*(3), 377–396.

Baum, M., Ernst, E., Lejeune, S., & Horneber, M. (2006). Role of complementary and alternative medicine in the care of patients with breast cancer: report of the European Society of Mastology (EUSOMA) Workshop, Florence, Italy, December 2004. *European Journal of Cancer, 42*(12), 1702–1710.

Best, D. L., & Puzio, A. R. (2019). Gender and culture. In D. Matsumoto & H. C. Hwang (Eds.), *The handbook of culture and psychology* (pp. 235–291). Oxford University Press. https://doi.org/10.1093/oso/9780190679743.003.0009

Bird, P., Omar, M., Doku, V., Lund, C., Nsereko, J. R., Mwanza, J., & MHaPP Research Programme Consortium. (2011). Increasing the priority of mental health in Africa: findings from qualitative research in Ghana, South Africa, Uganda and Zambia. *Health policy and planning, 26*(5), 357–365.

Boakye, Maxwell Kwame, Pietersen, D. W., Kotzé, A., Dalton, D.-L., & Jansen, R. (2015). Knowledge and uses of African pangolins as a source of traditional medicine in Ghana. *PLoS One, 10*(1), e0117199.

Bond, S. (2009). Couple and family therapy: The evolution of the profession with social work at its core. *Intervention, la revue de l'Ordre des travailleurs sociaux et des thérapeutes conjugaux et familiaux du Québec,, 131 ,* 128–138.

Bonye, S. Z., Wuollah-Dire, D., & Der Bebelleh, F. (2020). Socio-economic Contributions of Bride Price Payment and its Implications on Women's Access to, and Ownership of Land in Wa West District, Ghana. *ADRRI Journal (Multidisciplinary), 29*(1(6)), 143–166

Breuer, E., De Silva, M. J., Fekadu, A., Luitel, N. P., Murhar, V., Nakku, J., ... & Lund, C. (2014). Using workshops to develop theories of change in five low and middle income countries: lessons from the programme for improving mental health care (PRIME). *International Journal of Mental Health Systems, 8*(1), 1–13.

Brook, J. A. (1992). Freud and splitting. *International Review of Psycho-analysis, 19*, 335–350.

Cluver, L. D., Meinck, F., Steinert, J. I., Shenderovich, Y., Doubt, J., Romero, R. H., ... & Nzima, D. (2018). Parenting for lifelong health: a pragmatic cluster randomized controlled trial of a non-commercialized parenting program for adolescents and their families in South Africa. *BMJ global health, 3*(1).

Denborough, D. (2014). Retelling the stories of our lives: Everyday narrative therapy to draw inspiration and transform experience. W. W. Norton & Company.

Doherty, T., Tabana, H., Jackson, D., Naik, R., Zembe, W., Lombard, C., ... & Chopra, M. (2013). Effect of home based HIV counselling and testing intervention in rural South Africa: cluster randomised trial. *BMJ, 346.*

Ewuoso, C., & Hall, S. (2019). Core aspects of ubuntu: A systematic review. *South African Journal of Bioethics and Law, 12*(2), 93–103.

Ford, J. D., & Blaustein, M. E. (2013). Systemic self-regulation: A framework for trauma-informed services in residential juvenile justice programs. *Journal of Family Violence, 28*(7), 665–677.

Forgatch, M. S., & Patterson, G. R. (2010). Parent Management Training – Oregon Model: An intervention for antisocial behavior in children and adolescents. In J. R. Weisz & A. E. Kazdin (Eds.), *Evidence-based psychotherapies for children and adolescents* (pp. 159–177). The Guilford Press.

Glebova, T., Bolotina, N., & Kravtsova, N. (2014). Training across the Pacific: Women create an international family therapy program. *Women & Therapy, 37*(1–2), 24–35.

Gureje, O., Appiah-Poku, J., Bello, T., Kola, L., Araya, R., Chisholm, D., Esan, O., Harris, B., Makanjuola, V., & Othieno, C. (2020). Effect of collaborative care between traditional and faith healers and primary health-care workers on psychosis outcomes in Nigeria and Ghana (COSIMPO): a cluster randomised controlled trial. *The Lancet*, *396*(10251), 612–622.

Hart, C. (2009). In search of African literary aesthetics: Production and reception of the texts of Amos Tutuola and Yvonne Vera. *Journal of African Cultural Studies*, *21*(2), 177–195.

Hook, D. (2012). A critical psychology of the postcolonial: The mind of apartheid. Routledge.

Hosegood, V., McGrath, N., & Moultrie, T. (2009). Dispensing with marriage: Marital and partnership trends in rural KwaZulu-Natal, South Africa 2000–2006. *Demographic Research*, *20*, 279.

Hossain, M., Zimmerman, C., Kiss, L., Abramsky, T., Kone, D., Bakayoko-Topolska, M., ... & Watts, C. (2014). Working with men to prevent intimate partner violence in a conflict-affected setting: a pilot cluster randomized controlled trial in rural Côte d'Ivoire. *BMC Public Health*, *14*(1), 1–13.

Idang, G. E. (2015). African culture and values. *Phronimon*, *16*(2), 97–111.

Ikuenobe, P. (2016). Good and beautiful: A moral-aesthetic view of personhood in African communal traditions. *Essays in Philosophy*, *17*(1), 125–163.

Iliffe, J. (2017). Africans: The history of a continent (Vol. 137). Cambridge University Press.

Jithoo, V., & Bakker, T. (2011). Family therapy within the African Context. *Counseling people of African ancestry*, 142–154.

Johnson, S. (2019). Attachment in action – changing the face of 21st century couple therapy. *Current opinion in psychology*, *25*, 101–104.

Jordan, L. S., & Seponski, D. M. (2018). Public participation: Moving beyond the four walls of therapy. *Journal of Marital and Family Therapy*, *44*(1), 5–18.

Kabagenyi, A., Reid, A., Ntozi, J., & Atuyambe, L. (2016). Socio-cultural inhibitors to use of modern contraceptive techniques in rural Uganda: a qualitative study. *The Pan African Medical Journal*, *25*.

Kamwangamalu, N. M. (2013). Ubuntu in South Africa: A sociolinguistic perspective to a pan-African concept. In The global intercultural communication reader (pp. 240–250). Routledge.

Kamya, H. (2018). Harnessing spirituality within traditional healing systems: A personal journey. In *Engaging with spirituality in family therapy* (pp. 67–81). Springer, Cham.

Kaye, D. K., Mirembe, F., Johansson, A., Ekstrom, A. M., & Kyomuhendo, G. B. (2005). Implications of bride price on domestic violence and reproductive health in Wakiso District, Uganda. *African health sciences*, *5*(4), 300–303.

Kim-Appel, D., & Appel, J. K. (2015). Bowenian family systems theory: Approaches and applications. *Foundations of couples, marriage, and family counseling*, 185–213.

Knizek, B. L., Andoh-Arthur, J., Osafo, J., Mugisha, J., Kinyanda, E., Akotia, C., & Hjelmeland, H. (2021). Religion as meaning-making resource in understanding suicidal behavior in Ghana and Uganda. Frontiers in psychology, 12.

Koinange, J.W. (2004). Psychology in Kenya. In M. J. Stevens, & D. Wedding. (2004). *The handbook of international psychology* (pp 56–83). New York, NY: Brunner- Routledge.

Kyei, J. J., Dueck, A., Indart, M. J., & Nyarko, N. Y. (2014). Supernatural belief systems, mental health and perceptions of mental disorders in Ghana. *International Journal of Culture and Mental Health*, *7*(2), 137–151.

Lachman, J. M., Sherr, L. T., Cluver, L., Ward, C. L., Hutchings, J., & Gardner, F. (2016). Integrating evidence and context to develop a parenting program for low-income families in South Africa. *Journal of Child and Family Studies*, *25*(7), 2337–2352.

Lesch, E., de Bruin, K., & Anderson, C. (2018). A pilot implementation of the emotionally focused couple therapy group psychoeducation program in a South African setting. *Journal of Couple & Relationship Therapy*, *17*(4), 313–337.

Mafumbate, R. (2019, September). The Undiluted African Community: Values, The Family, Orphanage and Wellness in Traditional Africa. In *Information and Knowledge Management* (Vol. 9, No. 8, pp. 7–13).

Mason, J., & Shuda, S. (1999). The history of family therapy in South Africa. *Contemporary family therapy*, *21*(2), 155–172.

Mathibela, M. K., Egan, B. A., Du Plessis, H. J., & Potgieter, M. J. (2015). Socio-cultural profile of Bapedi traditional healers as indigenous knowledge custodians and conservation partners in the Blouberg area, Limpopo Province, South Africa. *Journal of Ethnobiology and Ethnomedicine*, *11*(1), 1–11.

Mbaye, L. M., & Wagner, N. (2017). Bride price and fertility decisions: Evidence from rural Senegal. *The Journal of Development Studies*, *53*(6), 891–910.

Mbiti, J. S. (1970). Concepts of God in Africa.

McDowell, T., Brown, A. L., Kabura, P., Parker, E., & Alotaiby, A. (2011). Working with families in Uganda and the United States: Lessons in cross-cultural professional training. *Journal of Systemic Therapies*, 30(2), 65–80.

McDowell, T., Knudson-Martin, C., & Bermudez, J. M. (2017). Socioculturally attuned family therapy: Guidelines for equitable theory and practice. Routledge.

Metz, T. (2010). African and Western moral theories in a bioethical context. *Developing World Bioethics*, 10(1), 49–58.

Miller, J. K. (2011). International issues in clinical practice and training. *Journal of Systemic Therapies*, 30(2), 41.

Minuchin, S. (1974). Families and family therapy. Cambridge, MA: Harvard University Press. Routledge.

Mnyaka, M., & Motlhabi, M. (2005). The African concept of Ubuntu/Botho and its socio-moral significance. *Black Theology*, 3(2), 215–237.

Morgan, E., Wieling, E., Hubbard, J., & Dwanyen, L. (2020). Perceptions of War Trauma and Healing of Marital Relations Among Torture-surviving Congolese Couples Participating in Multicouple Therapy. *Family Process*, 59(3), 1128–1143.

Morgan, E., Wieling, E., Hubbard, J., & Dwanyen, L. (2020). Perceptions of War Trauma and Healing of Marital Relations Among Torture-surviving Congolese Couples Participating in Multicouple Therapy. *Family Process*, 59(3), 1128–1143.

Morgan, E., Wieling, E., Hubbard, J., & Kraus, E. (2018). The development and implementation of a multi-couple therapy model with torture survivors in the Democratic Republic of the Congo. *Journal of Marital and Family Therapy*, 44(2), 235–247.

Morton, K., Mhlakwaphalwa, T., Msimango, L., Van Heerden, A., Ngubane, T., Joseph, P., ... & McGrath, N. (2021). Optimising a couples-focused intervention to increase couples' HIV testing and counselling using the person-based approach: a qualitative study in Kwa-Zulu Natal, South Africa. *BMJ open*, 11(12), e047408.

Mtika, M. M. (2007). Political economy, labor migration, and the AIDS epidemic in rural Malawi. *Social Science & Medicine*, 64(12), 2454–2463.

Mugisha, J., Hjelmeland, H., Kinyanda, E., & Knizek, B. L. (2013). Religious views on suicide among the Baganda, Uganda: A qualitative study. *Death Studies*, 37(4), 343–361.

Muhorakeye, O., Biracyaza, E. (2021). Exploring Barriers to Mental Health Services Utilization at Kabutare District Hospital of Rwanda: Perspectives From Patients. *Frontiers In Psychology*, 12, 1–13. www.frontiersin.org/articles/10.3389/fpsyg.2021.638377/full

Muruthi, B. A., Bermudez, J. M., Chou, J., & Farnham, A. (2015). Neither here nor there: Working with transnational immigrant families in marriage and family therapy. *Family Therapy Magazine*, 14(3), 12–17. Retrieved August 8, 2023, from: http://hdl.handle.net/10919/74444

Nandutu, W. (2017). Cultural explanations of depression in children among the Baganda. Unpublished thesis. Makerere University.

National Institute of Statistics of Rwanda (NISR) [Rwanda], Ministry of Health (MOH) [Rwanda], and ICF. 2021. Rwanda Demographic and Health Survey 2019–20 Final Report. Kigali, Rwanda, and Rockville, Maryland, USA: NISR and ICF.

National Population Commission – NPC/Nigeria and ICF. 2019. Nigeria Demographic and Health Survey 2018. Abuja, Nigeria, and Rockville, Maryland, USA: NPC and ICF.

Ngugi, wa Thiong'o (1972). Homecoming: Essays on African and Caribbean Literature, Culture and Politics. London: Heinemann

Nichols, M. P. (2013). Family therapy: Concepts and methods. Pearson Education, Inc, tenth edition.

Nkrumah, K. (1970). Consciencism: Philosophy and Ideology for De-colonization. New York and London: Monthly Review Press.

Nwadiora, E. (1996). Therapy with African families. *The Western Journal of Black Studies*, 20(3), 117.

Nwoye, A. (2001). History of family therapy: The African perspective. *Journal of Family Psychotherapy*, 12(4), 61–77.

Nwoye, A. (2006). A narrative approach to child and family therapy in Africa. *Contemporary Family Therapy*, 28(1), 1–23.

Nwoye, A. (2018). Family therapy and the pedagogy of the oppressed: Therapeutic use of songs in apartheid South Africa. *Australian and New Zealand Journal of Family Therapy*, 39(2), 200–217.

Ojagbemi, A., & Gureje, O. (2020). The importance of faith-based mental healthcare in African urbanized sites. *Current Opinion in Psychiatry, 33*(3), 271–277.

Okocha, A. A., & Alika, I. H. (2012). Professional counseling in Nigeria: Past, present, and future. *Journal of Counseling & Development, 90*(3), 362–366.

Olaoba, O. B., Anifowose, R., Yesufu, A. R., & Oyedolapo, B. D. (2010). African traditional methods of conflict resolution. National Open University of Nigeria.

Osafo, J., Akotia, C. S., Andoh-Arthur, J., & Puplampu, B. M. (2021). The Role of Religious Leaders in Suicide Prevention in Ghana. A Qualitative Analysis. *Pastoral Psychology, 70*(5), 525–539.

Osafo, J., Knizek, B. L., Akotia, C. S., & Hjelmeland, H. (2013). Influence of religious factors on attitudes towards suicidal behaviour in Ghana. *Journal of Religion and Health, 52*(2), 488–504.

Patel, V., Chowdhary, N., Rahman, A., & Verdeli, H. (2011). Improving access to psychological treatments: lessons from developing countries. *Behaviour research and therapy, 49*(9), 523–528.

Patterson, J. E., Edwards, T. M., & Vakili, S. (2018). Global mental health: a call for increased awareness and action for family therapists. *Family Process, 57*(1), 70–82.

Paul, I. A. (2019). An Expository Study of Witchcraft among the Basoga of Uganda. *IJHSSE: International Journal of Humanities Social Sciences and Education, 6*(12), 83–96.

Peprah, P., Gyasi, R. M., Adjei, P. O.-W., Agyemang-Duah, W., Abalo, E. M., & Kotei, J. N. A. (2018). Religion and Health: exploration of attitudes and health perceptions of faith healing users in urban Ghana. *BMC Public Health, 18*(1), 1–12.

Pohoață, G. (2019). Dignity, Democracy, Diversity XXIX World Congress of the International Association for Philosophy of Law & Social Philosophy. *Cogito-Multidisciplinary Research Journal 3*, 7–11.

Princewill, C. W., Wangmo, T., Jegede, A. S., Riecher-Rössler, A., & Elger, B. S. (2019). Bride price payment and women's autonomy: Findings from qualitative interviews from Nigeria. *Women & Health, 59*(7), 775–788.

Puffer, E. S., Friis-Healy, E. A., Giusto, A., Stafford, S., & Ayuku, D. (2021). Development and implementation of a family therapy intervention in Kenya: A community-embedded lay provider model. *Global Social Welfare, 8*(1), 11–28.

Rautenbach, C. (2015). Legal reform of traditional courts in South Africa: Exploring the links between Ubuntu, restorative justice and therapeutic jurisprudence. *J. Int'l & Comp. L., 2*, 275.

Roberts, J., Abu-Baker, K., Diez Fernández, C., Chong Garcia, N., Fredman, G., Kamya, H., ... & Zevallos Vega, R. (2014). Up close: Family therapy challenges and innovations around the world. *Family Process, 53*(3), 544–576.

Rosenberg, N. E., Mtande, T. K., Saidi, F., Stanley, C., Jere, E., Paile, L., ... & Hosseinipour, M. (2015). Recruiting male partners for couple HIV testing and counselling in Malawi's option B+ programme: an unblinded randomised controlled trial. *The lancet HIV, 2*(11), e483-e491.

Rummun, N., Neergheen-Bhujun, V. S., Pynee, K. B., Baider, C., & Bahorun, T. (2018). The role of endemic plants in Mauritian traditional medicine–Potential therapeutic benefits or placebo effect? *Journal of Ethnopharmacology, 213*, 111–117

Sall, A. O. (2009). Multilinguism, linguistic policy, and endangered languages in Senegal. *Journal of Multicultural Discourses, 4*(3), 313–330.

Semrau, M., Alem, A., Ayuso-Mateos, J. L., Chisholm, D., Gureje, O., Hanlon, C., ... & Thornicroft, G. (2019). Strengthening mental health systems in low-and middle-income countries: recommendations from the Emerald programme. *BJPsych Open, 5*(5).

Sensoy, Ö., Culham, J. C., & Schwarzer, G. (2020). Do infants show knowledge of the familiar size of everyday objects? *Journal of Experimental Child Psychology, 195*. https://doi.org/10.1016/j.jecp.2020.104848

Seponski, D. M., Bermudez, J. M., & Lewis, D. C. (2013). Creating culturally responsive family therapy models and research: Introducing the use of responsive evaluation as a method. *Journal of Marital and Family Therapy, 39*(1), 28–42.

Seponski, D. M., Lewis, D. C., Bermudez, J. M., & Sotelo, J. M. (2020). Cambodian therapists' perspectives of western-based psychotherapy models: Addressing the challenges for service providers. *Journal of Family Psychotherapy, 31*(1–2), 36–55.

Shah, A., Wheeler, L., Sessions, K., Kuule, Y., Agaba, E., & Merry, S. P. (2017). Community perceptions of mental illness in rural Uganda: An analysis of existing challenges facing the Bwindi Mental Health Programme. *African Journal of Primary Health Care & Family Medicine, 9*(1), 1–9.

Shambare, B. (2021). The Ubuntu Parenting: Kairos Consideration for the 21st Century Dynamics and Globalization. In *Parenting- Challenges of Child Rearing in a Changing Society*. IntechOpen.

Shenderovich, Y., Ward, C. L., Lachman, J. M., Wessels, I., Sacolo-Gwebu, H., Okop, K., ... & Cluver, L. (2020). Evaluating the dissemination and scale-up of two evidence-based parenting interventions to reduce violence against children: study protocol. *Implementation Science Communications*, 1(1), 1–11.

Sim, T., & Sim, C. (2020). Global contexts for the profession of systemic family therapy. In K. Wampler & A. Blow's (Eds.), *The handbook of systemic family therapy*, (Vol. 1) (pp. 51–77). New York, NY: WIley-Blackwell.

Sliep, Y., Weingarten, K., & Gilbert, A. (2004). Narrative Theatre as an Interactive Community Approach to Mobilizing Collective Action in Northern Uganda. *Families, Systems, & Health*, 22(3), 306.

Sluzki, C. E. (2017). The impact of authoritarian regimes on families... and on therapists. *Australian and New Zealand Journal of Family Therapy*, 38(3), 398–404.

Smit, R. (2001). The impact of labor migration on African families in South Africa: Yesterday and today. *Journal of Comparative Family Studies*, 32(4), 533–548.

Sodi, T., Esere, M. O., Gichinga, E. M., & Hove, P. (2010). Marriage and Counselling in African communities: challenges and counselling approaches. *Journal of Psychology in Africa*, 20(2), 335–340.

Tenkorang, E. Y. (2021). Women as perpetrators of intimate partner violence in Ghana. *Journal of Gender-based Violence*, 5(1), 75–94.

Tenkorang, E. Y., Asamoah-Boaheng, M., & Owusu, A. Y. (2021). Intimate partner violence (IPV) against HIV-positive women in Sub-Saharan Africa: a mixed-method systematic review and meta-analysis. *Trauma, Violence, & Abuse*, 22(5), 1104–1128

Theresa, A. (2014). *Methods of Conflict Resolution in African Traditional Society*. 8(33), 138–157.

Tomita, A., & Ramlall, S. (2018). A nationwide panel study on religious involvement and depression in South Africa: Evidence from the South African National Income Dynamics Study. *Journal of Religion and Health*, 57(6), 2279–2289.

Tuwe, K. (2016). The African oral tradition paradigm of storytelling as a methodological framework: Employment experiences for African communities in New Zealand. In African Studies Association of Australasia and the Pacific (AFSAAP) Proceedings of the 38th AFSAAP Conference: 21st Century Tensions and Transformation in Africa. Deakin University.

Umubyeyi, B., & Mtapuri, O. (2019). Approaches to marital conflict resolution: a perspective of democratic Republic of Congo migrants living in Durban, South Africa. *Journal of Family Issues*, 40(8), 1065–1085.

Umubyeyi, B., Mtapuri, O., & Naidu, M. (2020). The role of religion and religious leaders in marital conflict resolution: a perspective of congolese migrants' families living in Durban, South Africa. *The Family Journal*, 28(4), 413–419.

UNHCR. (2020). *UNHCR Global Report 2020*. Global Focus UNHCR Operations Worldwide. https://reporting.unhcr.org/globalreport2020

Van Duijl, M., Nijenhuis, E., Komproe, I. H., Gernaat, H. B., & De Jong, J. T. (2010). Dissociative symptoms and reported trauma among patients with spirit possession and matched healthy controls in Uganda. *Culture, Medicine, and Psychiatry*, 34(2), 380–400.

Van Dyk, G. A. J., & Nefale, M. C. (2005). The Split-Ego Experience of Africans: Ubuntu Therapy as a Healing Alternative. *Journal of Psychotherapy Integration*, 15(1), 48.

Vessel, E. A., Starr, G. G., & Rubin, N. (2013). Art reaches within: aesthetic experience, the self and the default mode network. *Frontiers in Neuroscience*, 7, 258.

wa Thiong'o, N. (1980). *Devil on the Cross* (English translation of Caitaani mutharaba-Ini). Nairobi, Kenya.

Walker, J. A. (2012). Early marriage in Africa-trends, harmful effects and interventions. *African Journal of Reproductive Health*, 16(2), 231–240.

Ward, C. L., Wessels, I. M., Lachman, J. M., Hutchings, J., Cluver, L. D., Kassanjee, R., ... & Gardner, F. (2020). Parenting for Lifelong Health for Young Children: a randomized controlled trial of a parenting program in South Africa to prevent harsh parenting and child conduct problems. *Journal of Child Psychology and Psychiatry*, 61(4), 503–512.

White, M., Wijaya, M., & Epston, D. (1990). Narrative means to therapeutic ends. W. W. Norton & Company.

Wieling, E., Mehus, C., Möllerherm, J., Neuner, F., Achan, L., & Catani, C. (2015). Assessing the feasibility of providing a parenting intervention for war-affected families in Northern Uganda. *Family & Community Health, 38*(3), 252–267.

Williamson, D., & Williamson, J. (2020). Family Counseling in Uganda. In Intercultural Perspectives on Family Counseling (pp. 22–35). New York, NY: Routledge.

Wilson, D., & Williams, V. (2013). Ubuntu: Development and framework of a specific model of positive mental health. *Psychology Journal, 10*(2).

Wissing, M. P., Wilson Fadiji, A., Schutte, L., Chigeza, S., Schutte, W. D., & Temane, Q. M. (2020). Motivations for relationships as sources of meaning: Ghanaian and South African experiences. *Frontiers in Psychology, 11,* 2019.

World Health Organization. (2013). *Global and regional estimates of violence against women: prevalence and health effects of intimate partner violence and non-partner sexual violence.* World Health Organization.

Yaya, S., Odusina, E. K., & Bishwajit, G. (2019). Prevalence of child marriage and its impact on fertility outcomes in 34 sub-Saharan African countries. *BMC International Health and Human Rights, 19*(1), 1–11.

Zacarias, A. E., Macassa, G., & Soares, J. J. (2012). Women as perpetrators of IPV: The experience of Mozambique. *Journal of Aggression, Conflict and Peace Research, 4*(1), 5–27. https://doi.org/10.1108/17596591211192966.

13

THE DEVELOPMENT OF CAMBODIAN FAMILY THERAPY

Bernhild Pfautsch

Background

Over the last decade several international scholars have shown a longstanding commitment to provide concepts of family therapy for Cambodian students (Miller et al., 2018; Seponski & Jordan, 2018). However, up to now, family therapy has not been part of tertiary education as a whole course program in Cambodia (Miller et al., 2019). The Southeast Asian country is still dealing with the legacy of the Pol Pot regime from 1975–1979, the following decade of civil war, and the associated traumatization of an entire generation (Chandler, 2003). In order to forcefully enforce the new ideology, Pol Pot's apparatus dismantled social pillars such as religion, art, and in some cases also family structures (van Schaack & Chhang, 2011). Forced marriages conducted at that time are still a stigma for the families concerned and lead to identity and loyalty conflicts of the descendants (Langis et al., 2014). Children were pressured to denounce their parents, and families were brutally torn apart and assigned to separate labor camps. In addition to the destruction of economic structures and the health and education systems, the Khmer Rouge era also left disintegrated families and communities behind. Against this background, it becomes clear that in any counseling with Cambodian families, the aftermath of the traumatic past must be taken into account (Boehnlein & Kinzie, 2011). Medical treatment gradually became available again in the 1980s (Somasundaram et al., 1999), but access to mental health services remains very limited to this day (Jegannathan et al., 2015). The need of those services is illustrated by the findings of the Cambodian Mental Health Survey (Schunert et al., 2012), referring to the high prevalence of anxiety disorder, posttraumatic stress disorder, and suicide attempts in the general population.

Reconstruction of Higher Education in Cambodia

The psychology department of the Royal University of Phnom Penh (RUPP) was supported in the post-Khmer-Rouge era by various western scientists on site and the Bachelor degree in psychology started as early as 1994. The Master's program in Clinical Psychology and Counseling followed in 2009 with a curriculum in which several local psychologists and

DOI: 10.4324/9781003297871-15

a number of international academics worked, often staying with the university for long periods of time (Miller et al., 2019; Seponski & Jordan, 2018). This program has been supported by the Civil Peace Service (CPS) of the German Corporation for International Cooperation (GIZ) since 2009. The CPS program in Cambodia works in the context of the Khmer Rouge Tribunal for reconciliation and dealing with the past (GIZ, 2021). Psychosocial services are supported, and this was the context for my job as a psychologist at RUPP from 2015 to 2018. At the Royal University I was working with my Cambodian colleagues in terms of Capacity Development (GIZ, 2013) on the further development of curricula, and carried it out with Cambodian co-lecturers.

Systemic family therapy approaches are practiced occasionally by non-governmental organizations (NGOs) (Miller et al., 2019), but there is a growing interest in family therapy (Seponski et al., 2014), and the systemic approach is considered to be of high relevance for psychosocial care in low-and-middle-income countries (Patterson et al., 2018). After a thorough discussion with my local colleagues, the students and key people at the university, I was able to get the family therapy training off the ground, with the support of Anna Huisman, a Dutch social worker and transcultural family therapist on site. Before I continue to share about implementing systemic family training in Cambodia, I would like to shed the light on significant overarching themes.

Internationalization of Family Therapy

Marcela Polanco (Polanco, 2016) points out that with the internationalization of professional knowledge from the field of family therapy (e.g., when Western experts carry out further education and training in a global context or advise educational institutions on the creation of their curricula) a reflection on a potentially colonizing agenda of the content is indispensable.

A multilateral fair trade of knowledge between different cultures contributes to the integrity of all those involved and secures internationalization, especially for therapists who do not identify themselves with the Euro-American paradigm. In cultures outside of this paradigm, it is important to rethink the (Euro-American) foundations for family therapy training and to bring them more in line with one's own cultural location and that of their clients (Polanco, 2016). I learned from my Cambodian colleagues how to consider family hierarchy not only in the therapy session but also as a cultural frame of mind, challenging my highly valued (individualistic) views of equity within the family. Furthermore, Cambodian professionals have understood very well the great empowering potential of seeing the client as the expert. However, they also know the very demand and expectation of their clients to get advice for a quick fix. Listening to their creative solutions to bridge that gap has taught me a lot about the unquestionable importance of indigenous knowledge.

Implications for a Global Transfer of Knowledge

Making professional knowledge culturally suitable across cultural borders requires the analysis of the content to be conveyed in terms of its universality or the necessary transformation into the local context. This calls for indigenous knowledge (McDowell et al., 2017) provided in close cooperation by local partners (Charlés & Bava, 2020; Seponski & Jordan, 2018). In Cambodia, Euro-American mental health therapy modules have been introduced and a growing need for adaption to resonate well within the context is acknowledged

(Seponski et al., 2020). Moreover, the taught models are expected to theoretically and technically comply with the unique needs of the addressed population (Seponski et al., 2013). Bearing these necessities in mind, I could refer to previously presented systemic family therapy content in some of my psychology courses for the master students at RUPP and the respective discussions. These experiences were incorporated in the planning of the training together with my Cambodian colleagues, searching for family therapy models that address the challenges on multiple systemic levels in Cambodia (Seponski et al., 2020). The teaching units were critically reflected in de-briefings. Feedback from the participants and observations from local colleagues were discussed and documented (McDowell et al., 2011). In the second and third round of the training, Cambodian colleagues were more intensively involved and were then responsible for the modification, relating to their own training experience. The local specialists (therapists) are currently faced with the task of continuing the local knowledge production in accordance with their cultural values and traditions (Polanco, 2016).

Knowledge Fair Trade

The family therapists Laurie Charlés and Gameela Samarasinghe (2016), who work in global contexts, focus on international knowledge transfer as the trade of knowledge across borders. All sides should benefit equally from this trade. The authors ask about the implications when – in the context of international humanitarian aid – knowledge is brought mainly from countries with high incomes to countries with low or middle incomes. Do the channels of knowledge transfer play a role? What infrastructure does this knowledge apply to? What capacities are there for the application? Can there be an unintentional, unfair distribution of knowledge and resources? How does the knowledge transfer intervene in local structures? Working closely on a daily basis with my colleagues at the university in Phnom Penh I had the opportunity to build trustful relationships that have proven to be resources for deeper insights in culture and context, particularly to answer the aforementioned questions. My hierarchical role as an international expert implies power imbalance, and my colleagues initially refrained from open criticism or sharing own controverse ideas. Further, many of the trainees who were sent to be trained by the employing organization often found themselves pressured by conflicting schedules due to working requirements during training modules. Balancing the need to keep up with the requirements (e.g., for attendance) and well-founded exceptions was an ongoing challenge, especially considering that most of the trainees were juggling several jobs and family duties.

First Steps: Training Design

The knowledge transfer in family therapy training must be based on the conditions and needs within the given context (Charlés & Samarasinghe, 2016). In Cambodia, the limited access to education and healthcare among other injustices related to poverty (Seponski et al., 2014) needed to be considered. The few professionals in the psycho-social field have to bear enormous responsibilities and are confronted with various expectations regarding their professional role (Jordan et al., 2019). The training curriculum for mental health professionals (psychologists and social workers as well as counselors) with at least two years of professional experience was put together under these premises.

Conceived as a basic course, key concepts of systemic work are presented in theory and its respective practice in the Cambodian context. In its current framework as a basic course, the training comprises four teaching modules, each lasting 2 or 2.5 days, as well as the graduation module, and extends over 7–8 months. The components of the course are intended to promote reflective practice related to professional and personal development (Aponte & Kissil, 2016). Immediate practical transfer of the newly acquired knowledge is stimulated by practical assignments and its reflective logging between teaching modules in order to build skills from the interplay of theoretical knowledge, its practical application and reflection (Hilzinger & Henrich, 2020). Accordingly, peer group work and group supervision (Ebbecke-Nohlen, 2015; Proctor, 2008) comprising also role play (Natrajan-Tyagi et al., 2016) and casework (Bauer, 2020) are part of the curriculum in addition to the teaching modules.

Learning by Doing: The Course Reality

The first Postgraduate Certificate in Family Therapy and Systemic Practice started at the RUPP's Psychology Department in spring 2017 (GIZ Cambodia, 2017). So far, three groups, each with 10–12 participants, and four Cambodian psychologists have been trained as trainers.

Taking into account the contextual and cultural background requires consideration of the educational imprint and qualification level of the participants (Weinhardt, 2020). We as international specialists were not fluent enough in Khmer to present the training in the native language of the trainees, therefore the communication took place mainly in English, which posed a barrier to follow the teaching conversation for some trainees. Moreover, historically many of the technical terms from western therapeutic concepts had no equivalent terms in Khmer. The Cambodian translators (and now trainers) were essential to clarify for the trainees and provide feedback to us as lecturers. Language transports discourses in a social-constructionist conception of language (Anderson, 1997; Gergen, 2009) reality is constituted by individual understanding. When the use of language is reflected in the context of knowledge transfer and international training, it is not only about the linguistic use of terms but also about the discourses contained therein, and thus about the translation and interpretation of ideas. Language shapes perspectives and guides practices; certain perspectives and practices are included or excluded through language. In addition to the content, a viable translation must also focus on the context – what meaning is ascribed to certain terms in the current context. Subtext can be lost in literal translation, and a good cooperation with interpreters who are familiar with both the local and the professional context is essential for the quality of communication (Charlés & Bava, 2020). As interpreter for our trainings served colleagues from the psychology department with whom a warm and trustful collaboration was already established and who were acknowledged as experts by the trainees. Both aspects have been proven effective for the training.

Adapting New Learning Culture

The students were accustomed to frontal teaching, memorizing of content, and final repetition for exams (Brehm & Aktas, 2020). This rote learning or memorization as a complex construct is deeply interwoven in East Asian culture (Po Li, 2011) and must be taken into account as a cultural difference related to learning and teaching when designing the training. It needs to be acknowledged that, in addition to the content-related requirements of the training, the participants also needed to establish new unfamiliar learning strategies. In the professional exchange with Cambodian colleagues, it became clear that the culturally new learner-oriented methods of knowledge formation are, from their point of view, indispensable for the desired competency development of the participants, but require a careful and step-by-step introduction. For instance, the requirements of reflective practice seemed to be a huge challenge for most Cambodian trainees, both in terms of the reflective tasks as well as the respective writings. They were asked to create a learning portfolio in which peer and group supervision meetings as well as the practical application of at least eight interventions in their professional practice were reflected. The use of the portfolios promoted self-organized learning by the Cambodian participants, ensure the documentation of the learning processes, and offer an opportunity to assess the learning progress of the participants (Gläser-Zikuda & Hascher, 2007). The Cambodian trainers discovered that the task, being so different from previous learning experience, needed much more clarification than we had expected. Therefore, the tasks and written instructions for the portfolio were linguistically simplified.

Learning from Peers

In the graduation module, the participants were required to present their final project, the documentation of the application of a therapeutic intervention from their field of work. This demand was met with incomprehension at first. Besides the common reluctance to expose oneself, the trainees didn't consider their own contributions as being instructive enough for their peers in the first place. These concerns were rebutted by the impressive presentations and lively discussions in the group during the graduation module. As intended, systemic case understanding was promoted, and practical knowledge was established by peer learning (Bauer, 2020). Outstanding trainees were invited to present their work at the symposia "Working with Families in Cambodia" organized by RUPP's psychology department in 2017 and 2019. The provision of supervision by international trainers needs sensitive consideration (Seponski & Jordan, 2018). The future provision of supervision by Cambodian professionals is planned; to train these colleagues remains a crucial task.

Beyond reflection on experience made in this first phase of curriculum development, qualitative research on aspects of culturally and contextually adapted family therapy education was conducted to support further development. As an academic from the global north, socialized in the knowledge base of western human science, I came to a country affected by European colonization (Chandler, 2003) to conduct research – a background that requires fundamental considerations described below.

Decolonial Research Practice

The global expansion of Europe took place not only militarily, economically, and politically, but also had a profound influence on culture and the tradition of thought (Brunner, 2016). Eurocentric knowledge has established itself worldwide in the course of colonialism and still outlasts it. This is where the argument comes in to decolonize knowledge and to dissolve the dominance of the Eurocentric canon (Brunner, 2016). The approach of decolonial research is committed to this critical practice, which assumes that Western research ideology is associated with certain values, biases and practices that influence the production of knowledge and were influenced by them (Bermúdez et al., 2016).

Research

I pursued questions about the cultural and contextual adaptation of existing concepts of systemic family therapy in a mixed methods study. The data presented here come from expert interviews with 18 Cambodian (9 female/"CF" and 9 male/"CM") as well as 7 international (4 female/"EF" and 3 male/"EM") specialists in Phnom Penh in spring 2019.

The cross-cultural Multidimensional Ecosystemic Comparative Approach (MECA) (Falicov, 2017) as a postmodern concept for a culturally adapted family therapy based on the empowerment approach served as a theoretical framework for the evaluation of my data using the qualitative content analysis according to Mayring (Mayring & Fenzl, 2019).

Referring to the interplay from theories of family therapy and traditional, spiritual belief systems I use particularly the MECA dimension of ecological context for analysis of the respective data. This MECA domain examines the diverse living conditions of families within the immediate as well as broader socio-political realities. Ethnic and religious affiliation, working and living conditions as well as educational opportunities and access to social institutions are explored. In this domain, power imbalances and the psycho-social consequences of marginalization and discrimination are examined (Falicov, 2017). Attitudes with regard to health, illness, and religion as well as the relation to spirituality or magical ideas are relevant in order to be able to consider with the view of the clients when it comes to modern medical care, psychotherapy and the involvement of traditional healers. Attitudes on personal responsibility as well as cultural coping strategies in dealing with personal impairments are important; these also include spiritual and health resources available from parishes, priests (Falicov, 2009), or Buddhist monks in the immediate vicinity. In addition to these institutionalized religions and a mainstream understanding of medical treatment, traditional healing rituals are used in many ethnic groups. Traditional healers are sought out for help with psychological or interpersonal problems (Falicov, 2016).

Findings

Statements from the interviewees about the importance of religion and spiritual practice and their influence on family counseling and therapy revealed a manifold mosaic of respective aspects. The significance of Buddhism, the influence of different religions and spiritual belief systems found in all generations as well as the multifaceted nature of religious practice with its influence on the understanding of mental health and the treatment of mental or family problems were found. The Cambodian counselors described their own attitudes to assimilate and acknowledge religious and spiritual practices of their clients. Further, the still strong restrictions of stigma related to mental health and counseling were exemplified.

Buddhism being of great importance for the people of Cambodia was described. Buddhist monks are treated with reverence, and many young men still choose to live in the pagoda for a period of one to two years. With the culture of seniority being rooted in Buddhism, hierarchical structures are religiously legitimized. Buddhism in Cambodia is historically interwoven with various spiritual belief systems, such as Hinduism, the worship of ancestors, and the strong belief in animism and its magic practices.

In our house we have like the spirit of our ancestor to stay in the house "to keep the house happiness" something like that. So, we prepare the food and we like/we pray to our ancestors

(2CF)

The growing influence of a more modern Buddhism can be observed. Monks are active in social media, and are invited to schools and can thus represent their reading of the religion. Some of the interviewees described the practice of religion as a cultural tradition and less as an active religious practice, at least the younger people. They stated that it is mostly older people who are interested in the issues of the next life. There are also a small but growing number of Christians and Muslims in the country.

"And They Really Deeply Believe in That Kind of Thing"

The practice of religious practice is omnipresent. The belief in magic influences many life decisions.

> *They to go to traditional healer or drink traditional medicine or go to fortune teller and they really deeply believe in that kind of thing.*
>
> (6CF)

If children cause a lot of problems, they are given new names on the advice of the temple priest, and pregnancies are scheduled so that the birthday falls under a lucky sign. Some conflicts are attributed to unfortunate star constellations and marriages are divorced for this reason. Black magic practices are common, especially in the countryside. The fear of evil spirits is widespread among all generations and young people also go to the pagoda to ensure happiness with water blessings. However, some of the interviewees also described a trend of diminishing influence of religion – people who are doing well might not be interested, or rather religion may only come into play when people feel desperate. Also, people no longer just believe in fate, but have started to think more from a scientific framework.

"They Gonna Burn the Spirit out of Them"

Spiritual explanations for mental disorders and even for conflict are common. Mentally ill people might have bad karma because of misconduct in a previous life, might be possessed by angry ancestors, or might have been cursed by black magic. That is why the mentally ill are feared. Even if a child is born with a physical disability or epilepsy, it is often seen as bad karma as a result of the mother's or ancestors' actions.

> *A lot of people until now still think that mental illness (is) not a problem that occurs by themself or by the chemical factor or by the neuron something like that. They only believe that this is the third power I mean that it's rather related to the traditional sector [...] from magic or from the Kruh, something like that.*
>
> (14CM)

Help is sought from traditional healers, fortunetellers, and monks. Special sacrifices are made to appease the ancestors. Treatment by traditional healers is frequently harmful and costs people a lot of money. Examples were described, whereby attempts were made to cast out evil spirits by beating with clubs. The consumption of dubious substances would be prescribed.

This time last year there was one girl who had terrible necrosis of her face and they were told to put dung on it. And it's still you know "go and get some battery acid and put on your burn" there is still this belief that the Cambodian witch doctors know best.

(21EF)

Without question, the supporting influences of religion were also named and considered as a means of support and healing.

Buddhism that's good because it's peaceful/I mean every religion give you a benefit of be in peace, not harm to others. But here especially for self-awareness, meditation, I really like Buddhism. And I would really love every family would practice meditation.

(8CF)

The interviewees referred to the meditation practice from Buddhism with its positive, also scientifically confirmed, effects. The rituals of the monks such as the chanted prayers and the water blessing were described as helpful. The Christian doctrine of mutual love and respect as well as unconditional divine acceptance and forgiveness was mentioned as conducive to well-being.

But (it is) the problem also, you know some people believe in karma. When they have problem, they didn't want to solve. They just believe it's their karma in their previous life or something.

(16CM)

The belief system of good and bad karma, which comes from Hinduism, is intertwined with Buddhism in Cambodia. Practitioners know the negative aspects such as passive fatalism and scapegoat thinking, which should be carefully questioned. However, they also acknowledge that the idea of good karma, which is earned through good deeds, can also act as a positive drive and a coping mechanism. For example, for victims of the Khmer Rouge regime, the belief that perpetrators will have to face the consequences of their actions in the future is a reason not to seek revenge themselves.

"That's a Form of Family Therapy That Has Been Practiced for Ages"

So the first thing, I think we can go like we can try to reconcile anything – the family first. They come to seek the advice to bring the older people who have more power to help to reconcile in the family first. And then if not possible, they can go to the village chief to help them to reconcile, or they might put like a filing the complaint for divorce something like that.

(2CF)

Attempts have been made to solve family problems within the family first; advice is sought from the elderly, who can use their influence for an arbitration. If that is not possible, the mayor or some other leader in the municipality would be the next person visited for help. One of the interviewees characterized this very practice as a traditional form of family therapy. Additionally, the traditional spiritual counselors – the healers, magicians, monks, priests, and fortunetellers – are consulted in the case of family problems.

Kruh Khmer refer to like the person who can help to solve problem like you know they listen the family problem and then they can give advice and also they can give some herbs.

(16CM)

"Not to Challenge It, But Just to Understand"

Because even now we are living in the city but the most family still when [...] something went wrong in their family the first thing they would like to meet with the monk or with the fortune teller or with someone that/about the spiritual.

(1CF)

The professional specialists know that in the case of psychological and family problems, traditional helpers have usually already been consulted, since they are a well-known source for such support. These include spiritual healers who have broad knowledge of traditional herbal medicine, Buddhist priests, spiritual mediums, masters of black magic, and professional fortunetellers. A lot of money is often spent on their advice and treatment. Professional advice and therapy is usually only sought if nothing else has worked.

But of course, we have to be careful as a therapist whether it is an extreme attitude or extreme belief or not. We have to find a way in the middle.

(8CF)

Even though the therapists stated that severe mental disorders cannot be treated successfully by spiritual healers, it is important for the professionals interviewed to be aware of the influence of traditional belief systems. Therapists pointed out that exploring the respective religious attitudes of the clients and a cultural understanding are important. Therefore, they claim that the modern biomedical paradigm should not be imposed on clients. Rather it is a matter of respecting the religious attitudes of the clients instead of discrediting them, which is not conducive to the healing process. The goal is coexistence and recommending additional information and offering modern treatment methods and at the same time appreciating the traditional methods of treatment.

And whatever your fit or your belief system (is) I think to support the person in being who they are and where they belong it/that's where it begins, we don't bring in our own, we support them where they are and their belief system is.

(20EF)

"I Can See It's Useful, Because It's the Faith or Belief of the People"

Belief systems and religious ceremonies can also be actively incorporated into treatment. A number of examples were given for this. The concepts of mindfulness, self-respect, and moral action anchored in Buddhism are beneficial. Breathing exercises and meditation are an integral part of the counseling. Existing ceremonies can be reconnected with therapeutically relevant topics and in this way be healing on a deeper level. This type of healing is already being used in connection with trauma treatment. It is also conceivable to use the great influence of traditional healers or monks to spread more knowledge about mental illnesses. There are already monks who regularly refer clients for psychiatric treatment. The aim is to help clients reflect on the advantages and disadvantages of traditional methods and offer them new concepts, but also warn of harm and treatment errors.

> *So, people sell the cows, sell their land, give to monks. We warn against that kind of malpractice – traditional but malpractice. So, accept: ok, go, pray, they put water for the children, so is fine.*

(22EM)

"It Helps People to Have a Sense of Belonging"

Rituals and holidays are traditionally associated with diverse religious ceremonies. Weddings and funerals are of great importance, but cermonies with monks, prayers, offerings, and meals for relatives are also common. Birthday parties for children and the celebration of school leaving certificates and exams are new.

> *I think, it's rooted in their traditions and cultures and I guess it's identity and during the Khmer Rouge people lost their identity and were/there were such atrocities and trauma that I think, it helps built the nation back up and have it's own identity [...] I think, it's important that Cambodia still has it's own and it's special time together it helps people have a sense of belonging and a value and meaning in life and who they are and where they fit.*

(20 EF)

Traditional ceremonies convey identity and belonging. Suppressed during the Khmer Rouge period, cultural and religious values became an important part of stabilizing society after this period. Against this background, a renewed uprooting of traditions may be perceived as a threat.

The high holidays of Khmer New Year and Pchum Ben, the commemoration of the dead, are of paramount importance to Cambodian families. Adult children return to their parents' homes and are expected to bring gifts. Many people otherwise have little time to relax; the holidays are often the only days off during the year and a precious time for families to get together.

"Are You Going to Work With the Crazy People?"

Mental health problems and illnesses are associated with being insane and are associated with a high degree of stigmatization. The word for crazy is one of the worst swear words in the Khmer language. Families with mentally ill members are avoided, and marrying into such a family is discouraged. A career choice in the psychosocial area is also not encouraged by parents.

My parents they were so surprised, and they didn't know anything about psychology as well [...] but the first reaction was: "Are you going to work with the crazy people?"
(9CM, Seg.42)

Thus, visiting psychologists and counselors for mental health help is associated with shame and fear and being labeled as crazy, since this could affect job security – especially with state employers – as well as the reputation of the family. This prevents people from taking advantage of counseling and therapy services, even if they are free.

Every time when we are going to the treatment like to see the counselor for the mental health something like that, is not really recommended or very good looking or they are like a stigma seen on this people.

(2CF)

It is therefore important to formulate the designation of these offers in an appropriately unobjectionable way, a direct translation of "Therapy" or "Mental Health" into Khmer is negatively associated with mental illness. Many of the interviewees stated that there is little knowledge about mental health and understanding of therapy and counseling in the population.

The concept of professional family therapy or other psycho-social counseling offers is not known to many; existing counseling offers are not used for this reason. In the cities, people would rather orientate themselves towards medical care.

People prefer quick fix, they prefer medicines and being told what to do than being empowered and enabled to make informed decisions.

(20EF)

When a therapist or counselor is consulted, however, one expects a quick solution or clear instructions on what to do next. Problems of children, including school problems, are commonly the reason to take advantage of counseling offers. These also represent apoint for therapists to work on underlying family dynamics with the parents. The concept of counseling should be advertised through various media and also in schools along with psychoeducation to support the mentally ill. Stigmatization must be counteracted through education, and the key leaders in the municipalities should be educated.

Conclusions

Religion, Spirituality, and Rituals

Spirituality is often deeply interwoven with all aspects of family life (Walsh, 2009). The data show the strong and omnipresent influence of religion in Cambodia. Khmer Buddhism, a combination of ancient animist and former Hindu traditions with Buddhism (Agger, 2015), is commonly practiced. The interviewees expressed their concern regarding harmful animistic practices (see Eisenbruch, 2018). The questions about how to integrate religious practices into therapeutic process puzzled some of the interviewees. Also, in discussions with my students, I got the impression they were more prone to leave the premodern concepts behind in favor for "real scientific knowledge." I share the view of Seponski et al.

(2020), questioning the role of educational colonization. However, religion and spiritual practices such as ceremonies and rituals are seen also as resources.

In all religions, important life events – such as births, entering adulthood, marriage, or death – are celebrated with traditional rituals (Walsh, 2009) and on deep emotional levels (Imber-Black, 2009). Especially in traditional, strongly spiritual contexts like in Cambodia, the inclusion or at least the observance of existing spiritual/religious rituals is important for therapeutic work (Eisenbruch, 2018).

New rituals for the needs of individuals, families, and communities can also be created and with therapeutic intent (Imber-Black, 2012). Within the teaching modules during the trainings, we started and ended the day with a newly created ritual. After conferring with Cambodian colleagues for appropriate symbols – like lotus blossoms or colorful fabrics, candles, or symbolic objects to symbolize important elements of the ritual – we gathered in a circle and shared thoughts on a particular topic. According to our evaluation, the Cambodian trainees highly valued this practice, which was intended to set the atmosphere but also to serve as a model for how to create new meaningful therapeutic rituals with a more holistic approach (see Stewart et al. cited in Seponski et al., 2020).

Dealing with Stigma

In Cambodia, mental disorders cause strong stigmatization (Jegannathan et al., 2015). In accordance with Seponski et al. (2020) the data show that seeing a counselor or even pursuing a career in the psycho-social field is stigmatized and a cause of shame for individuals and families and thus more psychoeducation is needed to educate people on modern mental health resources.

The concept of face, in collectivist societies as an expression of a sociocentric self-image, is primarily derived from assessment by others (Hinton A. L., 1998), and needs to be thoroughly considered in counseling trainings in Cambodia. Honor and prestige give "face" in socially degrading situations. At the same time, there is a loss of face conveyed through shame and humiliation. Due to a collective obligation, everyone in the group is shamed if one of its members violates social rules or conventions (Hofstede et al., 2010). Stigma can lead to extreme sanctions such as chaining or locking up the ill person, which is still practiced in rural areas in Cambodia (Miller et al., 2019) to protect the individual from self-harm but also to prevent community rejection and isolation for the whole family (Thornicroft et al., 2008).

Therefore, the affiliation of the training to the highly regarded university is of great importance. In addition, advocating events for mental health and its providers by the university are important measures to counteract stigmatization. Local specialists play a key role in finding specific terms for the content and concerns of mental health and systemic family therapy that prevent stigmatization.

Transmodern Practice

Psychotherapy has been developing in Western Europe for around 120 years. Emlein (2018, p. 4) calls it "the younger half-sister of pastoral care," because "the individual accompaniment of people in difficult situations can be traced back to antiquity. It was the task of religion." Under the new premises of modernity, bringing those seeking advice is no longer sufficient – social work, counseling, and psychotherapy emerged accordingly (Emlein, 2018).

Counselors and therapists come into contact with very different worldviews, and students also bring very different worldviews with them to the training courses (Gonzales & Faubert, 2019). In doing so, the premodern understanding of the world can meet the logical positivism of modernity, which can see itself challenged by postmodern deconstruction. In Cambodia, for many students the modern worldview seems to be the preferred frame of reference.

A collaborative-dialogical practice (Anderson, 2020) requires the therapist to be able to see the world from the perspective of her clients. In order to be able to enter into this collaborative dialogue, the process of self-reflection on the part of the therapist about one's own location (Aponte & Kissil, 2016; Falicov, 2014a) must certainly precede. This is exactly where a transmodern approach can help everyone involved – loyal to their own values and identity – to participate in the dialogue.

Effective counseling must establish a connection with the client's world – meeting people where they are and respecting their worldview (Falicov, 2014a). Like the majority of people in Cambodia, 85% of the global population incorporates various beliefs in supernatural powers into their life practice (Pew Forum, 2017, cited in Gonzales & Faubert, 2019). Counselors face complex combination of premodern, modern, and postmodern beliefs. The introduction of a transmodern perspective (worldviews from different thought traditions are valued; emotional and spiritual commitments to community are met with mindfulness) (Rodriguez Magda, 1988, cited in Gonzales and Faubert, 2019) in family therapy training in Cambodia appears to be a helpful orientation. This enables local students to leave a dichotomous point of view with which knowledge categories were viewed as "unscientific/scientific" (premodern/modern) knowledge – regardless of whether it comes from the category "premodern," "modern," or "postmodern" – is anchored in cultural history.

Then local students could approach any knowledge – foreign, western, as well as local – courageously with their own convictions. The students decide for themselves which knowledge is important or resonates with their clients. They also decide for themselves which discourses of knowledge they want to integrate into their own worldview. In any case, a collaborative-dialogical practice requires adopting the transmodern perspective when working with clients (Gonzales and Faubert, 2019).

As discussed above, Celia Falicov (2014a) developed the MECA model as a concrete reflection framework for self-reflection of one's own ecological niche – and thus the location in premodern/modern/postmodern worldviews – as well as for reflection for the clients. The Cambodian professionals interviewed for my research described this necessity as being crystal clear. They shared valuable strategies for how to work with the spiritual beliefs and practices of their clients and their own professional knowledge.

Take up Local Knowledge Production

As explained in this chapter – the approach of only developing faithful adaptations to the local culture for Western family therapy practices falls short. Rather, the underlying family theories must be placed in their Euro-American geographical and political context. The implicit values, traditions, and intentions should be revealed, and their differences should be considered in the current context. This seemingly unusualness of the theories brought with them should be clearly marked and presented in such a way that the training participants see themselves as people asked to take up their own transformed, local know-ledge production outside the Euro-American paradigm in therapy (Polanco, 2016). This emphasizes the role of reflective practice within the courses and its careful guidance. An ongoing conversation with the Cambodian trainers is yet requested to foster the development of local supervision capacities.

References

Agger, I. (2015). Calming the mind: Healing after mass atrocity in Cambodia. *Transcultural Psychiatry*, *52*(4), 543–560. https://doi.org/10.1177/1363461514568336

Anderson, H. (1997). *Conversation, language, and possibilities: A postmodern approach to therapy* (1st ed.). BasicBooks. www.loc.gov/catdir/enhancements/fy0832/96017802-b.html

Anderson, H. (2020). Collaborative-dialogic practice: A relational process of inviting generativity and possibilities. In S. McNamee, M. M. Gergen, C. Camargo-Borges, & E. F. Rasera (Eds.), *The Sage handbook of social constructionist practice* (pp. 132–139). SAGE Inc.

Aponte, H. J., & Kissil, K. (2016). *The Person of the Therapist Training Model: Mastering the Use of Self*. Taylor and Francis. http://gbv.eblib.com/patron/FullRecord.aspx?p=4332643

Bauer, P. (2020). Systemisch denken lernen – systemische Kompetenzentwicklung als Lernen am Fall. In P. Bauer & M. Weinhardt (Eds.), *Systemische Kompetenzen entwickeln: Grundlagen, Lernprozesse und Didaktik* (pp. 188–202). Vandenhoeck & Ruprecht.

Bermúdez, J. M., Muruthi, B. A., & Jordan, L. S. (2016). Decolonizing Research Methods for Family Science: Creating Space at the Center. *Journal of Family Theory & Review*, *8*(2), 192–206. https://doi.org/10.1111/jftr.12139

Boehnlein, J. K., & Kinzie, J.D. (2011). The Effect Of The Khmer Rouge On The Mental Health Of Cambodia And Cambodians. In B. van Schaack (Ed.), *Documentation series/Documentation Center of Cambodia: Vol. 17. Cambodia's hidden scars: Trauma psychology in the wake of the Khmer Rouge; an edited volume on Cambodia's mental health*. Documentation Center of Cambodia (DC-Cam).

Brehm, W., & Aktas, F. (2020). All education for some? International development and shadow education in Cambodia. *International Journal of Comparative Education and Development*, *22*(1), 66–81. https://doi.org/10.1108/IJCED-01-2019-0005

Brunner, C. (2016). Das Konzept epistemische Gewalt als Element einer transdisziplinären Friedens- und Konflikttheorie. In W. Wintersteiner & L. Wolf (Eds.), *Friedensfoschung in Österreich: Bilanz und Perspektiven* (pp. 38–53). Drava Verlag. https://doi.org/10.25595/146

Chandler, D. P. (2003). *A history of Cambodia* (3. ed.). Westview Press; Silkworm Books.

Charlés, L. L., & Samarasinghe, G. (Eds.). (2016). *AFTA SpringerBriefs in Family Therapy. Family Therapy in Global Humanitarian Contexts: Voices and Issues from the Field*. Springer International Publishing. http://gbv.eblib.com/patron/FullRecord.aspx?p=4558182 https://doi.org/10.1007/978-3-319-39271-4

Charlés, L., & Bava, S. (2020). Systemic Family Therapy and Global Mental Health: Reflections on Professional Development and Training. In K. S. Wampler, M. Rastogi, & R. Singh (Eds.), *The Handbook of Systemic Family Therapy* (Vol. 4, pp. 550–565). Wiley.

Ebbecke-Nohlen, A. (2015). *Einführung in die systemische Supervision* (3. Aufl.). *Compact*. Auer.

Eisenbruch, M. (2018). Violence Against Women in Cambodia: Towards a Culturally Responsive Theory of Change. *Culture, Medicine and Psychiatry*, *42*(2), 350–370. https://doi.org/10.1007/s11013-017-9564-5

Emlein, G. (2018). Die Evolution entlässt ihre Kinder: Psychotherapie als "devotio moderna." *Systemische Notizen* (2).

Falicov, C. J. (2009). Religion and Spiritual Traditions in Immigrant Families: Significance for Latino Health and Mental Health. In F. Walsh (Ed.), *Spiritual resources in family therapy* (2nd ed., pp. 156–173). Guilford Press.

Falicov, C. J. (2014a). *Latino families in therapy* (Second edition). The Guilford Press.

Falicov, C. J. (2016). The Multiculturalism and Diversity of Families. In Sexton, T., Lebow, J. (Ed.), *Handbook of family therapy* (pp. 66–85). Routledge.

Falicov, C. J. (2017). Multidimensional Ecosystemic Comparative Approach (MECA). In J. Lebow, A. Chambers, & D. C. Breunlin (Eds.), *Encyclopedia of Couple and Family Therapy* (Vol. 34, pp. 1–5). Springer International Publishing. https://doi.org/10.1007/978-3-319-15877-8_848-1

Gergen, K. J. (2009). *Relational Being: Beyond Self And Community.* Swartmore College. https://works.swarthmore.edu/fac-psychology/213

GIZ Cambodia. (2017). *Future Family therapists started training at Department of Psychology RUPP.* https://giz-cambodia.com/page/5/

GIZ. (2013). *giz2018-de-orientierungsrahmen-capacity-development.* Bonn und Eschborn. GIZ.

GIZ. (2021, June 10). *Ziviler Friedensdienst: Kambodschas Vergangenheit aufarbeiten.* www.giz.de/de/weltweit/17322.html

Gläser-Zikuda, M., & Hascher, T. (Eds.). (2007). *Lernprozesse dokumentieren, reflektieren und beurteilen: Lerntagebuch und Portfolio in Bildungsforschung und Bildungspraxis.* Klinkhardt. https://d-nb.info/983484155/04

Gonzales, E., & Faubert, M. (2019). Transmodern and Collaborative-Dialogic Practice: an Integration. *International Journal of Collaborative-Dialogic Practices* (9), 143–156.

Hilzinger, R., & Henrich, M. (2020). Implizite Wissensbildungsprozesse von systemischen Therapeutinnen und Therapeuten. In P. Bauer & M. Weinhardt (Eds.), *Systemische Kompetenzen entwickeln: Grundlagen, Lernprozesse und Didaktik* (pp. 103–120). Vandenhoeck & Ruprecht.

Hinton A. L. (1998). Why Did You Kill? The Cambodian Genocide and the Dark Side of Face and Honor. *The Journal of Asian Studies*(1), 93–122.

Hofstede, G., Hofstede, G. J., & Minkov, M. (2010). *Cultures and organizations: Software of the mind; intercultural cooperation and its importance for survival* (Rev. and expanded 3. ed.). McGraw-Hill.

Imber-Black, E. (2009). Rituals and Spirituality in Family Therapy. In F. Walsh (Ed.), *Spiritual resources in family therapy* (2nd ed., pp. 229–246). Guilford Press.

Imber-Black, E. (2012). The Value of Rituals in Family Life. In F. Walsh (Ed.), *Normal family processes: Growing diversity and complexity* (pp. 483–497). The Guilford Press.

Jegannathan, B., Kullgren, G., & Deva, P. (2015). Mental health services in Cambodia, challenges and opportunities in a post-conflict setting. *Asian Journal of Psychiatry*, *13*, 75–80. https://doi.org/10.1016/j.ajp.2014.12.006

Jordan, L. S., Seponski, D. M., & Armes, S. (2019). "Oh, it is a special gift you give to me …": a phenomenological analysis of counsellors in Cambodia. *Asia Pacific Journal of Counselling and Psychotherapy*, *10*(2), 146–158. https://doi.org/10.1080/21507686.2019.1629470

Kriz, J. (2001). *Grundkonzepte der Psychotherapie* (5., vollst. überarb. Aufl.). *Schlüsselbegriffe.* Beltz PVU. http://d-nb.info/961412135/04

Langis, T. de, Strasser, J., & Kim, thida, Taing, Sopheap. (2014). *" 'Like Ghost Changes Body': A Study on the Impact of Forced Marriage under the Khmer Rouge Regime."* Phnom Penh. Transcultural Psychsocial Organisation of Cambodia.

Mayring, P., & Fenzl, T. (2019). Qualitative Inhaltsanalyse. In N. Baur & J. Blasius (Eds.), *Handbuch Methoden der empirischen Sozialforschung* (pp. 633–648). Springer Fachmedien Wiesbaden. https://doi.org/10.1007/978-3-658-21308-4_42

McDowell, T., Brown, A. L., Kabura, P., Parker, E., & Alotaiby, A. (2011). Working with Families in Uganda and the United States: Lessons in Cross-Cultural Professional Training. *Journal of Systemic Therapies*, *30*(2), 65–80. https://doi.org/10.1521/jsyt.2011.30.2.65

McDowell, T., Knudson-Martin, C., & Bermudez, J. M. (2017). *Socioculturally Attuned Family Therapy: Guidelines for Equitable Theory and Practice* (1st ed.). Taylor and Francis. https://ebookcentral.proquest.com/lib/gbv/detail.action?docID=5160941

Miller, J. K., Platt, J., & Conroy, K. (2018). Single-session therapy in the majority world: Addressing the challenge of service delivery in Cambodia and the implications for other global contexts. In M. F. Hoyt, M. Bobele, A. Slive, J. Young, & M. Talmon (Eds.), *Single-session therapy by walk-in or appointment: Administrative, clinical, and supervisory aspects of one-at-a-time services* (116–114). Routledge.

Miller, J. K., Platt, J., & Nhong, H. (2019). Psychological Needs in Post-Genocide Cambodia: The Call for Family Therapy Services and the Implications for the "Majority World" Populations. *Journal of Family Psychotherapy*, *30*(2), 153–167. https://doi.org/10.1080/08975353.2019.1613610

Natrajan-Tyagi, R., Gutierrez, N. S., Elizalde, M., Phan, V. M., Christensen, J. F., Crossley, L., Drollinger, K., Faulk, M., Garcia, R., & Meng, C. (2016). Using a Constant Family in Role-Plays for Training MFTs. *The American Journal of Family Therapy*, 44(5), 221–233. https://doi.org/10.1080/01926187.2016.1223564

Patterson, J. E., Edwards, T. M., & Vakili, S. (2018). Global Mental Health: A Call for Increased Awareness and Action for Family Therapists. *Family Process*, 57(1), 70–82. https://doi.org/10.1111/famp.12281

Po Li, T. (2011). Towards a Culturally Sensitive and Deeper Understanding of "Rote Learning" and Memorisation of Adult Learners. *Journal of Studies in International Education*, 15(2), 124–145.

Polanco, M. (2016). Knowledge Fair Trade. In L. L. Charlés & G. Samarasinghe (Eds.), *AFTA SpringerBriefs in Family Therapy. Family Therapy in Global Humanitarian Contexts: Voices and Issues from the Field* (pp. 13–25). Springer International Publishing.

Proctor, B. (2008). *Group supervision: A guide to creative practice* (2nd ed.). *Counselling supervision.* Sage. http://site.ebrary.com/lib/alltitles/docDetail.action?docID=10392708

Schunert, T., Khann, S., Kao, S., Pot, C., Saupe, L. B., Lahar, C. J., Sek, S., & Nhong, H. (2012). *Cambodian mental health survey.* Royal University of Phnom Penh.

Seponski, D. M., & Jordan, L. S. (2018). Cross-cultural supervision in international settings: experiences of foreign supervisors and native supervisees in Cambodia. *Journal of Family Therapy*, 40(2), 247–264. https://doi.org/10.1111/1467-6427.12157

Seponski, D. M., Bermudez, J. M., & Lewis, D. C. (2013). Creating culturally responsive family therapy models and research: Introducing the use of responsive evaluation as a method. *Journal of Marital and Family Therapy*, 39(1), 28–42. https://doi.org/10.1111/j.1752-0606.2011.00282.x

Seponski, D. M., Lewis, D. C., & Megginson, M. C. (2014). A responsive evaluation of mental health treatment in Cambodia: Intentionally addressing poverty to increase cultural responsiveness in therapy. *Global Public Health*, 9(10), 1211–1224. https://doi.org/10.1080/17441692.2014.947302

Seponski, D. M., Lewis, D. C., Bermudez, J. M., & Sotelo, J. M. (2020). Cambodian Therapists' Perspectives of Western-based Psychotherapy Models: Addressing the Challenges for Service Providers. *Journal of Family Psychotherapy*, 31(1–2), 36–55. https://doi.org/10.1080/08975353.2020.1759018

Somasundaram, D. J., van de Put, W. A.C.M., Eisenbruch, M., & Jong, J. T.V.M. de (1999). Starting mental health services in Cambodia. *Social Science & Medicine*, 48(8), 1029–1046. https://doi.org/10.1016/S0277-9536(98)00415-8

Thornicroft, G., Brohan, E., Kassam, A., & Lewis-Holmes, E. (2008). Reducing stigma and discrimination: Candidate interventions. *International Journal of Mental Health Systems*, 2(1), 3. https://doi.org/10.1186/1752-4458-2-3

van Schaack, B., & Chhang, Y. (2011). Cambodia's Hidden Scars: Trauma Psychology in the Wake of the Khmer Rouge. *SSRN Electronic Journal*. Advance online publication. https://doi.org/10.2139/ssrn.2758130

Walsh, F. (Ed.). (2009). *Spiritual resources in family therapy* (2nd ed.). Guilford Press.

Weinhardt, M. (2020). Systemische Professionalisierung als Lern- und Bildungsprozess: Fachliche Entwicklungsaufgaben lösen, Professionalisierungskulturen gestalten. In P. Bauer & M. Weinhardt (Eds.), *Systemische Kompetenzen entwickeln: Grundlagen, Lernprozesse und Didaktik* (pp. 121–133). Vandenhoeck & Ruprecht.

14

TAIWANESE COUPLES AND FAMILIES

Current Treatment Perspectives

Chi-Fang Tseng and Pei-Fen Li

Introduction

Taiwan is known as one of the "Four Asian Little Dragons" (along with South Korea, Hong Kong, and Singapore) because it has undergone rapid industrialization since 1960. Taiwan's economy has continued to grow, and it is now considered a high-income country (United Nations, 2014). As of 2021, Taiwan has a population of about 23 million people (Department of Household Registration Affairs, 2021). The average household size has decreased from 4.8 persons in 1980 to 3.0 persons in 2010 and 2.8 persons in 2020 (Department of Household Registration Affairs, 2021). Taiwan also has the lowest birth rate worldwide, with an estimated 1.07 children per woman aged 15–45 (Statista, 2021). It has become common in Taiwanese society to postpone traditional timelines of marriage and childbearing. The share of people who marry at age 30–39 increased from 26% in 2000 to 47% in 2020 (Ministry of the Interior Taiwan, 2021). The average age at first childbirth has also increased from 26.74 years in 2000 to 31.09 years in 2020 (Ministry of the Interior Taiwan, 2021).

The rapid economic change has affected Taiwanese family structure and household composition (Wang & Yang, 2019). The nuclear family household is still the dominant household structure in Taiwan, but there has been a significant decline in the share of nuclear family households. In 1990, 50.9% of households were comprised of couples with unmarried children; in 2020, this group accounted for just 30.6% of households. This decline can be attributed to an increase in couple-only households from 6.9% in 1990 to 13.3% in 2020, as well as an increase in single-person households from 13.4% in 1990 to 26.0% in 2020. As Taiwan continues to progress and thrive, these economic and societal changes challenge traditional family organizations and lead to more liberal and open mindsets, which in turn opens opportunities for diverse family structures (Yi et al., 2019) and western cultures and perspectives. Even though Western values have influenced Taiwanese culture, several Taiwanese scholars have argued that traditional values still exist in the country and affect the couple and family dynamics in subtle ways (Li, 2012; Li & Hsiao, 2016). In other words, traditional cultural values, such as Confucianism, still influence Taiwanese couples' daily practices, while western cultural values also shape their perspectives.

DOI: 10.4324/9781003297871-16

Specific Cultural Characteristics of Taiwanese Families/Couples and Clinical Implications

With the mixed influences of Chinese and Western cultures, couples and families in Taiwan face unique challenges in balancing different cultural discourses that inform their practice and formation of couple and family relationships. Therefore, therapists should recognize how these Taiwanese cultural characteristics influence couples' dynamics and interactions. This section will provide an overview of some traditional values of Taiwanese families and couples, such as filial piety, enqing, sacrifice, and tolerance.

Filial Piety

According to Confucian values, filial piety is the core virtue for people (Hwang & Han, 2010). The concept of filial piety includes several values that one should follow, including the obligation to provide and care for parents, gratitude toward parents' sacrifices and care, obedience to parents, continuation of family blood, and maintenance of good behavior that will bring honor to the family (Ho, 1996; Yeh & Bedford, 2003). Filial piety affects how people prioritize relationships when and after they are married. In this context, marriages are seen as the joining of two extended families, and a couple is expected to care for both sets of their parents. This practice reflects the traditional value of *Xiao* (filial piety), which is defined as obligation and respect for one's parents (Wu et al., 2016; Yeh & Bedford, 2003). In Western culture, married couples are the most central unit of the family, whereas in Taiwanese culture, couples' relationships with their own parents and children are viewed as equally important units in the family (Shweder et al., 2003; Lam et al., 2016).

In a comparison of marriage ideals in Taiwan and the United States, researchers found that ideals regarding stable financial resources and care for extended families were more strongly held by Taiwanese couples than U.S. couples (Lam et al., 2016). Western married couples tend to develop firm boundaries with their families of origin (Bryant et al., 2001; Epstein et al., 2005). Filial piety offers a different lens through which to consider couple and family relationships that differ from those prevalent in Western culture, and therapists working with Taiwanese couples should be aware of this concept and the ways in which it affects the dynamic of not only a couple unit but also the couple's extended families.

Enqing

Li and Chen (2002) examined differences in intimacy and affection between Western and Chinese cultures. They found that, in addition to the intimacy component of couple relationships, another component called "enqing" was characteristic of relationships among couples in Chinese cultures, such as Taiwan. Enqing is defined as "one person's feelings of indebtedness, gratitude, and appreciation for what the other has done in the marriage" (Li & Chen, p. 407). In the past, couples in Taiwan used to enter marriage without having the opportunity to foster intimacy and affection since their marriages are arranged. The main purpose of marriage was to produce offspring, and Taiwanese society considered the newlywed couple an extension of the husband's parents' family (Epstein et al., 2005; Chen & Li, 2007).

With the rapid economic and social development and Westernization of Taiwan in the last few decades, couples now have the autonomy to choose their own partners and emphasize love and intimacy as the foundation of their marriages (Epstein et al., 2005; Chen & Li, 2007). However, Li and Chen (2002) confirmed that although Western concepts have impacted couples' relationships, traditional Chinese concepts such as enqing have not disappeared. In research on this topic, Li and Chen (2002) found that couples with children had a lower level of marital satisfaction but no less enqing with their partners than couples without children. Additionally, men had higher enqing for their wives than their wives did for them (Chen & Li, 2007; Li & Chen, 2002). Researchers have also found that when couples express more enqing to their partners and appreciate their partners' efforts in marriage, their partners' depression levels decrease (Li et al., 2019).

Sacrifice

The concept of enqing is interrelated with sacrifice, which is an essential characteristic in Chinese culture. In Chinese culture, sacrifice in couple relationships is defined as one's willingness to give up personal interests and desires to maintain harmony, family function, and unity (Chen & Li, 2007; Van Lange et al., 1997). This cultural virtue echoes with Collectivism that individuals often prioritize groups' needs over theirs. In studies of Taiwanese couples, men were found to perceive more sacrifice from their partners than their partners perceived from them; additionally, the level of perceived sacrifice among men significantly predicted their level of enqing toward their partners (Chen & Li, 2007). Li and colleagues (2019) also found that Taiwanese men who had higher enqing toward their wives were more willing to make sacrifices than their peers with lower enqing. Li and Wickrama (2014) also found that Taiwanese couples use sacrifice as a coping strategy (e.g., willingness to sacrifice their needs and listen to the other's opinions) to handle distressful marital situations, and this coping strategy in turns enhances the marital satisfaction.

Tolerance

Tolerance in relationships is another characteristic that is highly appreciated in the Chinese cultural context. Chang et al. (2020) found that tolerance is often used to repress negative emotions to maintain harmony among Taiwanese couples. Tolerance is important because it helps to maintain harmony, even by sacrificing one's own needs. Chen and Li (2007) found that tolerance predicts an individual's own marital satisfaction and their partner's supporting behaviors. Huang (2009) pointed out that in a culture that emphasizes Confucian values, such as Taiwanese culture, people are expected to use tolerance to maintain harmony as their initial reaction when conflicts and disagreements arise. Tolerance doesn't solely entail individuals calming down; it also involves generating and considering alternative solutions to a problem (Huang et al., 2008).

The concepts of enqing, sacrifice, and tolerance have specific clinical implications in relationships among Taiwanese couples. Therapists working with Taiwanese couples should be aware that some concepts that may be considered malfunctional or unhealthy in Western cultures (e.g., suppressing one's needs, avoiding conflicts) are culturally acceptable coping strategies among couples in Taiwan. Therapists should also observe couples' negotiations between specific traditional values and their own desires. For example, in one Taiwanese couple in the first author's clinical practice, the female partner had used sacrifice and tolerance in the relationship to maintain harmony for the sake of the family. This female partner had sacrificed her career and decided to care for her children at home, and her sacrifice was supported by the male partner and his extended family. During therapy, the female partner identified struggles and confusion regarding her choice. Part of her wanted to return to work because her work gave her a sense of accomplishment, but part of her felt selfish about choosing work over her children. Her desire to return to work was not supported and empowered by her husband or in-laws because they considered it normal for a mother to stay at home instead of pursuing career goals. As a therapist, it is important to explore this female partner's struggles and empower her to identify her desires, even if this exploration leads her to not follow the traditional values her society expects of her. It is also essential to invite the couple to be aware of how Taiwanese traditional and current cultural values have shaped and influenced their perceptions and emotions regarding this personal career and relational struggles. Throughout this exploration, the couple can understand and validate each other's perspective and sacrifice in enhancing the family's wellbeing. It is especially beneficial for their relationship if the male partner can express his acknowledgement and gratitude toward female partner's sacrifice in a changing patriarchal society (Li & Wickrama, 2014). The female partner might feel more heard and supported and have more space to challenge traditional cultural values of her role in their marriage and family.

Common Relationship Issues Among Taiwanese Heterosexual Couples

Taiwanese couples face specific challenges in their relationships that are unique to their cultural expectations and characteristics. For example, raising children is the most reported problem among Taiwanese couples, whereas it is the least reported problem among U.S. couples (Su et al., 2015). This phenomenon may be explained by Confucian values, which prioritize the parent-child relationship over the couple relationship (Su et al., 2015). This finding is consistent with Pfeifer and colleagues' (2013) finding that the most commonly reported problems among Taiwanese couples are related to raising children, communication, relationships with parents/in-laws, intimacy, and finances.

Based on these findings, couples and families in Taiwan and the United States may perceive their relationships differently such that the presenting problems of Taiwanese couples are more likely to be related to parenting than to the couple relationship (Su et al., 2015). However, this does not necessarily mean that therapists should not focus on common relationship issues, such as intimacy or sexual satisfaction. Therapists should be aware of how parenting and the prioritization of parent-child relationships may become the focus of Taiwanese couples' problems. Researchers have also suggested that Taiwanese couples may choose to come to couple and family therapy for parent-focused issues, including children's academic or behavioral problems (Akutsu & Chu, 2006; Sze et al., 2011). The focus on problems related to children may mask more core relational issues between couples, including problems related to communication, intimacy, and relationship satisfaction. As the previous section mentioned, tolerance may play a role in maintaining couples' relationships. Avoiding communication issues and focusing on children can distract a couple from directly dealing with other relationship issues, which corresponds with the Confucian value that individuals should maintain harmonious relationships by avoiding conflict and negative self-disclosure (Zhang et al., 2012). Considering this cultural influence, when working with Taiwanese couples, the therapist should first join with couples by carefully listening to their perception of the presenting problems (e.g., the child's behavioral issues). A therapist can then further assist the couple in identifying similar and different parenting strategies and highlighting their shared goal of achieving the child's best interests.

A therapist also helps the couple in acknowledging how each person contributes to the child's issue (e.g., their communication or relational power issues in parenting). Gradually, this might shift the couple's original focus from the child to their relationship issues.

Different Forms of Couplehood and Their Clinical Implications

Although couples with unmarried children are still the dominant family structure in Taiwan, there has been a recent increase in small households, including couple-only households and single-individual households (Ministry of the Interior Taiwan, 2021). Additionally, the growing Western influence in Taiwan has given rise to a greater acceptance of diverse family structures, such as households headed by same-sex couples and those comprised of transnational partners. The increase in diverse forms of couplehood has led to more diverse family structures in Taiwan, as well as the coexistence of traditional and modern values.

Singlehood and Childlessness

According to social demographic transition theory, demographic trends in high-income countries such as Taiwan tend to emphasize personal needs and desire over child-centered family structures (Lesthaeghe, 2010). This transition leads to greater social approval of individuals who decide to adopt singlehood and childlessness (Tsai et al., 2021). In Taiwan, marriage is still considered an important life event, but people have become more mindful of the costs and sacrifices of marriage (Cheng & Yang, 2021). In their study of Taiwanese attitudes toward marriage from 1985–2015, Cheng and Yang (2021) found that attitudes toward marriage have shifted from traditional to more liberal values, including the belief that individuals can enjoy a satisfactory life without marriage. Compared to all men, women with a high level of education and highly skilled jobs more strongly support choices of singlehood and childlessness (Tsai et al., 2021). However, this transition challenges traditional core family values, such as family lineage continuity and filial piety (Tsai & Wang, 2019; Chen & Chen, 2014).

Same-Sex Couples

Taiwan legalized same-sex marriage on May 24, 2019, and as of 2022, it is the only Asian country in which same-sex marriage is legal. However, discrimination and stigma toward same-sex couples persists, in part because traditional Chinese patriarchal values continue to affect Taiwanese attitudes toward relationships and families. In a study of Taiwanese gay and lesbian coming out processes, Shieh (2009) found that women tend to introduce their same-sex partners to family and friends as a friend or a roommate, whereas men tend to avoid the topic or simply say that they have a girlfriend. The emphasis on marriage, carrying on the family lineage, and filial piety (i.e., not disappointing your parents) has impacted same-sex Taiwanese couples' decisions regarding coming out and marriage. Yu (2020) found that before same-sex marriage was legalized in Taiwan, lesbian couples focused on their own relationships and their parents often treated their children's partners as friends. Since same-sex marriage was legalized, parents have been more likely to view their children's lesbian relationships using heterosexual norms. Yu proposes that parents need time to adjust and build relationships with their daughters' same-sex partners (Yu, 2020).

Like other countries that have legalized same-sex marriage, Taiwan faces ongoing challenges regarding transnational same-sex marriages, reproductive autonomy, and justice for same-sex couples (Smith, 2005). For example, Taiwan only recognizes transnational same-sex marriages if the non-Taiwanese partner is from a country in which same-sex marriage is legal (Ministry of Justice, 2019). Moreover, Huang and colleagues (2021) found that gay and bisexual men considered childbearing less important after marriage was legalized in Taiwan. This phenomenon may be explained by insufficient and unfair access to childbearing options, including surrogacy and adoption, for same-sex couples. Under the Assisted Reproduction Act in Taiwan, assisted reproductive technologies are only allowed for heterosexual married couples; the law excludes same-sex couples and single or unmarried couples (Ministry of Health and Welfare, 2018). This restriction forces same-sex couples who want to have children to seek a surrogate outside of Taiwan, which leads to issues, including those related to cost and language barriers (Chen, 2019). There is an urgent need to modify current policy and laws regarding adoption, assisted reproductive technologies, and surrogacy to ensure equity among same-sex couples in Taiwan (Chan et al., 2022).

Therapists who work with same-sex couples must be aware of the institutional barriers and discrimination that might impact the well-being of same-sex couples in Taiwan. Therapists should also be sensitive to the effect of Confucian values and family values on same-sex couples' relationship satisfaction and well-being. Couples may want to come out and marry, but they may also have concerns about how family members view them as a couple unit and worry about the possible challenges of coming out to family members. Without support and understanding from family, same-sex couples in Taiwan may face unique challenges despite the recognition of their marriages under the law.

Transnational Couples

From 1987–2015, 89% of married transnational heterosexual couples in Taiwan were comprised of a female immigrant who was not Taiwanese, and the majority of these immigrants were from China (64.70%), Vietnam (18.31%), Indonesia (5.63%), and Thailand (1.68%; Ministry of the Interior National Immigration Agency, 2022). This surge in transnational marriages has been observed not only in Taiwan but also in other countries in Asia, such as Singapore and Korea (Jongwilaiwan & Thompson, 2013; Yeung & Mu, 2020). This section mainly focuses on women immigrants from China and Southeast Asia, whose marriage experiences are often different from those of immigrants who marry their partners voluntarily. In Taiwan, most non-voluntary transnational marriages are facilitated by marriage agencies through which men can arrange marriages with foreign brides (Lien et al., 2021). Women often migrate from developing countries with low socioeconomic status and are in a vulnerable economic position, hoping to advance their socioeconomic status by marrying men who can improve their families' economic situations (Tseng, 2010; Yeoh et al., 2013). Jongwilaiwan and Thompson (2013) describe transnational marriage as a complicated phenomenon involving gender, power, and race issues. Marriages without a foundation of intimacy often face challenges, and in transnational marriages, these challenges intersect with other adaptation and acculturation issues, such as language barriers, age gaps, cultural differences, and differences in marriage goals (e.g., husbands marry for childbearing and family lineage, whereas wives marry for stable financial support for their families of origin; Chung et al., 2010).

Immigrant women who are in multiple vulnerable positions often experience power differentials in their marriages, including verbal or physical violence from their husbands and families (Chang et al., 2005). The lack of intimacy in marriage and social support in Taiwan may further deteriorate the well-being of immigrant women. Moreover, women from Southeast Asia often immigrate alone and live with their husband's family upon arriving in Taiwan. They are often expected to take care of children and their husbands' families, learn Mandarin, adjust to the Taiwanese culture, and learn how to cook Taiwanese meals for their families (Li & Yang, 2020; Lien et al., 2021).

Therapists who work with transnational couples and immigrant families should provide resources to assist them in acculturating to the host culture and their marriages and to empower immigrant women (Lien et al., 2021). Immigrant women who have access to legal institutions, religious organizations, and social networks with people from their home countries tend to be happier than those who do not have access to these supportive networks (Li & Yang, 2020). Therapists also need to be aware of the complexity of couple dynamics, which may involve gender, class, race, and power issues that affect the well-being and marital satisfaction of immigrant women. When working with women immigrants in Taiwan, Wang (2020) suggests that therapists: 1) be aware of how the language barrier affects the client's motivation in accessing therapy services, 2) take into account both Taiwanese culture and the client's native culture in relation to the presenting issues, 3) enhance therapists' cultural sensitivity, 4) empower women to identify their strengths and support autonomy, and 5) collaborate with social workers to identify resources to offer clients. For husbands in transnational marriage, a therapist can invite them to acknowledge and appreciate their partner's efforts and sacrifice in cultural adaptions and acculturation in a foreign country. Even though transnational couples might have different goals in starting their marriage, it does not mean that they do not have common interests in maintaining and continuing their marriage. A therapist should encourage the transnational couple to explore their personal and relational interests while paying attention to how each partner's multiple social locations (e.g., gender, race, SES class, nations) shape the power dynamics in defining these matters.

The Current State of Couple and Family Therapy (CFT) Development in Taiwan

In Taiwanese culture, there is a strong emphasis on valuing family relationships and harmony, treating the family as a unit. It emphasizes the family as a unit. The emphasis on family and harmonious relationships between family members aligns with systemic thinking, which is the main concept of couple and family therapy. Several empirical studies conducted in Taiwan have found that couples' well-being is interrelated such that one partner's mental health affects the other partner's mental health in a dyadic relationship (Kubricht et al., 2017). Thus, leveraging couple and family therapy to address and improve couple and family relationships can play a critical role in Taiwan.

The stigma of receiving health treatment has decreased over time in Taiwan; however, individual therapy still dominates the field and is considered the norm (Tseng et al., 2020). In Taiwan, there is no regulation or evaluation of CFT practice, nor is there an accreditation licensure for CFT practitioners (Tseng et al., 2020). Therapists who practice CFT in Taiwan are mostly licensed counseling psychologists, clinical psychologists, social workers, or psychiatrists (Tseng et al., 2020). Therapists often receive CFT training and information from translated CFT books or workshops and trainings. Such workshops are conducted by foreign-trained instructors or local instructors who have received formal CFT training in other countries (Tseng et al., 2020).

As Tseng and colleagues (2020) suggest, increasing public awareness of CFT plays a critical role in advancing the field of CFT. If more people are aware of the advantages of CFT, therapists will be motivated to train in systemic thinking and use CFT in their practices. It is also critical for therapists to recognize that CFT is not just about learning skills, techniques, and theories; rather, it is about thinking and conceptualizing problems in a systemic framework. Chao and Lou (2018) developed the Taiwan Family Therapist Core Competencies by adapting the competencies developed by the American Association of Marriage and Family Therapy. As part of this work, they proposed three competencies that could be particularly helpful for therapists who practice CFT in Taiwan: (1) recognize and comprehend cultural norms, beliefs, and customs in local ideas of family and marriage and appreciate cultural differences; (2) be capable of tolerating tension and conflict; do not hasten to reconcile; and (3) have insight into/be conscious of how the self can be influenced/impacted by the system in the therapeutic process, and can enhance therapeutic goals (Chao and Lou, 2018, p. 15).

Taiwan has taken the first steps toward establishing the discipline of CFT. Moving forward, the development and success of CFT can be ensured by establishing accreditation and licensure regulation, increasing public awareness of CFT, and having more CFT trainers who are acquainted with the cultural norms and values of Taiwan. These steps would enable more Taiwanese couples and families to receive appropriate and effective treatment (Tseng et al., 2020).

The Future of Couple and Family Therapy in Taiwan: Reflections on Likely Future Advancements in the Research Agenda

As more therapists train in CFT in Taiwan, it is critical to ensure that this training is culturally appropriate and responsive to the needs of Taiwanese couples and families. Chao (2011) suggests a need for more clinical research to support therapists in understanding the cultural dynamics of Taiwanese couples and families and developing treatment plans that are tailored to these clients.

There is also a need for effectiveness studies and clinical process research of CFT with Taiwanese couples and families to ensure that CFT treatment can be effectively applied in the Taiwanese context. To date, only one effectiveness study has been conducted in Taiwan to evaluate the effectiveness of Emotionally Focused Therapy among Taiwanese couples (Tseng et al., under review). Most CFT research on Taiwanese couples and families has been limited to case studies, case conceptualizations, or qualitative studies (e.g., Liu & Hung, 2019; Sun, 2019; Wang & Wang, 2015). Without effectiveness studies or clinical process research, the appropriateness of CFT or specific interventions in the Taiwanese population is uncertain, as most CFT approaches are based on Westernized concepts and have been developed in Western countries. It is also important to use culturally sensitive scales in conducting effectiveness studies in Taiwan. Developing culturally sensitive scales and testing them with Taiwanese populations is another important research agenda that could further the development of CFT in Taiwan.

Three Key Takeaways

1. Taiwanese couples and families face unique challenges due to the influences of traditional Confucian values and post-industrialization modern and Western values. Therapists should be mindful of how these values are embedded within couples' cultural contexts and affect their presenting problems.
2. Democratization and progression of liberal values have led to diverse family structures in Taiwan, including an increase in singlehood, childless couples, same-sex couple households, and transnational couple households. Taiwan is the first country in Asia to legalize same-sex marriage.
3. Therapists should be mindful of the specific cultural norms and values of Taiwan and should not apply Western treatment approaches to Taiwanese couples and families without carefully examining the cultural differences and adapting treatment approaches accordingly.

Resources and Further Reading

Chao, W., & Lou, Y. (2018). Construction of core competencies for family therapists in Taiwan. *Journal of Family Therapy, 40*(2), 265–286.

Lam, B. C. P., Cross, S. E., Wu, T. F., Yeh, K. H., Wang, Y. C., & Su, J. C. (2016). What Do You Want in a Marriage? Examining Marriage Ideals in Taiwan and the United States. *Personality and Social Psychology Bulletin, 42*(6), 703–722. https://doi.org/10.1177/0146167216637842

Li, P. F., Wickrama, K., Worch, S. M., & Muruthi, B. (2019). Marital Enqing and Depression in Taiwanese Couples: The Mediating Role of Active and Passive Sacrifice. *Marriage and Family Review, 55*(3), 199–215. https://doi.org/10.1080/01494929.2018.1458009

Li, T., & Hsiao, Y. (2016). Implicit affection in Taiwanese couples: gratitude, forbearance, and marital satisfaction. *Indigenous Psychological Research in Chinese Societies, 45*, 93–128. https://doi.org/10.6254/2016.45.93

Li, T. S. (2012). Ren (Forbearance) in couple relationship and how it is related to marital satisfaction. *Formosa Journal of Mental Health, 25*(3), 447–475.

Tseng, C., Wittenborn, A. K., Blow, A. J., Chao, W., & Liu, T. (2020). The development of marriage and family therapy in East Asia (China, Taiwan, Japan, South Korea, and Hong Kong): Past, present, and future. *Journal of Family Therapy, 42*, 477–498.

Yi, C. C., Lin, W. H., & Kuo-Hsun Ma, J. (2019). Marital Satisfaction Among Taiwanese Young Married Couples: The Effects of Resources and Traditional Norms. *Journal of Family Issues, 40*(14), 2015–2043. https://doi.org/10.1177/0192513X19863212

References

Akutsu, P. D., & Chu, J. P. (2006). Clinical problems that initiate professional help-seeking behaviors from Asian Americans. *Professional Psychology: Research and Practice, 37*(4), 407–415. https://doi.org/10.1037/ 0735-7028.37.4.407.

Bryant, C. M., Conger, R. D., & Meehan, J. M. (2001). The influence of in-laws on change in marital success. *Journal of Marriage and Family, 63*, 614–626.

Chan, C. H. Y., Huang, Y. Te, So, G. Y. K., Leung, H. T., Forth, M. W., & Lo, P. Y. I. (2022). Examining the demographic and psychological variables associating with the childbearing intention among gay and bisexual men in Taiwan. *Journal of Ethnic and Cultural Diversity in Social Work*, 1–11. https://doi.org/10.1080/15313204.2022.2027313

Chang, K. L., Teng, Y. H., & Jao, J. Y. (2005). Domestic violence in transnational marriage. *Chung Shan Medical Journal, 16*, 169–176.

Chang, S. C., Chang, J. H. Y., Low, M. Y., Chen, T. C., & Kuo, S. H. (2020). Self-regulation of the newlyweds in Taiwan: Goals and strategies. *Journal of Social and Personal Relationships, 37*(8–9), 2674–2690. https://doi.org/10.1177/0265407520929762

Chao, W. (2011). Review and reflections on 40 years of family therapy development in Taiwan. *Journal of Family Therapy, 33*(4), 415–428. https://doi.org/10.1111/j.1467-6427.2011.00550.x

Chao, W., & Lou, Y. C. (2018). Construction of core competencies for family therapists in Taiwan. *Journal of Family Therapy, 40*(2), 265–286. https://doi.org/10.1111/1467-6427.12204

Chen, C. (2019). A same-sex marriage that is not the same: Taiwan's legal recognition of same-sex unions and affirmation of marriage normativity. *Australian Journal of Asian Law, 20*(1), 1–10.

Chen, F. M., & Li, T. S. (2007). Marital enqing: An examination of its relationship to spousal contributions, sacrifices, and family stress in Chinese marriages. *Journal of Social Psychology, 147*(4), 393–412. https://doi.org/10.3200/SOCP.147.4.393-412

Chen, Y. H., & Chen, H. (2014). Continuity and changes in the timing and formation of first marriage among postwar birth cohorts in Taiwan. *Journal of Family Issues, 35*(12), 1584–1604. https://doi.org/10.1177/0192513X14538026

Cheng, Y. A., & Yang, C. W. (2021). Continuity and changes in attitudes toward marriage in contemporary Taiwan. *Journal of Population Research, 38*(2), 139–167. https://doi.org/10.1007/s12546-021-09259-z

Chung, F. J., Chao, S. R., Wang, S. C., & Wu, Y. L. (2010). Immigrant family: service and practice. Taipei: Chuliu Publisher (in Chinese). Department of Household Registration Affairs (2021). *Demographic information.* www.ris.gov.tw/app/portal/346

Epstein, N. B., Chen, F., & Beyder-Kamjou, I. (2005). Relationship standards and marital satisfaction in Chinese and American couples. *Journal of Marital and Family Therapy, 31*(1), 59–74. https://doi.org/10.1111/j.1752-0606.2005.tb01543.x

Ho, D. (1996). Filial piety and its psychological consequences. In M. H. Bond (Ed.), *The handbook of Chinese psychology* (pp. 155–165). Hong Kong and New York: Oxford University Press

Huang, K. K. (2009). *Confucius Relationships: Philosophy, theory construction, and evidence research.* Taipei: Psychology Publisher.

Huang, L., Cheng, W. J., & Huang, K. K. (2008). Pathways toward voicing: Ren (forbearance) and self-transformation in the context of vertical relations. *Indigenous Psychological Research in Chinese Societies, 29,* 3–76.

Huang, Y. T., Lau, B. H. P., Forth, M. W., & Gietel-Basten, S. (2021). *Does same-sex marriage legalization invoke childbearing desire in gay and bisexual men in Taiwan: A panel study.* www.researchsquare.com/article/rs-673609/latest.pdf

Hwang, K. K., & Han, K. H. (2010). Face and morality in Confucian society. In M. H. Bond (Ed.), *The Handbook of Chinese Psychology* (pp. 479–498), New York, NY: Oxford University Press.

Jongwilaiwan, R. & Thompson, E.C. (2013). Thai wives in Singapore and transnational patriarchy. *Gender, Place and Culture, 20* (3), 363–381. https://doi.org/10.1080/0966369X.2011.624588

Kubricht, B. C., Miller, R. B., Li, T. S., & Hsiao, Y. L. (2017). Marital conflict and health in Taiwan: A dyadic longitudinal analysis. *Contemporary Family Therapy, 39*(2), 87–96. https://doi.org/10.1007/s10591-017-9404-3

Lam, B. C. P., Cross, S. E., Wu, T. F., Yeh, K. H., Wang, Y. C., & Su, J. C. (2016). What do you want in a marriage? Examining marriage ideals in Taiwan and the United States. *Personality and Social Psychology Bulletin, 42*(6), 703–722. https://doi.org/10.1177/0146167216637842

Lesthaeghe, R. (2010). The unfolding story of the second demographic transition. *Population and Development Review, 36*(2), 211–251. https://doi.org/10.1111/j.1728-4457.2010.00328.x

Li, C. H., & Yang, W. (2020). Happiness of female immigrants in cross-border marriages in Taiwan. *Journal of Ethnic and Migration Studies, 46*(14), 2956–2976. https://doi.org/10.1080/1369183X.2019.1585015

Li, P. F., & Wickrama, K. (2014). Stressful life events, marital satisfaction, and marital management skills of Taiwanese couples. *Family Relations, 63,* 193–205.

Li, P. F., Wickrama, K., Worch, S. M., & Muruthi, B. (2019). Marital enqing and depression in Taiwanese couples: The mediating role of active and passive sacrifice. *Marriage and Family Review, 55*(3), 199–215. https://doi.org/10.1080/01494929.2018.1458009

Li, T. S. (2012). Ren (Forbearance) in couple relationship and how it is related to marital satisfaction. *Formosa Journal of Mental Health, 25*(3), 447–475.

Li, T. S., & Chen, F. M. (2002). Affection in marriage: a study of marital enqing and intimacy in Taiwan. *Journal of Psychology in Chinese Societies, 3*(1), 37–59.

Li, T., & Hsiao, Y. (2016). Implicit affection in Taiwanese couples: gratitude, forbearance, and marital satisfaction. *Indigenous Psychological Research in Chinese Societies, 45*, 93–128. https://doi.org/10.6254/2016.45.93 (In Chinese)

Lien, M. H., Huang, S. S., & Yang, H. J. (2021). A pathway to negative acculturation: marital maladjustment mediates the relationship between the length of residency and depressive symptoms in immigrant women in Taiwan. *BMC Women's Health, 21*(1), 1–9. https://doi.org/10.1186/s12905-021-01334-0

Liu, T., & Hung, S.-T. (2019). The clinical practice of Emotionally Focused Couple Therapy with an in-expressive partner: A case example. *The Archive of Guidance and Counseling, 41*(2), 57–77. (In Chinese)

Ministry of Health and Welfare (2018). Assisted Reproduction Act. https://law.moj.gov.tw/ENG/LawClass/LawAll.aspx?pcode=L0070024

Ministry of Justice (2019). Act for Implementation of J.Y. Interpretation No. 748. https://law.moj.gov.tw/ENG/LawClass/LawAll.aspx?pcode=B0000008

Ministry of the Interior National Immigration Agency (2022). *Statistics.* www.immigration.gov.tw/5385/7344/7350/8887/

Ministry of the Interior Taiwan (2021). *Demographic information.* www.moi.gov.tw/cl.aspx?n=3951&page=1&PageSize=10

Pfeifer, L., Miller, R. B., Li, T. S., & Hsiao, Y. L. (2013). Perceived marital problems in Taiwan. *Contemporary Family Therapy, 35*(1), 91–104. https://doi.org/10.1007/s10591-012-9233-3

Shieh, W. Y., Hsiao, Y. L., & Tseng, H. Y. (2009). A comparative study of relationship quality of same-sex couples and married couples in Taiwan. *The Archive of Guidance & Counseling, 31*(2), 1–21.

Shweder, R. A., Balle-Jensen, L., & Goldstein, W. (2003). Who sleeps by whom revisited. In R. A. Shweder (Ed.), *Why do men barbecue?* (pp. 46–73). Cambridge, MA: Harvard University Press.

Smith, M. (2005). The politics of same-sex marriage in Canada and the United States. *Political Science and Politics, 38*(2), 225–228.

Statista (2021). *The 20 countries with the lowest fertility rates in 2021.* www.statista.com/statistics/268083/countries-with-the-lowest-fertility-rates/

Su, L. P., Miller, R. B., Canlas, J. M., Li, T. S., Hsiao, Y. L., & Willoughby, B. J. (2015). A cross-cultural study of perceived marital problems in Taiwan and the United States. *Contemporary Family Therapy, 37*(2), 165–175. https://doi.org/10.1007/s10591-015-9337-7

Sun, S.-H. (2019). The experiences of Emotionally Focused Couple Therapy for unmarried couples. *Research in Applied Psychology, 71*, 137–182. https://doi.org/10.3966/156092512019120071005 (In Chinese)

Sze, Y. T., Hou, J., Lan, J., & Fang, X. (2011). Brief report: Profiling family therapy users of a therapy center in Beijing. *American Journal of Family Therapy, 39*, 299–306. doi:10.1080/01926187.2010.542073

Tsai, M. C., Peng, S. C., & Kuo, W. Ben. (in press). Singlehood and childlessness: an age-period-cohort analysis of changing attitudes toward family in Taiwan (2005-2020). *Journal of Family Studies.* https://doi.org/10.1080/13229400.2021.2004912

Tsai, M., & Wang, Y. (2019). Intergenerational exchanges in East Asia: A new look at financial transfers. *Comparative Sociology, 18*(2), 173–203.

Tseng, C. F., Wittenborn, A. K., Blow, A. J., Chao, W., & Liu, T. (2020). The development of marriage and family therapy in East Asia (China, Taiwan, Japan, South Korea and Hong Kong): past, present and future. *Journal of Family Therapy, 42*(4), 477–498. https://doi.org/10.1111/1467-6427.12285

Tseng, C., Wittenborn, A. K., Morgan, P. C., & Liu, T. (under review). Exploring the effectiveness of Emotionally Focused Therapy (EFT) for depressive symptoms and relationship distress among couples in Taiwan: A single-arm pragmatic trial.

Tseng, Y. (2010). Marriage migration to East Asia: Current issues and propositions in making comparisons, in M. Lu and W. Yang(eds.), *Asian cross- border marriage migration: Demographic patterns and social issues* (pp. 31–48). Amsterdam: Amsterdam University Press.

United Nations (2014). *Country classification.* www.un.org › policy › wesp › wesp_current

Van Lange, P. A. M., Rusbult, C. E., Drigotas, S. M., Arriaga, X. B., Witcher, B. S., & Cox, C. L. (1997). Willingness to sacrifice in close relationships. *Journal of Personality and Social Psychology, 72*, 1373–1395.

Wang, W.-H., & Wang, C.-H. (2015). Exploring the attachment injury after experiencing Extramarital affair with EFT couple therapy. *Guidance Quarterly*, *51*(2), 14–20. (In Chinese)

Wang, Y. (2020). Exploring multicultural counseling practice experiences of counseling psychologists: the case of female new immigrant clients. *Chinese Journal of Guidance and Counseling*, *58*, 127–159.

Wang, Y. T., & Yang, W. S. (2019). Changes and trends in family structure in Taiwan, 1990 to 2010. *Journal of Family Issues*, *40*(14), 1896–1911. https://doi.org/10.1177/0192513X19863203

Wu, T. F., Cross, S. E., Wu, C. W., Cho, W., & Tey, S. H. (2016). Choosing your mother or your spouse: Close relationship dilemmas in Taiwan and the United States. *Journal of Cross-Cultural Psychology*, *47*(4), 558–580. https://doi.org/10.1177/0022022115625837

Yeh, K. H., & Bedford, O. (2003). A test of the Dual Filial Piety model. *Asian Journal of Social Psychology*, *6*(3), 215–228. https://doi.org/10.1046/j.1467-839X.2003.00122.x

Yeoh, B. S. A., Hen, L. C., Thi, K. D. V., & Cheng, Y. (2013). Between two families: The social meaning of remittances for Vietnamese marriage migrants in Singapore. *Global Networks*, *13*(4), 441–458.

Yeung, W. J., & Mu, Z. (2020). Migration and marriage in Asian contexts. *Journal of Ethnic and Migration Studies*, *24*(14), 2863–2879.

Yi, C. C., Lin, W. H., & Kuo-Hsun Ma, J. (2019). Marital satisfaction among Taiwanese young married couples: The Effects of resources and traditional norms. *Journal of Family Issues*, *40*(14), 2015–2043. https://doi.org/10.1177/0192513X19863212

Yu, W. (2020). *The first year since the legalization of same-sex marriage in Taiwan: Experience of newlywed female couples* [Unpublished doctoral dissertation]. Shih-Chien University, Taiwan.

Zhang, S., Merolla, A. J., Sun, S., & Lin, S. (2012). The nature and consequences of topic avoidance in Chinese and Taiwanese close relationships. *Asian Journal of Social Psychology*, 1–10. http://doi.org/10.1111/j.1467-839X.2012.01367.x

15

BOSPHORUS CONNECTING EUROPE AND ASIA

Couple and Family Therapy in Turkey

Yudum Söylemez and Senem Zeytinoğlu Saydam

Introduction

If Turkey were a family (Akyıl & Aydın Erol, 2018), it would have similar dynamics as a multicultural family. At the crossroads of Europe and Asia, Turkey experiences both the advantages and the challenges of the complexity of meeting Western and Eastern worldviews. Turkey is the birthplace of both Rumi and Santa Clause. Covering a surface area the size of Texas, with triple its population, Turkey hosts Greeks, Armenians, Jews, Laz, Syrians, Circassians, Kurds, etc. Culturally, Turkish people speak many languages and dialects, and the country celebrates more than fifteen holidays. Although most of the population is Muslim (99%), there is great diversity in religious practices. Such diversity means Turkey harbors the richness of traditions, coping mechanisms, healing stories, and remedies of many ancient and modern cultures.

On the one hand, Turkey faces challenges in maintaining unity due to the segregation caused by hierarchies in power. As Elif Şafak wrote in *The Bastard of Istanbul*, we're stuck between the East and the West, between the past and the future (Şafak, 2007). There has been a divide between the secular and traditional sections of the society, western modernization versus religious conservatism. Atatürk, the founder of the Turkish Republic in 1923, said, "We want to modernize our state. If we want civilization, we need to turn to the West" (Atatürk's Discourses and Speeches, 2010). On the other hand, the religious and conservative party coming to power in 2002 and still having one third of all votes in the country prioritizes traditional and religious customs and values in conventional family life. These opposing views sometimes lead to polarization, which makes it harder to reach a state of solidarity. In a qualitative study with liberal parents, it was found that although some of these parents were raised by religious parents themselves, they did not transmit religious values to their children (Akyıl, Prouty, Blanchard, & Lyness, 2014). Parents reported that although they wanted to balance traditional and modern values in their families, as religious doctrines are imposed on them (such as the restrictions on alcohol use), the meaning of religion has changed from spiritual to dogmatic.

Being close to the midpoint on the collectivistic side of Individualism-Collectivism classification by Hofstede (1980) and a complex cultural structure where different geographic,

DOI: 10.4324/9781003297871-17

religious, and socioeconomic segments of the society meet, Turkey serves as an excellent laboratory to observe social change, family dynamics, gender roles, and the evolution of couple and family therapy. It is a rapidly changing country with a high growth and urbanization rate and a young population (median age: 32.7, Turk stat, 2021). The rapid social change can easily be observed in marriage and divorce rates. From 2018 to 2019, marriage rates went down 2.3%, and divorce rates climbed to 8%.

Kağıtçıbaşı, a pioneer social psychologist, defined Turkey as a "culture of relatedness" and families as "close-knit" (1996) even though she also proposed that independence is on the rise among young people in Turkey, especially in urban areas (Kağıtçıbaşı & Ataca, 2005). The self is not readily separable from conceptions of others in the family (Fişek, 1991), which may resemble enmeshment from a western point of view, but as Fişek argues the negative connotation of enmeshment would be inappropriate for Turkish culture and suggests the term "individualized/familial self" instead. Furthermore, recent findings indicate that when Turkish millennials are compared to their Generation Xer and Boomer counterparts, they are less collectivistic, more self-enhancing, and less self-transcending (Marcus, Ceylan, & Ergin, 2017). Patriarchal hierarchy, where control is based on age and gender, is being replaced by nurturant order where the parents have the power in the family system with their protective and caring role (Fişek, 2002).

Gender roles in a traditional Turkish family are clear: men are breadwinners and women are in charge of housework and childcare (Poyrazlı, 2003). As women's employment has increased, men have started to participate in childcare in the last three decades, and women have more say in family decisions (Eraslan et al., 2012). However, in a recent report, half of the women thought household and child-rearing were their primary responsibilities (Family Value Research in Turkey, 2010), wives should not argue with their husbands (Institute of Populations Studies, 2015), and many Turkish men believed that one of women's roles was to meet their husband's sexual needs (Laumann et al., 2006). Premarital sex is not condoned, especially for women (Boratav & Çavdar, 2012). Not surprisingly, in *The Global Gender Gap Reports*, among 144 countries, Turkey had shallow scores, ranking 105th in 2006 and 131st in 2017.

The Need for a Comprehensive Mental Health Law

One of the most significant challenges for mental health professionals in Turkey is mental health law. The field of mental health has been regulated by a law that was first issued in 1928, namely the Law on the Practice of Medicine and its Branches/Related Fields (Tababet ve Şuabatı San'atlarının Tarzı İcrasına Dair Kanun, 1928). The Law on Practice of Medicine conceptualizes "therapy" as medical treatment. It will only allow mental health professionals without a medical degree to practice under the supervision and oversight of a medicine specialist (Turkish Psychological Association, Türk Psikologlar Derneği, 2008). This means that couple and family therapists and other mental health professionals cannot practice psychotherapy independently.

In 2011, an additional law was issued for clinical psychology (Bazı Kanun ve Kanun Hükmünde Kararnamelerde Değişiklik Yapılmasına Dair Kanun, 2011) that enables individuals who either earned a master's degree or doctoral degree in clinical psychology to be recognized as clinical psychologists. A caveat does exist, as such individuals can only work with clients who have no official diagnosis. Furthermore, the original mental health law excluded couple and family therapists and other mental health professionals. To combat the exclusion of couple and family therapists and other mental health practitioners, the Mental Health Platform-Turkey (MHPT) was established in 2006 when fifteen mental health organizations (including ÇATED, CFT Association) in the country came together as a taskforce to improve mental health services in Turkey and work on the proposal of the law that includes a definition of psychotherapy and psychotherapist, as well as client rights preventive measures, etc. (Türkiye Psikiyatri Derneği, 2017; Türk Psikolojik Danışma ve Rehberlik Derneği, 2017).

Unfortunately, couple and family therapy (CFT) is not included in the mental health laws in Turkey. This might be because CFT is not yet viewed as an independent profession. Instead, CFT is recognized as a subspecialty of clinical psychology. Additionally, the focus on legislative issues and CFT's bourgeoning status as a newer academic discipline has hampered inclusion into mental health laws in Turkey. In 2007 and 2009, Social Services and Child Protection Institution issued a regulation on family counseling centers (Gerçek Kişiler ve Özel Hukuk Tüzel Kişileri ile Kamu Kurum ve Kuruluşlarınca Açılacak Aile Danışma Merkezleri Hakkında Yönetmelik, 2009) with the government's aim to protect the "family institution" and reduce divorce rates in the country. This required certified clinicians to work in these centers. Rapidly, a 100-hour family counseling training popped up for psychologists, social workers, psychological counselors, child development specialists, doctors, and nurses (Konuk, Akyıl, Arduman & Sarimurat Baydemir, 2011), and over 25,000 people graduated as family counselors. The Couple and Family Therapy Association (ÇATED) revised training hour requirements from 100 to 450. Supervision was also implemented. Most programs, however, still need improvement in trainer competency and the oversight of clinical and supervision hours. Some of these certificate programs have been approved by the Ministry of Education, permitting the certificate owners to open up their family counseling practices. However, there is no accrediting body that specializes in CFT education.

Another area of conflict within the CFT field in Turkey centers around the debate about whether to use the terms "family therapy" or "family counseling." Since therapy is a medical procedure and can only be conducted by medical doctors, government institutions prefer to use the term "counseling" rather than "therapy" (Roberts et al., 2014). However, this is a problem since it opposes the need for CFT to be recognized as a separate profession and denies individuals who graduated from qualified CFT programs the right to call themselves "couple and family therapists."

Development of CFT in Turkey

The building blocks for the development of CFT in Turkey began in the 1980s by the great pioneers in social psychology such as Çiğdem Kağıtçıbaşı and Diane Sunar and clinical psychologists with a specific interest in family dynamics such as Güler Fişek. In the 1990s, several clinicians, mostly the students of these pioneers, went to the United States to study CFT in Mental Research Institute or Ackerman Institute and came back to Turkey to start their training programs. In 1999 a disastrous earthquake occurred, which displaced and had a detrimental effect on many families in the region. Professionals from different disciplines from other countries had to collaborate to address the needs of the survivors (Arduman, 2013).

At the beginning of the millennium, Turkey hosted the International Family Therapy Association (IFTA, 2004) and the European Family Therapy Association (EFTA,

2013) conferences. The 2009 IFTA conference in Portoroz was another milestone in establishing family therapy in Turkey by connecting therapists from Turkey and IFTA to train supervisors and form a cohesive training program. (Kafescioğlu & Akyıl, 2018). Eventually, these professionals founded the Couple and Family Therapy Association (Çift ve Aile Terapisi Derneği, ÇATED) in 2012, and now, the association has over 500 members. This was the second association after the AETD (Association of Family and Marriage Therapies, 1997).

Research also supports that the Turkish population has embraced a systemic perspective in the last 20 years. A study by Korkut in 2001 found that 75% of clinicians worked with families, but only 12.5% of that group used the systemic perspective. However, in 2015, this percentage went up to 63% (Akyıl, Üstünel, Alkan & Aydın, 2015). The latter study also shows a post-modern trend in clinical work, recognizing solution-focused ideas that enable absolute truths to be challenged and alternative hypotheses to be explored.

Training Programs

In 2010, the first CFT master's program was established at Doğuş University in Istanbul by Yudum Söylemez and Nilüfer Kafescioğlu. Söylemez and Kafescioğlu both earned Ph.D. degrees in CFT and collaborated with Sibel Erenel, a U.S.-licensed couple and family therapist and faculty member with a Ph.D. in family studies, Aslı Çarkoğlu. After this program was closed due to some problems with the university administration, the faculty members moved to other universities and established CFT programs at their new institutions. In 2013, one of the university-based certificate programs, the Istanbul Bilgi University certificate program, became a part of the clinical psychology master's program as a CFT track. The CFT program offered an adult and child/adolescent track in which the first author of this chapter coordinated.

Currently, there are two master's programs in CFT (Istanbul Bilgi University and Özyeğin University). The International Accreditation Commission accredits both programs for Systemic Therapy Education (IACSTE) because they meet the theoretical and clinical criteria for installing competent supervision and faculty, maintaining clinical and leadership hour requirements, a well-equipped clinic with one-way mirrors, and recording equipment. These clinics offer affordable individual, couple, and family therapy for university students and the surrounding communities and enabled the first CFT psychotherapy research in the country.

Aside from the MA programs, certificate programs offer programs meeting IFTA and EFTA criteria for CFT education. Some of these programs are certified by the Ministry of Education. Most of the founders of these programs are also co-founders of ÇATED.

Backgrounds of Professionals Practicing Couple and Family Therapy in Turkey

To better understand the current picture of the CFT profession in Turkey, a descriptive study was conducted by the members of ÇATED Research Committee (Akyıl, Üstünel, Alkan & Aydın, 2015) in which demographic characteristics, educational background, and clinical practices of professionals who work with couples and families in Turkey were investigated. Results revealed that, like their American counterparts, most of the clinicians working with couples and families (87%) were women (Beaton, Dienhart, Schmidt, & Turner, 2009).

However, compared to the United States, the Turkish clinicians were younger (25–30 years old vs. 47–52 years old) and less experienced (5 years vs. 13–15 years). Only 57% of the sample had a graduate degree (U.S.: 75%, Morris, 2007), out of which only 15% had a graduate degree in CFT. Twenty percent of the participants had no specialized training in CFT or had very little theoretical and clinical training and supervision. Thirty four percent of the participants worked without any supervision, especially in cities other than Istanbul.

Most clinicians identified themselves as psychologists or psychological counselors rather than as couple and family therapists, which can be explained by the lack of recognition of the CFT profession within the mental health field and the public. The need for well-structured standards and guidelines for practicing family therapy cannot be understated. Participants from the association have made efforts to acknowledged and recognized the profession within the mental health community.

Although the participants felt competent in working with child-parent relationships, couple relational issues, anxiety, and depression, they felt inadequate in working with domestic violence, sexual problems, and addictions. This finding reveals that there is a need for special education in curriculums. Unfortunately, many of the certificate programs in CFT mainly focus on specific techniques but lack components that give an overall systemic perspective to address a variety of individual, couple, and family issues. One book written by interns in the CFT program at Istanbul Bilgi University called "Couple and Family Therapy: Fundamental Issues and Interventions" aimed to fill this gap by highlighting CFT issues from a systemic perspective (Söylemez, 2021).

The study mentioned above also underlined that in the last fifteen years (Akyıl et al., 2015; Korkut, 2001) a systemic approach has become more prominent for clinicians working with couples and families, and solution-focused and emotionally focused therapies gained interest in Turkey. This could be associated with the emergence of structured training, supervisions and seminars, and social media posts by associations that make specific approaches more visible. Also, a post-modern trend in clinical work in Turkey where common cultural beliefs are to be challenged and alternative ideas to be explored is on the rise, similar to the rest of the world (Beaton et al., 2009).

Development of Specific Models and Specialties in Turkey

Multiple systemic treatment modalities are in use in Turkey. Masters' programs offer courses on various CFT models but focus primarily on ecological systems theory where individualism is embedded in developmental, familial, cultural, and chronological contexts (Bronfenbrenner, 1989). Common factors lens, intergenerational approaches, structural therapy, narrative therapy, experiential therapy, emotionally focused therapy are commonly used and recently self of the therapist issues have become more prominent. The post-modern culture in both programs encourages a strength-based and collaborative learning environment where students can incorporate their existing knowledge and experience into their theoretical and clinical training.

CFT faculty mainly emphasize the models that they were trained and experienced in. A qualitative examination of the experiences of U.S.-based trained CFTs in Turkey pointed out that training was relevant and applicable in Turkish culture with some modifications in therapeutic approaches (Güvensel, 2015). Some faculty integrate different models to adapt to the needs of their populations. For example, the first author of this chapter incorporated her play therapy training with CFT and gave courses on family play therapy. She has also designed a family game Bizbize (Just Us) that can be played both by therapists and families themselves (Akyıl, 2017). The second author incorporated her training and experience in person of the therapist model and emotionally focused therapy and has been giving training and supervisions on the integration of these two models.

Certificate programs vary in the modalities they offer. Some programs train in different CFT approaches and let students choose the model they want to specialize in. Some programs are affiliated with institutes or associations and represent specific models such as Satir's Experiential Family Therapy, Narrative Therapy, and Emotionally Focused Therapy (EFT).

Although CFT training implements systemic approaches, we give a few examples of how specific models have evolved in the last decade.

Emotionally Focused Therapy

As the EFT trainer in Turkey, the second author would like to describe the development of this model here, its current state, and future directions. The authors of this chapter started organizing EFT training in Turkey in 2014. There are many EFT training seminars given in Turkey by trainers who have questionable knowledge and qualifications to teach the model. Thus, we wanted the training to be internationally accredited and conducted by a credible trainer. For this reason, we got approval from the International Center for Excellence in Emotionally Focused Therapy (ICEEFT) to conduct activities in Turkey, and we had the first training in April 2014. Since then, we have been organizing at least one training a year. The second author became a local trainer in 2019, and is currently offering training in Turkish. As of now, we have two ICEEFT-approved supervisors and one trainer-in-training. The Turkish community of emotionally focused therapy became an association in 2019 and has continued to grow ever since. The association supports the community by conducting bi-weekly supervision meetings by ICEEFT-approved supervisors. ICEEFT-certified trainers worldwide also provide online training on emotionally focused individual therapy, family therapy, and other special topics with trainers worldwide via Zoom. Three hundred people over the years have been trained. For future directions, the goal is to teach in different cities in Turkey, research the effectiveness of EFT in the Turkish context, and improve the number of certified therapists and supervisors.

Medical Family Therapy

Medical family therapy has been growing in Turkey, even though it is still a subspecialty of family therapy. Currently, we have one couple and family therapist who completed a certification training in medical family therapy, another one receiving her doctorate, and one Ph.D. in medical family therapy. There are even studies on individuals coping with physical illness (Gürtekin, 2019), the focus on the family and relationships in research and clinical practice is rare. When mental health professionals working with individuals coping with physical illness were asked to complete a survey about their adherence to medical family therapy principles, the findings showed that couple and family therapists include family members more in the treatment process and focus on strengthening the emotional bonds among family members. The same study also showed that a significant number of respondents reported that their training did not include any materials about mental health experiences of individuals and families coping with physical illness (Kaytan, 2016).

These findings highlighted the necessity of introducing an approach that will help mental health professionals in aiding their clients and their families in coping with illness. For this reason, medical family therapy was presented at a ÇATED conference in 2018. The second author called all interested parties to join a subcommittee that was going to be formed by the second author under ÇATED's umbrella. In the same year, the subcommittee of medical family therapy was formed. Since then, this committee has been working very actively to broaden the knowledge and application of medical family therapy in Turkey. Furthermore, the second author and her colleagues wrote a manual for medical family therapy and trained mental health professionals working in municipalities to provide services for their clients. They later introduced the ÇATED's medical family therapy subcommittee members to offer the same training to interested parties under ÇATED's umbrella. Future goals include improving the application of medical family therapy among Turkish mental health professionals and researching systemic aspects of coping with illness.

Person of the Therapist Model

There is a consensus in couple and family therapy about incorporating self-of-the-therapist work. This issue becomes even more significant as we supervise the next generation of therapists as part of our training (Lee & Nelson, 2014). Yet, there is a need for an integrated approach with a clear philosophical foundation and practical tools to meet this need. The Person of the Therapist model was developed by Dr. Harry Aponte (Aponte, 1982; 1994; Aponte & Winter, 2013; Aponte & Kissil, 2016) to improve the clinical skills of therapists through assisting them in effectively using themselves. This model has been implemented in training and supervision in clinical and academic settings for more than 30 years (Kissil & Nino, 2018).

In Turkey, this model was introduced in the training of graduate students by the authors of this chapter through supervision, in-class activities, and research. With the establishment of the Aponte Institute for Person of the Therapist Development, our goal is to fully incorporate the model into graduate school curriculums.

Feminist Family Therapy (FFT)

In a 2018 study, 38% of men and 42% of women said they had not heard the word "feminism" before (O'Neil & Çarkoğlu, 2018). Additionally, many participants believed that feminism advocated man-hating (21%) and dominance of women (43%). Although women's movements in Turkey have been active almost synchronously with the western world, psychology and psychotherapy have yet to be influenced by feminism (Bolat-Boratav, 2011). Psychology master's theses written between 1978 and 2009 at Boğaziçi University (one of the top universities in Turkey), only 28 out of 264 had words such as "sex," "sex role," or "gender," and "feminism" or "feminist."

Similar to CFT in general, feminist family therapy practices and literature in Turkey are 50 years behind most western countries (there are only three articles, one book chapter, and some oral presentations). One study examined the effectiveness of a feminist-informed relationship enhancement program and found it was influential on the power-sharing, self orientations, and dyadic adjustment of married couples (Arıcı-Şahin, 2017). A recent qualitative study aimed to explore the experiences of CFTs in gender-related topics in therapy and the ways they incorporate feminist ideas in their clinical practices (Kılıçer, Gürçağ,

Civan, Akyıl, & Prouty, 2021). The results showed that even the participants who identified themselves as a feminist did not use feminist ideas in therapy to protect their neutrality and therapeutic alliance with men and believed they should not exercise their values in medicine. These results were interpreted as sexism because therapists may feel unsupported to practice FFT in a gendered society due to the sexist ideology ingrained in culture; there is an immense need for intensive training, ongoing supervision, and peer groups to discuss ideas. In 2021, a Gender Studies committee was founded at ÇATED that collaborates with other institutions to advocate on critical gender-related topics, advise other committees regarding gendered language in social media posts, and organize seminars.

Collaborations with Social Services/NGOs

Systemic culture leads CFTs to think in a multilayered fashion regarding clinical, academic, and social relationships. Socially responsible CFTs cannot deny their role as advocates for their clients, students and supervisees, and the public; therefore, they cannot limit themselves in a therapy room or a university office. This ecosystemic culture can also be observed in Turkey. Most of us, as CFT professionals and academicians, conduct collaborative projects with NGOs (social services and foster care, domestic violence prevention, etc.), ministries of health and education. We also give feedback on family regulations, advocate for CFT to be acknowledged as a mental health profession and play an active role in natural disasters and collective trauma.

The pandemic has been an example of how systemic therapists joined forces to help families stuck at home dealing with anxiety, depression, and relationship problems. As we have transitioned to online therapy in our privacy practices, we have developed rules and regulations at the university clinic for the supervisees; we published an online CFT manual, which is in the process of being a chapter in a teletherapy book that will be published soon. Additionally, we have organized talks in the CFT association on how to keep relationships safe during Covid and provided interviews with health workers. Tele-ÇAT (Tele-CFT) was initiated in ÇATED, where our members volunteered to work in a brief solution-focused approach with almost 100 families from many different cities.

Publications and Research

Most of the literature on couples and families in Turkey reviews articles on team and parent-child relationship dynamics, psychotherapeutic techniques, and movie analyses. There are also scale adaptation studies such as the adaptation of the BARE scale (Zeytinoğlu-Saydam, Erdem & Söylemez, 2021); multi-cultural studies on sexuality (Leavitt, Lefkowitz, Akyıl & Serduk, 2019), technology and CFT (Akyıl, Üstünel & Bacigalupe, 2017), feminist family therapy supervision during Covid-19 (Maier, Prouty & Söylemez, 2022).

Face to Face: Couple and Family Therapy Stories from Turkey is a book co-edited by the first author and a chapter penned by the second author (Akyıl, 2016). The research committee of ÇATED planned this book and ten CFTs authored case studies from different approaches. Two other projects conducted by the research committee were the Public Perception of CFT and Experiences in Close Relationships During Corona Times (ÇATED, 2021). Besides research publications and case studies, ÇATED has a Systemic Bulletin (now online) published a couple of times a year that includes updates on research, training, professional developments, and committee activities.

With an academic uptrend in CFT in the last decade, the systemic worldview has been influential in psychology and psychotherapy research in Turkey. As opposed to the field's medical and quantitative culture, CFT's participatory, post-modern, collaborative, and strength-based approach led to qualitative and mixed-method designs. Similarly, a jump in qualitative study publications in the United States occurred in the early 1990s (Faulkner et al., 2002).

Although the most common tradition within qualitative studies in CFT is grounded theory in the United States (Gehart et al., 2001; Beitin, 2008), since most CFT research in Turkey is being conducted by master's students, and grounded theory requires a higher number of participants, phenomenology is the most common method. In terms of most commonly studied issues in CFT, the experiences in couple and family relationships such as being from diverse cultures (jews, Armenians, family buildings, etc.), in different life-cycle stages (having the first baby, etc.), going through challenging life experiences (chronic illness, extradyadic relationships, etc.).

Another common research area is psychotherapy or intervention research that includes fathers in family therapy, play in couples therapy, attachment-focused approaches in working with foster families, etc. A study with 23 women who attended systemic treatment (individual, couple, and family) for three months indicated that couple satisfaction increased at the end of the therapy process in all modalities (Araç, 2019).

Single-subject designs such as Hermeneutic Single-case Efficacy Design (HSCED; Elliot, 2002) that utilize quantitative and qualitative measures to gather evidence of the effectiveness of a therapy process have also been suitable to use in university clinics since most therapy sessions are being recorded. One study exploring the online couple therapy process and outcomes during Covid-19 found that together with extra-therapeutic factors, a sixteen-session experiential couple therapy increased couple satisfaction (Söylemez & Gürmen, 2021, unpublished manuscript).

In September 2020, two of the MA programs in CFT joined a practice research network (MFT-PRN) based in Brigham Young University, Utah (Johnson, Miller, Bradford, & Anderson, 2017). This system is designed to collect clinical data via an online platform that facilitates clinical, supervisory, and research data use and aims to build an international professional community. In PRN, individual, couple, and family clients fill out online questionnaires regularly during their therapy process. They rate their progress in their presenting problem, personal wellbeing, couple satisfaction, family functioning, and therapeutic alliance. Ongoing assessments give the clinicians a chance to follow their clients' progress and the process of therapy and provide direct feedback to their clients, which increases the effectiveness of treatment (Karam & Sprenkle, 2010). Moreover, the intern therapists' owning their therapy process as part of a research team allows them to keep client goals and change processes in their focus at all times. In the coming years, we plan to publish clinic outcomes, compare two clinics, and make cross-cultural comparisons with other MFT-PRN sites.

Conclusion and Future Directions

The developments in the CFT field in Turkey are promising; however, as Roberts and colleagues (2014, p. 561) stated, "family therapy in Turkey is in its infancy." The biggest challenge for the profession is the lack of standards for family therapy training (Korkut, 2001, 2007; Akyıl et al., 2015). This is not a new problem when we look at the history of the development of the profession in the United States, and is parallel to the search for and development of core competencies in CFT (Kaslow, Celano, & Stanton, 2005; Miller, Todahl, & Platt, 2010; Nelson, Chenail, Alexander, Crane, Johnson, & Schwaillie, 2007). The adoption of core competencies into the system in Turkey will be helpful for the future of CFT in the Turkish mental health professional context.

Moreover, professional organizations and governments need to reach a consensus regarding mental health laws in general and family therapy regulations, in particular, to form and enforce the standards in family therapy training. Instead of increasing the number of programs to meet the increasing demand for CFT training, improving the program's quality should be the focus. Even though there are newly emerging master's programs in CFT aligned with international standards, there are no Ph.D. programs in CFT in Turkey. Only seven trainers in Turkey have doctoral degrees in CFT (6 PhDs and 1 PsyD). We, as the authors of this chapter, are two of them. We collaborate with other CFTs a great deal. However, there is a need for more professionals with doctoral degrees who can teach master's or doctoral level CFT programs in Turkey. Doctoral programs would contribute to the development of the field as a separate discipline (separate from clinical psychology or counseling) and research in the area and training of future trainers and supervisors. In addition, having doctoral programs in CFT offered at universities in Turkey would eliminate the need to live abroad to get postgraduate degrees in CFT and allow us to have academics in our discipline who obtained their education in our own culture.

Improving the quality of the training programs will also require an accrediting and supervising body such as COAMFTE. Currently, the number of CFT supervisors is deficient and concentrated in bigger cities in Turkey and mainly in Istanbul. We need to develop ways to require and provide training for supervisors and create pathways to spread supervision to the rest of the country. Due to the pandemic and the accessibility of online training and supervision, the opportunity to train and offer supervision to practitioners in smaller cities in Turkey has been created.

There is no licensing process for any mental health field in Turkey, including CFT. When the assessment of trainees' competencies is considered, the master's programs apply their regular testing and assessment methods in their courses; however, certificate programs do not offer any evaluation to the trainees as far as we know. Eventually, there needs to be a licensing process for the CFT field and other mental health fields.

Until 2021, there have been no ethical codes specific to CFT in Turkey. Recently, as ÇATED, we have adapted AAMFT moral codes to cultural and legal norms in the country and published the Ethical Codes for CFTs in Turkey; we have selected an ethics committee and finalized the procedures for handling ethical matters our members.

"3 Keys"

1. Turkey, located at the center of both the richness of ancient civilizations and the tension of political conflicts, has the challenge to come to peace by sometimes integrating opposing values. A systemic view would benefit the country to conceptualize its problems without blame and unify the society to face the challenges together.
2. Although Turkish culture is very family-oriented, CFT has been growing as a profession in the last decade. Since 2010, three master's programs and one association opened the door for a systemic community by generating research studies, intervention programs, community work, a productive learning environment with training and supervision.

3. Now, we need a mental health law with specific regulations for the profession. Doctorate programs, a licensing process, a systemic peer-reviewed journal, branches of associations in different cities would be necessary to expand, strengthen and enrich CFT.

Resources and Further Reading

CFT Association: www.cated.org/
Emotionally Focused Therapies Association www.docat.org/
Akyıl, Y., Pham, B., & Cunningham, N. (2014). Concerns of a Beginning Therapist: Giving a Voice to the Therapist-In-Training. In R. Bean & M. Davey (Eds), *Clinical Supervision Activities for Increasing Competence and Self-Awareness*. New York: Wiley.
Hiebert, W. J., Alkanat, Ö., & Leblebici, Ç. (2014). Çift terapilerinde yapılandırılmış ilk görüşmeler. Pegem Akademi.
Zeytinoğlu, S., Akyıl, Y., Kissil, K. (2014). Supervising Foreign-born therapists in the United States: A Clinical Guide. In R. Bean & M. Davey (Eds), *Clinical Supervision Activities for Increasing Competence and Self-Awareness*. New York: Wiley.
Zeytinoglu Saydam, S. (2018). Cross-culturally responsive training of EFT: International experiences (Chapter 4). In Poulsen, S., & Allen, R. (Eds). *Cross-cultural responsiveness & systemic therapy: personal and clinical narratives*. Cham, Switzerland: Springer

References

Akyıl, Y. (2017). Aile Terapisinde Oyun. In A. Dost-Gözkân, N. Kafescioğlu, D. Tahiroğlu, *Gelişim psikolojisi ve terapi perspektifinden oyun*. İstanbul: Özyeğin Üniversitesi Yayınları.
Akyıl, Y., & Aydın Erol, T. (2018, March). Suppose Turkey was a Family: Systemic Conceptualization of a country going through Crises. IFTA Conference, Bangkok, Thailand.
Akyıl, Y., & Güven, N. (2016). *Yüzyüze: Türkiye'den çift ve aile terapisi öyküleri*. Pegasus Yayınları.
Akyıl, Y., Bacigalupe, G., & Üstünel, A. Ö. (2017). Emerging technologies and family: A cross-national study of family clinicians' views. *Journal of Family Psychotherapy*, 28(2), 99–117. https://doi.org/10.1080/08975353.2017.1285654
Akyıl, Y., Prouty, A., Blanchard, A., & Lyness, K. (2014). Parents' experiences of intergenerational value transmission in Turkey's Changing Society: An interpretative phenomenological study. *Journal of Family Psychotherapy*, 25(1), 42–65. https://doi.org/10.1080/08975353.2014.881690
Akyıl, Y., Üstünel, A. O., Alkan, S., & Aydın, H. (2015). Türkiye'de çift ve ailelerle çalışan uzmanlar: Demografik özellikler, eğitim ve Klinik uygulamalar. *Psikoloji Çalışmaları Dergisi*, 35(1), 57–84.
Aponte, H. J. (1982). The person of the therapist: The cornerstone of therapy. *Family Therapy Networker*, 46, 19–21.
Aponte, H. J. (1994). How personal can training get? *Journal of Marital and Family Therapy*, 20(1), 3–15. https://doi.org/10.1111/j.1752-0606.1994.tb01007.x
Aponte, H. J., & Kissil, K. (Eds.). (2016). *The person of the therapist training model: Mastering the use of self*. Routledge.
Aponte, H. J., & Winter, J. E. (2013). The person and practice of the therapist: Treatment and training. In M. Baldwin (Ed.), *The use of self in therapy* (3rd ed) (pp. 141–165). Routledge.
Araç, H. I. (2019). *Associations between dyadic adjustment and psychological symptoms: A preliminary study assessing therapeutic change for couples* [Master's Thesis]. İstanbul Bilgi University.
Arduman, E. (2013). A perspective on evolving family therapy in Turkey. *Contemporary Family Therapy*, 35(2), 364–375. https://doi.org/10.1007/s10591-013-9268-0
Arıcı Şahin, F. (2017). Feminist yaklaşıma dayalı ilişki geliştirme programının güç paylaşımı, benlik yönelimleri ve çift uyumuna etkisi (Doktora tezi). *Hacettepe Üniversitesi, eğitim Bilimleri Enstitüsü, Ankara*.
Baltalarlı, N., Şişman, Z., Cilmeli, E., Akınkoç, İ., Kızılırmak, K., Coklar, Ö., Bayraktar, G., & Mutlu, İ. (2021). *Close relationships in the times of Covid-19 research report*. Couple and Family Therapy Association Research Committee.

Bazı Kanun ve Kanun Hükmünde Kararnamelerde Değişiklik Yapılmasına Dair Kanun (2011). Resmi Gazete (Sayı: 27916). Retrieved June 24, 2017 from www.resmigazete.gov.tr/eskiler/2011/04/20110426-1.htm

Beaton, J., Dienhart, A., Schmidt, J., & Turner, J. (2009). Clinical practice patterns of Canadian couple/marital/family therapists. *Journal of Marital and Family Therapy*, *35*(2), 193–203. https://doi.org/10.1111/j.1752-0606.2009.00116.x

Beitin, B. K. (2008). Qualitative research in marriage and family therapy: Who is in the interview? *Contemporary Family Therapy*, *30*(1), 48–58. https://doi.org/10.1007/s10591-007-9054-y

Bolak-Boratav, H. (2011). Searching for feminism in psychology in Turkey. In A. Rutherford, R. Capdevila, U. Vindhya & I. Palmary (Eds.), *Handbook of international feminisms* (pp. 17–36). Springer.

Boratav, H. B., & Çavdar, A. (2012). Sexual stereotypes and practices of university students in Turkey. *Archives of Sexual Behavior*, *41*(1), 271–281. https://doi.org/10.1007/s10508-011-9811-8

Bronfenbrenner, U. (1989). Ecological systems theory. *Annals of Child Development*, *6*, 187–249.

Eraslan, V. (2012). Türkiye İşgücü Piyasasında Ücret Seviyesinde Cinsiyet Ayrımcılığı: Blinder-Oaxaca Ayrıştırma Yöntemi. [Gender wage discrimination in the Turkish labor market: A Blinder-Oaxaca decomposition method]. *İstanbul Üniversitesi, İktisat Fakültesi Mecmuası*, *62*(1), 231–248.

Faulkner, R. A., Klock, K., & Gale, J. E. (2002). Qualitative research in family therapy: Publication trends from 1980–1995. *Journal of Marital and Family Therapy*, *28*(1), 69–74. https://doi.org/10.1111/j.1752-0606.2002.tb01174.x

Fişek, G. O. (1991). A cross-cultural examination of proximity and hierarchy as dimensions of family structure. *Family Process*, *30*(1), 121–133. https://doi.org/10.1111/j.1545-5300.1991.00121.x

Fişek, G. O. (2002). Bende bir ben var ailemden içeri. Paper presented at the XII National Congress of Psychology, September 11–13. Ankara.

Gehart, D. R., Ratliff, D. A., & Lyle, R. R. (2001). Qualitative research in family therapy: A substantive and methodological review. *Journal of Marital and Family Therapy*, *27*(2), 261–274. https://doi.org/10.1111/j.1752-0606.2001.tb01162.x

Gerçek Kişiler ve Özel Hukuk Tüzel Kişileri ile Kamu Kurum ve Kuruluşlarınca Açılacak Aile Danışma Merkezleri Hakkında Yönetmelik (2009). Resmi Gazete (Sayı:27152). Retrieved June 24, 2017 from www.resmigazete.gov.tr/eskiler/2009/02/20090225-4.htm

Gürtekin, D. B. *The relationship between the gain of resources and burden of care in caregivers to cancer patients* [Master's Thesis]. İstanbul Bilgi University.

Hofstede, G. (1980). *Culture's consequences*. SAGE.

Institute of populations studies. (2015). *Türkiye'de kadına yönelik aile içi şiddet araştırması.* [Domestic violence against women in Turkey] Ankara: Elma Teknik Basım Matbaacılık. www.hips.hacettepe.edu.tr/KKSA-TRAnaRaporKitap26Mart.pdf

Johnson, L. N., Miller, R. B., Bradford, A. B., & Anderson, S. R. (2017). The Marriage and Family Therapy Practice Research Network (MFT-PRN): Creating a perfect union between practice and research. *Journal of Marital and Family Therapy*, *43*(4), 561–572. https://doi.org/10.1111/jmft.12238

Kafescioglu, N., & Akyıl, Y. (2018). Couple and family therapy training in the context of Turkey. In. *Focused Issues in Family Therapy*. Springer (135–148). https://doi.org/10.1007/978-3-319-71395-3_9

Kağıtçıbaşı, Ç. (1996). *Family and human development across cultures. Mathway*. Lawrence Erlbaum Publ.

Kağıtçıbaşı, C., & Ataca, B. (2005). Value of children and family change: A three-decade portrait from Turkey. *Applied Psychology*, *54*(3), 317–337. https://doi.org/10.1111/j.1464-0597.2005.00213.x

Karam, E. A., & Sprenkle, D. H. (2010). The research-informed clinician: A guide to training the next-generation MFT. *Journal of Marital and Family Therapy*, *36*(3), 307–319. https://doi.org/10.1111/j.1752-0606.2009.00141.x

Kaslow, N. J., Celano, M. P., & Stanton, M. (2005). Training in family psychology: A competencies-based approach. *Family Process*, *44*(3), 337–353. https://doi.org/10.1111/j.1545-5300.2005.00063.x

Kaytan, B. (2016). *Mental health professionals' use of systemic principles when working with individuals with a physical illness and disability: A survey study with a sample from Turkey* [Master's Thesis]. İstanbul Bilgi University.

Kissil, K., & Niño, A. (2018). The Person-of-the-Therapist Training's state of affairs: Evaluating research and implementation of the model. *Journal of Family Psychotherapy, 29*(4), 318–335. https://doi.org/10.1080/08975353.2018.1477383

Konuk, E., Akyıl, Y., Arduman, E., Erenel, S., & Sarımurat Baydemir, N. (2011). Ekim. *Türkiye'de çift ve aile terapisi: Yasal düzenlemeler ve eğitim standartları.* Oral presentation presented at VI. Ulusal Aile ve Evlilik Terapileri Kongresi. [Cuople and family therapy in Turkey: Legal regulations and education standards].

Korkut, Y. (2001). Aile danışmanlığı ve aile terapisi hizmetleri. *Psikoloji Çalışmaları Dergisi, 22*, 111–133.

Laumann, E. O., Paik, A., Glasser, D. B., Kang, J. H., Wang, T., Levinson, B., Moreira, E. D., Nicolosi, A., & Gingell, C. (2006). A cross-national study of subjective sexual well-being among older women and men: Findings from the Global Study of Sexual Attitudes and Behaviors. *Archives of Sexual Behavior, 35*(2), 145–161. https://doi.org/10.1007/s10508-005-9005-3

Leavitt, C. E., Lefkowitz, E. S., Akyıl, Y., & Serduk, K. (2019). A cross-cultural study of mid-life relational and sexual health: Comparing Ukraine to the US and Turkey. *Sexuality and Culture,* 1–22

Lee, R. E., & Nelson, T. (Eds.). (2014). *The contemporary relational supervisor.* Routledge.

Maier, C. Prouty, A. & Söylemez (2022). Zooming into Feminist Family Therapy TeleSupervision: Experiences of Supervisors During Covid-19. Manuscript in preparation.

Marcus, J., Ceylan, S., & Ergin, C. (2017). Not so "traditional" anymore? Generational shifts on Schwartz values in Turkey. *Journal of Cross-Cultural Psychology, 48*(1), 58–74. https://doi.org/10.1177/0022022116673909

Miller, J. K., & Todahl, J. L. (2010). The core competency movement in marriage and family therapy: key considerations from other disciplines. *Journal of Marital and Family Therapy, 36*, 59–70

Ministry of Family and Social Policies (Turkey). (2010). Turkey Family and Social Policies Ministry Research Center'de aile değerleri araştırması [Family values research in Turkey] Ankara: Manas Medya Planlama Reklam Hizmetleri San. Tic. Ltd. (2010). *Sti.*

Morris, J. (2007). Characteristics and clinical practices of rural marriage and family therapists. *Journal of Marital and Family Therapy, 33*(4), 439–442. https://doi.org/10.1111/j.1752-0606.2007.00043.x

Nelson, T. S., Chenail, R. J., Alexander, J. F., Crane, D. R., Johnson, S. M., & Schwallie, L. (2007). The development of core competencies for the practice of marriage and family therapy. *Journal of Marital and Family Therapy, 33*(4), 417–438. https://doi.org/10.1111/j.1752-0606.2007.00042.x

O'Neil, L. M. & Çarkoğlu, A. (2018). Kadir Has University, Gender and Women Studies Research Center. (2018). Türkiye'de toplumsal cinsiyet ve kadın algısı araştırması. [Gender and Women's perception in Turkey research.] Unpublished manuscript, Department of Psychology, Kadir Has University, İstanbul, Turkey. https://gender.khas.edu.tr/sites/gender.khas.edu.tr/files/inline-files/GenderKHAS_Activity%20%20Report%202018-2019.pdf

Poyrazlı, S. (2003). Validity of Rogerian therapy in Turkish culture: A cross-cultural perspective. *Journal of Humanistic Counseling, Education and Development, 42*(1), 107–115. https://doi.org/10.1002/j.2164-490X.2003.tb00172.x

Roberts, J., Abu-Baker, K., Diez Fernández, C., Chong Garcia, N., Fredman, G., Kamya, H., Martín Higarza, Y., Fortes de Leff, J., Messent, P., Nakamura, S., Torun Reid, F., Sim, T., Subrahmanian, C., & Zevallos Vega, R. (2014). Up close: Family therapy challenges and innovations around the world. *Family Process, 53*(3), 544–576. https://doi.org/10.1111/famp.12093

Şafak, E. (2007). *The bastard of Istanbul.* Viking Press.

Söylemez, Y., & Gürmen, S. (2021). *Online couple therapy during Covid-19: An HSCED application* [Unpublished manuscript].

Tababet, San'atlarının Tarzı, Ş., & Kanun, İ. D. (1928). Retrieved June 24, 2017. www.mevzuat.gov.tr/MevzuatMetin/1.3.1219.pdf

Türk Psikologlar Derneği (2008). *Meslek yasası çalışmaları.* Retrieved June 24, 2017. www.psikolog.org.tr/ozluk-haklari/Meslek-Yasasi-Calismalari-1975-2008.pdf

Türk Psikolojik Danışma ve Rehberlik Derneği (2017). (Mart 24 2017). Retrieved June 24, 2017. www.turkpdristanbul.com/ruh-sagligi-yasa-tasarisi-toplantisi-24-mart-2017/. *Ruh Sağlığı Yasa Tasarısı Toplantısı.*

Türkiye Psikiyatri Derneği (2017). *Ruh sağlığı yasası çalışmaları sürüyor.* Retrieved June 24, 2017. www.psikiyatri.org.tr/1729/ruh-sagligi-yasasi-calismalari-suruyor

Zeytinoğlu-Saydam, S., Erdem, G., & Söylemez, Y. (2021). Psychometric properties of the brief accessibility, responsiveness, and engagement scale in a community sample of Turkish adults. *Family Relations, 70*(2), 557–574. https://doi.org/10.1111/fare.12446

16

THE THERAPEUTIC DANCE OF BOWENIAN THERAPY AND SOUTH ASIAN FAMILIES

Issues to Consider

Gita Seshadri and Shruti Poulsen

Murray Bowen has been said to have been "one researcher who was able to take a step back [to analyze process amidst family chaotic interactions] and to discover that there was indeed an order and predictability to human relationships" (Kerr and Bowen, 1988, p. 4). Bowenian family therapy and family processes are key to an advanced understanding of family functioning, family dynamics, intergenerational experiences, and patterns of functioning in systems. Thus, Bowen's contributions to couple and family therapy (CFT), and clinical application of the intergenerational lens to working with family systems, is well documented in the CFT literature and scholarly work to date (Gehart, 2018). Bowen Family Systems is one of the hallmark foundational systemic models for clinical work with individuals, couples, and families, and is a focus of CFT training and supervision across CFT training programs. What is less evident in the literature pertaining to Bowen Family Systems approaches is a focus on cross-cultural applications and adaptations in applying this approach with diverse client populations. In general, Bowen's contributions of differentiation, multigenerational transmission, chronic anxiety, and impacts on marital satisfaction were empirically supported; however, other concepts like triangling and those marrying of similar differentiation levels were not empirically supported (Miller, Anderson, & Keals, 2004). This brings us to the conundrum of how a theory that has been empirically supported in some ways but continually critiqued for lack of attention to gender (Knudson-Martin, 1994; Leupnitz, 1988) and culture (Carter & Mcgoldrick, 1988; Carter and Mcgoldrick, 1980; Mcgoldrick, 2011). We also ask how we would apply these concepts with South Asian families.

In this chapter, the authors' goal is to present the elements of Bowen Family Systems and clinical work more broadly, but with a focus on how this approach can be a good fit for working with diverse client groups such as South Asians, and more specifically Indian families from the South Asian diaspora. This chapter will highlight aspects of South Asian family experiences and characteristics, primarily focusing on Indian families and their context of immigration, family life in the United States, experiences of cultural adjustment

DOI: 10.4324/9781003297871-18

and adaptation in the United States, and the experiences of connection with, and differentiation from their country of origin and the United States (Inman, Howard, Beaumont, & Walker, 2007). This chapter will also focus on describing clinical work from a Bowen Family Systems approach in working with South Asian-Indian families, and elucidate the relevance of this model in working with diverse family systems. Through clinical examples and descriptions of applications of the Bowen Family Systems approach, its theoretical conceptualizations, interventions, and techniques, the authors hope to provide support for the use of this model across cultural contexts and diverse clinical markets, globally as well as in working with South Asian families in the US.

South Asian-Indian Families

South Asian-Indian families are a large and diverse group of people who come from varied experiences of language, religion, regional differences, cultural values, cultural practices, and immigration and migration experiences. South Asian-Indian families also have diverse family structures ranging from the nuclear family to larger extended family structures. Immigrant South Asian-Indian families may experience a range of connections, emotional and physical, to their country-of-origin and family-of-origin (Inman et al., 2007). While one can generalize to some degree about the experiences and characteristics that are applicable to many South Asian-Indian families, it is important to remember that these families also represent a great deal of diversity as well based on region, caste, religion, and other factors.

South Asian-Indians have been part of the US immigration landscape since the late 1800s and early 1900s. Immigration of East Indians to the United States began in the late 1800s and early 1900s to engage in employment in agricultural and railroad development in the west (Gibson, 1988; Farwer, Bhadha, & Narang, 2002). During these early periods of Indian immigration to the United States, mostly poor and uneducated Punjabi laborers immigrated to be part of the logging and railroad industries in the west (Das Gupta, 1997). South Asian-Indian immigration to the United States during this period was generally short-term and temporary with many immigrant men leaving their families back home, in the care of extended family members. The 1965 US Immigration and Naturalization Act significantly changed Indian immigration patterns by allowing families to reunite in the United States. Opening up immigration to others from the Indian diaspora at this time allowed mostly educated, financially secure, and English-speaking Indians to immigrate (Das Gupta, 1997). As a result, South Asian-Indian immigrants to the United States over the past several decades have been from professional and educated, financially stable, mostly English-speaking backgrounds. While South Asian-Indian immigrants continue to migrate to places around the globe, including Great Britain, increasingly immigration for higher education and professional opportunities in the United States continues to be a major trend (Poulsen, Karuppawamy, & Natrajan, 2005).

While South Asian-Indian families and their experiences are diverse and varied, some experiences and characteristics can be observed across different groups of Indians (Poulsen, 2009). Values such as religious and spiritual practices and beliefs, connections to family-of-origin, and country-of-origin are significant for South Asian-Indian families. Traditions such as speaking their native language at home, actively practicing religious rituals, and promoting a sense of cultural heritage and community among family members are key parts of daily family life for Indians (Inman et al., 2007) . Many South Asian-Indians may also actively participate in organizations and larger systems such as cultural organizations and associations that help them support and promote their cultural and religious traditions through outside engagement for their family system. Connections within the nuclear family system are often valued, with boundaries for this system often seemingly rigid and impervious to outside, "foreign," and western influence. Socialization that does not include educational or professional settings outside of the family system may be restricted to similar cultural and ethnic groups. Given that ethnic and cultural identity are important components of the Indian immigration experience, there is the expectation that Indian families will socialize with each other alone, and that much of the socialization will be across multiple generations. Values such as collectivism, interconnectedness, and interdependence within one's own family and community are predominant across many South Asian-Indian families (Bhattacharya, Cleland, & Holland, 1999; Dugsin, 2001).

Life-span developmental concerns and experiences are particularly salient for South Asian-Indian families (Carter, McGoldrick, & Garcia-Preto, 2010). Life cycle stages such as raising young children and adolescents, preparing young adult children for partner selection and career choices, beginning and caring for own families, and ultimately the transition into old age are impacted by ethnic identity and cultural values to which South Asian-Indian families adhere (Hines, Garcia Preto, McGoldrick, Almeida, & Weltman, 2005). Values such as intergenerational obedience, filial piety, and multigenerational patterns and expectations are often viewed as the key to professional and personal success in life. East Indian cultural norms such as individual development and preferences taking a backseat to family well-being and the welfare of the whole often conflict with the American-born adolescent's desire to achieve differentiation and independence based on a culturally different set of norms (Ungar & Mahalingam, 2003). Some South Asian-Indian families may adopt what may be considered as more western values related to independence and personal autonomy; these shifts in values and expectations may lead to some conflict, instability, and challenges within the family system and across multiple generations. Attempts at independence and differentiation may be viewed and experienced as disloyalty, disrespect, a cutting off from family and identity, and may be experienced with shame and a sense of dishonor towards the family.

Even into adulthood and the lifespan developmental stages of intimate partnering and marriage, South Asian-Indians relationship between generations continues to be paramount (Carter, McGoldrick, & Garcia-Preto, 2010). Marriage is viewed as a partnership not just between two individuals, but between entire family systems. The purpose and primary focus of marriage is less frequently about the intimate, emotional connection between the partners, and much more focused on childbearing and parenting the next generation of family members. Parenthood and parenting is the primary goal of marriage in many South Asian-Indian families. Raising children who will then follow specific norms and expectations for life experiences such as profession, education and career success, own partner selection and marriage, and developing belief systems is a major focus and purpose in South Asian-Indian intimate partnered life (D'Cruz & Bharat, 2001). A key aspect and focus of marriage is the parenting of children well into adulthood with attention paid to issues such as the marriageability of adult children and the timeline for their marriage. A frequent query facing young adults in their early to late twenties from well-meaning family members and parents is "why aren't you married yet?" Other queries and pressure from family include input on career choices with parents often wanting their adult children to choose more "mainstream" careers such as becoming a doctor, engineer, or businessperson. Other parenting concerns may revolve around day-to-day mundane issues such as how the child and even adult child dresses, what and how much they eat, and whether they are getting enough rest to facilitate their focus on their studies, careers, and daily functioning tasks, which is meant to be demonstrated as care and participating in their life versus a lack of boundaries. Developing independence and autonomy overall is not the primary focus of parents and their married partnership (Gupta, 2011). Individuality, autonomy, and romantic love in partner selection is generally less valued, with the emphasis in married life placed on intergenerational relationships and harmony, raising and nurturing future generations, and promoting similar values and expectations across multiple generations.

Although the concept of mental health services and resources is becoming more acceptable and less stigmatized across all cultural groups, South Asian-Indian families typically struggle to reach out for such resources and support (Hines et al., 2005). Often, when South Asian-Indian families do reach out for mental health treatment, they are more likely to seek out medical care such as psychiatry rather than family therapy, listing physical symptoms vs. emotional symptoms, and therefore further carrying generational anxiety (Shariff, 2009). However, there are some important considerations and implications for family therapists working with these families and this is where a family therapy modality such as Bowen family therapy could be of great value and utility in engaging South Asian-Indian families in treatment.

Applicable Bowen Concepts

Bowenian Family Therapy is in general terms a "theory of people" – how families function, what they experience in terms of connection, individual needs, communication patterns, emotional expression, etc. In this next section, we describe how each Bowenian-based concept is applied to South Asian families, along with the description of each concept.

Differentiation of Self

Bowen was interested in how the family was an emotional unit and the level of differentiation of each member in the family because it was an indication of how they handled their anxiety in triangles, the family of origin, and their current family (the nuclear family). He created a scale from 1 to 100 to distinguish different levels of anxiety in relationship to autonomy and closeness.

Differentiation is:

> the difference between people at the various points on the scale the degree to which they are able to distinguish between the feeling process and the intellectual process. Associated with the capacity to distinguish between feelings and thought is the ability to choose between having one's functioning guided by feelings or thoughts.
>
> (Kerr & Bowen, p. 97)

More specifically, differentiation is the heart of Bowen's model and guides how human beings relate to one another. He contrasts thoughts and feelings in that he places higher emphasis on emotional regulation and distance. However, this differentiation scale is a continuum in that the extremes are at both the higher and lower ends of the scales. Bowen describes this scale as a metaphorical emotional temperature of a person's level of anxiety and how they make their relationship decisions; in addition, he also described family members being of similar differentiation levels. Low levels of differentiation indicated the development of symptoms in people, when they presented for therapy. For example, a 35-year-old South Asian female, identifying as a lesbian, and despite also having a significant other could be cut off from her family of origin (high anxiety, low differentiation) due to family pressures of traditional marriage and not knowing how to negotiate with her low differentiating parents with high emotionality. In the end, both the 35-year-old and her parents have the choice of whether or not they choose to increase their differentiation through personal work, or risk passing on low differentiation (i.e., high anxiety, distance, high emotional, and/or a pseudo self with low self esteem). This may include family discussions around how the daughter may carry on cultural traditions and values of the family while exercising her autonomy; if willing, in family therapy or with the use of the elders (e.g., the parents, or grandparents), using them to help the family to support the greater good of the family, once they can come together to agree upon this vision.

Emotional Triangles

Triangles depict the relationships between three people along with the level of stability that they share; they each have their role to maintain the triangle, and therefore anxiety is managed. Typically, Bowen described the use of triangles in a negative way. It is the connection between the three people within the triangle that maintains an aura of stability. However, if one person steps out of this emotional triangle, chaos ensues. Bowen characterizes a triangle to have different processes when there are "calm periods and anxious periods" (Kerr and Bowen, 1988, p. 136). The anxiety is bound within the triangles, and because of this, the insider's relationships become eroded. More specifically, a third member is recruited so that the other two members can maintain what they believe is a harmonious relationship, and this keeps anxiety within the system. For example, though this is cultural, it is not an uncommon practice for a South Asian married couple to focus on their children through the lifespan of the marriage, instead of the marriage. An extreme example of this is the couple bringing their children to their anniversary dinner to balance the emotional energy within the couple. This can also be exemplified in a husband triangling with his work (workaholism) and his wife; even though the work is not a person, the emotional energy and anxiety is displaced on the work, so that the relationship with his wife is stabilized. This contributes to the overall emotional climate in the relationship as well as others in the nuclear family.

Nuclear Family Emotional Process

The nuclear family emotional process describes the process of how unexpressed anxiety shows up in individuals, the family process, and implications over future generations, through differentiation levels. This is transmitted through attitudes, patterns, beliefs, values, and other emotional forces across the lifespan. Examining this process includes paying attention to moments of change, which include marriage, illness, graduation, etc., because how the family responds to each of these changing events is influenced by their level of differentiation and influences their level of differentiation. Further, attention to patterns of relationship are also reflective of this concept; dysfunction and impairment are shown through fusion (i.e., extreme closeness) and distance. This shows up through conflict, dysfunction in one spouse, and projection to children (Kerr & Bowen, 1988). In addition, this may show up in pursuer-distancer patterns or overfunctioning-underfunctioning relationships. For example, a couple who has an arranged marriage, which goes awry, because the bride moves in with her in-laws (a cultural expectation) who treat her poorly because in their eyes she doesn't meet their perfectionistic standards. She also must take care of the sick uncle, while pleasing her husband's parents; this impacts the extended family, the marriage, how she is treated entering this new system, how she treats them, and it also influences how all the family members participate in this system. Inevitably, all those who participate in the family contribute to the emotional climate of the family as well as influencing each other.

Family Projection Process

Family projection process refers to adults and/or parents projecting their own anxiety, problems, immaturity, and lack of differentiation upon their children or other family members (Gehart & Tuttle, 2003). The process of projection is similar to the following: the parent focuses on a child out of fear that something is wrong with the child, then the parent interprets the child's behavior as confirming the fear, and then the parent treats the child as if something is wrong with the child. According to Bowen, the chosen child to receive this projection receives assistance from:

> ... .Traumatic events that disrupt the family during the pregnancy or about the time of birth, and special relationships with sons or daughters..[and] is one of the most emotionally attached to the parents and the one who ends up with the lower differentiation of self.
>
> (Bowen, 1978, p. 381)

These patterns inevitably transmit through the generations in a multigenerational transmission process. In South Asian families, this may manifest in a mother's desire to cherish her son's role, based on his gender, or other family positioning, or both. She may decide to be emotionally fused to him, so much that she doesn't allow him to be independent, take care of himself emotionally or physically, controls him in that she even caters to his every need including doing his chores, meals, etc.; she may even choose his wife. In this scenario, his mother fuses her anxiety on her son, which influences his differentiation level. Thus, the son may marry someone of a similar differentiation level and will eventually pass on his mother's differentiation level and anxiety to his marriage, the maritial relationship, the wife, and their future children through multigenerational transmission process.

Multigenerational Transmission Process

The multigenerational transmission process is the transmission of coping styles and emotional processes and patterns through the family and throughout generations. This can be seen through differentiation levels, patterns of fusion, distance, cutoffs, and nodal events (e.g., marriage, death, illness, addiction, pregnancy, etc.). Although multigenerational transmission processes typically track negative events, more neutral topics and patterning can be tracked within culture, sex, spirituality, or any other contextual process. For example, one can track the impact of South Asian values of education/degrees and how this influences differentiation level and related emotional conflict/relationship dynamics that were created.

Sibling Position

Sibling position refers to the characterization of emotional processes based on a child's birth order because of the "concept of functioning position, if family systems theory predicts that every family emotional system generates certain functions" (Kerr and Bowen, 1988, p. 315). Expanding on the first example, let's look at an eldest South Asian daughter who chose to drop out of college to pursue acting rather than pursuing the reins for the family business in their medical practice. As the eldest, she is expected to take on the role that her parents expect for her either through marriage or employment. Bowen also describes sibling position in terms of *fixed personality trait*s; as the eldest daughter she is expected to lead based on the parents' values, and not have *her own mind* (Gilbert, 2021). If she and her nuclear family are at an impasse and decide to cut off, this has multigenerational repercussions.

Emotional Cutoff

Emotional cutoff is done in an effort to reduce pain and anxiety from relational rupture (Gilbert, 2021). There are societal and contextual elements and how they impact the emotional environment of the family that produce this type of distance. For example, if a son chooses to defend his mother in a marital conflict between his father and mother, he could be threatened with emotional cutoff. In this example, there is also a triangle, but the one cutting off is not always deemed the differentiated one; all must work on emotional reactivity, the unresolved issues, anxiety, and differentiation, or this unexpressed anxiety will be passed onto future generations. The appearance of superficial independence and emotional distance often turns into immaturity, if there is no processing around these events and feelings then it becomes a reflection of parental attachment (Bowen, 1978; Gilbert, 2021).

Societal Emotional Process

The societal emotional process is not directly related to the family; however, it is considered an external context in relationship to understanding the family. More specifically, Bowen believed that the societal emotional process was a reflection of how societal behavior impacts the family (The Bowen Center, 2021). Depending on what happens in society, it can raise or lower societal differentiation, and in turn impact the family. Within this concept, stereotypes, gender, culture, inequality, class, and other social locations can be examined (McGoldrick, 2011). For example, immigrant South Asian parents may increase pressure on their children regarding their grades and employment prospects based on the current climate around immigration practices, in an effort to achieve the American dream and be successful.

Treatment Plan

How does a therapist work with a South Asian family using Bowen family therapy concepts if the family is willing to do Bowenian family therapy? First, after establishing the therapeutic relationship through joining, the goals for therapy would include the following (in no particular order):

- maintain neutrality
- reduce anxiety and other non-productive emotions

- help clients to have better emotional regulation
- increase differentiation
- deepen connection and reduce anxiety
- understand the family dynamics/interactions/problem in the context of the multigenerational system
- discover interlocking and unproductive triangles
- explore projection within the family and societal context
- adapt goals depending on presenting problem, system, or subsystem of focus (intergenerational sensitivity)
- increase autonomy

The Bowenian therapist's role is well-regulated, where the therapist has worked on their own differentiation, is able to manage one's own anxiety, and can model adaptive, functional behaviors and ways of interacting as a coach, supporter, or outside observer. Often the therapist is seen as an expert. Oftentimes South Asians, if they consider therapy, look towards the therapist as *the expert*; this matches the Bowenian therapist's stance. In an effort to move the family and/or the individual forward, a Bowen therapist would use the following techniques.

Interventions

Genogram. A genogram is a detailed family tree designed to show the dates of marriage, deaths, and divorces of each family member in the last three generations. Other important information includes separations, cutoffs, and distanced individuals. Genograms also highlight emotional patterns such as closeness, fusion, distance, cutoffs, estrangements, and abuse. Genograms can also reflect life-stage events and living patterns, or are centered around a certain theme (e.g., sex, anger, communication). Genograms can also be a way to track triangles as well. Genograms can also open the door for the therapist to ask process questions in relationship to the family tree or even in therapeutic dialogue. For example, the therapist can ask "what happens to you when your mothers says you make her feel jealous?"

Displacement stories. Displacement stories are the use of similar stories of the current family or client to gain a different perspective on the process of their current problem. Some use film, movies, media, music, or even asking them how they would approach a friend with a similar issue. In this way, the therapist operates as a coach.

Pursuer/distancer. In pursuer-distancer, the goal is to help the pursuer maintain their own anxiety in relation to their distancer. By default, the distancer will always back up; by helping the pursuer to hold themselves back from continuing to pursue (i.e., teaching the pursuer to hold back from pursuing temporarily), this creates anxiety in the distancer because it is different than the normal pattern, and therefore, will come forward towards the pursuer. The goal is to help those in this type of relationship to do the opposite of their partner, while taking care of their own anxiety, and in turn, giving them what they desire.

De-triangling. Detriangling includes not taking sides, having neutrality, having a lack of defensiveness, and contact with those involved in emotionally involved issues (Papero, 2014). Even in a therapeutic triangle, the therapist must maintain a sense of neutrality so that the family/client anxiety is not taken on by the therapist. A therapist can maintain this by having a non-anxious presence and not becoming emotionally reactive during client conflict (Gehart & Tuttle, 2003).

Going home. With this intervention, the client is asked to be in contact with family members whether it be physically contacting them or visiting them in person. The goal for the client is to be non-reactive, or not participate in old emotional ways while being in their presence. This can also be a reflection of areas of strength and growth after some therapy has transpired.

Increasing differentiation/I statements. Through the therapist's non-anxious presence, the client can practice increasing their level of differentiation through raising their own personal awareness of their family and how they can be less emotionally reactive to their family. They can also practice using I statements to develop more of an individual self. For example, the client can say "I feel hurt when I am accused of making you jealous" instead of "you made me feel jealous." Other ways of increasing differentiation include finding ways to reduce blame, increasing accountability, and focusing on relationship building acts. It is also appropriate that boundaries are set within abusive and toxic relationships. The goal here is reducing emotional reactivity towards that person regardless of if they are in your life or not.

Healthy Functioning

With South Asian families, there needs to be a balance between connection and autonomy that appears less rigid with fewer triggering/escalated interactions. The goal is for the family and each member to gain insight about themselves and their family patterns and how this may transmit through the generations. Further, regulating and processing their emotions more productively with thought, awareness, and action while managing stress (within and from outside the family system) differently can help get one's individual needs met while attuning to the needs and welfare of the whole system simultaneously and changing the overall anxiety and emotional climate in the family.

Clinical Example/Application

Arun and Sneha have been married for over 10 years. They have a 10-year-old daughter and an 8-year-old son. They had an arranged marriage and are seeking therapy because they both feel that their marriage is in trouble. Through the course of therapy you discover that there is a lot of unspoken resentment on Sneha's part, because she holds her feelings in, and when she can't take it anymore, she explodes. Arun is busy with his tech job that has him working 60 to 70 hours a week, on a good week. What brings them into therapy is the following argument: though they both immigrated to the United States as children, should they celebrate both South Asian and American holidays with their children? Though this may seem like a surface issue, the therapeutic issues are deeper within the anxiety of the family relationships. This has made the issue become divisive, as Arun sees it as a threat to his identity and Sneha just wants the children to enjoy with their friends and not be set apart.

Treatment plan. After establishing a therapeutic relationship, the goal would be to map out the family of origin patterns and how they are playing out in the current marriage. Through the work of the genogram, it is discovered by the therapist for Arun that his father passed away when he was 8 years old, which propelled his avoidant nature to focus on himself and his aspirations (i.e., work). For Sneha, her development was different in that she was the youngest child and had everything done for her by her elder siblings. This seems to highlight her resentment for always having to be in charge. Further, the therapist could help Sneha reduce her resentment by helping her communicate I statements once Arun moves out of his distancer positioning, so he is able to hear her without being emotionally reactive or defensive. The therapist also needs to address and assess potential triangles with the kids and the couple, and also the triangle between the couple and Arun's work. With all this, the therapist can also look at nodal events for the couple and how lifespan challenges have impacted the couple dynamic. Lastly, the therapist can explore how societal processes have affected the couple, while incorporating their traditions. This might include exploring the process-based meaning for the couple about celebrating American holidays vs. South Asian and if there are any emotional or generational messages behind this.

Clinical and Research Implications

Bowen family therapy has historically been critiqued as lacking in cultural sensitivity and applicability to culturally diverse client populations. Although there is little empirical evidence for the efficacy of one therapy model over another when considering clinical work with South Asian-Indian families, some recommendations can be made. Given the different realities and experiences these families may experience across multiple generations, Bowenian family therapy can be a model particularly suited to these families and their cultural context. According to Dasgupta (1998), neither generation can afford to deny each other's realities and experiences. Parents cannot deny the differing realities experienced by their American-born children, while the younger generation cannot denounce their parents' values without losing a sense of identity and connection to their parents, extended family, and to their culture. Culturally relevant and sensitive Bowenian family therapy could be of value in creating understanding, empathy, and connection across multiple generations while also honoring many of the values and beliefs that South Asian-Indian families bring to their experience of parenting, marriage, and other lifespan developmental transitions (Ungar & Mahalingam, 2003).

Bowenian family therapy prioritizes the regulation of emotional processes and reactivity so that clear communication between parents, their children, and between generations can occur. A Bowenian approach that is sensitive to cultural factors and lifespan developmental experiences could prepare families to understand developmental challenges, normalize and reframe the stress experienced during lifespan transitions, and find creative and culturally appropriate ways to support each other through these stages while remaining connected (Hines et al., 2005). Hines et al. pointed out that South Asian-Indian families who do seek therapy are often likely to enter treatment through referrals by physicians and organizations such as schools; the authors suggested several areas of exploration for therapists working with these families. First, they suggested exploring with the family their lifestyle and family structure prior to coming to the United States, the similarities and differences, and their overall immigration experience. In addition, they suggested that therapists may want to engage the parental subsystem in an exploration of their own experiences growing up in India, coming of age and adulthood, and entering life transitions such as education, career, partner selection, and their own family life (Gupta, 2011). A tool, such as the genogram may be used with these families, to explore issues such as their household composition; organization and expectations; religious affiliation and its importance in day-to-day functioning; experiences and expectations around partner selection, dating, and arranged marriage; and finally, family members' sense of identity in relation to gender considerations, social class issues, and issues related to autonomy and interdependence. Baptiste (1990) recommends that therapists develop self-awareness of their own feelings, attitudes, and beliefs about immigrants and working with immigrant families; this self-of-the-therapist work can effectively be done through Bowenian-based methods such as the genogram and the cultural genogram (McGoldrick, Gerson, & Petry, 2008). Additional recommendations include understanding the family's experience of the immigration process and where different family members are in terms of their acculturation and comfort level within this process.

Bowenian family therapy offers techniques and interventions that can be flexible and practical, and resonate for South Asian-Indian families. Given that immigration can be both a regenerative and a painful process for many immigrant families (Poulsen et al., 2005), it is important to consider both the strengths and the areas of growth needed for South Asian-Indian families to successfully traverse the cross-generational challenges they face in raising their American-born family members. Working clinically with these families may need to include creating a safe, healing environment that creates a bridge between multiple generations and between parents' experiences that are more closely aligned with the home country and their children and adult children's world of school, peers, and the U.S. culture (Dugsin, 2001). Although Asian Americans are typically less likely to turn to mental health resources in the case of family problems (Carter, McGoldrick, & Garcia-Preto, 2010; Durvasula & Mylvaganam, 1994), they are a growing population in the United States. Therefore, it is imperative that therapists consider the applicability and relevance of models such as Bowenian family therapy in working with these families as they increasingly seek out mental health services.

Research considerations and implications may include further exploring the use of foundational models such as Bowenian family therapy, cross-culturally (Segal, 1991). How scholars and clinicians are using such models and adapting them in ways to be culturally responsive are areas of future research that would contribute to the gaps in the field of couple and family therapy. Additional research implications may include developing an understanding of Bowenian classical concepts and interventions and their applicability and relevance across diverse client populations.

Resources and Further Reading

Additional resources and reading for understanding of Bowenian family therapy include the classic texts by Kerr and Bowen, *Family Evaluation* (1988), *Family Therapy in Clinical Practice* (Bowen, 1978), and McGoldrick's work on genograms and family life cycle transitions (McGoldrick, 2011; McGoldrick, Gerson, & Petry, 2008). These texts provide in-depth exploration of Bowen's model and its application in clinical work, focusing on techniques such as the genogram and on contextual factors such as the experience of life cycle transitions. Contemporary resources such as Gilbert's (2021) recently revised text, *Extraordinary Relationships: A New Way of Thinking about Human Interactions*, offers the reader a overview of Bowenian family therapy, its contributions and innovations, and how Bowenian family therapy and systems theory can be applied to all areas of life such as family and couple relationships, work relationships, the global arena, and relationship with one's self. Gilbert and Jacobs' (2018) book, *The Eight Concepts of Bowen Theory*, provides a concise and applicable understanding of basic Bowenian concepts and techniques that are easy to understand and to apply to one's clinical work. Framo's self-of-the-therapist focused book, *Coming Home Again: A Family-of-Origin Consultation* (Framo, Weber, & Levine, 2003), provides readers with a candid and personal insider's experience of applying Bowenian concepts and theory to the exploration of self and connections to one's family-of-origin.

Resources focusing on the cross-cultural applications of Bowenian family therapy include authors such as M. Daneshpour (2017) who includes a chapter in her book, *Family Therapy with Muslims*, focusing on Bowenian family therapy with Muslim families specifically. McGoldrick and Hardy's recently revised text, *Revisioning Family Therapy: Addressing Diversity in Clinical Practice* (2019), is an additional resource for understanding the application of Bowenian family therapy across diverse populations. Bowenian family therapy has been written about widely in texts and in scholarly journals; however, there continues to be a need for developing resources specific to the application of Bowenian family therapy in culturally responsive ways and with attunement to diversity in client populations.

Three Important Takeaways

This chapter focused on the utility, utility, applicability, and relevance of Bowenian family therapy with South Asian families. Bowenian family therapy has not been a major focus of cross-cultural responsiveness and application to culturally diverse family systems. This chapter provided the reader with information on Bowen family therapy systems theory, concepts, techniques, and interventions, and how they may be used in working with South Asian-Indian families. The chapter also provided an understanding of South Asian-Indian families, their structure, commonalities, unique aspects, and their mental health concerns and needs from an intergenerational perspective and lens. And finally, a third primary "takeaway" of this chapter is on providing the reader with clinical adaptations and considerations when using a foundational systemic model such as Bowenian family therapy that takes into account cross-cultural responsiveness and sensitivity.

References

Baptiste, D. (1990). The treatment of adolescent immigrants and their families in cultural transitions: Issues and recommendations. *Contemporary Family Therapy, 12*, 3–20.

Bhattacharya, G., Cleland, C., & Holland, S. (1999). Peer networks, parental attributes, and drug use among Asian-Indian adolescents born in the United States. *Journal of Immigrant Health, 1*, 145–154.

Bowen, M. (1978). *Family therapy in clinical practice*: Jason Aronson Inc.

Carter, E., & McGoldrick, M. (1980). *The Family life cycle: A framework for family therapy.* New York, NY: Gardner Press.

Carter, E., & McGoldrick, M. (1988). *The changing family life cycle* (2nd ed). New York, NY: Gardner Press.

Carter, E., McGoldrick, M., Garcia-Preto, N. (2010). *The Expanded Family Life Cycle* (4th ed.). Prentice Hall.

D'Cruz, P. Bharat, S. (2001). Beyond joint and nuclear: The Indian family revisited. *Journal of Comparative Family Studies, 32*, 167–194.

Daneshpour, M. (2017). *Family Therapy with Muslims*. New York, NY: Routledge.

Das Gupta, M. (1997). "What is Indian about you?" A gendered, transnational approach to ethnicity. Gender & Society, *11*, 572–596.

Dugsin, R. (2001). Conflict and healing in family experience of second[1]generation emigrants from India living in North America. *Family Process, 40*, 233–241.

Durvasula, R. S., & Mylvaganam, G. A. (1994). Mental health of Asian Indians: Relevant issues and community implications. *Journal of Community Psychology, 22*, 97–108.

Farwer, J. M., Bhadha, B. R., & Narang, S. K. (2002). Acculturation and Psychological Functioning in Asian Indian Adolescents. *Social Development, 11*(1).

Framo, J., Weber, T., & Levine, F. (2003). *Coming Home Again: A Family-of-Origin Consultation*. New York, NY: Brunner-Routledge.

Gehart, D. & Tuttle, A. (2002). *Theory based treatment planning for marriage and family therapists*. New York, NY: Brooks Cole

Gehart, D. (2018). Intergenerational & Psychoanalytic Family Therapies. *Mastering Competencies in Family Therapy: A Practical Approach to Theories & Clinical Case Documentation* (pp. 263–307). Boston, MA: Cengage Learning.

Gibson, M. A. (1988). Punjabi orchard farmers: An immigrant enclave in rural California. *International Migration Review, 22*, 28–50.

Gilbert, R. (2021). *Extraordinary relationships: A new way of thinking of human interactions* (2nd ed): Leading Systems Press.

Gilbert, R., & Jacobs, G. (2018). *The Eight Concepts of Bowen Theory*. Peabody, MA: Leading Systems Press.

Gupta, R. (2011). Emotional autonomy in a collectivistic culture: A relationship perspective. *Indian Journal of Community Psychology, 7*(2), 231–240.

Hines, P. M., Garcia Preto, N., McGoldrick, M., Almeida, R., & Weltman, S. (2005). *Culture and the life cycle*. In B. Carter & M. McGoldrick (Eds.), *The expanded life-cycle: Individual, family & social perspectives* (pp. 69–83). Boston, MA: Allyn & Bacon.

Inman, A. G., Howard, E. E., Beaumont, R. L., & Walker, J. A. (2007). Cultural Transmission: Influence of Contextual Factors in Asian Indian Immigrant Parents' Experiences. *Journal of Counseling Psychology, 54* (1), 93–100. https://doi.org/10.1037/0022-0167.54.1.93.

Kerr, M. E., & Bowen, M. (1988). *Family evaluation: An approach based on Bowen theory*. New York, NY: W. W. Norton & Co.

Knudson-Martin, C. (1994). The female voice: Applications to Bowen's family systems theory. *Journal of Marital and Family Therapy, 20*, 35–46. https://doi.org/10.1111/j.1752- 0606.1994.tb01009.x

Leupnitz, D (1988). *The family interpreted*: Basic Books

McGoldrick, M. (2011). *The genogram journey: Reconnecting with your family*. W. W. Norton & Company.

McGoldrick, M., & Hardy, K. (2019). *Re-visioning Family Therapy: Race, Culture, & Gender in Clinical Practice*. New York, NY: Guilford Press.

McGoldrick, M., Gerson, R., & Petry, S. (2008). *Genograms: Assessment & Intervention*. New York, NY: W. W. Norton & Company.

Miller, R. B., Anderson, S., & Keals, D. K. (2004). Is Bowen theory valid? A review of basic research. *Journal of Marital and Family Therapy, 30*, 453–466. https://doi.org/10.1111/j.1752-0606.2004.tb01255.x

Papero, D. V. (2014). Assisting the two-person system: An approach based on the Bowen theory. *Australian and New Zealand Journal of Family Therapy, 35*(4), 386–397. https://doi.org/10.1002/anzf.1079

Poulsen, S. S. (2009). East Indian Families Raising ABCD Adolescents: Cultural and Generational Challenges. *The Family Journal: Counseling & Therapy for Couples & Families, 17*(2), 168–174. https://doi.org/10.1177/1066480709332715.

Poulsen, S. S., Karuppawamy, N., & Natrajan, T. (2005). Immigration as a dynamic experience: Personal narratives & clinical implications for family therapists. *Contemporary Family Therapy, 27*(3), 403–414. https://doi.org/10.1007/s10591-005-6217-6.

Segal, U. A. (1991). Cultural variables in Asian Indian families. *The Journal of Contemporary Human Services*, *11*, 233–242.

Shariff, A. (2009). Ethnic Identity and Parenting Stress in South Asian Families: Implications for Culturally Sensitive Counselling. *Canadian Journal of Counselling*, *43*(1), 35–46.

The Bowen Center for the Study of the Family (2021). *Societal emotional process*. The Bowen Center. www.thebowencenter.org/societal-emotional-process

Ungar, L. R., & Mahalingam, R. (2003). "We're not speaking any more": A cross-cultural study of intergenerational cut-offs. *Journal of Cross-Cultural Gerontology*, *18*, 169–183.

SECTION III

Specific Applications with International Populations

17
MEDICAL FAMILY THERAPISTS WORKING WITH CULTURALLY DIVERSE PATIENTS USING THE BIO-PSYCHOSOCIAL-SPIRITUAL MODEL WITH CHRONICALLY AND TERMINALLY ILL PATIENTS AND THEIR FAMILIES

Vaida Kazlauskaite and Elena Angelkova

Introduction

Health is extremely important to us all. Burroughs wrote "When you have your health, you have everything. When you do not have your health, nothing else matters at all" (2003, p. 121). Some people do not value health until they get diagnosed with an illness, with each person going through their own unique subjective experiences. Health is multifaceted and complex. According to the World Health Organization (WHO, 2022), health is an integration of physical, mental, and social well-being, not just the absenteeism of disease. As humans go through life, our health can be affected by numerous factors, resulting in drastic changes to lifestyles.

Disease, often considered the opposite of health, is the divergence from a strong biological homeostasis; illness, on the other hand, is the meaning that the person attaches to the disease, including cultural, social, and psychological dynamics (Boyd, 2000). In other words, illness and death are normalized experiences in our world, and personal beliefs and values about illness vary throughout different cultures (Williams-Reade & Trudeau, 2018). An illness accompanies a sequence of progression that creates psychosocial duties and challenges at each stage (Zaider & Steinglass, 2018). Medical family therapists trained in systems theory are systemic thinkers who know that a disease and illness do not only influence the person who has the disease, but also influence the various systems a patient identifies with. For example, illness can influence the microsystem (e.g., immediate family members), mesosystem (e.g., work, friends), exosystem (e.g., neighborhoods, extended family), and macrosystem (e.g., laws, economic system, and culture) (Bronfenbrenner, 1979).

Purpose

Navigating conversations around illness can be challenging, with many factors influencing the communication efforts (e.g., illness, who is ill, age of family members, culture). Families that have an ill family member and are seeking mental health services want their providers to be culturally competent (Dias et al., 2003). As systems-trained clinicians, medical family therapists (MedFTs) are well positioned to work with families who are coping with the vast spectrum of illness across a wide variety of cultures, regions, and populations. MedFTs work intentionally with clients and their families, paying special attention to the physical, psychological, social, and spiritual worlds and their influences on each member of the family (Hodgson et al., 2018). Using the BPSS model, MedFTs gain a holistic picture of the presented problem and pay specific attention to the cultural dynamics that will affect the meaning-making from the client as well as balancing their sense of agency and communion. Thus, MedFTs have expertise in working with families whose cultural or ethnical background may influence the meaning-making of illness and how it is communicated. This chapter focuses on how MedFTs can work with culturally diverse clients who are facing an illness. Efforts of MedFTs are highlighted and examples are provided of what working with ill clients may look like in different contexts.

Medical Family Therapy

MedFTs are systems-trained clinicians, specifically working with patients and their family members who are coping with physical health problems (Finney & Tadros, 2019). MedFTs utilize the bio-psycho-social-spiritual model (BPSS) and systems theory when working with clients. One goal of MedFTs working with patients and their families is to increase agency and communion. Agency focuses on the ability to be autonomous and actively engaged in decisions needing to be made around care (McDaniel et al., 2014). Communion focuses on the connection the patient has to others (Williams-Reade et al., 2014). When MedFTs interact with patients and their families, it is important to have patient-centered communication and create narratives of mutual significance of the illness between the practitioners, patients, and family members (Rajaei & Jensen, 2020). It is also critical to have open dialogues on the impact the illness will have on the patient and the family (Hodgson et al., 2018). When engaging in these conversations, a MedFT can gain an understanding of the family's meaning making, necessities, and boundaries surrounding the illness. When MedFTs interact with patients and families, they also interact with the patient's and family's cultural familial background, which may influence the patient and family on how they perceive the diagnosis and the decisions they make surrounding the illness.

Cultural Influences on Illness

Culture is defined as a person's sense of belonging in society, including their ethnicity, gender, social class, family beliefs, religion, language, sexual orientation, socioeconomic status, nationality, age, race, and education. A person views their world through cultural lenses (Williams-Reade & Trudeau, 2018). Culture can influence a person's beliefs surrounding illness and disease, ranging from influences to one's spirituality/religion to values and customs. It may impact a person's decision-making process around healthcare choices (Betsch et al., 2016). Medical healthcare practitioners habitually struggle to understand cultural differences, and may obstruct the patient's ability to receive efficient and adequate health care (Betsch et al., 2016). The beliefs around illness and disease are culturally informed, governing how a person labels, monitors, describes their symptoms, and even the patterns of behavior associated with the illness (Osokpo, et al., 2022). Ultimately, culture has a significant impact in dictating the treatment plan, care, and recovery from illness and disease.

The viewpoints people have about illnesses can vary drastically in different cultures. A healthcare system that does not account for cultural differences results in more life-threatening illnesses (Shaw et al., 2008). Culture may influence the decisions regarding the diagnosis, treatment options available, care team, and whom to involve during the trajectory. For example, Chinese families may interpret a chronic disease as a possession and choose not to treat it. Further, they people might disregard an epilepsy diagnosis and not engage in treatment, because they do not want to be taken out of school or work settings. Japanese people might view cancer as the patient having a death sentence, and might shun these people from the living, which in return might influence the patient's outcome. Historically, Japanese doctors and the patient's family may refrain from giving the patient their diagnosis (Turner, 1996). See below for more descriptive examples on cultural impacts on both chronic and terminal illness.

Agency and Communion: A Global Perspective

As mentioned above, agency and communion are often a focus and goals of MedFTs working with clients. However, agency and communion will vary among different cultures. It is important for the MedFT to understand what is important to their patients. For example, in the United States, emphasis is placed on including the patient in the treatment plan, thus agency is very relevant to American patients. They are active members in deciding which medication, treatment, and even who is part of their treatment team. They are active during decision-making processes regarding their health. Western countries, like the United States, are viewed as individualistic societies and therefore are more likely to be independent and rely on their abilities to make decisions on their own. Additionally, in the United States' emphasis is placed on communion – connecting patients to family members, social circles, and support groups to reduce a sense of isolation. In eastern countries, however, such as Japan, people are viewed as collective societies and therefore more emphasis is placed on pursuing harmony with others (Hirokawa & Dohi, 2007). A MedFT working with patients who are from Asian descent must reconngize the importance to them to be connected with their families, community, and surroundings, and thus may need more assistance than those who come from western countries (Tseng et al., 2020).

In a study that focused on terminally ill African-Americans, findings showed that patients often do not want to burden their family members and place much emphasis on maintaining control over their health care (Nath et al., 2008). Additionally, when it comes to communicating with their healthcare providers, research illustrates that individuals from minority groups are more likely to experience hardship (Duffy et al., 2006). Therefore, it is important for MedFTs to pay special attention to minorities and assist in increasing their involvement, voice, and interactions with the medical care team (i.e., agency).

While the goals of MedFTs are to increase communion and agency, it is vital that these goals align with the cultural beliefs of the family. For example, there are cultures that do not view children and adolescents as autonomous human beings and thus may not want to share the diagnosis with them. Middle Eastern cultures tend to avoid sharing medical information with the children in order to protect them (Rosenberg et al., 2017). Thus, it is important to assess what the patients' goals are for themselves and their families to help reach agency and communion in a culturally sensitive manner.

Experience of Chronic Illness Across Different Cultures

Chronic illnesses are rising and overwhelming healthcare spending (Newman et al. 2004). Chronic illness is defined as a physical condition that is gradual in development, sustained, seldomly cured, and frequently connected with functional limitations (Osokpo et al., 2022). According to the U.S. Center for Disease Control and Prevention (CDC, 2022), chronic diseases are illnesses that have a duration of one year or more and demand continuous medical assistance. Six in ten adults in the United States are diagnosed with a chronic disease, and four in ten adults have a diagnosis of two or more (CDC, 2022). There are over 100,000 identified chronic illnesses in modern society, but some examples are heart disease, diabetes, arthritis, and asthma. People living with chronic illnesses are viewed as "missing voices", due to a shortage of research on this topic (Larsson & Grassman, 2012). Across the world, one in three adults live with more than one chronic condition, or multiple chronic conditions (Hajat & Stein, 2018). Fifteen percent of people live with two or more chronic conditions in Australia, 14% in the UK, and 22% in Canada (Tikkanen & Abrams, 2022).

People who have lived with a chronic illness for most of their life, starting in early childhood, view their chronic illness as part of their identity, whereas people acquiring a chronic illness in adulthood or later life view it as catastrophic and unsettling (Larsson & Grassman, 2012). As a chronic illness becomes a part of someone's everyday life, there are a multitude of concerns and changes that arise. This varies from fear of complications to the known/diagnosed chronic illness to the continuous worry of physical and/or mental deterioration as the illness runs its course (Larsson & Grassman, 2012). Rural southern African-Americans do not go to the doctors for high blood pressure, with doctors calling it the "silent disease" amongst this population. African-American people make their decisions based on their cultural background and experiences of the disease, including symptomology like headaches, nose bleeds, and hallucinations (Shaw et al., 2008). Asians perceive stress differently than Americans, and are less likely to report stress regarding chronic illnesses, portraying how stress can vary amongst different cultures as well. Latinos have the highest rate of chronic illnesses, but due to their lack of understanding, they have a hard time moderating their chronic illness.

There is also a variety of ways people want to treat their chronic illness. For example, in the Vietnamese culture, people incorporate traditional healing practices for chronic illnesses, like oil steam inhalation, making themselves bleed, using herbal remedies and acupuncture to treat asthma (Shaw et al., 2008). Puerto Ricans include conventional practices for asthma, like specific breathing exercises and rubbing the chest area with herbal medicines (Hajat & Stein, 2018). It is important for the MedFT to have cultural conversations with the patient and their family members about what cultural practices they would like to incorporate in their treatment, with the MedFT providing an open-minded, validating, and nonjudgmental stance.

In certain cultures, chronic pain can be discussed openly amongst patients, family members, and healthcare professionals, while in other cultures it may not. For example, in Iranian and Arab culture, the patient might express their pain loudly and very expressively, while in Japanese and East Asian cultures, the patient may be very stoic, and it is important to look for nonverbal signs (Tseng et al., 2020). In Filipino culture the patient might express chronic pain as "cold" or "hot". In Ghanain culture, pain might be described as emotional or spiritual (Givler et al., 2021). In Native American cultures, chronic pain might be undertreated, and the patient suffering from chronic pain might only express it in private to their family members or close friends (Givler et al., 2021).

Living in a world that is culturally diverse means healthcare workers must increase their cultural competence and cultural humility in conversations regarding the patient's treatment plan (Givler et al., 2021). Chronic disease involves the management of pain, which is often a challenge. Patients that have a chronic illness typically have comorbid symptomatology of mental health struggles, with the most common being depression and anxiety (Harsh & Bonnema, 2018). Therefore, MedFTs in various settings are beneficial to patients and their families alike.

MedFT Responses to Chronic Illness

As systemic thinkers, MedFTs understand that if one family member has a diagnosis of an illness it affects the entire family unit. The family unit goes through a series of behaviorial and psychlogical changes (Harsh & Bonnema, 2018). Family relationships can greatly impact how the individual perceives their diagnosis, and how they express their symptomatology, bearing in mind their familial cultural background (Sperry, 2007). Westernized medicine, for example, focuses on creating a treatment plan that is intended to manage and/or cure an illness. It is intended to alleviate physical symptoms, rather than enhance the experience of the individual's subjective experience of the illness (Sperry, 2007). Communication amongst family members about the individual's symptoms can improve or impair the outlook on the illness, highlighting the importance of the individual's perception of the illness. It is important that the MedFT working with the patient addresses who should have access to their medical and mental health information before they begin working with the identified family members, to avoid any personal and private information to be revealed without consent (Brown et al., 2016).

The disease itself does produce symptoms in the individual's body, but there are other factors as well, like the individual's anticipations, cultural beliefs, temperaments, sociocultural status, family dynamics, and overall life circumstances (Sperry, 2007). A MedFT can guide these conversations with the patient and their family members through a cultural lens. The MedFT can ask the patient and their family about the meaning of the illness, and what cultural factors they would like to embody in the treatment plan. The MedFT guides conversation with the family on what dynamics need to be altered, and which ones can stay the same. Some of these include childcare, caregiver roles, daily routines, diet, weight, amount of sleep, relational satisfaction, sexual intimacy, managing stress levels, etc., providing a sense of a new normalcy for the family (Marlowe & Hodgson, 2014). Exploring the patient's and family members' emotions regarding the illness can be beneficial to adapting to a new homeostasis. Providing the family with the emotional and physical space to share, giving each member a voice, all-the while respecting their cultural boundaries is vital for the therapeutic process.

When a person experiences a chronic illness, their experience is frequently an outcome of the relationship between physiological and psychological factors (Gatchel & Oordt, 2003). People do have a subjective experience of chronic pain. There are a series of psychological, emotional, and socioeconomic elements that are present in addition to the physical symptomatology. Chronic illnesses also create changes in family dynamics. This is where the MedFT can incorporate the usage of psychoeducation to explain to the patient some of the potential psychosocial stressors that may occur, and how to effectively problem solve the stressors (Marlowe & Hodgson, 2014). For example, if a patient has diabetes, the MedFT and patient can problem solve on how the patient can productively explain to their loved ones that they do not feel aided in the process of them changing their diet and exercise routine, because their loved ones keep eating cake around them. A MedFT can also guide the patient and their family on how to constructively bring up certain concerns about their illness to their medical provider. They can also help the patient and their family with anxiety, through relaxation techniques and mindfulness. This gives the patient a sense of agency and active voice in their illness, by increasing their knowledge of the illness, decreasing any anxieties they might be experiencing, and by providing them with a sense of power (Marlowe & Hodgson, 2014). When it comes to the socioeconomic elements of the illness, a MedFT can have conversations with the patient and their family on the financial responsibilities they will encounter (Marlowe & Hodgson, 2014). If the patient and family members need financial medical assistance, the MedFT can connect them with the resources they need to make the life adjustments necessary to hopefully have the best possible outcomes regarding the illness, providing them with community resources to increase communion, which may include Medicaid, dental services, and substance abuse facilities (Marlowe & Hodgson, 2014).

Experience of Terminal Illness Across Different Cultures

A terminal illness is defined as an ailment that will most likely reduce an individual's life span (Orford et al., 2016). Common examples of terminal illness include, but are not limited to, cancer, chronic liver disease, Amyotrophic Lateral Sclerosis (ALS), dementia, and pulmonary disease. Illnesses that are terminal may impact the patient and their family members in several ways. For example, families may have to adjust to role changes in the family system, assume new responsibilities, and/or adapt their daily routines to accommodate the ill family member.

Some cultures prefer that the ill person is not incorporated in conversations about their illness because of the belief that it would only add to their pain, and maybe even accelerate death (Williams-Reade & Trudeau, 2018). For example, in Japan, a terminal diagnosis is often not shared with the patient because of beliefs that it will burden them and take away any type of hope. In China much emphasis is placed on harmony of the family and thus sharing a terminal disease with family members would threaten the harmony. In Turkey, the strongest member of the family is often seen as the guardian and protector of cancer patients and therefore makes the decision around treatments. In families of Latin descent, often the man is seen as the head of the household and therefore carries the burden to receive information about the illness and share it accordingly with family members. If the spouse is deceased, the responsibility falls onto the children, not the patient themselves. There are also religious factors that can influence the way a patient and family make decisions regarding their illness. For example, Jehovah's Witnesses do not allow their members to have blood transfusions. They view this as defiant behavior and discourteous of God (Williams-Reade & Trudeau, 2018). Members of the Hmong culture often believe that only God holds the power to determine when someone's time is up on this Earth, and thus if a healthcare professional suggest imment death, family members may view this as a threat (Williams-Reade & Trudeau, 2018). Different cultures also have different inclinations concerning end-of-life decisions including those relating to drug treatments, the usage of breathing machines, and the location of where the patient dies (Williams-Reade & Trudeau, 2018).

In African cultures and contexts, when a person is diagnosed with a terminal illness, it is believed that that illness was caused by the devil's doing, or by supernatural beings, coming in the form of spiritual strikes, or through other human beings that curse or poison the person who has the illness (Agom et al., 2019). People in Africa, specifically Nigeria, often want to wait for divine interference, while simultaneously praying and engaging in spiritual rituals that they feel will heal them, asking for forgiveness (Agom et al., 2019). This has given the Nigerian people facing a terminal illness the chance to feel psychological peace by implementing religious and spiritual practices that make the dying process special and distinctive. This impacts the patient's and family's decision-making process regarding treatment plans and options for the patient, with some choosing not to receive medical care (Agom et al., 2019). This is why it is so important for healthcare professionals to incorporate health education but also give patients the freedom to express themselves spiritually and religiously.

MedFT Responses to Terminal Illness

The way terminal illness is understood, accepted, adjusted to, and shared with patients as well as how it is talked about with family members differs across different parts of the world and thus people from different cultures, ethnicities, and backgrounds. The prognosis and severity of a terminal diagnosis specifically can alter the way it is accepted, communicated about, and adjusted to. MedFTs working with terminally ill patients and their family members may focus on comfort care and death itself. End-of-life (EoL) conversations have been found to relieve stress and provide support for family members (Bernacki & Block, 2014). Family members who do not engage in EoL conversations have been found to have increased feelings of remorse and prolonged grief (Beale et al., 2005). Cultural implications have to be considered as they may influence who is involved in the discussions around the illness (e.g., patient alone, patient and their family members, family members without patients). It may also impact decisions around treatment and medical interventions and EoL care (e.g., drug treatments, utilization of breathing devices, and location of death) (Barnato et al., 2007). Further, preferences regarding what is to be talked about during EoL conversations varies by ethnicity and culture. For example, a study showed that Americans of Arab descent thought it was important to make peace with others as an important part of EoL decisions (Thomas et al., 2008). Within the Latino culture, topics of EoL such as assisted suicide and preferred comfort care are often influenced by the age of the patient (Kelley et al., 2010). Elder Latinos prefer to talk about less aggressive treatment options compared to younger ones.

MedFTs working with terminally ill patients and focusing on EoL decisions must have a basic understanding of the various beliefs, backgrounds, religions, and cultures and their effects on how death is perceived (Pentaris & Thomsen, 2020). It is also vital to remember that there will be differences in beliefs and practices within cultural groups specifically (Bloomer et al., 2013). Thus, MedFTs need to approach each client, and their family members, openly and respect individuality within the broad belief spectrums within cultures (Fang et al., 2016). It is a good idea to begin EoL conversations by asking questions around the impact the family's culture, beliefs, religions, etc., has on their meaning-making and understanding of the illness. This information can gauge who should be part of the conversation and what it should focus on.

Cultures also vary in ways that will influence the caregiving family members provide and view death. For example, in cultures that emphasize paying respect to parents and ancestors (e.g., Chinese cultures), it is important to listen to the dying wishes of the individual, particularly pertaining to treatment trajectories (Fang et al., 2015). Thus, the MedFT must address these wishes and talk to family members, assisting them in carrying them out. Within the Thai Buddhist cultures, end of life is a period for the dying individual and their family members to focus on their time together rather than suffering and pain (Kongsuwan et al., 2012). MedFTs may guide the conversation in remembering the good times and bringing family members together.

Culturally Sensitive Assessments Utilizing the Bio-Psycho-Social-Spiritual Model

The BPSS model sees the human body as complex and to be viewed in a holistic manner (Hodgson et al., 2018). There is a connection between the mind and body, which can influence the development and outcome of an illness. In the BPSS model, illness is the primary focus while considering the interaction that consists of the biological, psychological, social, and spiritual components; each component has an expression that is extremely multifaceted, and therefore never the same for two people (Gatchel et al., 2018; Rajaei & Jensen, 2020). The BPSS model has shown evidence-based efficacy in understanding the development and maintenance of chronic illness and chronic pain. The variety of subjective pain patients experience requires clinicians to provide an empathic atmosphere that comprises the patient's individualized preference of the treatment plan (Gatchel et al., 2018).

From the BPSS model, it is important to classify and recognize comorbid mental health disorders as an important component of chronic illness treatment, because of the individualized experiences of pain that can be amplified by comorbid psychiatric disorders, which in return prolongs the pain associated with a chronic illness in patients. There are specific negative emotions and mood disorders that are correlated with chronic illnesses and level of chronic pain experienced (Gatchel et al., 2018). Some examples are apprehension, rage, depression, difficulties, and anxiety. Stress and anger are emotions specifically interrelated with the preservation of chronic pain in chronic illnesses. Depression can play a role in intensifying pain and impeding the ability for a patient to cope in a healthy manner. It occurs at a significantly higher level amongst this population of patients, with 20% to 50% of chronic illness patients experiencing depressive symptoms (Mills et al., 2019).

Biological Dimension

At the beginning stages of working with a patient, it is important that the MedFT assess the patient's understanding of the disease. Assessment questions such as "Tell me what you understand about your illness" are important to gauge where the patient is with understanding and where they may need more information. Appropriate referral sources must be made if there are clarifications needed around the physiological aspect of the illness (i.e., paying attention to one's scope of practice). Once a therapeutic relationship has been established, moving on to more process questions such as "Tell me about what meaning-making you have created around your illness" and "How does your culture influence your understanding and meaning-making of your diagnosis?" will assist in having conversations around cultural impact.

It is also important to assess whom the patient wants to have part of their treatment team. Asking them specifically about their knowledge about the various healthcare providers as well as the importance (or not) of having family members be part of the team.

Biological Assessment Tools

When MedFTs utilize biological assessment tools, it is critical for them to understand their scope of practice, and refer out, when necessary, because there are multiple factors related to biological changes in the patient's body that MedFTs are not trained to treat. The Setting, Perception, Invitation/Information, Knowledge, Empathy, and Summarize/Strategize (SPIKES) model was created to navigate difficult conversations regarding the delivery of the unfortunate news to the patient and families in an empathic manner, where the knowledge of the disease is delivered through clear and concise language than can be comprehended by the patient and family and treatment choices are discussed (Baile et al., 2000). When engaging in these conversations, it is important to consider everyone's emotions towards the illness. A second assessment that can be utilized by MedFTs is the Prepare, Evaluate, Warning, Telling, Emotional response, Regrouping preparation (PEWTER) (Keefe-Cooperman et al., 2018; Keefe-Cooperman & Brady-Amoon, 2013). MedFTs need to collaborate with the medical provider, to gain an understanding of what has been discussed regarding the illness with the family, and what the patient and family know already before meeting with the patient and family.When meeting with the family, it is important to disclose that the conversation will be serious and heavy. When the information is being discussed amongst the MedFT, patient, and family members, it is important for the MedFT to use comprehensible and translucent language, giving small bits of information, and making sure that the patient and family understand what is happening, and that the information being disclosed is tracked and comprehended (Keefe-Cooperman et al., 2018). If the patient and family members express certain emotions and reactions, it is important for the MedFT to address them. The ending of the conversation should give the patient and family members a depiction of hope and optimism, and that throughout every step of the way, they will be supported and taken care of (Keefe-Cooperman et al., 2018).

Psychological Dimension

A MedFT can explain to a patient how their philosophies and feelings are correlated to their actions, and how these actions are expressed either through active or passive coping mechanisms. This may be a patient incorporating a healthier sleeping schedule (active) or becoming a chronic alcohol user (passive) (Mendenhall et al., 2018). It is important to relay the information to patients on how their patterns of thinking, emotions, dynamics in families, occupations in society, socioeconomic statuses, accessibility to healthcare services, and their identity formation as a person with an illness all play a role in the management and treatment of their illness (Gatchel et al., 2018). It is meaningful for a MedFT to have open and honest conversations with the entire family system present in the patient's life, to assess the level of changes that will need to occur from each family member and to lessen anxieties (Mendenhall et al., 2018).

Having knowledge of the patient's projection and the level of extremity of a diagnosis can give the MedFT ideas of how to structure of the conversation (Kazlauskaite, 2021). Assessment questions such as "Have you noticed signs of mental health decline in yourself and/or your loved ones?", "How has your mental health been impacted due to your chronic/terminal illness?", "What is your culture's view on mental health, and how are your beliefs the same and/or different?", "Have you sought out mental health services or support groups?", "What mental health choices have you made thus far?", "Are you experiencing any suicidal thoughts or ideations of hurting yourself or others? If yes, how are you coping with it, and how severe are they on a scale of 1–10?". MedFTs can then move on to assess family dynamics more in depth. Asking questions such as "Have you had conversations with your loved ones about your illness? If so, how did it go and what did the structure of it look like?", "What family dynamics will change, and how can we all work on getting you there?", and "How has your diagnosis impacted your relationships with your partner(s), family members, and loved ones?" This should help the MedFT understand the patient's psychological beliefs towards their meaning making of the illness, including their cultural and ethnic backgrounds, and the level of impact the illness has had on the patient's and their family's mental health. It will also give MedFTs a chance to understand what family dynamics the family wants to change, and have an opportunity to create a treatment plan on how to do it most effectively.

MedFTs should utilize psychoeducation and place an emphasis on the importance of having the family system involved and educated on the disease, where everyone can gain an understanding of the illness and comprehend it at each individual person's developmental stage. For example, if a mother received a diagnosis of cancer, a MedFT can talk to her younger kids, and use statements like "Your parent will be sick for some time, and things at the house might change, where you might have to take on some more responsibilities. Your parent's sickness is not your fault, you did not do anything bad. However, they will appreciate your help so much". Using language that is congruent with the person's cognitive development is ideal when having these conversations.

Parents are advised to have discussions about family dynamic changes, and a genogram may be a beneficial intervention a MedFT can utilize (McGoldrick et al., 1999; Kazlauskaite, 2021). The genogram can illustrate where new boundaries and rules are needed, and where certain family roles might have to be adjusted. This can in return change the hierarchy of the family, which should be discussed as well (Kazlauskaite, 2021). A MedFT can ask assessment questions like "How can your family make it easier for you, where your level of negative emotions decrease, and your positive emotions increase?", "What kind of family dynamic changes will be occurring?", "How will this affect the family's mental health?", "How will culture impact the dynamic changes in the family?", "Will you have conversations with your family regarding mental health, and if so, what would that look like?", "How do you plan on creating a space where everyone is taking care of their mental health?" and "Who would you like to be involved in your treatment plan?" All these questions can assess the level of emphasis the patient and their family will place on mental health, and how their cultural backgrounds will influence their decision making. In the process of conducting verbal communication about the illness with the patient and their families, it is important to pay attention to certain cues like the tone of their voices and their speech rates. It is also crucial to be cognizant of non-verbal cues, including eye and body language (Kazlauskaite, 2021).

Psychological Assessment Tools

People that are living with a chronic illness are more likely to experience mood disorders, anxiety disorders, substance use disorders, sleep disorders, and suicidal ideation (Gatchel et al., 2018). All these factors increase chances of disruption and distress in the life of a person diagnosed with a chronic illness. There are a few assessment tools MedFTs can utilize to assess the level of disruption and impact the chronic illness has in a patient's everyday life.

One of them is the Pain Disability Questionnaire (PDQ), a calculation of subjective recognized disability. It encloses operative and psychosocial subscales from a holistic perspective on health with regard to patients diagnosed with chronic illnesses (Gatchel et al., 2018). A second assessment is the Fear-Avoidance Components Scale (FACS). This assessment tool identifies the impediments a patient experiences that are stopping them from managing and recovering. This includes the patient's engagement in pain catastrophizing, and showing strong psychometric markers for both psychosocial and physical dynamics (Gatchel et al., 2018). A third is the Patient-Reported Outcomes Measurement Information System (PROMIS) that assesses pain effect, pain behavior, pain restrictions, and level of pain, alongside psychosocial factors like sleep disruption patterns, lethargy, role gratification in society, anxiety, depression, and physical performance (Gatchel et al., 2018). A fourth assessment is a questionnaire called the Chronic Pain Acceptance Questionnaire (CPAQ) that focuses on the two main domains of pain and acceptance. The first one is the disposition to experience pain, and the second is the commitment to creating a life that incorporates valuable activities the patient enjoys despite the pain (Moore, 2018).

Social Dimension

Family members of ill patients will often assume responsibility for becoming a caregiver. Such caregivers are in need of social and professional support. Lack of such support can result in lack of knowledge and lack of accessing available resources, thus burdening family members and caregivers (Brazil et al., 2005). MedFTs working with patients and their families need to assess the support the members feel they have from various sources, such as extended family, social circles, communities, and even their medical care team. Research has positively correlated patients with higher social support and increased medication compliance (DiMatteo, 2004; Druley & Townsend, 1998; Hagedoorn et al., 2000). Thus, assessing and providing assistance in creating social connections is an important task for MedFTs.

Social Assessment Tools

A great way to understand the connection and support the family and patient has is to create a genogram (McGoldrick et al., 1999). Understanding social support can be helpful for the family as it may point out resources, they were not aware of before or illustrate the changes in perceived support and connection over the progression of the illness (Rempel et al., 2007). To begin, the MedFT may assess who is part of the patient's family and social circle. Questions such as "who is part of your immediate family? Who is part of your close social network?" can begin the conversation about perceived support. Continuing with questions that give insight on who else the patient feels connected to, such as "who else in the community do you feel you can go to for support?" can give the MedFT a fuller understanding of the social connection and support the client has.

Another method to assess social connectedness and support is to utilize the Three-Component Model of Social Relationships (Oxman & Berkman, 1990). This model assesses the a) structural and functional models of social networks, b) the type and amount of social support the networks provide, and c) the perceived adequacy of such support. The structural and functional components focus on identifying who is included in the social network and how often they rely on one another as well as geographic location. When assessing the type and amount of support a patient has, it is important to identify whether such support is emotional, physical, or tangible support. The third and final component focuses on understanding whether the patient perceives their support as helpful or harmful. This component has cultural implications to it, as various backgrounds can perceive the availability and helpfulness of support differently. Thus, it is important to address and assess how they perceive the support based on their cultural background (McCauley, 1995).

Finally, it is important for MedFTs to pose questions regarding patients' perceived support from their medical care team and help facilitate connections if needed. For example, asking "Do you feel like you are receiving enough time and information from all your providers?" may provide detail on the connection between patient and care teams. In addition, questions around who from their family has been or needs to be connected to the medical team ensures inclusivity and can help the patient feel respected and heard.

Spiritual Dimension

MedFTs working with patients who are chronically or terminally ill may focus on topics such as quality of life, psychological suffering, loss, meaning-making, and spirituality (Williams-Reade & Trudeau, 2018). Exploring the family's meaning-making around terminal illness, for example, can start conversations around spiritual, religious, and existential questions. Aspects influencing meaning making include the individual's personal life experience, characters, social context, as well as their culture. It is important for MedFTs to explore these aspects when working with their patients and family members.

Conversations about spirituality in Westernized medical societies can be unpleasant, but spirituality does impact how an individual copes with an illness and how they respond to it (Dyer, 2011). About 72% of patients that have a terminal illness disclosed that their spiritual needs were scarcely supported by the medical system, or not supported at all, and 47% disclosed that they did not feel supported religiously (Bussing & Koenig, 2010). Spirituality is complex and can encompass religion, but not necessarily. Spirituality and religion do have benefits for the individual with the disease, which can be feasibly rationalized through science, through the intercessions of the immune system (Dyer, 2011). Spirituality and religion can consist of a multitude of rituals, including individual or community prayers, meditation, worship, etc. Participating in these rituals has certain benefits to the body, consisting of enhanced physical health from the illness, a drop in depressive and anxious symptomatology, increased family stability, and decreased social seclusion (Mendenhall et al., 2021). The biggest advantage of MedFTs having clinical conversations with their patients and family members is that it helps the family create meaning-making, while simultaneously portraying cultural humility and competence (Mendenhall et al., 2021). MedFTs should be trained and have a level of competence regarding spirituality, by acquainting themselves with the five most shared religions (Christianity, Buddhism, Hinduism, Judaism, and Islam) (Mendenhall et al., 2021).

Spiritual Assessment Tools

Understanding a person's spiritual dimension can aid in fostering a supportive and holistic approach to working with clients who are ill (Williams-Reade & Trudeau, 2018). Assessing spiritual influences on how the new medical diagnosis is understood and accepted is vital. Various assessment tools have been established to assist MedFT in their assessment of spiritual influences of their clients. For example, FACIT-Sp (Functional Assessment of Chronic Illness Therapy-Spiritual Well-Being; Peterman et al., 2002) assesses meaning-making and faith. Another example is FICA (Faith, Importance/Influence of beliefs, Community involvement, and Addressing issues in providing care; Puchalski, 2006), which focuses on a person's faith and beliefs and their impact on coping with disease. A third assessment tool that can be beneficial for MedFTs to use in having spiritual conversations with their patients and family members is HOPE Questions (H=source of Hope, meaning, consolation, etc.; O= Organized religion's role for the patient and their loved ones; P= Personal spiritual practices; E= Effects of spiritual beliefs and values on treatment decisions and other processes related to patient's treatment) (Mendenhall, et al., 2021). Krakowiak and Fopka-Kowalczyk (2015) recommend asking questions such as "Do you consider yourself spiritual or religious?", "Do you have spiritual beliefs that help you cope with stress?", and "What importance does your faith or belief have in your life?" (p. 127) to learn more about the spiritual elements of the client. Spirituality can be present for patients in their everyday life, or can be present predominantly during times of hardship and discomfort, and MedFTs should be competently receptive (Mendenhall et al., 2021).

Assessment Availability in Different Languages

Some of the assessment tools provided below are available in other languages. The PDQ is available in Spanish and Korean. The FACS is available in Spanish, French, and Serbian. PROMIS is obtainable in Spanish, French, Korean, and German, and is in the works for other languages like Dutch, Mandarin Chinese, Portuguese, and Hebrew. The CPAQ is available in Chinese, Danish, Finnish, German, Greek, Italian, Japanese, Korean, Norwegian, Persian, Portuguese, Russian, Spanish, Swedish, and Turkish. The FACIT-SP is accessible in Arabic, Bengali, Burmese, Chinese, Croatian, Czech, Danish, Dutch, Farsi, French, German, Greek, Hebrew, Hindi, Hungarian, Indonesian, Italian, Japanese, Korean, Lithuanian, Malay, Marathi, Norwegian, Polish, Portuguese, Sinhalese, Spanish, Slovak, Slovene, Swedish, Tamil, Telugu, Thai, Turkish, and Vietnamese. Lastly, a genogram can be utilized in all languages, as long as it is properly explained to the patient along with the purpose of the genogram.

Case Example

Luis, a 24-year-old Mexican American, migrated to the United States five years ago with his family from Mexico, and currently lives in Texas. Luis recently got diagnosed with stage

II pancreatic cancer, which has changed many aspects of his and his family's life. Some of the changes that have occurred for Luis are his decreased overall quality of life, inlcuding reduced hours at work, taking on less responsibilities around the house, and taking a leave of absence from college courses. His family members have had to change their daily routines as well, by switching schedules at their jobs to be at the house more and be available for Luis to help him. They have also had to delegate the responsibilities of the house amongst family members in a different manner, with each of them doing more than usual. The medical doctors at Memorial Hermann Cancer Center created a treatment plan that consists of radiation and chemotherapy, and if no improvements are seen within the next three months, surgery will be scheduled to take out part of the cancer. Luis and his family are also working with a *curandero* (traditional healer), who believes Luis and his family have been cursed and that they are victims of the evil eye. The traditional healer treated him with herbs, rituals, and prayers. Luis and his family consider themselves Roman Catholic, and attend mass at a local church every Sunday. Luis and his family are extremely close, and do everything together as a family. However, Luis's mom, Maria, has not shared Luis's diagnosis with any extended family members, because she fears they would blame her for it.

Luis attends his radiation and chemotherapy regularly at the medical center, while also following the herb regiment the healer prescribed. Out of a fear of being judged, he does not share his herb regiment with his medical providers. Luis and his family consistently pray for him, and believe that God will give them a miracle and cure Luis. After a few months, Luis's cancer progressed, and he was hospitalized. Luis stated "I used to be angry at God at first, but now I believe that he would not give anything to anyone that they could not handle. My family and I plan to continue to pray intensely and I hope that helps, but I also believe that God cannot cure me anymore, only medicine can".

At the hospital, Luis gets introduced to an interdisciplinary team, consisting of his oncologists, nurses, the MedMFT, radiologists, and the anesthesiologist. Ezra, the MedFT, introduces herself and gives a brief summary of her credentials and what her role includes. She tells Luis and the family that she has been in the field of MedFT for ten years now, and that she is going to address all of the domains of the BPSS model with Luis and his family. She explains to Luis and his family that her role as a MedFT is to take a holistic approach to Luis's illness. She explains that when an illness is diagnosed, it has an impact on the patient, but also on the family system, focusing on the changes biologically (physically), psychologically, socially, and spiritually. She elaborates on how the utilization of the BPSS model has been integrated into healthcare settings, showing positive results in patients and their families. Luis discloses feeling reluctant to share everything he and his family believe and think about his illness, out of a fear of being judged. Ezra expounds that she is extremely open-minded, and has a nonjudgmental stance, as long as it is not harmful to Luis or anyone else. She encourages Luis and his family to be their authentic selves with her. She clarifies that her role is to support and advocate for Luis and his family throughout this difficult process, and to develop a sense of agency and communion to improve Luis's overall well-being.

Biological Domain

Ezra utilizes the SPIKES model with Luis and his family in order to navigate the difficult conversations that need to happen amongst the family members about the illness. Ezra looks over Luis's medical records from the hospital about his disease and asks Luis and his family,

"When the medical doctors explained your diagnosis, did you feel like you understood the language they were using?". Luis and his family explain how the medical doctors used medical terms that were clear to a certain extent, but that they still were confused about specific aspects of the diagnosis and the treatment plan, and felt some anxiety towards it. Ezra asked Luis and his family, "Could you please explain to me what you do understand about your diagnosis this far?" After they answer, Ezra uses clear and concise language that could be comprehended by Luis and his family. She also explains that specific details about the biological aspects of the disease will need to be discussed collaboratively with a medical doctor, elaborating that she is not one. Ezra then asks who Luis would like to have included in his treatment plan, and he states that it would be both of his parents, and that that is extremely important to him. When she utilizes the SPIKES assessment tool, she took into consideration everyone's emotions about the diagnosis. Luis's parents explain how they did not appreciate the medical doctors informing Luis on his disease and current condition without them being present. Ezra validated their emotions regarding this, she thanks them for their honesty, and tells them that she would speak with the medical doctors about including them in any future conversations about the diagnosis. Luis tells the MedFT that his culture is extremely important to him, and that he wants to make all of his treatment decisions collectively with his family members.

Psychological Domain

Ezra has a discussion with the family on what individual changes need to be made from each family member to create a new homeostasis, by stating, "What changes in the family do you believe need to happen and how do you think we can get you there together as a team?" She utilizes a genogram to assist with creating new boundaries in the family and addresses any anxieties each member in the family might be experiencing regarding Luis and his illness. Then Ezra focuses on Luis specifically, and asks him a more specific question, stating "How has your mental health been impacted by your illness and how have you been coping?" She utilizes the Patient-Reported Outcomes Measurement Information System (PROMIS) to assess the level of psychological impact the illness has made on Luis and his family as a whole. Ezra asks Luis and his family about the effects the physical pain of the diagnosis is causing on their behavior, the level of anxiety, depression, and fatigue each person is experiencing. Creating coping skills and increasing life satisfaction is something Ezra discusses with Luis and his family, by utilizing SFBT and creating goals and actions for how to adhere to coping skills and increase overall well-being.

Social Domain

Ezra assesses the patient's perception of available support. She does this by asking Luis questions such as "Who have you felt the most supported by?", "Are you connected to any support groups?", "What can others do or say to make you feel supported?", "What does it mean to be supported?", "What are your thoughts/feelings about your relationship with your medical care team?", and "How can I be of assistance to build your support group?" Through these questions Ezra can gain a sense of Luis' perceived and actual support, as well as how connected he wants to be with the community, support groups, and his medical care team. Ezra also includes questions about Luis's cultural background and how connected or independently difficult situations are handled and coped with within his family. This will provide Ezra with the knowledge of whom to include or exclude when considering Luis's social connections.

Spiritual Domain

Ezra encourages Luis and his family to talk about spirituality, asking them if they are religious, and what their religion means to them surrounding Luis's illness. Ezra asks them "How does your religion/spirituality affect the meaning you create regarding the illness, and how does it help you cope?", explaining to Luis and his family that spirituality might be helpful to Luis in coping with the illness. She utilizes psychoeducation in helping the family understand the physical and mental benefits of participating in meaningful rituals, whatever that may look like to Luis and the family. Ezra uses the HOPE Questions assessment tool in aiding conversations around spirituality, especially focusing on the effects Luis's and his family's spiritual beliefs have on treatment decisions and/or treatment options. Ezra also asks Luis if his spiritual beliefs differ from his parents and family, and he answers yes. Ezra then proceeds to ask Luis, "Since your spiritual beliefs differ from those of your family, how would you like for me to approach topics about spirituality when they are present?". By giving him this option, she is increasing his level of autonomy. She is also giving him control and power in one aspect of his illness.

Implications for Clinicians

A MedFT can help the family in a multitude of ways. They can assist in writing a treatment plan that adheres to the patient's and family's needs and goals, using a systemic and BPSS lens (Mendenhall et al., 2018). The individual and family should become familiar with an illness genogram that can give the family a sense of comfort and control, provide insight, and decrease anxiety. A MedFT should encourage the patient to choose a family member that will be involved in goal formation and the plans for achieving those goals. Motivational Interviewing (MI) is one form of an evidence-based psychological intervention a MedFT can use to gather motivational elements in a person's life surrounding the illness and put them into action (Mendenhall et al., 2018). Using reflective hearing, open-ended questions, motivational affirmations, and change and solution talk (Solution-Focused Brief Therapy (SFBT)) can increase the feelings of agency in the patient, and provide a sense of hope for the future (Mendenhall et al., 2018). Cognitive-Behavioral Therapy (CBT) has also shown high efficacy amongst MedFTs. CBT has been shown to help patients with anxiety, depression, side effects from medicine, chronic illness management, and parent management proficiencies of child patients (Mendenhall et al., 2018). Physicians and MedFTs should strive to decrease distress and preserve or progress the quality of life of the patient and their family. Illness is characterized by all-embracing self-management; the patient must take the responsibility of monitoring and managing their illnesses, by the regulation of cognitive, emotional, and behavioral feedback, to be able to obtain overall well-being (Newman et al., 2004).

MedFTs can utilize certain psychotherapeutic theories, models, and interventions to help patients and their family system live with illness and manage it to the best of their abilities. CBT is an evidence-based model that has been proven to help patients with anxiety and depression, and it was recently approved for treatment of chronic illnesses and pain (Moore, 2018). Pain management and the creation of coping skills is incorporated through the CBT lens. Mindfulness also is scientifically proven to be advantageous (Moore, 2018). Mindfulness helps patients be present and slow down their nervous system, while simultaneously decreasing physical and psychological symptoms associated with the chronic illness. A third theory is Acceptance and Commitment Therapy (ACT). A MedFT can instruct the patient to engage in acceptance-aligned tactics to counteract the pain and psychological distress, by creating personal values and goals that can increase productivity and quality of life (Moore, 2018).

Conclusion

The way a family understands, accepts, talks about, and adapts to a new medical diagnosis can be influenced by their cultural background. When a MedFT works with patients and their family members, it is important that they assess the extent they are influenced by their culture. The Biopsychosocial-Spiritual model can help MedFTs help the patient and their family members in a holistic way. Utilizing the various inventories outlined above, MedFTs can gauge how cultural and ethical backgrounds may impact the way a patient's illness is perceived, talked about, and adapted to. They can also assist in understanding who needs to be included in the sessions to provide physical and emotional space to process the new diagnosis, receive psycho-education, and adapt to the lifestyle changes that often accompany a medical illness.

References

Agom, D. A., Neill, S., Allen, S., Poole, H., Sixsmith, J., Onyeka, T. C., & Ominyi, J. (2019). Construction of meanings during life-limiting illnesses and its impacts on palliative care: Ethnographic study in an African context. *Psycho-Oncology (Chichester, England)*, 28(11), 2201–2209. https://doi.org/10.1002/pon.5208

Baile, W., Buckman, R., Lenzi, R., Glover, G., Beale, E., & Kudelka, A. (2000). SPIKES- A six-step protocol for delivering bad news: Application to the patient with cancer. *The Oncologist, 5*, 302–311. https://doi.org/10.1634/theoncologist.5-4-203

Barnato, A., Herndon, B., Anthony, D., Gallagher, P., Skinner, J., Bynum, J., & Fisher, E. (2007). Are regional variations in end-of-life care intensity explained by patient preference? *Medical Care, 45*, 386–393. https://10.1097/01.mlr.0000255248.79308.41

Beale, E., Baile, W., & Aaron, J. (2005). Silence is not golden: Communicating with children dying from cancer. Journal of Clinical Oncology, 23, 3621–3629. https://doi.org/10.1200/JCO.2005.11.015

Bernacki, R. E. & Block, S. D. (2014). Communication About Serious Illness Care Goals: A Review and Synthesis of Best Practices. *JAMA Internal Medicine*, 174(12), 1994–2003. https://doi.org/10.1001/jamainternmed.2014.5271

Betsch, C., Böhm, R., Airhihenbuwa, C. O., Butler, R., Chapman, G. B., Haase, N., Herrmann, B., Igarashi, T., Kitayama, S., Korn, L., Nurm, Ülla-K., Rohrmann, B., Rothman, A. J., Shavitt, S., Updegraff, J. A., & Uskul, A. K. (2016). Improving Medical Decision Making and Health Promotion through Culture-Sensitive Health Communication. *Medical Decision Making, 36*(7), 811–833. https://doi.org/10.1177/0272989X15600434

Bloomer, M.J., Endacott, R., Ranse, K., & Coombs, M.A. (2017). Navigating communication with families during withdrawal of life-sustaining treatment in intensive care: A qualitative descriptive study in Australia and New Zealand. *Journal of Clinical Nursing, 26*, 690–697. https://doi.org/10.1111/jocn.13585

Boyd. K.M. (2000). Disease, illness, sickness, health, healing and wholeness: exploring some elusive concepts. *Medical Humanities*, 26(1), 9–17. https://doi.org/10.1136/mh.26.1.9

Brazil, K., Bedard, M., Abernathy, T., Lohfeld, L., & Willison, K. (2005). Service preferences among family caregivers of terminally ill. *Journal of Palliative Medicine, 8,* 69–87. https://doi.org/10.1089/jpm.2005.8.69

Bronfenbrenner, U. (1979). *The ecology of human development: Experiments in nature and design.* Harvard University Press.

Brown, S., Aboumatar, H., Francis, L., Halamka, J., Rozenblum, R., Rubin, E., Sarnoff Lee, B., Sugarman, J., Turner, K., Vorwaller, M., & Frosh, D. (2016). Balancing digital information-sharing and patient privacy when engaging families in the intensive care unit. *Journal of the American Medical Informatics Association, 23,* 995–1000. https://doi.org/10.1093/jamiaa/ocv182

Burroughs, A. (2014). *Dry.* Atlantic Books.

Center for Disease Control and Prevention (2022). National Center for Chronic Disease Prevention and Health Promotion. www.cdc.gov/chronicdisease/index.htm

Dias, L., Chabner, B., Lynch, T., & Penson, R. (2003). Breaking bad news: A patient's perspective. *The Oncologist, 8,* 587–596. https://doi.org/10.1634/theoncologist.8-6-587

DiMatteo, R. (2004). Social support and patient adherence to medical treatment: A meta-analysis. *Health Psychology, 23,* 207–218. https://10.1037/0278-6133.23.2.207

Druley, J. A., & Townsend, A. L. (1998). Self-esteem as a mediator between spousal support and depressive symptoms: A comparison of healthy individuals and individuals coping with arthritis. *Health Psychology, 17,* 255–261. https://doi.org/10.1037/0278-6133.17.3.255

Duffy, S., Jackson, F., Schim, S., Ronis, D., & Fowler, K. (2006). Racial/ethnic preferences, sex preferences, and perceived discrimination related to end-of-life care. *Journal of American Geriatric Society, 54,* 150–157. https://doi.org/10.1111/j.1532-5415.2005.00526.x

Fang, M., Malcoe, L., Sixsmith, J., Wong, L., & Challender, M. (2015). Exploring traditional end-of-life beliefs, values, expectations, and practices among Chinese women living in England: Informing culturally safe care. *Palliative & Support Care, 13,* 1261–1274. https://doi.org/10.1017/S1478951514001126

Fang, M., Sixsmith, J., Sinclair, S., & Horst, G. (2016). A knowledge synthesis of culturally – and spiritually – sensitive end-of-life care: Findings from a scoping review. *BMC Geriatrics, 16,* 1–14. https://doi.org/10.1186/s12877-016-0282-6

Finney, N. & Tadros, E. (2019). Medical family therapy in home-based settings: A case application. *The Family Journal, 28,* 210–233. https://doi.org/10.1177/0032885521991109

Gatchel, R. J. & Oordt, M. S. (2003). *Clinical health psychology and primary care: practical advice and clinical guidance for successful collaboration* (1st ed.). American Psychological Association.

Givler, A., Bhatt, H., & Maani-Fogelman, P. (2021). The importance of cultural competence in pain and palliative care, *In StatPearls.* StatPearls Publishing.

Hagedoorn, M., Kuijer, R. G., Buunk, B., DeJong, G., Wobbes, T., & Sanderman, R. (2000). Marital satisfaction in patients with cancer: Does support from intimate partners benefit those who need it most? *Health Psychology, 19,* 274–282. https://doi.org/10.1037/0728-6133.19.3.274

Hajat, & Stein, E. (2018). The global burden of multiple chronic conditions: A narrative review. *Preventive Medicine Reports, 12,* 284–293. https://doi.org/10.1016/j.pmedr.2018.10.008

Harsh, J. & Bonnema, R. (2018). Medical Family Therapy in Internal Medicine. In *Clinical Methods in Medical Family Therapy* (Eds.) (pp. 87–110). Springer.

Hirokawa, K. & Dohi, I. (2007). Agency and communion related to mental health in Japanese young adults. *Sex Roles, 56,* 517–524. https://doi.org/10.1007/s11199-007-9190-8

Hodgson, J., Lamson, A., Aamar, R., & Limon, F. (2018). Medical Family Therapy in Community Health Centers. In *Clinical Methods in Medical Family Therapy* (Eds.) (pp. 357–400). Springer.

Hodgson, J., Trump, L., Wilson, G., & Garcia-Huidobro, D. (2018). Medical Family Therapy in Family Medicine. In *Clinical Methods in Medical Family Therapy* (Eds.) (pp. 17–59). Springer.

Kazlauskaite, V. (2022). Navigating difficult conversations with children when parents are ill: How Medical Family Therapists can assist. *Contemporary Family Therapy, 44,* 55–66. https://doi.org/10.1007/s10591-021-09628-z

Keefe-Cooperman, K., & Brady-Amoon, P. (2013). Breaking bad news in counseling: Applying the PEWTER model in the school setting. *Journal of Creativity in Mental Health, 8,* 265–277. https://doi.org/10.1080/1/54-1383.2013.821926

Keefe-Cooperman, K., Savitsky, D., Koshel, W., Bhat, V., & Cooperman, J. (2018). The PEWTER study: Breaking bad news communication skills training for counseling programs. *International Journal for the Advancement of Counseling, 40,* 72–87. https://doi.org/10.1007/s10447-017-9313-z

Kelley, A., Wnger, N., Sarkisian, C. (2010). Opiniones: End-of-life care preferences and planning of older latinos. *Journal of American Geriatric Society, 58,* 1109–1116. https://doi.org/10.1111/j.1532.2010.02853.x

Kongsuwan, W., Chaiptetch, O., & Matchim, Y. (2012). Thai Buddhist families' perspective of a peaceful death in ICUs. *Nursing in Critical Care, 17,* 151–159. https://doi.org/10.1111/j.1478-5153.2012.00495.x

Larsson, A. T. & Grassman, E. J. (2012). Bodily changes among people living with physical impairments and chronic illnesses: biographical disruption or normal illness? *Sociology of Health & Illness, 34*(8), 1156–1169. https://doi.org/10.1111/j.1467-9566.2012.01460.x

Marlowe, & Hodgson, J. (2014). Competencies of Process: Toward a Relational Framework for Integrated Care. *Contemporary Family Therapy, 36*(1), 162–171. https://doi.org/10.1007/s10591-013-9283-1

McCauley, K. (1995). Assessing social support in patients with cardiac disease. *Journal of Cardiovascular Nursing, 10,* 73–80. https://doi.org/10.1097/00005082-199510000-00007

McDaniel, S., Doherty, W., & Hepworth, J. (2014). *Medical family therapy and integrated care* (2nd ed). American Psychological Association.

McGoldrick, M., Gerson, R., & Shellenberger, S. (1999). Genograms: Assessments and interventions. Norton.

Mills, E., Nicolson, K., & Smith, B. (2019). Chronic pain: A review of its epidemiology and associated factors in population-based studies. *British Journal of Anaesthesia, 132,* 273–283. https://doi.org/10.1016/j.bja.2019.03.023

Moore, R. J. (2018). *Handbook of Pain and Palliative Care Biopsychosocial and Environmental Approaches for the Life Course* (2nd ed. 2018.). Springer International Publishing: Imprint: Springer.

Nath, S., Kirschman, K., Lewis, B., & Strumpf, N. (2008). Place called life: Exploring the advance care planning of African-American PACE enrollees. *Social Work Heatlh Care, 47,* 277–292. https://doi.org/10.1080/00981380801985432

Newman, S., Steed, L., & Mulligan, K. (2004). Self-management interventions for chronic illness. *Lancet, 364*(9444), 1523–1537. https://doi.org/10.1016/S0140-6736(04)17277-2

Orford, N., Milnes, S., Lambert, N., Berkeley, L., Lane, S. E., Simpson, N., Elderkin, T., Bone, A., Corke, C., Bellomo, R., & Bailey, M. (2016). Prevalence, goals of care and long-term outcomes of patients with life-limiting illness referred to a tertiary ICU. *Critical Care Resuscitation, 18,* 181–188.

Osokpo, O. H., Lewis, L. M., Ikeaba, U., Chittams, J., Barg, F. K., & Riegel, B. (2022). Self-Care of African Immigrant Adults with Chronic Illness. *Clinical Nursing Research, 31*(3), 413–425. https://doi.org/10.1177/10547738211056168

Oxman, T., & Berkman, L. (1990). Assessment of social relationships in elderly patients. *International Journal of Psychiatry Medicine, 20,* 65–84. https://doi.org/10.2190/G6CX-YCGL-HAB3-8BMC

Pentaris, P., & Thomsen, L. (2020). Cultural and religious diverstiy in hospice and palliative care: A qualitative cross-country comparative analysis of the challenges of health care professionals. *Journal of Death and Dying, 81,* 648–669. https://doi.org/10.1177/0030222818795282

Rajaei, & Jensen, J. F. (2020). Empowering Patients in Integrated Behavioral Health-Care Settings: A Narrative Approach to Medical Family Therapy. *The Family Journal, 28,* 48–55. https://doi.org/10.1177/1066480719893958

Rempel, G., Neufeld, A., & Kushner, K. (2007). Genograms and ecomaps in family caregiving research. *Journal of Family Nursing, 13,* 403–419. https://doi.org/10.1177/1074840707307917

Rosenberg, A., Starks, H., Unguru, Y., Feudtner, C., & Diekema, D. (2017). Truth telling in the setting of cultural differences and incurable pediatric illness. *Journal of the American Medical Association, Pediatrics, 171,* 1113–1119. https://doi.org/10.1001/jamapediatrics.2017.2568

Shaw, Huebner, C., Armin, J., Orzech, K., & Vivian, J. (2008). The Role of Culture in Health Literacy and Chronic Disease Screening and Management. *Journal of Immigrant and Minority Health, 11*(6), 460–467. https://doi.org/10.1007/s10903-008-9135-5

Sperry, L. (2007). Utilizing a Family-Sensitive Cognitive Behavioral Intervention With Chronic Illness: The Impact of Family Dynamics and Therapy on Medical Symptoms. *The Family Journal (Alexandria, Va.), 15*(1), 56–61. https://doi.org/10.1177/1066480706294791

Thomas, R., Wilson, D., Justice, C., Birch, S., & Sheps, S. (2008). A literature review of preferences for end-of-life care in developed countries by individuals with different cultural affiliations and ethnicity. *Journal of Hospice & Palliative Nursing, 10,* 142–163. https://doi.org/10.1097/01.NJH.000 0306740.10636.64

Tikkanen, R., & Abrams,M. (2022). *U.S. Health Care from a Global Perspective, 2019: Higher Spending, Worse Outcomes?.* https://doi.org/10.26099/7avy-fc29

Tseng, Wittenborn, A. K., Blow, A. J., Chao, W., & Liu, T. (2020). The development of marriage and family therapy in East Asia (China, Taiwan, Japan, South Korea and Hong Kong): past, present and future. *Journal of Family Therapy, 42*(4), 477–498. https://doi.org/10.1111/1467-6427.12285

Turner, D.C. (1996). The Role of Culture in Chronic Illness. *The American Behavioral Scientist (Beverly Hills), 39*(6), 717–728. https://doi.org/10.1177/0002764296039006008

Williams-Reade, J., & Trudeau, S. (2018). Medical Family Therapy in Palliative and Hospice Care. In *Clinical Methods in Medical Family Therapy* (Eds.) (pp. 263–293). Springer.

Williams-Reade, J., Freitas, C., & Lawson, L. (2014). Narrative-informed medical family therapy: Using narrative therapy in practices in brief medical encounters. *Families, Systems, & Health, 32,* 416–425. https://doi.org/10.1037/fsh0000082ltl

World Health Organization (2022). WHO remains firmly committed to the principles set out in the preamble to the Constitution. www.who.int/about/governance/constitution

Zaider, T., & Steinglass, P. (2018). Medical Family Therapy in Oncology. In *Clinical Methods in Medical Family Therapy* (Eds.) (pp. 207–230). Springer.

18

SOLUTION-FOCUSED BRIEF THERAPY

Global Practices

Sara Smock Jordan and Benjamin T. Finlayson

Introduction

The application of solution-focused brief therapy (SFBT) occurs across presenting problems and many cultural groups. From substance abuse to physical therapy, the solution focused model provides a framework for helping individuals develop their preferred future. In the last decade, more literature has become available on the application of the model to various cultures and in various modalities (e.g., psychotherapy, medicine, etc.) all over the world. In 2014 John Kim published his edited book entitled Solution-focused brief therapy: A multicultural approach, which applies the model to a variety of populations. This was the first book of its kind providing a rationale for the use of SFBT with ethnic/racial minorities, gender/sexual minorities, disabled individuals, those from lower SES backgrounds, and spiritual/religious clients.

SFBT offers a culturally sensitive approach to psychotherapy, coaching, business, and medicine. Its use internationally is evidence of its ability to adapt to the background, culture, and values of clients and patients alike. This chapter will explore how SFBT is a culturally sensitive approach due to its philosophical underpinnings, its view and use of language through the co-construction process, and evidence-based international data.

SFBT as a Culturally Sensitive Approach

SFBT was developed by de Shazer and Berg as a model of dialogue that honors the client. Respect and belief in the client's ability to know what's best for them are core values of the approach. In addition to these values, several philosophical underpinnings of SFBT provide support in the models' ability to meet the needs of various cultures.

Theory. Most psychotherapy models have a theory from which techniques and interventions are based. From a cultural perspective, these theories contain biases from the culture in which they are developed. For example, "people have trust issues due to attachment injuries" or "cognitive distortions lead to depression." De Shazer had a different definition of "theory." He stated that "theory, as I use the term, is not meant as an 'explanation' [i.e., inferences] but rather as a coherent 'description' of specific sequences of events

DOI: 10.4324/9781003297871-21

within a specific context [i.e., a description of the therapist interacting with the client in the therapy setting] (1988, p. xiv). In other words, de Shazer didn't have preconceived ideas about why a client might be doing a specific behavior/having a specific problem. Causation of why people act or respond a certain way was not part of his model. Rather, de Shazer's "theory" lied in the process of doing therapy (1988). The use of theory of SFBT is unique and makes its application across cultures possible.

Social constructionism. Social constructionism serves as the meta framework for the SFBT "theory"/model/approach. Gergen (1992) states that social constructionism is a process by which people explain or describe the world they live in. This perspective allows for individuals from a variety of backgrounds and cultures to preserve their cultural meanings, allowing for culturally competent care. Multiple realities can exist from this framework. Recent research shows co-construction occurs through dialogue in the following ways: questions contain assumptions (McGee, Del Vento, & Bavelas, 2005), therapists summarize and transform client language in a directed manner (i.e., model based; Korman, Bavlas, & DeJong, 2013), and clients tend to follow the topic choice of the therapist in dialogue (Smock Jordan, Froerer, & Bavelas, 2013). While the therapist and client are influenced by one another, the *meaning* of the words spoken lies within the speaker's head.

Not knowing approach. Using a not knowing approach is another strength of SFBT's multicultural strength (Kim, 2014). In this stance, the therapist approaches dialogue with curiosity. For example, asking "I wonder what it would look like the day after your miracle occurred" allows the client to provide details about how *they* see their preferred future. Regardless of the client's background or culture, the therapist never knows what is ideal or best for the client. Thus, using a not knowing approach opens up possibilities for various outcomes.

Resource Based. SFBT often gets labeled as a strength based approach. According to the SFBT treatment manual (Bavelas et al., 2013), SF is a resource-based approach because all clients have resources, even if they lack skill, knowledge, and/or power. For example, a homeless man might not have "strengths" but he has the resources to keep himself alive. These resources may include seeking shelter under a bridge, gathering food from trashcans, etc. Acknowledging that all persons have resources empowers clients in an realistic and practical way.

Client is the expert. SFBT relies on the client as the expert of their life. This is a helpful stance when working with clients from various cultures because culture plays a big role in expectations that clients have for change. This stance relies on the concept "leading from one step behind" (Cantwell & Holmes, 1994; De Jong & Berg, 2013. One myth in SFBT is that the therapist is not an expert. In SFBT, while the client is the expert of themselves and their preferred future, the therapist is the expert in the interviewing process. This allows for the culture and values of the client to lead the content of the conversation while the therapist directs, from behind, the process.

Views of Problems and Solutions. Problems in SFBT exist because the client can image life in a better way. Thus, problems are not objective in nature (de Shazer, 1991). Problems are contextual. For example, if a person struggles with waking up on time for work, it is only a *problem* if the client can see a better path to starting their day. Waking up "late" isn't a problem for someone who is retired and doesn't have a set schedule. From a cultural perspective, the concept of "late" is relative and not problematic. The same goes for solutions. One's preferred future, solution, may not even be connected to the problem (de

Shazer 1991). For example, for a mom who experiences problematic drinking, having the goal of getting her kids back from CPS becomes her "solution" to managing her drinking.

Language is reality. In de Shazer's 1994 book *Words Were Originally Magic*, Steve describes the *language* from a philosophical stance. "Language is reality" means that words and the meaning of those words are constructions created by the speaker (p. 9). For example, the term "depression" means something unique to every person. The same for "we're having communication problems" as stated from one partner about their marriage. Poststructuralism (de Shazer, 1991; de Shazer & Berg, 1992) means that the meaning of words varies, opposite from structuralism which means words have universal meanings. From a SFBT perspective, meaning is negotiated through conversation (de Shazer, 1994).

Importance of Language in SFBT and in Culture

Co-construction

So how does culture fit into meaning making in conversations? To answer this question, we must first discuss the building blocks of dialogue. Clark (1996) developed a *collaborative model* conversation which depicts how both speaker and listener contribute information that develops into a mutually agreed-upon narrative. Each speaker contributes their ideas, thoughts, experiences, and perspectives into the conversation, including culture. For example, in a therapy session where the client says, "I want to have a good marriage," each speaker's "having a good marriage" influences the conversation. Culture is part of our experiences and schemas, and thus our conversations. Culture and language go hand in hand.

de Shazer stated on many occasions that SFBT is a model for having a useful conversation. Since we can never truly understand the meaning that another person associates with words, the focus should be on the meaning that is co-constructed within the conversation. De Jong and Berg (2013) describe the process of co-constructing in SFBT as listen, select, and build. This sequence involves the therapist *listening* for evidence of exceptions to the problem, or the client's preferred future. For example, a client might say "It's been a really hard week. I lost my job and got in a fight with my spouse ...I really need next week to be better." The therapist listens for an opportunity "really need next week to be better" to comment on. The next step involves selecting. The therapist can respond by saying "yes, it sounds like you really do need next week to be better." Here the therapist *selects* this piece of the client's language to rephrase and formulate. In step three, the therapist continues their utterance of "yes, it sounds like you really do need next week to be better" but adds "so what would that look like, if next week was better for you?." This is the *build* step. This process continues throughout the dialogue.

While the process of listen, select, and build is helpful in teaching SFBT, it focuses entirely on the therapist. Since SFBT is a collaborative model, it seems useful to think about therapy as a collaborative process. The linguists Clark & Schaefer (1987) are known for their testing of dialogue as a collaborative process. The speaker can be the therapist or client, changing positions throughout the conversation, and information is shared. This view of conversation fits with the philosophy of SFBT and with the idea that meaning is made through the process of dialogue.

Myself (SJ), along with my colleagues Peter De Jong, Sara Healing, and Jennifer Gerwing, conducted a study to illustrate how speakers' *ground* or collaborate to create mutual understanding (Clark & Schaefer, 1987). We used Bavelas et al's (2017) model of *calibrating* to quantify the co-construction process (De Jong, Jordan, Healing, & Gerwing, 2020). In essence, *calibration* occurs when meaning is co-constructed through dialogue when a three-step process occurs: the speaker shares new information, the addressee responds to the speaker in a way that lets the speaker know they understand the speaker, then the speaker demonstrates that the addressee's response was sufficient. This co-constructive process occurs in all dialogues, not just therapeutic conversations.

During calibration, several elements contribute to the meaning-making process. As a SFBT therapist, choices are made about what questions to ask, what words to summarize, and what to drop. This section focuses mainly on what therapists and clients do in response to one another, including what parts of the dialogue they drop. For example, the previous utterance of "It's been a really hard week. I lost my job and got in a fight with my spouse ...I really need next week to be better" includes both negatives about the recent past and hope for a better future. A solution-focused therapist is focused on creating a preferred future rather than dwelling or digging into the nature of the problem. In this example, "It's been a really hard week. I lost my job and got in a fight with my spouse" is dropped. What isn't restated/questioned is just as important as what is stated by the therapist.

Elements of Dialogue

Over the years, my (SJ) research team has produced several studies and papers to examine the elements within dialogue. These include, but are not limited to, questions, formulations, and topic choice. Other elements of dialogue include gestures, tone, generic listener responses, acknowledgements, and gaze. The latter list informs the context of the words used within questions, formulations, and topic choice.

Questions. The literature on questions finds that presuppositions, assumptions within questions, are contained in any question (McGee et al., 2005). For example, "how late did you arrive to work today?" assumes 1) you arrived late, 2) there is a variable time in which you were late, and 3) you made it to work today. Questions are never value free. Given this fact, the types of questions and how we word our questions need to be carefully constructed. Carefully constructing questions is especially important in SFBT and when being a culturally competent therapist. Clients may ask a variety of questions to their therapist like "do you have children?" or "do you have experience working with trauma?." The therapist, in their role, makes choices about the questions they ask based on their model and/or curiosity. A SFBT therapist often begin sessions with "how can I be helpful today?" or "what's been better since the last time we've met?" These questions possess assumptions: that the therapist can be helpful, that the client knows what is helpful to them, that things have been better since their last session, and that the client has recognized improvements since the last session. These assumptions promote a resources-based, culturally sensitive approach. In fact, in my (SJ) opinion, the assumptions within SFBT questions are some of the most respectful in nature.

Formulations. Formulations occur when the speaker summarizes in some form pieces of what the previous speaker said. For example, in the previous example "yes, it sounds like you really do need next week to be better" is the therapist's formulation of what the client previously said. The words "really" and "need next week to be better" are examples of preserving the exact words from the client. Other types of formulations include preserved in altered form and using dietetics (i.e., it, they; Korman et al., 2013). The words that a therapist chooses to summarize or alter from a client depict the values of the therapist. For example, if a client says "I've had a really hard time opening up to people and talking because of negative experiences I've encountered" the therapist has several choices. They can choose to wait for more content then respond with a formulation or question, they can follow-up immediately with a question, or they can formulate this utterance. If the therapist responds with "so you have a hard time opening up to people?" that is a formulation within a question. This question assumes that the client has difficulty opening up to people. Another option for the therapist is "sounds like you've had some negative experiences that have closed you off." This assumes that the client is closed off and because of bad experiences. When considering cultural sensitivity in what to formulate, it is important to think about the meaning that is created in the summary. By formulating a negative aspect or experience from the client, the client may be viewed in a negative light. SFBT is culturally sensitive in its use of formulations because it *selects* pieces that focus on the client's preferred future.

Topic Choice. Topic choice is the type of content the speaker chooses to use, whether of a positive, negative, or neutral nature. Positive topic choices include "questions, statements, formulations, suggestions, etc., by the therapist (or client) that focused the client on some positive aspect of the client's life" (e.g., a relationship, trait, or experience in the past, present, or future) (Smock Jordan, Froerer, & Bavelas, 2013, p. 50).

> Negative topic choice included "questions, statements, formulations, suggestions, etc., by the therapist that focused the client on some negative relationship, trait, or experience in the past, present, or future. Examples of negative therapist content included a bad situation (e.g., other people, lack of money), the client's helplessness, the client's feeling out of control, the client's lack of agency, generalizing the problem or seeing no exceptions, and negative presuppositions in questions.
> (Smock Jordan, Froerer, & Bavelas, 2013, p. 52)

Neither positive nor negative topic choice is used as a category when the content does not fit into "positive topic choice" nor "negative topic choice." It is important to note that "positive" or "negative" do not contain value. Positive is not equal to good and negative is not equal to bad.

Positive is about the nature of the content, whether it is positive to the client within the context of the conversation. For example, if a client says, "I had a good day," that statement would be considered positive because it relates to a positive aspect of the client's life. Sometimes it is impossible or hard to tell whether the content is a positive or negative situation outside of the context of the conversation. Thus, it is imperative that the determination of the type of topic choice is determined within its context. In SFBT, positive topic choice is used to point the client in the direction of their preferred future in a way that honors their culture.

Negative topic choice is when the content refers to the above listed circumstances. For example, a therapist could say "you've had a really hard time managing your anxiety this week huh?" This would be negative because it addresses a bad situation about the client. If the uses negative topic choice about the client in a manner that is not respecting the client, it can be harmful. In SFBT, negative topic choice is not avoided but used in a way that does not 1) disrespect the client, 2) dig into the root of the problem, or 3) go against any of the philosophical underpinnings mentioned in the section above.

Neither positive nor negative content occurs in instances such as when the client says "yeah" or "I wore a green shirt yesterday." These statements do not appear to fit the definition of positive nor negative in the above section.

So how does a quantifiable model of co-construction apply to SFBT as a culturally sensitive approach? Therapists are given choices all along the way about what to respond to, the way to respond, and what not to respond to. In SFBT, the focus is on the client and their expertise about their life – including their culture, values, and experiences. SFBT therapists make meaning through calibration by listening to, selecting, and building from what the client brings to the dialogue. Both are active participants in co-creating meaning. The therapist, just as the client, has choices to make about what questions to ask, what formulations to use, and the topic choice they select. While the client makes these choices too, the therapist leads from behind in a culturally sensitive manner, honoring the client, towards a path that is preferred, as defined by the client.

International Application of SF Tenants

The global practice of SFBT anecdotally speaks to its adaptability across varying cultural groups, spiritualities, and languages. The international practice of SFBT demonstrates the active utilization of highlighting and building into "what works" in SF conversations. Though the model utilizes what the client brings, adaptation of the SF model requires a therapist that practices cultural humility and attunes to the client's dialogue use. For example, attunement to cultural scripts and dynamics might mean focusing more on solutions are than rumination on past insight or the client might value clearly defining their presenting issue with the therapist. The goal is to listen to what the client wants, honoring their cultural values and background. At the risk of generalizing a region's cultural/spiritual experiences by presenting SF international research by geography, the authors present international research by what process of SF was utilized, how and why the adaptation was useful for this population.

Resource-Based

Listening for and repeating back the measurable and visible client resources the therapist hears is a cornerstone practice of solution-focused therapy. In an international study of Hungarian teens, a program utilizing non-formal education emphasized unique skillsets of individual participants through reflection and direct experiences (Barnai & Soregi, 2021). The aim of solution-focused experiential education empowered Hungarian teenagers that were unhoused, without family or abandoned (Barnai & Soregi, 2021). The focus was implementing solution-focused experiential learning to promote the cultural heritage of impoverished communities who were dealing with unstable housing, discrimination, and trauma (Barnai & Soregi, 2021). Deidel and Hedley (2008) found that examining client resources can impact the self-reported severity of a problem across age and economic status of adults. Among Mexican older adults, context-related age difficulties, such as lower economic status, were perceived as less significant among participants after receiving SFBT therapy and showed improvement in their reported outcome (Seidel & Hedley, 2008). Utilization of client resources in SF highlights client agency to work through and over social and cultural filters in a co-collaborative, community-based and driven program.

Exceptions

Global practice of solution-focused therapy tailors to cultural scripts that may center on the desire to emphasizes solutions rather than insight into what may have created or maintained the problem (Neipp & Beyebach, 2022). The emphasis is on moments of disruption to the problem.

A Spanish study of solution-focused group therapy demonstrated a significant decrease in anxiety and depression compared to clients receiving treatment as usual (Carrera et al., 2016). The solution-focused group therapy focused on exceptions, interrupting problematic patterns, and paradoxical interventions (Carrera et al., 2016). However, the solution-focused group therapy did not utilize more common techniques such as the miracle question and scaling questions.

Elements of Dialogue

Adaptations of solution-focused dialogue across the globe highlight a particular emphasis on cultural dialect and importance in language. A study in the Czech Republic emphasized the utilization of client metaphor as a driving force for clients engaging in solution-focused treatment (Zatloukal et al., 2019). The process of using metaphors in therapy and the choice between client-driven and therapist-driven metaphor had particular importance when matching client dialogue. Like the process of listen, select, and build, therapists listen to listen to the client's metaphor, then "capture" and "explore" the metaphor (Zatloukal et al., 2019). Zatoukal et al. stress the explicit importance of client's language and to take language at face value. The syntax of dialogue may shift across understandings and utilization of language.

Syntax, grammar, and the utility of abstract and concrete language may impact the therapist's understanding of what is important to clients, or if their clients understand what is asked of them. Suitt et al. (2019) utilized thirteen Spanish-translated solution-focused tools to understand the cultural application and utility of linguistically modified solution-focused practice. Establishing linguistic modifications mirrors similar solution-focused processes of co-construction in which the therapist and client may reiterate statements until mutual understanding has been reached. In some instances, modifications across culture involved expanding condensed solution-focused questioning. For example, Suitt et al. (2019) expands the question of pre-session change based on participant response to "What things related to the issue you came here about have improved/been between since you scheduled gave you the appointment with me?" (Adaptations were originally in Spanish adapted to English for publication.) Other adaptations involve a more direct utilization of language such as, "How would you like things to be when the problem does not exist?" (Suitt et al., 2019, p.112). In a language-based model that centers on the utilization of dialogue, it is important for the therapist to understand how and in what way the implementation of SFBT might shift based on varying cultural and geographic application; an understanding of client-centered will only go as far as the therapist's willingness to know the client and client context.

Cultural Attunement

Solution-focused emphasis on strengths, resources, and dialogue allows the client to tap into what is culturally and appropriately salient to their experience (Reddy et al., 2022). Doing so allows the therapist to curiously engage the client system in their therapeutic process. This cultural attunement demystifies the process of therapy and lessens the hierarchy in the therapeutic relationship by allowing the client active voice to share what may or may not be working. Cultural attunement is practiced through the incorporation of filial piety in Taiwanese/Chinese utilize of solution-focused therapy (Hsu & Wang, 2011). Filial piety impacts inter- and intrapersonal behaviors. Filial piety identifies the individual self in reference to family and relationships. Hsu and Wang (2011) introduce an integrative model that incorporates practices of SFBT and filial piety: positive opening and problem description, transformation of problem into hopeful and preferred future prospects, exploration and utilization of exceptions, recycling of counseling components, and consolidation of counseling progress to subsequent life situations. This model highlights unique cultural considerations: positive reframing at the conceptualization level, promotion of relationship-based perspectives, and facilitation of pragmatic solutions via the counseling process (Hsu & Wang, 2011). Consistent with the focus and priority of interpersonal relationships, solution-focused therapy has been adapted and implemented across global contexts through a deliberate and purposeful understanding of how the client(s) show up to therapy and the context that surrounds the therapeutic lens.

Future Research Directions

The future of SFBT, and its application internationally, includes more writing and research on the co-construction process. For almost two decades, the process of having a solution-focused dialogue has been noted more in the literature. Previously, SFBT techniques were the main focus. The shift in studying dialogue occurred near the end of Steve de Shazer and Insoo Kim Berg's lives when they reconnected with Janet Bavelas, a communication researcher. Both Steve and Insoo believed that the focus of SFBT training needed to include closely examining dialogue. After their deaths (2005 and 2007), Janet Bavelas' method of microanalysis became the premier mechanism for understanding "what's different" in SFBT conversations.

As we move forward, additional research on the components of SFBT conversations should occur. This can include more detailed studies about what makes solution-focused talk different from non-solution-focused talk to train the next generation on the model. For example, Fredrike Bannink of the Netherlands views SFBT and *positive* CBT to be more similar than different (Bannink, 2013). This claim differs from the research conducted by Smock Jordan et al (2013) in North America where we (SJ) found that the negative topic choice in CFT sessions was significantly higher when compared to SFBT sessions. The positive topic choice content was also significantly higher in SFBT sessions when compared to CBT sessions. Does culture and language play a role in model differences?

Another way to study SFBT dialogue is by examining the cultural nuances within language. When the culture of the therapist and client differ, more precise calibrating may need to occur. For example, SFBT is very future focused. Some cultures are past or present focused by nature. When the time orientation of the therapist and client differ, modifications of traditional SFBT questions may need to occur. Another example of this might include differences in cultural values and religion. The "miracle question" is a good example. In some cultures and/or religions, "miracle" takes on a Judeo-Christian meaning. Kayrouz and Hansen (2019) conducted a study looking at the various cultural adaptations of the miracle question. Substitutes included "fresh start, dreams, at your best, harmony with people and life, click your fingers, something big is possible, and on track." They provide a framework for deciding the best "fit" in altering this classic SFBT question.

Finally, analyzing non-English SFBT dialogues will provide insight into solution-building conversations. For example, Gonzalez Suitt et al (2019 conducted the first linguistic transformation of the model in Latin America. Her study found that some language modifications of SFBT needed to occur when working with her sample. More studies like this one are needed to understand the cultural adaptations needed when applying the model to various populations.

Resources and Further Reading

Bavelas, J. B. (2020). Face-to-face dialogue: theory, research, and applications. Oxford University Press.

Brokerick, N. (2017). From solving problems to finding solutions. In D. Hogan, D. Hogan, J. Tuomola, & A. K. L. Yeo. (Eds.) Solution Foccused Practic in Asia, 105–109. Routledge.

Cauffman, L. (2006). The solution tango. Marshall Cavendish Limited & Cyan Communications Limited.

De Jong, P., & Kim Berg, I. (2013). Interviewing for solutions. (4th edition). Cengage Learning.

de Shazer, S. (1988). *Clues: Investigating solutions in brief therapy*. New York: Norton.

de Shazer, S. (1994). *Words were originally magic*. Norton.

Dierolf, K., Hogan, D., van der Hoorn, S., & Wignaraja, S. (Eds). Solution focused practice around the world, Routledge, New York.

Froerer, A. S., Cziffra-Bergs, J. V., Kim, J. S., & Connie, E. E. (2018). Solution-focused brief therapy with clients managing trauma. Oxford University Press.

Furman, B., & Abola, T. (1992). Solution talk: hosting therapeutic conversations. Norton & Company.

Gilligan, S., & Price, R. (1993). Therapeutic conversations. Norton & Company.

Kayrouz, R., & Hansen, S. (2019, December 23). I Don't Believe in Miracles: Using the Ecological Validity Model to Adapt the Miracle Question to Match the Client's Cultural Preferences and Characteristics. Professional Psychology: Research and Practice. Advance online publication. http://dx.doi.org/10.1037/pro0000283

Kim, J. S. (2014). Solution-focused brief therapy: a multicultural approach. Sage Publications Inc.

Lethem, J. (1994). Moved to tears, moved to action: Solution focused brief therapy with women and children. BT Press.

Miller, S. D., Duncan, B. L., & Hubble, M. A. (1997). Escape from babel: toward a unifying language for psychotherapy practice. Norton & Company.

Milner, J., Myers, S. (2017). Working with violence and confrontation using solution focused approaches: creative practice with children, young people and adults. Jessica Kingsley Publishers.

Nelson, T. S. (2019). Solution-focused brief therapy with families. Routledge.

Ouer, R. (2016). Solution-focused brief therapy with the LGBT community: creating futures through hope and resilience. Routledge.

Preston, J., & Johnson, J. (2020). Clinical psychopharmacology made ridiculously simple. (9th edition). MedMaster Inc.

Reddy, S. M., Naseh, M., Panisch, L. S., Rafieifar, M., O'Gara J. L., Cervantez, C. (2022). Solution-focused brief therapy in Iran: A scoping review of the outcome literature. *Journal of Evidence-Based Social Work*, 19, 493–508.

Suitt, G. K., Franklin, C., Cornejo, R., Castro, Y., & Jordan, S. S. (2019). Solution-focused brief therapy for Chilean primary care patients: Exploring a linguistic adaptation. *Journal of Ethnicity in Substance Abuse*. 18, 103–128.

Zatloukal, L., Zakovsky, D., & Bezdickova, E. (2018). Utilizing metaphors in solution-focused therapy. *Contemporary Family Therapy*, 41, 24–36.

References

Bannink, F. (2013). Are you ready for positive cognitive behavioral therapy? The journal of happiness & well-being, *1*(2), 61–69.

Barnai, A. & Soregi, V. (2021). Facing new challenges using a solution focused approach. In Yusuf, D. (ed.) The Solution Focused Approach with Children and Young People, 130–139. Routledge.

Bavelas, J. B., Gerwing, J., & Healing, S. (2017). Doing mutual understanding. Calibrating with micro-sequences in face-to-face dialogue. Journal of Pragmatics, 121, 91–112.

Cantwell, P. & Holmes, S. (1994). Social construction: A paradigm shift for systemic therapy and training, The Australian and New Zealand Journal of Family Therapy, 15, 17–26.

Carrera, M., Cabero, A., Gonzalez, S., Rodriguez, N., Garcia, C., Hernandez, L., & Manjon, J. (2016).

Clark, H. H. (1996). Using language. Cambridge, UK: Cambridge University Press.

Clark, H. H., & Schaefer, E. F. (1987). Collaborating on contributions to conversations. Language and Cognitive Processes, 2(1), 19–41.

De Jong, P., & Berg, I. K. (2013). Interviewing for solutions (4th ed.) [DVD]. Brooks/Cole, Cengage Learning.

De Jong, P., Jordan, S. S., Healing, S., & Gerwing, J. (2020). Building miracles in dialogue: Observing co-construction through a microanalysis of calibrating sequences. Journal of Systemic Therapies, *39*(2), 84–108.

de Shazer & Berg, (1992) Doing therapy: A poststructual revision (article). Journal of Marital and Family Therapy, 18(1), 71–81. https://doi.org/10.1111/j.1752-0606.1992.tb00916.x

de Shazer, S. (1991). Putting difference to work. Norton.

Gergen, K. J. (1992). The social constructionist movement in modern psychology.

Hsu, W., & Wang, C. D. C. (2011). Integrating Asian clients' filial piety beliefs into solution-focused brief therapy. International Journal of Advanced Counseling, *33*, 322–334. DOI: 10.1007/s10447-011-9133-5

Jordan, S. S., Froerer, A., & Bavelas, J. (2013). Microanalysis of positive and negative content in solution-focused brief therapy and cognitive behavioral therapy expert sessions. Journal of Systemic Therapies, *32*, 46–59. https://10.1521/jsyt.2013.32.3.46

Korman, H., Bavelas, J. B., & De Jong, P. (2013). Microanalysis of formulations in solution focused brief therapy, cognitive behavioral therapy, and motivational interviewing. Journal of Systemic Therapies, 32(3), 31–45.

McGee, D., Del Vento, A., & Bavelas, J. B. (2005). An interactional model of questions as therapeutic interventions. Journal of Marital and Family Therapy, 31, 371–384.

Neipp, M. C., & Beyebach, M. (2022). The Global Outcomes of Solution-Focused Brief Therapy: A Revision. *The American Journal of Family Therapy*, ahead-of-print(ahead-of-print), 1–18. https://doi.org/10.1080/01926187.2022.2069175

Seidel, A. & Hedley, D. (2008). The use of solution-focused brief therapy with older adults in Mexico: A preliminary study. The American Journal of Family Therapy, *36*, 242–252. DOI: 10.1080/01926180701291279

19

BRIDGING TRAINING AND EXPERIENCES

Expanding Clinical Practices with Latinx Communities

Melissa M. Yzaguirre and Andres Larios Brown

Introduction

Studies have shown the negative impact on Latinx family's well-being due to the increase of immigration policy in the United States in the last several years (Rayburn et al., 2021; Torres et al., 2018; Vespa et al., 2018). Unfortunately, the racist, xenophobic, and anti-immigrant societal cultures, values, and structures maintained in the United States have left Latinx parents and children vulnerable to institutional racism and discrimination (Perreira et al., 2006; Rayburn et al., 2021; Torres et al., 2018). These negative ideologies trickle down to impact various life contexts for Latinx families such as the workplace, health care, and local government (Andrade et al., 2021; Bronfenbrenner, 1979; Viruell-Fuentes et al., 2012). The diverse contextual challenges Latinx families are exposed to leave them susceptible to adverse mental health outcomes such as psychological distress, depression, anxiety, and substance abuse (Alegría et al., 2008; Stein et al., 2012; Torres et al., 2018).

Parents are left to find necessary coping strategies when exposed to discrimination in these interrelated systems, ultimately influencing the protective response strategies they will pass down to their children (Cross et al., 2020; Else-Quest & Morse, 2015; Hughes, 2003). For instance, Latinx parents' desire to inculcate cultural values has shown to be a protective factor as their children positively adapt and acculturate to U.S. mainstream culture (Bouza et al., 2018; Cross et al., 2020; Parra-Cardona et al., 2012). Growing evidence suggests that ethnic-racial socialization (i.e., parent messages regarding race and ethnicity to children) is a key contributor to supporting Latinx family's resilience and coping with the effects of ethnic-racial discrimination (Ayón et al., 2020; Hughes et al., 2006). To support Latinx families in therapy, there is a need to acknowledge and understand the different ethnic-racial and cultural considerations of being a Latinx parent in the United States and how this impacts child development (e.g., Ayón, 2016; Bernal & Sáez-Santiago, 2006; Stein et al., 2016).

There has been an increase in research dedicated to promoting culturally informed practices across mental health disciplines to help meet the needs of different ethnic-racial

DOI: 10.4324/9781003297871-22

groups (e.g., García Coll et al., 1996; Griner & Smith, 2006; Rotheram & Phinney, 1987; Stevenson, 1994; Sue, 1998). Given the growing Latinx population in the United States and the need for comprehensive culturally inclusive mental health care, it is critical to understand therapists' application of relevant practices and considerations when working with Latinx families (Cross et al., 2020). The conceptual and theoretical efforts in Western family therapists' practices to bolster inclusion in therapeutic approaches have demonstrated great benefits for positive mental and behavioral health outcomes, and the promotion of positive parent-child relationships (Ayón, 2016; Bermúdez et al., 2010; Parra-Cardona et al., 2012). Further, the attention to the ethnic-racial background and culture-specific circumstances has been shown to resonate more with families and address unique issues with which they struggle, thereby increasing the effectiveness of treatment (Coard et al., 2004; Domenech-Rodríguez & Wieling, 2004; Parra-Cardona et al., 2019; PettyJohn et al., 2020; Turner et al., 2004).

This chapter provides an overview of therapeutic considerations and practices to support therapists trained in the United States who work with domestic and international Latinx populations. A literature synthesis includes the contextual considerations (e.g., immigration, socialization, acculturation) and potential impacts on Latinx families. Informed by Hook and colleagues' (2017) definition of cultural humility, we encourage the reader to consider the cultural and social similarities and differences they share with their clients in treatment as a means to promote personal and professional growth as a therapist. Further, to remain open-minded and curious about the *humanity* of working with ethnic/racial minority groups. As family therapists based in the United States, we mirror these efforts through our lived experiences as clinicians who have worked with Latinx individuals, couples, and families through case examples. Recommendations are provided to further social advocacy efforts and keep therapists cognizant of structural influences when working with Latinx populations.

Inclusive Language

The field of couple/marriage and family therapy has been dedicated to honoring diversity, social justice, and multicultural awareness since its inception in the 1960s. One meaningful aspect regarding culture is the consideration of *language* (including native tongue, mannerisms, idioms, and nuances). For instance, the broad and largely politized pan-ethnic terms "Hispanic" and "Latino" are often used interchangeably in the United States to describe populations of Latin American or Spanish-speaking descent (Hayes-Bautista & Chapa, 1987; Martinez & Gonzalez, 2021; U.S. Census Bureau, 2021). Recent adjustments to the terms "Latino" such as "Latino/a," "Latinx," and "Latine" have gained momentum in academic literature and activist groups in an attempt to raise awareness and inclusivity to the gender binaries encoded in the Spanish language (Logue, 2015; Salinas, 2020; Vidal-Ortiz & Martinez, 2018). The use of Hispanic/Latino/a/x/e brings forward the complexities and heterogeneity encompassing a person's Latin American culture and identity.

The use of "x" in Latinx as a marker of inclusion is debated among scholars. Some advocate that the shift is an essential signal of safety, inclusion, and liberation to those who have been marginalized and oppressed in many ways, while others suggest that the term is narrow and stems from ivory tower frameworks (Dame-Griff, 2021; Scharrón-del Río, & Aja, 2015; Scharrón-del Río & Aja, 2020). Language is a powerful and deeply meaningful part of a culture that carries social understandings, symbols, political positions, and power

(Kramsch, 2014). Thus, there is great attention needed to empower the diverse voices represented in scholarly writing in a way that captures self-identity to ethnic-racial identity, country of origin, class, cultural heritage, and migration history (Taylor et al., 2006). As authors, we hold a great deal of privilege to provide readers with important information and facts that may be used to inform clinical practice. As such, we have a responsibility to our stakeholders (i.e., Hispanic/Latino/a/x/e populations) to ensure accurate representation is put forward on their behalf.

Where We Stand

Much like previous literature, this chapter does not seek to challenge the coined terms that are largely used in academic literature or bind individuals to a "label" or "box." Instead, it aims to raise awareness of the importance of justification and explanation for using specific terminology in the therapeutic context. To model transparency and intentionality, we predominantly use the term Latinx to refer to populations that include persons who self-identify with Latin American culture and identity. Additionally, efforts will be dedicated to appropriately corresponding matching language used when identifying specific Latinx groups (e.g., Mexican, Cuban, Puerto Rican) as an added measure to honor the unique complexities associated with their ethnic and cultural backgrounds. Our hope is, moving forward, for family therapists to be mindful of the potentially harmful outcomes that come with over-generalizing or making assumptions about their clients' backgrounds or origins. Instead, it is important to embrace the complexities of these groups and affirm the experiences of all Latinx identities grounded in their respective cultural background.

Encompassing the Uniqueness of Latinx Culture

For Latinx families, the ability to socialize their children with an affirming sense of their cultural heritage and racial-ethnic identity has been shown to be a protective factor in children's behavioral and academic outcomes (Hughes et al., 2006; Umaña-Taylor et al., 2004). Despite the increased focus on Latinx families and immigration-related outcomes, less work has aimed to equip therapists with approaching immigration-related conversations inclusively and sensitively in the therapeutic context (Ayón et al., 2020; Torres et al., 2018). It is critical that therapists' efforts to understand and support Latinx families be attuned to the disparities and discrimination facing ethnic-racial minority groups and their families.

Culturally adapted practices are especially effective in improving therapeutic outcomes among Latinx parent populations. Cultural adaptation encourages therapist practices "to consider language, culture, and the context in such a way that it is compatible with the client's cultural patterns, meanings, and values" (Bernal et al., 2009, p. 362). Without disrupting fidelity or diminishing model integrity, culturally adapted treatment approaches improve existing models to be culturally relevant to historically marginalized communities (e.g., Castro et al., 2004; Bernal & Sáez-Santiago, 2006). Further, cultural adaptation practices among Latinx communities can be used as therapeutic tools to strengthen parenting practices and parent-child relationships. We acknowledge that no intervention or approach can (or is meant to) capture all the unique considerations of working with Latinx families. Instead, we offer examples of interventions and practices that have captured the positive application of culture by encompassing the uniqueness of a person's *language* (including native tongue, mannerisms, idioms, and nuances), *worldviews* (i.e., values, customs, beliefs, and traditions exemplified by values of family obligations, respect for adults), and broader social and economic *context* (e.g., coping with discrimination, migration phases, acculturative stress, social support availability, or relationship to one's country of origin) (Bernal & Saez-Santiago, 2006).

For example, scholars such as Parra-Cardona and colleagues (2012) have culturally adapted an evidence-based parenting intervention called "Criando con Amor, Promoviendo Armonia y Superacion" (CAPAS; Raising Children with Love, Promoting Harmony, and Self-Improvement; Parra-Cardona et al., 2012). The intentional efforts to preserve cultural values and attend to considerations like immigration status were at the forefront of this intervention adaptation, extending prior initial research focused on linguistic translation and attention to culture (Bernal & Sáez-Santiago, 2006). This work promotes the importance of linguistic, immigration status considerations, and cultural appropriateness when working with Latinx families and ensuring programs understand the importance of cultural sensitivity (Parra-Cardona et al., 2012; Parra Cardona et al., 2019). Despite great progress, more research is needed to examine therapists' abilities to engage actively and work effectively when incorporating these culturally relevant practices in treatment (Ayón et al., 2020; Soto et al., 2018). Given the increased representation of diverse racial and ethnic populations in the United States, conformity to therapeutic approaches traditionally created for a White American society is no longer a standard for treatment. Thus, promoting inclusive practices in therapy can provide therapists with the necessary tools to effectively work with Latinx families.

Though tremendous progress in culturally adapted interventions continues, not all therapists are trained in or engage in these interventions. Therapists each have their unique approaches to how they view a presenting problem, ultimately guiding their course of treatment. Rather than narrowing it down to a therapeutic approach, we offer social contextual considerations for therapists working with Latinx populations in the United States For example, Hughes and colleagues (2006) identify ethnic-racial socialization (ERS) as the transmission of ethnic-racial information, values, and perspectives from parents to children. The four major dimensions of ERS are cultural socialization, preparation for bias, promotion of mistrust, and egalitarianism (Hughes et al., 2006; Umaña-Taylor & Hill, 2020). The dimensions of ERS may be relevant for therapists working with diverse populations and seeking to integrate ethnic-racial background and culture in their practice.

Recently, Ayón and colleagues (2020) published the first systematic review focused on empirical literature targeting ERS strategies (i.e., cultural socialization, preparation for bias, promotion of mistrust, and egalitarianism) specifically with Latinx families, which resulted in 68 identified studies. Interestingly, *immigration-related socialization* was discussed as a new strategy not previously identified as an ERS dimension, but a rising discussion among Latinx families due to immigration policies (see Ayón, 2016; Ayón et al., 2020). Several empirical studies have highlighted the reoccurring weight parents hold to address the painful realities of discrimination and ethnic-racial bias (e.g., immigration) encounters their children are likely to be exposed to (Ayon et al., 2020; e.g., Ayón, 2016; Ayón et al., 2019; Else-Quest & Morse, 2015; Park et al., 2019). One example includes Huguley and colleagues' (2019) meta-analysis that included 68 U.S.-based studies with youth between kindergarten and college ages to investigate the effects of parental ERS on the ethnic-racial identity of children of color. The results revealed that pride and heritage socialization were most positively associated with youth ethnic-racial identity. Further, Latinx families held the highest positive associations between parental ERS and youth's ethnic-racial identity

(Huguley et al., 2019). Additionally, implications found across studies in the systematic review emphasized the need for therapists to incorporate ERS strategies and measures in practice in order to support and empower families who come up against discrimination (Ayón et al., 2020; Hughes et al., 2006; Umaña-Taylor et al., 2004; Viruell-Fuentes et al., 2012).

Holistic Advocacy as an International Family Therapist

Cultural humility describes a therapist's ability to hold "an accurate perception of their cultural values as well as maintain an other-oriented perspective that involves respect, lack of superiority and attunement regarding their own cultural beliefs and values" (Hook et al., 2017, p. 29). Since its recent incorporation into mental health practices, cultural humility has been shown to increase culturally relevant processes and identity self-reflection for therapists to consider when working with diverse populations (Davis et al., 2016; Fisher-Borne et al., 2015; Foronda, 2020). Although similar existing approaches aim to enhance therapists' knowledge and skills when working with diverse clients (e.g., multicultural competence, cultural competence), cultural humility holds a greater emphasis on a therapist's way of being with their clients by incorporating self-awareness and reflection about their personal values and beliefs (Ahluwalia et al., 1999; Gushue et al., 2008; Sue, 1978; Sue et al., 2009). Further, cultural humility extends related culturally relevant practices in that therapists can never fully account for all there is to know about cultural similarities and differences shared with their clients (Hook et al., 2013; Hook et al., 2017).

Cultural humility is considered an ever-growing process meant to help therapists self-reflect using an other-oriented perspective and reduce oppressive barriers which may prevent optimal treatment outcomes (Davis et al., 2016). Further, cultural humility identifies learning about culture and diversity as a lifelong growing process, not a destination meant to be reached (Hook et al., 2013; Hook et al., 2017). In essence, cultural humility captures both the importance of culturally relevant skills and self-reflection that come with therapists' different identities and influences carried over when working with diverse ethnic-racial populations. Therapists with higher levels of cultural humility refuse an expert stance when working with diverse populations. Instead, the use of self-evaluation helps therapists push back on potentially stereotyping biased interpretation behavior and allow room for a more open understanding about the encounters their clients have through their own lived experiences. To provide effective treatment, these practices are necessary and beneficial for therapists working with Latinx populations facing unique cultural disparities in the United States (Cooper et al., 2020; Soto et al., 2018; Taylor et al., 2006).

Clinical Case Example

A therapist's self is a foundational aspect of therapeutic work, often accounting for the utility of therapeutic interventions (Asay & Lambert, 1999). While there are a number of therapeutic modalities and frameworks from which a therapist can work, Satir's human growth and human transformation philosophy explicitly names self-of-the-therapist as a tool for therapeutic practice (Satir et al, 1991; Satir, 1972 & 1964). As such, each therapist that operates from a Satir lens will weave in aspects of self to the work they do (Satir et al, 1983). Thus, therapeutic interventions within the following examples will differ, where

Melissa offers a more traditional approach, and Andres demonstrates embracing a sense of self, education about cultural background/beliefs, and therapeutic intuition.

Authors Reflection Statement

Melissa Marie Yzaguirre (She/Her/Ella). I am a cisgender, heterosexual female, bilingual second-generation Mexican American, and first-generation college graduate. I am the third youngest of six children born in California and raised in a diverse, non-traditional household in Nevada. As a family therapist based in the United States, I have provided individual, couple, and family treatment for clients of diverse backgrounds (e.g., gender, sexual orientation, race/ethnicity, and language), including services for English and Spanish speaking Latino/a/x populations. I focus heavily on building a strong therapeutic alliance with clients by prioritizing inclusive approaches throughout my practice. Specifically, I use processes such as cultural humility (Hook et al., 2013; Hook et al., 2017), intersectionality (Crenshaw, 1989, 1991), and experiential therapy (Satir et al., 1991) to address the various positions my clients and I hold at the forefront of treatment. I remain active and flexible in learning from the differences and similarities we bring in the therapy room.

By stating some of the same positions I have identified in this introduction, I have experienced stronger therapeutic alliances and depth to the clients' presenting problems to the treatment room. These practices are also used in supervision. The information I learn from clients guides my therapeutic approaches to ensure they are culturally relevant to their needs. I have come to understand in my therapeutic experience that theories and frameworks gained from training are meant to provide us with different perspectives to view presenting problems. While no one theory or approach can (or should) be used to capture the complexity of a client's diverse background, I use the various identities and experiences everyone brings to the therapy room to influence the best treatment approach. Remaining in the position as a life-long learner allows me to remain open to the expertise my clients bring to treatment and identify points of adaptation necessary to support them in reaching their therapeutic goals.

Case Description

Following the events of the 2016 election, I worked with the Villatoro family, who are composed of mother (Joanna) who is 42 years old and daughter (Roselyn) who is 17 years old (pseudonyms were used to protect client identity). The identified patient of the family was Roselyn, with Joanna reporting that Roselyn was unable to focus on schoolwork and was concerned with her recent change in behavior. Joanna and Roselyn were born in Mexico and moved to the United States when Roselyn was roughly four years old.

In acknowledging their migration to the United States, I took this opportunity to position myself as a second-generation bilingual therapist. I posed the question of language preference early on. Joanna reported that she preferred to speak Spanish, and Roselyn preferred to speak English. To this day, I recall the immediate shift in the room by posing this question. I could feel a sense of comfort from Joanna as she asked, "¿Y de dónde son tus padres?" or "where are your parents from?" I took this as another opportunity to strengthen the therapeutic relationship and gain valuable information from the family. I responded with my mother's hometown in Mexico and shared that she migrated to the

United States when she was a teenager. During the following sessions, I worked with Joanna and Roselyn to gather information about their concerns about the presenting problems.

During one session, I noticed the conversation about immigration policies continued to come up, and I noticed Roselyn's discomfort as she sat in her chair. Given the recent political shift, I took a moment to re-discuss confidentiality with Roselyn and explain that anything she wanted to share related to immigration would remain private. As it turns out, Roselyn shared that she was in the United States under the Deferred Action for Childhood Arrivals (DACA) policy, an administrative relief from deportation. Immediately, she became frustrated and shouted, "people just don't understand!" I allowed for a moment of silence as tears slowly ran down her cheeks. Joanna wiped Roselyn's tears and said, "está bien hija" or "it's alright daughter."

Rather than assume in that moment what Roselyn could have meant in stating that others don't understand, I validated her bravery to "let it out." I then told her, "I can see you are hurting right now. I can feel the heavy weight in your statement about no one understanding. I appreciate you letting it out because it must be exhausting to be in your position right now." She nodded in agreement and remained silent. I followed up with, "I hear you and want to acknowledge that you have two people in this room right now who want to understand. If it is alright with you, I would like to ask you to give us that chance."

At that moment, Joanna grabbed Roselyn's hand to reassure her daughter that she had the support she needed in the room. Roselyn went on to describe that she was scared about what her and her mother's future would look like. She had always worked hard to maintain good grades with hopes of going to college. Roselyn also felt she had owed it to her mother to go to college and have a successful career. She wanted to prove that her mother's sacrifices in coming to the United States was not for nothing. As a first-generation, she longed for "the American dream." Following news of the 2016 election, she had no idea if that would be a possibility anymore. She went on to share her fear of being deported and losing everything. This was the only home she knew, and with her future left in a completely unknown stage, she shared, "so what is the point?" Here, she referred to losing interest in schoolwork. To this end, Joanna posed the question, "¿Es por eso que has estado actuando tan diferente?" or "is this why you have been acting so different?" It was also an eye-opening moment for Joanna to realize the amount of pressure Roselyn had been putting on herself, even prior to the results of the election.

As I was not aware of explicit practices for approaching the topic of immigration prior to this point, I allowed Roselyn to take the expert stance in the room. I owned that there were no "tricks or trainings" that could help me get this conversation "right." I also acknowledged that getting it "right" was not the point of the conversation. Instead, by approaching the conversation with empathy and curiosity, I was able to understand the extent of the systemic impact the recent political current events had on her. Instead of trying to solve the problem, we shifted the focus to the emotional experience shared by Joanna and Roselyn. Their vulnerability with each other allowed space to connect on a deeper level and helped to strengthen the parent-child relationship.

Authors Reflection Statement

Andres Larios Brown (They/He/Elle). Therapeutic training can often ask us to distance ourselves from the work we are doing, attempting to remove bias through the notion of neutrality. The discussion as to whether neutrality is possible given the influence that our values have in every facet of our work is one of philosophy and worldview (Barton & Bishop, 2014). As a post-modern, social constructionist, and intersectional feminist therapist and healer, it is my position that not only can I not remove my full bias, but that lived experience adds depth and human connection to the incredibly human process of therapy and healing. These ideas are further articulated by Acosta (2018), who states the importance of looking to how queer, feminists of color have used *theory of the flesh* – lived experience fueled politics, activism, and scholarship – as a tool for creating theory (Acosta, 2018). As a Queer & Non-Binary m*escla bella* (beautiful mix) of a father who immigrated from Guatemala and a mother who is an American citizen with Western European roots who are divorced, my experience of navigating the complexity of personal identity development in the context of colonization, immigration, internal and external racism and bias have provided me with an understanding of the many nuanced ways in which our role as systemic therapists demands that we understand our own complex identities and values, as well as the identities and values of those we work with. This ongoing understanding is present in my scholarship focusing on queer identity development among collectist and community-focused cultures as well as my clinical work at Encircle Therapy, a non-profit that works with LGBTQIA+ people and families from religiously conservative cultures. I feel honored to be a healer, and believe that we are truly whole when we are in authentic connection and community with others, and seek to bridge the gap between research and clinical practice.

Case Description

I had the honor of healing with Elena (pseudonyms were used to protect client identity). Elena came to see me while she was finishing up her graduate degree in business at a Predominantly White Institution (PWI) in the United States. She had sought me out specifically because I had been invited to talk with a group of Latinx parents about trauma, parenting, and identity development. She told me that one of her parent's friends told her that there was "uno de nosotros" or that there was a therapist in our community that was "one of us." She told me that she had avoided therapy for years due to fear of being misunderstood, distrust of "colonizers," and difficulty in "always having the right words in English."

> *Therapist Reflections: I have read in many chapters the collectivist nature of Latino communities. My own experiences increased my understanding that for many Latino/a/x/es populations, community and shared identities are important factors in building trust. I had specifically advocated for larger group meetings and trainings, educational nights to connect with and build rapport with the entire community. I had hoped that I would be able to share WHO I am with the communities, in an effort to communicate that seeking therapy would not be another instance of interacting with cultures where we feel disempowered. Elena coming to see me could be tied to that effort.*

In our first session, we talked about Elena's presenting concerns, her history, her family of origin, her current positions, and her identities. Elena shared that she had immigrated to the United States from a pueblito (small town) in central America when she was a young mother and had raised her 3 children mostly on her own. She shared how she had always struggled with romantic relationships because she was a "strong woman" and that many of her partners were intimidated by her. We cried together as she shared her immigration story, as well as her experiences with being mistreated by people due to her skin color and her gender. We continued to cry as she shared experiences of sexual assault, abuse, and fear. Elena reported a significant amount of trauma. She shared with me some of her current symptoms (i.e., experiencing nightmares, flashbacks, anxiety/panic attacks, and self-harm), which seemed to be getting worse.

Therapist Reflections: Elena has many identities and experiences that are connected to my own. We covered a lot of ground in our initial meeting, much of which was done in a fluid conversational style. As she shared each part of her story, I was able to connect with not only the information she was sharing, but the EXPERIENCE she was sharing. To do this, I had spent years unpacking my own concepts of machismo (Binary Gender hierarchy and power differentials), navigating micro/macro aggressions at PWI's and throughout my life, experiences of trauma, healing family ruptures and cultural differences, and honing my therapeutic self. This work showed up in me being able to tap into my experiences for empathy, but not have those experiences take center stage in myself or the session. By so doing, Elena was able to show up in her full self and feel me with her in her story.

Elena and I spent just under a year together doing what she referred to as "sanando mi alma" or "healing my soul." Elena expressed experiences of dreams that were significant, which we explored together in session. Many of the dreams involved catholic saints and indigenous imagery, some as guides and protectors, and some as evil spirits. Elena and I processed experiences of abuse, tapping into those protective imagery and colors. On days when we were deepening into the wounds, Elena and I would bring stones, blankets, and clothing that represented protection, strength, and power. Elena and I would co-create the space of "limpiando" or "cleansing" using scents and other adjustments to the environment. As Elena would share her trauma, she would begin to become dissociated. Rather than doing a simple breathing exercise, a practice I often help people stay within the window of tolerance, Elena and I would breathe in the color of "safety" or would ask our guardian angels to walk with us through the pain.

Therapist Reflections: I approach therapy with the lens of collaboration- honoring and utilizing each person's "expertise" in experience as well as my training and therapeutic intuition. I am rooted in Satir's human growth model and philosophy, which offered me the agility to use each session as an experiential space for healing. I utilized a number of therapeutic interventions (e.g., parts work, increasing sense of self, understanding physiological responses to danger and trauma, reducing activated stress responses, and increasing capacity) to honor and respond to needs. Given Elena's culture and spirituality, I framed our work in terms and concepts that made sense to her. Rather than doing "interventions," we practiced "rituals."

During one session, Elena shared a dream where she was begging her saint for protection, and he was unresponsive. Elena shared that she was covered in purple flowers, and that she felt abandoned once again by a male protector, a theme in her trauma. As Elena and I explored this, she began to experience an incredible amount of distress in session, and she began to weep and speak only in Spanish. Up to this point, much of our sessions were

Spanglish (a mixture of Spanish and English). The emergence of Spanish only signaled to me that we were in early trauma, and that the pain was experienced in a brain and a world that spoke and understood Spanish. Instead of jumping in to save or "protect" Elena from her pain, my response was to say "Tienes todo lo que necesitas. El poder eres tu. El poder eres tu" or "You have all that you need. You are the power. The power is you." As I spoke, Elena breathed in deeply, and repeated "Soy el poder. El poder soy yo" or "I am the power. The power is me." I invited her to access her inner power and describe what color it was. She shared that it was a purple cloud, and that it was filled with flowers. As she focused on that purple, her body became more empowered, and her tears softened, and she held herself with warmth and compassion.

She later shared that the next night, she dreamt that she had a conversation with her guardian saint, during which he shared with her that he wasn't abandoning her, but that "tienes todo lo que necesitas. El poder eres tu. El poder eres tu" "You have all that you need. You are the power. The power is you." We talked about how she had been looking to others to protect her, and that her power had been taken from her. She shared that since that experience, she had found that purple was her "self-power color" and that she was reclaiming her "poder" or "power." We discussed the process of reclaiming, and the ways in which she could tap into her inner healer and seek wisdom from her innate sense of self.

After that session, Elena's symptoms reduced significantly and in a consistent way. Elena began to sleep throughout the nights and decorated her room with purple.

Therapist reflections: This healing experience did not come from a textbook. There is no EBT model that orients us to engage with dream saints, colors, and switch languages. The phrasing is not a step in a manualized treatment. Instead, I tapped into my own internal wisdom. I had been collecting understanding of Elena's world from the very beginning and honoring it as essential for our healing journey. While I do not have a personal familiarity with Catholic saints and symbols, I do have access to people who do. I spent some time reading and researching angels, saints, colors, and imagery. Some of this framework came from my training in IFS, EMDR, and experiential therapies. However, the actual enactment of the session was less about following a script, and more about attuning to not only her experience of pain, but also her capacity to heal.

Three Key Takeaways

- First, it is important to broaden the understanding of the social contexts influencing Latinx populations well-being. This will ultimately result in more opportunities to be of service and to fullky understand the complexities which affect patient mental health.
- Second, therapists must consisder how their own positionality and influence treatment when working with Latinx populations.
- Finally, therapists working with the Latinx populations must identify opportunities in treatment to remain flexible and adapt practices with personal experience.

Conclusion

As systemic therapists, we are trained to pay attention to contexts in which our clients are exposed to. While understanding our client's contexts is essential to our work, there is also importance in understanding our own contexts. The training practices we are exposed to are meant to support our therapeutic approaches. However, this does not take away from the experiences we bring into the treatment room. As such, there is a balance that is needed that showcases both our knowledge as therapy experts and the humility that comes from working with clients of diverse ethnic-racial backgrounds. Moving forward, we encourage therapists working with Latinx populations to expand their use of *language* and reflect on the shared humanity they hold with their clients. As the world continues to diversify and grow, so must our practices. Thus, we are challenged to take what we have learned and add to them.

References

Acosta, K. L. (2018). Queering family scholarship: Theorizing from the borderlands. *Journal of Family Theory & Review*, 10(2), 406–418.

Ahluwalia, J., Baranowski, T., Braithwaite, R., & Resnicow, K. (1999). Cultural sensitivity in public health: defined and demystified. *Ethnicity & Disease*, 9(1), 10–21.

Alegría, M., Chatterji, P., Wells, K., Cao, Z., Chen, C. N., Takeuchi, D., ... & Meng, X. L. (2008). Disparity in depression treatment among racial and ethnic minority populations in the United States. *Psychiatric services*, 59(11), 1264–1272. https://doi.org/10.1176/appi.ps.59.11.1264

Andrade, N., Ford, A. D., & Alvarez, C. (2021). Discrimination and Latino health: A systematic review of risk and resilience. *Hispanic Health Care International*, 19(1), 5–16. https://doi.org/10.1177/1540415320921489

Asay, T. P., & Lambert, M. J. (1999). The empirical case for the common factors in therapy: Quantitative findings.

Ayón, C. (2016). Talking to Latino children about race, inequality, and discrimination: Raising families in an anti-immigrant political environment. *Journal of the Society for Social Work and Research*, 7(3), 449–477. https://doi.org/10.1086/686929

Ayón, C., & García, S. J. (2019). Latino immigrant parents' experiences with discrimination: Implications for parenting in a hostile immigration policy context. *Journal of Family Issues*, 40(6), 805–831. https://doi.org/10.1177/0192513X19827988

Ayón, C., Nieri, T., & Ruano, E. (2020). Ethnic-racial socialization among Latinx families: A Systematic review of the literature. *Social Service Review*, 94(4), 693–747. https://doi.org/10.1086/712413

Barton, A. W., & Bishop, R. C. (2014). Paradigms, processes, and values in family research. *Journal of Family Theory & Review*, 6(3), 241–256.

Bermúdez, J. M., Kirkpatrick, D., Hecker, L., & Torres-Robles, C. (2010). Describing Latinos families and their help-seeking attitudes: challenging the family therapy literature. *Contemporary Family Therapy: An International Journal*, 32(2). https://doi.org/10.1007/s10591-009-9110-x

Bernal, G., & Sáez-Santiago, E. (2006). Culturally centered psychosocial interventions. *Journal of Community Psychology*, 34(2), 121–132. https://doi.org/10.1002/jcop.20096

Bernal, G., Jiménez-Chafey, M. I., & Domenech Rodríguez, M. M. (2009). Cultural adaptation of treatments: A resource for considering culture in evidence-based practice. *Professional Psychology: Research and Practice*, 40(4), 361–368. https://doi.org/10.1037/a0016401

Bouza, J., Camacho-Thompson, D. E., Carlo, G., Franco, X., Coll, C. G., Halgunseth, L. C., & White, R. M. B. (2018). The science is clear: Separating families has long-term damaging psychological and health consequences for children, families, and communities. *Society for Research in Child Development*, 20.

Bronfenbrenner, U. (1979). Contexts of child rearing: Problems and prospects. *American psychologist*, 34(10), 844.

Castro, F. G., Barrera, M., & Martinez, C. R. (2004). The cultural adaptation of prevention interventions: Resolving tensions between fidelity and fit. *Prevention Science*, 5(1), 41–45.

Coard, S. I., Wallace, S. A., Stevenson, H. C., & Brotman, L. M. (2004). Towards culturally relevant preventive interventions: The consideration of racial socialization in parent training with African American families. *Journal of Child and Family Studies*, 13(3), 277–293. https://doi.org/10.1023/B:JCFS.0000022035.07171.f8

Cooper, D. K., Wieling, E., Domenech Rodríguez, M. M., Garcia-Huidobro, D., Baumann, A., Mejia, A., ... & Acevedo-Polakovich, I. D. (2020). Latinx mental health scholars' experiences with cultural adaptation and implementation of systemic family interventions. *Family Process*, 59(2), 492–508. https://doi.org/10.1111/famp.12433

Crenshaw, K. (1989). Demarginalizing the intersection of race and sex: A Black feminist critique of antidiscrimination doctrine, feminist theory, and antiracist politics. The University of Chicago Legal Forum, 1989(8), 138–167.

Crenshaw, K. W. (1991). Mapping the margins of intersectionality, identity politics and violence against women of color. *Stanford Law Review*, 43(6), 1241–1300. https://doi.org/10.2307/1229039

Cross, F. L., Agi, A., Montoro, J. P., Medina, M. A., Miller-Tejada, S., Pinetta, B. J., ... & Rivas-Drake, D. (2020). Illuminating ethnic-racial socialization among undocumented Latinx parents and its implications for adolescent psychosocial functioning. *Developmental Psychology*, 56(8), 1458–1474. https://doi.org/10.1037/dev0000826

Dame-Griff, E. C. (2021). What do we mean when we say "Latinx?": Definitional power, the limits of inclusivity, and the (un/re) constitution of an identity category. *Journal of International and Intercultural Communication*, 1–13. https://doi.org/10.1080/17513057.2021.1901957

Davis, D. E., DeBlaere, C., Brubaker, K., Owen, J., Jordan, T. A., Hook, J. N., & Van Tongeren, D. R. (2016). Microaggressions and perceptions of cultural humility in counseling. *Journal of Counseling & Development*, 94(4), 483–493. https://doi.org/10.1002/jcad.12107

Domenech-Rodríguez, M., & Wieling, E. (2004). Developing culturally appropriate, evidence-based treatments for interventions with ethnic minority populations. *Voices of color: First person accounts of ethnic minority therapists* (pp. 313–333). https://doi.org/10.4135/9781452231662.n18

Else-Quest, N. M., & Morse, E. (2015). Ethnic variations in parental ethnic socialization and adolescent ethnic identity: A longitudinal study. *Cultural Diversity and Ethnic Minority Psychology*, 21(1), 54–64. https://doi.org/10.1037/a0037820

Fisher-Borne, M., Cain, J. M., & Martin, S. L. (2015). From mastery to accountability: Cultural humility as an alternative to cultural competence. *Social Work Education*, 34(2), 165–181. https://doi.org/10.1080/02615479.2014.977244

Foronda, C. (2020). A theory of cultural humility. *Journal of Transcultural Nursing*, 31(1), 7–12. https://doi.org/10.1177/1043659619875184

García Coll, C., Lamberty, G., Jenkins, R., McAdoo, H. P., Crnic, K., Wasik, B. H., & Vázquez García, H. (1996). An integrative model for the study of developmental competencies in minority children. *Child Development*, 67(5), 1891–1914.

Griner, D., & Smith, T. B. (2006). Culturally adapted mental health intervention: A meta-analytic review. *Psychotherapy*, 43(4), 531–548. https://doi.org/10.1037/0033-3204.43.4.531

Gushue, G. V., Constantine, M. G., & Sciarra, D. T. (2008). The influence of culture, self-reported multicultural counseling competence, and shifting standards of judgment on perceptions of family functioning of white family counselors. *Journal of Counseling & Development*, 86(1), 85–94. https://doi.org/10.1002/j.1556-6678.2008.tb00629.x

Hayes-Bautista, D. E., & Chapa, J. (1987). Latino terminology: conceptual bases for standardized terminology. *American Journal of Public Health*, 77(1), 61–68.

Hook, J. N., Davis, D. E., Owen, J., Worthington, E. L., & Utsey, S. O. (2013). Cultural humility: Measuring openness to culturally diverse clients. *Journal of Counseling Psychology*, 60(3), 353–366. https://doi.org/10.1037/a0032595

Hook, J. N., Davis, D., Owen, J., & DeBlaere, C. (2017). *Cultural humility: Engaging diverse identities in therapy*. American Psychological Association. https://doi.org/10.1037/0000037-000

Hughes, D. (2003). Correlates of African American and Latino parents' messages to children about ethnicity and race: A comparative study of racial socialization. *American Journal of Community Psychology*, 31(1–2), 15–33. https://doi.org/10.1023/a:1023066418688

Hughes, D., Rodriguez, J., Smith, E. P., Johnson, D. J., Stevenson, H. C., & Spicer, P. (2006). Parents' ethnic-racial socialization practices: A review of research and directions for future study. *Developmental Psychology*, 42(5), 747–770. https://doi.org/10.1037/0012-1649.42.5.747

Huguley, J. P., Wang, M. T., Vasquez, A. C., & Guo, J. (2019). Parental ethnic–racial socialization practices and the construction of children of color's ethnic–racial identity: A research synthesis and meta-analysis. *Psychological Bulletin*, 145(5), 437.

Kramsch, C. (2014). Language and culture. *AILA Review*, 27(1), 30–55. https://doi.org/10.1075/aila.27.02kra

Logue, J. (2015). Latina/o/x. Inside Higher Ed. www.insidehighered.com/news/2015/12/08/students-adopt-gender-nonspecific-term-latinx-be-more-inclusive

Martínez, D. E., & Gonzalez, K. E. (2021). "Latino" or "Hispanic"? The Sociodemographic Correlates of Panethnic Label Preferences among US Latinos/Hispanics. *Sociological Perspectives*, 64(3), 365–386.

Park, Irene J. K., Han Du, Lijuan Wang, David R.Williams, and Margarita Alegria. 2019. "The role of parents' ethnic-racial socialization practices in the discrimination-depression link among Mexican-origin adolescents." *Journal of Clinical Child and Adolescent Psychology*, 49(3), 391–404.

Parra Cardona, J. R., Domenech-Rodriguez, M., Forgatch, M., Sullivan, C., Bybee, D., Holtrop, K., ... & Bernal, G. (2012). Culturally adapting an evidence-based parenting intervention for Latino immigrants: The need to integrate fidelity and cultural relevance. *Family Process*, 51(1), 56–72. https://doi.org/10.1111/j.1545-5300.2012.01386.x

Parra-Cardona, R., López-Zerón, G., Leija, S. G., Maas, M. K., Villa, M., Zamudio, E., ... & Domenech Rodríguez, M. M. (2019). A culturally adapted intervention for Mexican-origin parents of adolescents: The need to overtly address culture and discrimination in evidence-based practice. *Family Process*, 58(2), 334–352. https://doi.org/10.1111/famp.12381

Perreira, K. M., Chapman, M. V., & Stein, G. L. (2006). Becoming an American parent: Overcoming challenges and finding strength in a new immigrant Latino community. *Journal of Family Issues*, 27(10), 1383–1414. https://doi.org/10.1177/0192513X06290041

PettyJohn, M. E., Tseng, C. F., & Blow, A. J. (2020). Therapeutic utility of discussing therapist/client intersectionality in treatment: When and how?. *Family Process*, 59(2), 313–327. https://doi.org/10.1111/famp.12471

Rayburn, A. D., McWey, L. M., & Gonzales-Backen, M. A. (2021). Living under the shadows: Experiences of Latino immigrant families at risk for deportation. *Family Relations*, 70(2), 359–373. https://doi.org/10.1111/fare.12534

Rotheran, M. J., & Phinney, J. S. (1987). Childrens ethnic socialization. *Children's Ethnic Socialization: Pluralism and Development. Beverly Hills, CA: Sage*.

Salinas Jr, C. (2020). The complexity of the "x" in Latinx: How Latinx/a/o students relate to, identify with, and understand the term Latinx. *Journal of Hispanic Higher Education*, 19(2), 149–168. https://doi.org/10.1177/1538192719900382

Satir, V. (1964). *Conjoint family therapy*. Palo Alto, CA. Science and Behavior Books, Inc.

Satir, V. (1972). *Peoplemaking*. Palo Alto, CA. Science and Behavior Books, Inc.

Satir, V., & Baldwin, M. (1983). *Satir Step by Step: A guide to creating change in families*. Palo Alto, CA. Science and Behavior Books, Inc.

Satir, V., Banmen, J., Gerber, J. & Gomori, M. (1991). *The Satir model: family therapy and beyond*. Palo Alto, California: Science and Behavior Books, Inc.

Scharrón-del Río, M. R., & Aja, A. A. (2015). The case FOR "Latinx": Why intersectionality is not a choice. *Latino Rebels*, 5.

Scharrón-del Río, M. R., & Aja, A. A. (2020). Latinx: Inclusive language as liberation praxis. *Journal of Latinx Psychology*, 8(1), 7–20. https://doi.org/10.1037/lat0000140

Soto, A., Smith, T. B., Griner, D., Domenech Rodríguez, M., & Bernal, G. (2018). Cultural adaptations and therapist multicultural competence: Two meta-analytic reviews. *Journal of Clinical Psychology*, 74(11), 1907–1923. https://doi.org/10.1002/jclp.22679

Stein, G. L., Gonzales, R. G., Garcia Coll, C., & Prandoni, J. I. (2016). Latinos in rural, new immigrant destinations: A modification of the integrative model of child development. In L. J. Crockett & G. Carlo (Eds.), *Rural ethnic minority youth and families in the United States: Theory, research, and applications* (pp. 37–56). Cham, Switzerland: Springer International. https://doi.org/10.1007/978-3-319-20976-0_3

Stein, G. L., Gonzalez, L. M., & Huq, N. (2012). Cultural stressors and the hopelessness model of depressive symptoms in Latino adolescents. *Journal of Youth and Adolescence*, 41(10), 1339–1349. https://doi.org/10.1007/s10964-012-9765-8

Stevenson Jr, H. C. (1994). Validation of the scale of racial socialization for African American adolescents: Steps toward multidimensionality. *Journal of Black Psychology*, 20(4), 445–468. https://doi.org/10.1177/00957984940204005

Sue S. (1998). In search of cultural competence in psychotherapy and counseling. *The American Psychologist, 53*(4), 440–448. https://doi.org/10.1037//0003-066x.53.4.440

Sue, D. W. (1978). Eliminating cultural oppression in counseling: Toward a general theory. *Journal of Counseling Psychology, 25*(5), 419. https://doi.org/10.1037/0022-0167.25.5.419

Sue, S., Zane, N., Nagayama Hall, G. C., & Berger, L. K. (2009). The case for cultural competency in psychotherapeutic interventions. *Annual Review of Psychology, 60*, 525–548. https://doi.org/10.1146/annurev .psych.60.110707.163651

Taylor, B. A., Gambourg, M. B., Rivera, M., & Laureano, D. (2006). Constructing cultural competence: Perspectives of family therapists working with Latino families. *The American Journal of Family Therapy, 34*(5), 429–445. https://doi.org/10.1080/01926180600553779

Torres, S. A., Santiago, C. D., Walts, K. K., & Richards, M. H. (2018). Immigration policy, practices, and procedures: The impact on the mental health of Mexican and central American youth and families. *The American Psychologist, 73*(7), 843–854. https://doi.org/10.1037/amp0000184

Turner, W. L., Wieling, E., & Allen, W. D. (2004). Developing culturally effective family-based research programs: Implications for family therapists. *Journal of Marital and Family Therapy, 30*(3), 257–270. https://doi.org/10.1111/j.1752-0606.2004.tb01239.x

Umaña-Taylor, A. J., & Fine, M. A. (2004). Examining ethnic identity among Mexican-origin adolescents living in the United States. Hispanic *Journal of Behavioral Sciences, 26*, 36–59. https://doi.org/10.1177/0739986303262143

Umaña-Taylor, A. J., & Hill, N. E. (2020). Ethnic–racial socialization in the family: A decade's advance on precursors and outcomes. *Journal of Marriage and Family, 82*(1), 244–271. https://doi.org/10.1111/jomf.12622

United States Census Bureau. (2021). *Improved race and ethnicity measures reveal U.S. population is much more multiracial.* The United States Census Bureau. Retrieved from: www.census.gov/library/stories/2021/08/improved-race-ethnicity-measures-reveal-united-states-population-much-more-multiracial.html

Vespa, J., Armstrong, D. M., & Medina, L. (2018). *Demographic turning points for the United States: Population projections for 2020 to 2060.* Washington, DC: U.S. Department of Commerce, Economics and Statistics Administration, U.S. Census Bureau.

Vidal-Ortiz, S., & Martínez, J. (2018). Latinx thoughts: Latinidad with an X. *Latino Studies, 16*(3), 384–395. https://doi.org/10.1057/s41276-018-0137-8

Viruell-Fuentes, E. A., Miranda, P. Y., & Abdulrahim, S. (2012). More than culture: structural racism, intersectionality theory, and immigrant health. *Social Science & Medicine* (1982), *75*(12), 2099–2106. https://doi.org/10.1016/j.socscimed.2011.12.037

20
RECOMMENDATIONS FOR WORKING WITH TRAUMA WITHIN INCARCERATED COUPLES AND FAMILIES

Eman Tadros and Sreevidya Nibhanupudi

Introduction

Considering both state and federal prison populations, the number of incarcerated people surpassed 1.2 million in 2020, a steep decline from the year before (Carson, 2021). A report by the Vera Institute of Justice showed that there was a high prevalence of victimization and health issues amongst incarcerated women, with 86% having experienced sexual assault, 32% having a serious mental illness, and 82% having a dependence on drugs or alcohol (Swavola et al., 2016). The lifetime prevalence of PTSD in the incarcerated population is 48%, compared to 8.7% in the general population (Piper & Berle, 2019). The purpose of this chapter is to provide information on the intersection of trauma and incarceration, advocate for incarcerated individuals and their families experiencing trauma, as well as provide recommendations for marriage and family therapists working with this population.

Impacts of Incarceration of Families

The literature has documented various impacts of incarceration on families, specifically children, coparents or caregivers, and romantic partners (Tadros et al., 2020; Tadros & Presley, 2022). These impacts include mental health issues (Tadros et al., 2021), financial problems (Bruns, 2017, 2019), and even health concerns (Turanovic et al., 2012). Given the severity and dynamic nature of these concerns, it is critical to view and work with this population systemically.

Children

Children of incarcerated parents are likely to experience changes in their living situations and face a higher risk of delinquency, an social behavior, and future incarceration

DOI: 10.4324/9781003297871-23

(Beckmeyer & Arditti, 2014). Children with incarcerated parents also experience adverse physical and mental health outcomes that are observed through increased health issues, academic concerns, and antisocial behaviors (Durante et al., 2022). In fact, children of incarcerated parents have higher chances of developing mental illnesses such as depression and anxiety than children whose parents are not involved with the criminal justice system (Kitzmiller et al, 2021). This adverse childhood experience can lead to an increased risk of experiencing psychological distress (Gifford et al., 2019). Families can help negate some of the symptomology children experience with incarceration by expressing empathy, sensitivity, and responsiveness to their children's emotional needs (Poehlmann-Tynan et al., 2017). Additionally, schools can also play a critical role in minimizing negative outcomes for children with incarcerated parents by implementing services focused on emotional counseling (Finkeldey & Dennison, 2020). Thus, suggesting the need for both emotional intelligence and connection when working with children of incarcerated parents.

Coparents and Caregivers

Due to parental incarceration, loved ones face consequences such as loss of income and more caregiving responsibilities (Arditti & Savla, 2015). These hardships serve to further encumber and traumatize caregivers (parents, grandparents, and coparents) of children left behind (Kitzmiller et al., 2021). When one parent is incarcerated, it often becomes the responsibility of the other parent to shoulder all responsibilities associated with childrearing. They are also tasked with trying to soften the emotional blow for their children. Other implications for caregivers and coparents of incarcerated individuals include negative mental health consequences and increased health risks, specifically, cardiovascular disease (Wildeman et al., 2019). Their ability to manage these new stresses will depend on the extent to which they can practice resiliency in terms of maintaining themselves (Dennison et al., 2020). Even families in which the incarcerated individual's presence created instability are negatively impacted by his absence (Wildeman & Western, 2010). Family support is one area that is critical for both family members and post-incarcerated individuals (Mowen et al., 2019). Families promote prosocial behaviors through emotional support and connectedness, and basic needs, such as housing, financial support, and caregiver roles (Mowen et al., 2019). Therefore, addressing the concerns of families impacted by incarceration from a systemic lens can help each member address the emotional, physiological, and tangible needs to produce the best outcomes for all members.

Romantic Partners

Romantic partners of incarcerated partners also experience an array of negative effects. Partners that are left behind when their significant other is incarcerated experience a number of emotional and mental health concerns that are exacerbated by external stressors such as physical distance and finances (Yeboaa et al., 2022). Partners of incarcerated individuals are also likely to experience higher rates of anxiety and depression (Tadros et al., 2022). In fact, the partner who stays at home also faces a great deal of shame about her situation, which may prompt her to keep the incarceration a secret. This secrecy can lead to isolation and depression (Wildeman & Western, 2010). The fluctuation of income can also be a significant challenge faced by non-incarcerated partners. To remedy the loss in household wages, the stationary partner may increase their hours at work or pick up a second job (Bruns, 2017). The incarceration of one partner negatively impacts the stability of the romantic relationship. One aspect of this is the sexual aspect of relationships, which yields great sex risk behaviors, resulting in higher rates of contracting sexually transmitted diseases (STIs) (Wildeman et al., 2019).

While there are risks for partners of incarcerated individuals during the time incarcerated, their partners also face concerns post-release. One of these includes risk of intimate partner violence, specifically, females with an incarcerated male partner may be more at risk for IPV, living in low income areas with minimal education and are likely to abuse post release due to being abused themselves, isolation, anger, and unemployment (Tadros & Vlach, 2022). Therefore, therapists working with incarcerated partners, both during and post incarceration, should address the needs of each individual partner, and address their concerns from a systemic approach.

The Intersection of Trauma and Incarceration

Trauma is commonly experienced in incarcerated populations, by both the incarcerated individual and by their children and other family members (Arditti, 2012; Arditti & Savla, 2015; Skinner-Osei & Levenson, 2018). Incarceration of a parent is considered an adverse childhood experience (ACE), with potential for both biological and psychosocial consequences throughout one's life (Arditti, 2012; Arditti & Savla, 2015; Levenson & Willis, 2019; Skinner-Osei & Levenson, 2018). ACEs can take the form of toxic stress, particularly when there are both unrelenting environmental threats and a lack of protective factors. These demands both require and result in the individual experiencing a prolonged stress response that leads to changes in endocrine and nervous system functioning (Levenson & Willis, 2019; Skinner-Osei & Levenson, 2018). This can lead to lasting changes in the architecture of a child's developing brain, particularly in the strengthening of brain regions involved in survival and the underdevelopment of regions responsible for executive functioning (Levenson & Willis, 2019).

The experience of having an incarcerated parent can also be traumatic for children from an attachment perspective (Arditti, 2012; Skinner-Osei & Levenson, 2018). Attachment theory is based on the notion that children need a safe, stable, and reliable relationship with a caregiver whom they share an emotional bond with for normal development. ACEs that involve the absence of a caregiver, as is common with incarceration, result in disruptions to attachment bonds, which has repercussions in terms of one's vulnerability to later adversity and their ability to form healthy relationships with others (Arditti, 2012; Skinner-Osei & Levenson, 2018). Arditti (2012) explains how parental incarceration can be considered a type of ambiguous loss for the child, in which the offending parent is still alive but is not physically present in the child's life, resulting in a lack of closure and loss of human connection with a loved one. They show how these effects are compounded by social stigma and accompanying attitudes that make it difficult to publicly acknowledge the loss, grieve for the loved one, or be supported by others in that grief.

Arditti (2012) identifies a few family processes that can influence the perception of incarceration as traumatic for the child. These include the pre-incarceration factors of both involvement of the incarcerated parent in the child's life and exposure to the incarcerated parent's arrest, the quality and stability of caregiving in the wake of the incarcerated parent's arrest and imprisonment, as well as the visitation experience. It is also important to remember that families with a parent in the criminal justice system are also often experiencing other harm and adversity, both in and outside of the home, such as exposure to community violence, poverty, and substance abuse (Skinner-Osei & Levenson, 2018). Parental incarceration is an ACE that often co-occurs with other such adversities, and it would therefore be beneficial to engage with children in a trauma-informed way.

Trauma is also woven into the experiences of the incarcerated parent. Many enter the prison system already having experienced adversity in childhood, and are therefore at risk of further traumatization and/or re-traumatization while in prison, due to the potential of having violent interactions with other incarcerated people (Levenson & Willis, 2019; Piper & Berle, 2019). This is quite likely given how widespread such violence is, with estimates of incident rates at 13 to 27 times higher than in the general population, as well as nearly 40% of incarcerated individuals reporting that they've experienced some type of physical violence (Piper & Berle, 2019). Young adults who are incarcerated also face the risk of experiencing trauma and victimization, due to being unaware of the social hierarchies that prisons have (Cochran et al., 2016). Overall, incarcerated populations have much higher rates of ACEs, potentially traumatic events (PTEs), and lifetime prevalence of PTSD than the general U.S. population (Levenson & Willis, 2019; Piper & Berle, 2019).

A systematic review and meta-analysis by Piper and Berle (2019) found a medium positive association between PTEs experienced during incarceration and the emergence of PTSD symptoms in the individual while in prison and/or at post-release, even when accounting for incarceration length or previous mental health concerns. This is an important consideration for care, as having PTSD can affect the re-entry experience and post-release outcomes for the incarcerated individual. Piper and Berle (2019) note that incarceration itself is a traumatic experience for many, with incarcerated people experiencing things like coercion, solitary confinement, and sexual/physical violence as a result of being in such an intense interpersonal environment. They also point out that the majority of incarcerated individuals have already experienced one such traumatic event prior to incarceration, so there is even greater risk for the development of PTSD. Protective factors, such as coping skills, may account for the apparent resilience of those incarcerated who also have cumulative traumatic and stressful experiences (Maschi et al., 2014). We advocate for services that look at trauma holistically; therefore, we will discuss providing medical family therapy and trauma-informed care in the following sections.

Medical Family Therapy

Medical Family Therapy (MedFT) is a biopsychosocial framework that applies systemic family therapy principles to treat mental and medical health conditions in patients and their families (Doherty et al., 2014; McDaniel et al., 2014; Mendenhall et al., 2018). This approach differs from traditional family therapy in that it explicitly embraces the mind, body, family, and community, as well as problems that are considered physical and mental health related (McDaniel et al., 2014). MedFT is a relatively new discipline in the work of trauma response, where members collaborate with other professionals to address the relational components of their fieldwork within their communities (Mendenhall et al., 2018). MedFTs work in various healthcare domains such as family medicine, pediatrics, obstetrics, gynecology, etc. (Doherty et al., 2014; Mendenhall et al., 2018). Part of their work includes developing treatment plans that coincide with the primary care team's, individual's, and the family's goals (Doherty et al., 2014). MedFTs implement their training in relational therapy to conceptualize, understand, and consult with patients and their providers around their issues and goals (Marlowe, 2013).

Taking a collaborative approach to creating a treatment plan allows the client and clinician to work as a team. Identifying goals of therapy allows the patient to reflect on his or her desired outcomes. This allows the patient to become more engaged in therapy and to understand the agency they have in the therapeutic process (McDaniel et al., 2014). MedFTs can enhance care beyond medical settings, such as in incarcerated areas (Marlowe, 2013; Rajaeil & Jensen, 2020), because they have the collaborative skillset and systems focus to bring people together, address community needs, and enhance population care in different settings (Rajaeil & Jensen, 2020). Following the guidelines set forth by the MedFT framework, a recent study identified that self-reported finances and the provision of counseling services were notable markers of physical health (Cappetto & Tadros, 2021). However, incarcerated facilities rarely employ MedFTs (Tadros et al., 2023). As such, advocacy is needed to bolster the availability of MedFTs where incarcerated individuals and their families need them.

Given the biopsychosocial framework for systems-based practice of MedFTS, we advocate for its usage to better understand the connection between trauma, health, and incarceration. Implementing a holistic approach to care for incarcerated people and their families could have a significant impact on their health and wellbeing. As MedFTs, we have the opportunity to let our clients tell us who they are – their histories, their goals, and their fears. We can then collaborate with clients to develop a plan that will address their physical health, emotional wellbeing, and healing from past and present traumas. We can also work with clients and their families to strengthen family relationships and to forge a clear path forward. MedFT theory contends that even though each client has experiences that have shaped them into who they are, they still possess the agency to build a brighter future (Rajaei & Jensen, 2019).

Trauma Informed Care

Based on the definition by the American Psychiatric Association, a traumatic event, or trauma, is a physically or psychologically threatening experience that is either observed or directly experienced and which overwhelms a person's ability to cope, often leading to difficult negative emotions such as shock, fear, and helplessness (Levenson & Willis, 2019). It should be noted that when not specified as an event, "trauma" is typically referring to the experiencing of a constellation of symptoms as part of the response to a stressor or event that the individual considers to be deeply distressing (or "traumatic"). Trauma-informed approaches are based on the understanding that traumatic events have an impact on the services that are needed by individuals seeking those services (Kulkarni, 2019). SAMHSA's trauma-informed care (TIC) approach involves understanding the effects, symptoms, and pervasiveness of trauma, and working to ensure that this understanding is incorporated into policies and procedures of correctional services, so that victims are not re-traumatized and are able to heal and grow (Levenson & Willis, 2019). SAMHSA outlines several components of TIC to achieve this, which are discussed below.

Communities burdened by incarcerational trauma typically are also those continuing to endure intergenerational effects of historical trauma, namely poverty, discrimination, and oppression (Levenson & Willis, 2019). It is important to understand the effects such experiences have on children and how they may contribute to future criminal behavior, as well as how they might have contributed to parental incarceration. Trauma-informed care can help incarcerated individuals, a population with higher rates of adversity and trauma than the general population, have more successful reentry into society and reduce the likelihood of recidivism (Levenson & Willis, 2019).

Trauma reactions range from hypervigilance to avoidance and should be seen as potentially adaptive responses to stressors that become maladaptive in the absence of those stressors (Piper & Berle, 2019). Individuals may engage in criminal behaviors while trying to meet their needs and cope with trauma, looking for social groups or activities that can help them feel like they belong and have power; however, new skills and ways of thinking about the world can be introduced through healthy therapeutic relationships that empower individuals (Levenson & Willis, 2019). TIC essentially involves shifting the focus from what is wrong with a person for them to have behaved that way, to what happened to a person for them to have engaged in that behavior. This is especially relevant when working with this population, where criminal behavior can also be thought of as adaptations to past hostile environments that are now maladaptive (Levenson & Willis, 2019). Therefore, disempowering dynamics, common in correctional settings and characterized by authoritative measures, may resemble early experiences with caregivers and inadvertently invoke and reinforce maladaptive coping methods in clients.

TIC is not a specific intervention or treatment program; rather, it is an approach to care that can be applied to a variety of treatment plans to help increase receptivity to and success of therapeutic interventions in strengthening the individual's independence, self-regulation, and coping skills in the context of the therapist-client relationship (Levenson & Willis, 2019). This is done through the inclusion of relational elements designed to improve client trust, respect, safety, and empowerment. Piper and Berle (2019) corroborate these recommendations in their review and meta-analysis, stating the need to avoid re-traumatizing prisoners, how trauma-informed care can achieve this, as well as the importance of having access to mental health care after release.

It should be noted, however, that while having access to care post-release is crucial, it may not always be the experience of formerly incarcerated individuals to have received it. Georgiou and Townsend (2019) analyzed annual reports of the Psychiatrists' Quality Network for Prison Mental Health Services (QNPMHS) to investigate any improvements or changes that have been made in the UK and Ireland since the program's start. Keeping service programs up to date and making advancements as needed is crucial to improving an incarcerated individual or their loved ones' physical and mental state. They discussed subsequent studies that reported some prisoners as receiving inappropriate or no treatment for their mental illness. Those incarcerated deserve the same standard of care and access to services as the general public.

As mentioned before, TIC principles can be flexibly applied to a vast set of treatments. CBT is one such treatment, and has been shown to be effective for incarcerated individuals (Tadros, 2022). The application of TIC in a juvenile justice setting showed that educating staff about the impacts of trauma on youth and development and their role in ameliorating those effects, as well as educating a significant fraction of youth in the facility about trauma, emotion coping, and communication, was associated with a decrease in violent incidents (Baetz et al., 2021). Finally, TIC principles can and should also be used when working with children of incarcerated parents (Skinner-Osei & Levenson, 2018). TIC is important because successful counseling outcomes are dependent on the quality of the therapeutic alliance, especially one that is "client-centered, empathic, and collaborative" (Levenson & Willis, 2019). For individuals with a history of trauma, it is crucial that therapists build and maintain trust, repair any ruptures in the relationship, and most importantly, ensure the individual's continued participation in treatment.

Clinical Implications

Formerly incarcerated individuals, as well as their children and romantic partners, face many challenges as they reintegrate back into society. A common challenge faced by formerly incarcerated individuals post-release include barriers to finding employment and housing due to their criminal record; reintegrating back into society with these and other challenges can increase the chances of recidivism (Tadros, 2022). Implications for families include subsequent impacts on romantic and parent-child relationships (Morgan-Mullane, 2018; Tadros, 2022; Tadros & Vlach, 2022). Within the romantic relationship, the incarcerated partner often experiences psychological changes as a result of needing to adapt to the demands of the incarcerated setting—an isolating, strict, and hostile environment—that can result in symptoms such as hypervigilance and distrust toward the non-incarcerated partner post-release (Tadros & Vlach, 2022). This is compounded by financial and occupational instability/role ambiguity that may result in conflicts between partners, or even IPV in some cases, which are correlated with the negative incarceration outcomes specified above (Tadros & Vlach, 2022).

There have recently been calls for an increased presence of Marriage and Family Therapists (MFTs) in incarcerated settings, due to the systemic approach and interpersonal lens they utilize, as they would be a beneficial addition to the criminal justice system (Tadros, 2022). Tadros (2022) identifies several barriers existing within the criminal justice system that are often experienced by incarcerated individuals and their families, ranging from communication between family members to financial difficulties; these are systemic barriers to achieving family connection by making it difficult to both maintain familial relationships while incarcerated and re-establish relationships after release. MFTs can help families learn how to support a loved one who has been incarcerated and who has experienced trauma (Tadros & Vlach, 2022). Studies indicate that improving marital and family satisfaction in this population is key to strengthening relationships and ensuring a successful reentry experience for the incarcerated individual; the inclusion of MFTs seems to help facilitate this (Tadros, 2021).

Barriers that MFTs might face when providing treatment to incarcerated individuals and their families include the inherent power imbalance that exists between the non-incarcerated therapist and incarcerated client, stigma typically associated with incarceration, their own biases or prejudices surrounding this population, and lack of knowledge around race-based traumatic stress that is pervasive in communities of color. When considering all of the personal barriers that a MFT might need to overcome to effectively work with the population of incarcerated individuals and their family members, it is clear that the ultimate goal is for MFTs to feel comfortable providing services and care to this population while also building rapport and strengthening the therapeutic alliance so that change and growth may be possible. The American Association for Marriage and Family Therapists (AAMFT) is the professional organization that can help to structure training so that MFTs are prepared to work with this clientele by better understanding their needs and experiences (Tadros, 2022).

MFTs must therefore be careful while working with clients not to perpetuate the stigma normally associated with incarceration in society, to be aware of how their beliefs may impact their interactions with a client, strive for cultural humility, and make space for what the client knows while refraining from inserting their own personal views into the conversation (Tadros, 2022). It is also crucial for MFTs and other mental health professionals to understand the long-term effects that race-based traumatic stress have on marginalized communities. Most of the current research looking at race-based traumatic stress in marginalized communities focuses on police interactions and the negative effects that come from those interactions (Bryant-Davis et al., 2017; Range et al., 2018; Williams et al., 2018).

One particular evidence-based treatment approach that has been shown to be successful in treating the children of an incarcerated parent and their formerly incarcerated parent is Trauma Focused Cognitive Behavioral Therapy, or TF-CBT (Morgan-Mullane, 2018). While there are a few studies looking at clinical treatments that could be effective in treating PTSD and trauma symptomatology in the children of incarcerated parents, TF-CBT has shown to be very promising due to its historical utilization in treating populations with similar presenting problems, including those impacted by the 9/11 terrorist attacks, as well as sexually abused children experiencing traumatic grief. An application of the treatment approach is explored in addition to how the three core phases of stabilization, trauma narrative, and integration and consolidation may prove effective in repairing ruptured parent-child relationships in the wake of an arrest and subsequent incarceration of the parent.

Theoretical techniques that MFTs can use when working with couples or families in this client population include those encapsulated by the Tadros Theory of Change, which emphasizes a strengths-based approach and client-centered change coupled with a variety of evidence-based treatments such as narrative, solution-focused, and structural family therapies (Tadros, 2022). It also encourages a holistic examination of concerns and uncovering of family interaction patterns, which is critical for positive change, as well as flexibility, so that client needs are prioritized. The aim is to empower clients and work collaboratively with them to set relevant goals for the future.

Stigma

Beyond the emotional trauma and financial adversity that incarceration of a family member brings, loved ones must also grapple with the stigma of having a child, parent, sibling, or romantic partner imprisoned. Stigma of incarcerated individuals has been exasperated not only socially, but legally through the strictness and unforgiveness of U.S. policies (Beckett et al. 2018). Romantic partners of incarcerated individuals may experience shame that the person they love committed a crime, which can reduce the closeness of individuals and the incarcerated person, as well as weaken the family bonds (Datchi et al, 2016). In some cases, the parent who is not incarcerated may choose to deepen the stigma of parental incarceration by attempting to hide the truth about what happened to the incarcerated parent (Gaston, 2016).

Children of incarcerated parents may internalize feelings of guilt for the crime that their parents committed. They may also become fearful of being associated with the offending parent, because that may in turn cause them to be seen in a negative light. These children may also socially isolate themselves if they genuinely come to believe that the incarcerated parent is a bad person and that others would not want to be around them (Luther, 2016).

Children of incarcerated parents may also experience difficulty engaging in social settings like school due to feelings of inferiority, humiliation, or ostracism. The correlation between parental incarceration and disruptions of symbols of financial stability such as permanent housing can also impact both children of incarcerated parents and also the coparents (Kremer et al., 2020). Children of incarcerated parents may also be unfairly compared to the incarcerated parent in terms of their morality. Further, teachers may lower their expectations for the academic performance of a child after his or her parent has become incarcerated. This is especially true for children of color, who are generally perceived as less competent than their white peers (Warren et al., 2019). Children of color comprise two-thirds of children who have an incarcerated parent (Gaston, 2016). These children, especially black children, are burdened with compounded trauma. Black children are much more likely than any other race to experience parental incarceration. Moreover, for a black child, the incarceration of a parent feeds into the generational trauma of the mass incarceration of black people that has taken place in the U.S. for centuries (Kitzmiller et al., 2021).

Future Directions

While the literature has progressed in researching incarcerated populations and their needs, there is still more work to be done to provide the families of incarcerated individuals with the most effective and competent care possible. One area that would be beneficial to study is determining ways to lessen the negative impact that children of incarcerated parents experience. As stated previously, the event of having a parent incarcerated traumatizes children and is considered to be an adverse childhood experience. Positive childhood experiences do not negate negative experiences, but can minimize the consequences of childhood trauma. Further examination of such positive childhood experiences could aim to target specific experiences that may buffer the impacts of parental incarceration (Kremer et al., 2020). Recent analysis has highlighted the ways in which structural family therapy can characterize the trauma that African American youth endure (Chappelle & Tadros, 2021). TIC can serve as a bridge for people of color who are reluctant to enter therapy. This framework can be especially useful for individuals who mistrust medical professionals or those who harbor apprehension toward systemic care.

Incarcerated individuals and their loved ones have the best outcomes if they receive adequate support during judicial proceedings and time away from home. These services include timely and competent responses to mental health crises that arise from experiencing the incarceration of a loved one. Enhanced awareness of mental health concerns is also imperative to increase positive outcomes for families of incarcerated populations. Further, services in which these feelings can be screened for and identified should be available (Georgiou & Townsend, 2019). MFTs should advocate not only for further training in working with this population, but for it to be accessible. Furthermore, advocacy work is needed to emphasize family members of the incarcerated as in need of and deserving of the care of MFTs.

References

Arditti, J. A. (2012). Child Trauma Within the Context of Parental Incarceration: A Family Process Perspective. *Journal of Family Theory & Review*, 4(3), 181–219. https://doi.org/10.1111/j.1756-2589.2012.00128.x

Arditti, J. A., & Savla, J. (2015). Parental Incarceration and Child Trauma Symptoms in Single Caregiver Homes. *Journal of Child and Family Studies, 24*(3), 551–561. https://doi.org/10.1007/s10826-013-9867-2

Baetz, C. L., Surko, M., Moaveni, M., McNair, F., Bart, A., Workman, S., Tedeschi, F., Havens, J., Guo, F., Quinlan, C., & Horwitz, S. M. (2021). Impact of a Trauma-Informed Intervention for Youth and Staff on Rates of Violence in Juvenile Detention Settings. *Journal of Interpersonal Violence, 36*(17/18), NP9463–NP9482. https://doi.org/10.1177/0886260519857163

Beckett, K., Beach, L., Knaphus, E., & Reosti, A. (2018). U.S. Criminal Justice Policy and Practice in the Twenty-First Century: Toward the End of Mass Incarceration? *Law & Policy, 40*(4), 321–345. https://doi.org/10.1111/lapo.12113

Beckmeyer, J. J., & Arditti, J. A. (2014). Implications of In-Person Visits for Incarcerated Parents' Family Relationships and Parenting Experience. *Journal of Offender Rehabilitation, 53*(2), 129–151. https://doi.org/10.1080/10509674.2013.868390

Bruns, A. (2017). Consequences of Partner Incarceration for Women's Employment. *Journal of Marriage & Family, 79*(5), 1331–1352. https://doi.org/10.1111/jomf.12412

Bruns, A. (2019). The third shift: Multiple job holding and the incarceration of women's partners. *Social Science Research, 80*(1), 202–215. https://doi.org/10.1016/j.ssresearch.2018.12.024

Bryant-Davis, T., Adams, T., Alejandre, A., & Gray, A. A. (2017). The Trauma Lens of Police Violence against Racial and Ethnic Minorities. *Journal of Social Issues, 73*(4), 852–871. https://doi.org/10.1111/josi.12251

Carson, E. A. (2021). *Prisoners in 2020 – Statistical Tables.* Bureau of Justice Statistics. https://bjs.ojp.gov/content/pub/pdf/p20st.pdf

Chappelle, N., & Tadros, E. (2021). Using Structural Family Therapy to Understand the Impact of Poverty and Trauma on African American Adolescents. *Family Journal, 29*(2), 237–244. https://doi.org/10.1177/1066480720950427

Cochran, J. C., Mears, D. P., Bales, W. D., & Stewart, E. A. (2016). Spatial Distance, Community Disadvantage, and Racial and Ethnic Variation in Prison Inmate Access to Social Ties. *Journal of Research in Crime & Delinquency, 53*(2), 220–254. https://doi.org/10.1177/002242781 5592675

Datchi, C. C., Barretti, L. M., & Thompson, C. M. (2016). Family services in adult detention centers: Systemic principles for prisoner reentry. *Couple and Family Psychology: Research and Practice, 5*(2), 89–104. https://doi.org/10.1037/cfp0000057

Dennison, S., Besemer, K., & Low-Choy, S. (2020). Maternal Parenting Stress FollowingPaternal or Close Family Incarceration: Bayesian Model-Based Profiling Using the HILDA Longitudinal Survey. *Journal of Quantitative Criminology, 36*(4), 753–778. https://doi.org/10.1007/s10 940-019-09430-z

Doherty, W. J., McDaniel, S. H., & Hepworth, J. (2014). Contributions of medical family therapy to the changing health care system. *Family Process, 53*(3), 529–543. https://doi-org/10.1111/famp.12092

Finkeldey, J. G., & Dennison, C. R. (2020). School-Based Resources as Protective Factors from the Influence of Parental Incarceration on Depressive Symptoms. *Social Currents, 7*(5), 402–423. https://doi.org/10.1177/2329496520921844

Gaston, S. (2016). The Long-term Effects of Parental Incarceration: Does Parental Incarceration in Childhood or Adolescence Predict Depressive Symptoms in Adulthood? *Criminal Justiceand Behavior, 43*(8), 1056–1075. https://doi.org/10.1177/0093854816628905

Georgiou, M., & Townsend, K. (2019). Quality Network for Prison Mental Health Services: reviewing the quality of mental health provision in prisons. *Journal of Forensic Psychiatry & Psychology, 30*(5), 794–806. https://doi.org/10.1080/14789949.2019.1637918

Gifford, E.J., Golonka, M., Kozecke, L.E. et al. (2019). Association of parental incarceration with psychiatric and functional outcomes of young adults. *JAMA Netw Open.* 2(8):e1910005. doi:10.1001/jamanetworkopen.2019.10005

Kitzmiller, M. K., Cavanagh, C., Frick, P., Steinberg, L., & Cauffman, E. (2021). Parental incarceration and the mental health of youth in the justice system: The moderating role of neighborhood disorder. *Psychology, Public Policy, and Law, 27*(2), 256. https://doi.org/10.1037/law0000274

Kjellstrand, J. M., & Eddy, J. M. (2011). Parental Incarceration During Childhood, Family Context, and Youth Problem Behavior Across Adolescence. *Journal of Offender Rehabilitation, 50*(1), 18–36. https://doi.org/10.1080/10509674.2011.536720

Kremer, K. P., Poon, C. Y. S., Jones, C. L., Hagler, M. A., Kupersmidt, J. B., Stelter, R. L., Stump, K. N., & Rhodes, J. E. (2020). Risk and Resilience among Children with Incarcerated Parents: Examining Heterogeneity in Delinquency and School Outcomes. *Journal of Child and Family Studies, 29*(11), 3239–3252. https://doi.org/10.1007/s10826-020-01822-1

Kulkarni, S. (2019). Intersectional Trauma-Informed Intimate Partner Violence (IPV) Services: Narrowing the Gap between IPV Service Delivery and Survivor Needs. *Journal of Family Violence, 34*(1), 55–64. https://doi.org/10.1007/s10896-018-0001-5

Levenson, J. S., & Willis, G. M. (2019). Implementing Trauma-Informed Care in Correctional Treatment and Supervision. *Journal of Aggression, Maltreatment & Trauma, 28*(4), 481–501. https://doi.org/10.1080/10926771.2018.1531959

Luther, K. (2016). Stigma Management among Children of Incarcerated Parents. *Deviant Behavior, 37*(11), 1264–1275. https://doi.org/10.1080/01639625.2016.1170551

Marlowe, D., Hodgson, J., Lamson, A., White, M. & Irons, T. (2013). Medical Family Therapy in a Primary Care Setting: A Framework for Integration. *Contemporary Family Therapy, 34*, 244–258. https://doi.org/10.1007/s10591-012-9195-5

Maschi, T., Viola, D., & Morgen, K. (2014). Unraveling Trauma and Stress, Coping Resources, and Mental Well-Being Among Older Adults in Prison: Empirical Evidence Linking Theory and Practice. *The Gerontologist, 54*(5), 857–867. https://doi.org/10.1093/geront/gnt069

McDaniel, S. H., Doherty, W.J. & Hepworth, J. (2014). Medical Family Therapy and Integrated Care, 2nd Ed. Washington DC: American Psychological Association Publications.

Mendenhall, T., Bundt, J., & Yumbul, C. (2018). Medical Family Therapy in disaster preparedness and trauma-response teams. In T. Mendenhall, A. Lamson, J. Hodgson, & M. Baird (1st ed., pp. 431–461), *Clinical methods in medical family therapy: Focused issues in family therapy.* Springer. https://doi.org/10.1007/978-3-319-68834-3_15

Morgan-Mullane, A. (2018). Trauma Focused Cognitive Behavioral Therapy with Children of Incarcerated Parents. Clinical Social Work Journal, 46, 200–209. https://doi.org/10.1007/s10 615-017-0642-5

Mowen, T. J., Stansfield, R., & Boman IV, J. H. (2019). Family matters: Moving beyond "if" family support matters to "why" family support matters during reentry from prison. *Journal of Research in Crime & Delinquency, 56*(4), 483–523. https://doi/10.1177/0022427818820902

Piper, A. & Berle, D. (2019). The association between trauma experienced during incarceration and PTSD outcomes: a systematic review and meta-analysis. *The Journal of Forensic Psychiatry & Psychology, 30*(5), 854–875. https://doi.org/10.1080/14789949.2019.1639788

Poehlmann-Tynan, J., Burnson, C., Runion, H., & Weymouth, L. A. (2017). Attachment in young children with incarcerated fathers. *Development and Psychopathology, 29*(2), 389–404. https://doi.org/2443/10.1017/S0954579417000062

Rajaei, A., & Jensen, J. F. (2019). Empowering Patients in Integrated Behavioral Health-Care Settings: A Narrative Approach to Medical Family Therapy. *The Family Journal, 28*(1), 48–55. https://doi.org/10.1177/1066480719893958

Range, B., Gutierrez, D., Gamboni, C., Hough, N. A., & Wojciak, A. (2018). Mass Trauma in the African American Community: Using Multiculturalism to Build Resilient Systems. *Contemporary Family Therapy: An International Journal, 40*(3), 284–298. https://doi.org/10.1007/s10 591-017-9449-3

Ruhland, E. L., Davis, L., Atella, J., & Shlafer, R. J. (2020). Externalizing Behavior Among Youth With a Current or Formerly Incarcerated Parent. *International Journal of Offender Therapy and Comparative Criminology, 64*(1), 3–21. https://doi.org/10.1177/0306624X19855317

Skinner-Osei, P., & Levenson, J. S. (2018). Trauma-informed services for children with incarcerated parents. *Journal of Family Social Work, 21*(4–5), 421–437. https://doi.org/10.1080/10522 158.2018.1499064

Swavola, E., Riley, K., Subramanian, R. (2016). *Overlooked: Women and Jails in an Era of Reform.* Vera Institute of Justice. www.vera.org/publications/overlooked-women-and-jails-report

Tadros, E. (2021). Treating Mental Illness and Relational Concerns in Incarcerated Settings. *Family Journal, 29*(3), 359–367. https://doi.org/10.1177/10664807211000083

Tadros, E. (2022). The Tadros Theory of Change with Incarcerated Populations. *The American Journal of Family Therapy, 50*(4), 366–388. https://doi.org/10.1080/01926 187.2021.1929560

Tadros, E. & Owens, D. (2021). Clinical Implications for Culturally Informed Counseling with Incarcerated Individuals. *The American Journal of Family Therapy, 49*(4), 344–355. https://doi.org/10.1080/01926 187.2020.1813659

Tadros, E. & Presley, S. (2022). "Fear of the Unknown": Coparenting with an incarcerated individual. *International Journal of Offender Therapy & Comparative Criminology.* https://doi.org/10.1177/0306624X221106335

Tadros, E. & Vlach, A. (2022). Conflictual couples: The impact of dyadic adjustment and depressive symptoms on conflict in incarcerated couples. *Journal of Family Trauma, Child Custody, and Child Development.* https://doi.org/10.1080/26904 586.2022.2041525

Tadros, E., Barbini, M., & Kaur, L. (2023). Collaborative healthcare in incarcerated settings. *International Journal of Offender Therapy and Comparative Criminology, 67*(9), 910–929. https://doi.org/10.1177/0306624X211058952

Tadros, E., Owens, D., & Middleton, T. (2021). Systemic Racism and Family Therapy. *The American Journal of Family Therapy.* https://doi.org/10.1080/01926 187.2021.1958271

Tadros, E., Fanning, K., Jensen, S., & Poehlmann-Tynan, J. (2021). Coparenting and mental health in families with jailed parents. *International Journal of Environmental Research and Public Health, 18*(16), 8705. https://doi.org/10.3390/ijerph18168705

Tadros, E., Durante, K. A., McKay, T., Barbini, M., & Hollie, B. (2022). Mental health, perceived consensus of coparenting, and physical health among incarcerated fathers and their non- incarcerated, romantic partners. *Families, Systems, & Health.* https://doi.org/10.1037/fsh0000671

Turanovic, J. J., Rodriguez, N., & Pratt, T. C. (2012). The collateral consequences of incarceration revisited: A qualitative analysis of the effects on caregivers of children of incarcerated parents. *Criminology, 50*(4), 913–959. https://doi.org/10.1111/j.1745-9125.2012.00283.x

Warren, J. M., Coker, G. L., & Collins, M. L. (2019). Children of incarcerated parents: Considerations for professional school counselors. *The Professional Counselor, 9*(3), 185–199. https://doi.org/10.15241/jmw.9.3.185

Wildeman, C., & Western, B. (2010). Incarceration in Fragile Families. *The Future of Children, 20*(2), 157–177. https://doi.org/10.1353/foc.2010.0006

Wildeman, C., Goldman, A. W., & Lee, H. (2019). Health consequences of family member incarceration for adults in the household. *Public Health Reports, 134*(1), 15S–21S. https://doi.org/10.1177/0033354918807974

Williams, M. T., Printz, D. M. B., & DeLapp, R. C. T. (2018). Assessing racial trauma with the Trauma Symptoms of Discrimination Scale. *Psychology of Violence, 8*(6), 735–747. http://dx.doi.org/10.1037/vio0000212

Yeboaa,P. A., Mbamba, C. R., & Ndemole, I. K. (2022): "Everything Has Turned Against Us": Experiences of Left-Behind Spouses of Incarcerated Persons. *Journal of Social Service Research, 48*(1), 1–8. https://doi.org/10.1080/01488376.2022.2042456

21

ADDRESSING TECHNOLOGY MISUSE IN RELATIONSHIPS

A Cross-Cultural Therapeutic Perspective

Katherine M. Hertlein

Introduction

Technology can be an incredibly positive tool for use in personal relationships. It has been demonstrated to provide a mechanism for the development of connection and intimacy couples and family members, whether they live together or are separated by geography (Abel et al., 2021; Bacigalupe & Lambe, 2011; Bacigalupe & Camara, 2012; Hampton et al., 2017; Hertlein & Ancheta, 2014; Murray & Campbell, 2015; Taipale, 2019; van Deursen & Helsper, 2018). Technology innovations such as texting, email, social media usage, and media apps assist romantic couples with the ability to experience different levels of problem solving within their relationship, create opportunities for communication throughout the day that may foster greater levels of intimacy, provide a mechanism for psychoeducation about the relationship, and create opportunities for expression of emotion (Billedo, Kerkhof, & Finkenauer, 2015; Hertlein & Ancheta, 2014; Hertlein & Chan, 2020; Janning et al., 2018). It also is a significant support in the development and maintenance of long-distance relationships in cultivating intimacy and eliciting a sense of commitment (Beck & Beck-Gernsheim, 2014; Belus et al., 2019; Hampton et al., 2017; Hertlein & Chan, 2020; Kolozsvari, 2015; Mok et al., 2010). This is especially true when a couple has established rules around cell phone usage in the relationship such as rules about relationship boundaries, rules around surveillance and monitoring, and if they did not have a rule about how often they can contact each other via cell phones (Miller-Ott et al., 2012).

Advancements in technology also help families strengthen relationships among its members and increase familial ties (Barakji et al., 2019; Fox & Rainie, 2014). Like the benefits to couples mentioned earlier, the use of technology allows for unique methods by which one can express affect and emotions (Felton, 2014). The flexibility of different apps allows multiple family members to select the tools that best fit each member's skills and preferences (Taipale, 2019; Taipale & Farinosi, 2018). Family members may also choose to use a common platform for the family to use. This platform can be accessed and used by all members with consideration of their skills (Siibak & Tamme, 2013; Taipale, 2019; Taipale & Farinosi, 2018). Further, the multiple methods of communication assist families in maintaining connectivity with the freedom to reach out to a family member when

DOI: 10.4324/9781003297871-24

it is convenient for them in both synchronous and asynchronous ways (Francisco, 2015; Madianou & Miller, 2011).

Technology, however, when misused can have a deleterious impact on personal relationships. For example, when relationships initially start and are characterized by frequent electronic communication, satisfaction tends to be higher; yet as electronic communication frequency dips, so does relational satisfaction and one's experience of closeness with their partner (Sullivan et al., 2020). Earlier studies have found an association between the presence of a phone in interpersonal situations and impairment in the develop of intimacy (Przybylski & Weinstein, 2012) and satisfaction (Campbell & Murray, 2015). Other studies have found that personal messaging through phone- and web-based technologies has a negative correlation with relational satisfaction in personal relationships (Goodman-Deane et al., 2016; McDaniel & Drouin, 2019).

The Role of Nuance and Culture in Perceived Technology Misuse

For many, technology has been considered an equalizer across various cultural groups, ethnicities, and regions. Because technology is so embedded in daily life, it is subject to cultural influences and interpretations into the meaning of its usage. These technologies have influenced the way we act and react to one another in social settings. How technology use is perceived is often informed by nuances. Specifically, people disclose online differently than they do in person, and those from collectivist cultures who are not identified as extroverts disclose the most audience-relevant, but least honest, information (Chen & Marcus, 2012).

The literature suggesting that the effects of technology use are not broad-based, but instead are influenced by the specific activities (Kim et al., 2011; Lin et al., 2015). For example, the relationship between how individuals perceive technology affecting their relationships is complicated by how much importance they place on online communication (Sullivan et al., 2020). For example, reducing time online does directly affect the perception of satisfaction or closeness in relationships, but is affected in a negative way by those who think online communication is important.

Whether technology use is helpful or harmful is often dependent on the context. Morgan et al. (2017) found that the intentions of using particular apps also made a difference in how the activity was perceived. In another example. David et al. (2018) found there was a general relationship between technology use and lowered levels of well-being; however, it was not until the analysis of individual apps were considered that the researchers were able to make sense of the well-being findings. In short, the types of apps that were used was more predictive of issues in couples than the fact that apps were being used at all. In other words, it is the context in which the media is used that is associated with the interpretation of its utility (Morgan et al., 2017). Number of children in the home for Americans dictates technology adoption (Hamill, 2011), while in Latin America, it is both the presence of younger people in the home fueling the adoption by older adults as more time is spent online by partners (Cáceres & Chaparro, 2017). Likewise, without younger people in the home, the adoption occurs at a slower rate (Taipale, 2019).

Considering context, the adoption of internet technologies as well as the perception of what is considered problematic internet use is culturally dependent. For example, contexts such as one's educational level and income level (specifically economic inequality) are both factors influencing technology usage (Blank & Lutz 2018; Scheerder et al., 2019; van Deursen & van Dijk 2011). In 2011, Hamill showed computer adoption in the United

States to be influenced not by money primarily, but by the presence or absence of children in the household (Hamill, 2011). Elsewhere, in Latin America, it was found that while the presence of young people in the households promoted older adults' internet adoption to begin with, the presence of their spouses or partners increased the time these adults spent online. Correspondingly, when family members do not share the same household, older family members appear to learn and adopt digital technologies far more slowly or reluctantly (Taipale et al., 2018).

Norms also dictate etiquette for technology use in social settings whose rules are often dependent on differences in regionality (Canton, 2012). According to Peters and Allan (2018), smartphones share four elements that intersect with regional and personal customs and values. One's technology use is often conceptualized as "value-laden" (Peters & Allan, 2018, p. 358) and reflects the users activities, social status, economic activities and status, preferences in leisure activities, and information about communication patterns and platforms (Bakardjieva, 2005; Calder-Dawe & Gavey, 2016). As a result, the way in which electronic media is used differently across cultures may result in or be a consequence of what norms are considered appropriate in relationships as it pertains to technology. For example, Facebook is perceived different by different cultures (Hong & Na, 2018). Another example often cited often in the literature is the concept of internet addiction, where different cultures have different definitions (Chen & Nath, 2016; Gmel et al., 2019). In fact, there is a relationship between one's personality, their culture, and their propensity toward meeting internet addiction criteria within their region (Sariyska et al., 2014).

Similarly, prevalence rates for social media addiction also vary based on culture, where individualist countries report a prevalence of 14% and collectivist cultures reporting 35% (Cheng et al., 2021). Another contextual factor as it relates to appropriateness of internet activities are norms that correspond with one's identity and roles in personal relationships. For example, the norms around how one communicates with families and partners now has changed drastically in the last 50 years, thus influencing the ways we connect with one another (Taipale, 2019). This is precisely how culture impacts the use of technology in relationships. The evaluation as to whether behavior is appropriate is dependent on the norms in one's social structure (Hertlein & Twist, 2019). One study examined technology and personal boundaries in romantic relationships in European couples. Their findings indicated that more boundary crossings were associated with lower levels of relationship satisfaction, but the study was unable to determine whether nationality made a difference in how boundaries were decided upon and enforced (Norton et al., 2018). In another study, however, Hertlein (in press) demonstrated that there were in fact differences in how Austrians and Americans perceive norms about technology use in relationships. The findings indicate that Austrians are more relaxed when it comes to establishing boundaries in their relationships, less likely to surveille their partners, and experience less distress when a breach in the relationship rules occurs.

Determining Cultural Effects of Technology on Relationships

Standardized Assessments

Several mechanisms are in place to determine at what point technology usage has a negative effect on relationships. One approach is to use standardized assessments dedicated to specific cultural groups (i.e., Laconi, et al., 2019). For example, one could use the Italian version of the Internet Disorder Scale (Monacis, Sinatra, Griffiths, & Palo, 2018), the Arabic version of the Internet Compulsive Use scale (Khazaal et al., 2011), a version with a Swiss population (Gmel et al., 2019), Korean population (Kim et al., 2014), and another developed for a Japanese population (Yong et al., 2017). There are also scales that focus on the use of the smartphone rather than the internet itself and are culturally dependent in their definitions such as problematic behaviors including the Problematic Smartphone Use scale for Spanish and French populations (Lopez-Fernandez, 2015). More have been developed to understand how the general Compulsive Internet Use Scale (Laconi et al., 2014) has fared in other populations including a Chinese population (Dhir et al., 2015); a Portuguese sample (Pontes et al., 2016), and Indian, Turkish, French, and Philippine samples (Fernendes et al., 2021; Khazaal et al., 2012).

This method, however, is fraught with challenges if one were to rely solely on these instruments. First, the bulk of the assessments is generally aimed at uncovering a level of dependence on technology (Lortie & Guitton, 2013) rather than highlighting the emergence of other internet technology interruptions and effects on relationships. One notable exception to the assessment of how technology affects relationships is the scale The Technology in Intimate Relationships Assessment (Campbell & Murray, 2015). This scale was developed based on the Couple and Family Technology Framework (Hertlein, 2012; Hertlein & Blumer, 2013) and two subscales (intimacy-enhancing behaviors and intimacy-reducing behaviors). Second, hey do not exclusively measure the effects of cell phone usage cross culturally.

Informal Assessment of Culturally Informed Impact on Structure and Process

The determination as to whether specific activities on the internet are interfering with relationship progress and satisfaction is likely to be found in the way in which it affects the structure and process of relationships. For example, it may be culturally appropriate in some circumstances to have rules in place where each partner gets permission to be able to make posts. In other cultures that type of rule or boundary might be considered restrictive and inappropriate. Again, it is not a specific set of behaviors that are universally deemed as problematic. It is the determination of the couple to identify how the boundaries and the rules that they see fit with their cultural norms, ideals, and expectations. A particular cultural group may have rules around contact with former partners while in a committed relationship. In the case of online technology that contact can be made relatively easily in that the individual may also be contacted by a former partner without necessarily inviting that former partner to do so. In other cultures, however, that rule may not be the case; the framework that we utilized does not dictate whether one rule is appropriate or not. The framework provides allowance for multiple perspectives and rules to be developed consistent with one's culture and then assess is whether those rules that have been developed have a positive negative or neutral effect on the relationship globally. In an exploration into phone usage and relationships in Mozambique, common issues included infidelity being facilitated over the phone and the intrusion of other people having access to you at many hours of the day and night, leading to questions from partners about who was messaging or calling and why (Archambault, 2011). The definition of infidelity in Mozambique may be different than the definition in other cultures, especially when trying to define emotional infidelity that is facilitated online (Morrissey et al., 2019). Another example is that mobile phones seem to be associated with more surveillance of husbands on their wives (Kenaw, 2012), perhaps more so than other cultures.

Bringing Couples Together in Establishing Technological Values

When couples are disparate in their cultural orientation, they may fall into one of four couple typologies: integrated, coexisting, singularity, and unresolved (Seshadri & Knudson-Martin, 2013). Independent of these typologies, however, there are some important principles that must be upheld in the process of negotiating difference. These include: (a) Creating a We, (b) Framing Differences, (c) Emotional Maintenance, and (d) Positioning themselves with family and societal contexts (Seshadri & Knudson-Martin, 2013). While not originally considered within the differences in cultures and technology use in relationships, these strategies can be applied to understanding the impact of technology on couple's lives. Below we list the adaptations we have made to these strategies specific to couples and technology.

Creating an "e-We." Creating a "We" means that the couple defines themselves not as a couple who experiences difference, but as a couple that is bonded and has a narrative about who they are that is characterized by shared meaning and togetherness rather than difference (Seshadri & Knudson-Martin, 2013). This strategy is characterized by friendship, commitment, shared time together, and common ground and shared goals. In the case of a "we" in technology, the couple can organize their technology usage in ways that demonstrate their commitment to one another and their friendship. For example, there may be cultural differences between individuals in a relationship on how (or whether) they should post information about themselves on their relationship with others. Depending on the cultural norms for a couple around posting, the therapist can conceptualize this as a strength for the couple in that they have a common agreement around how their rules about social media posting supports their connection to one another and their development of intimacy in their relationship. In cases where individuals in a couple are from disparate cultural backgrounds and report incompatible rules and values around posting, for example, the therapist can cultivate a "we" through exploring the motivations for decisions to post or not post, slowly moving the couple toward the motivation they had for posting.

For the purposes of this chapter, we translated this into creating an "e-We." This means that the couple can co-create their "e-version" of themselves and work toward agreement about how that "e-We" is communicated to others outside of the relationship. This can include communication of how photos are posted, whether certain people are tagged photos, how one responds to invitations from others outside of their relationship, who is included in text message changes (whether it is appropriate to include a new partner in text chains with family members or peers), etc.

Friendship can also be augmented by working with the couple to include technology as part of their norm in their relationship. For example, therapists can ask couples to share information, photos, or gifs via text or other messaging programs to move toward more self-disclosure and demonstrate commitment to one another. It demonstrates more disclosure by helping each person to really understand what makes the other tick and what the other finds interesting. It demonstrates commitment because one partner may feel that they are not important if texts do not come through when it is so easy to communicate. In fact, some research on technology and communication suggests that people who communicate over technology express higher degrees of commitment in their relationships than those who do not (Abbasi, 2019).

Framing Differences as Differences in Software, Not Hardware. Framing differences means that the couple decentralizes differences and instead emphasizes what they can learn from one another, how flexible they can be, and to utilize some of what is different (Seshadri & Knudson-Martin, 2013). In how they use technology as a strength, couples have the advantage of being able to pull from each of their cultures as to what might be the most advantageous ways to use technology in their relationship. To address framing difference is to convince the couple that, despite preferences in technology use, the difference is not as important as other people make it out to be. This includes focusing on the person and what the person can bring into the relationship rather than how that person uses technology.

In practice, we frame this as differences in software as opposed to differences in hardware. The rationale for this is that often couples experience their differences in how they use technology as akin to their personality (also viewed as immutable). To frame it as software suggests some flexibility and can be used with a metaphor to adapt or upgrade software, which will also translate into change more easily. One way we talk about it with couples is in terms of two seemingly disparate or competing operating systems: for example, one person's system may be described as an Apple and another as an IBM. Such a discussion can be used when the cultural difference exists between the members of the couple but can also be used when the couple agrees on their technology usage and the difference is between their use and the cultural context in which they are positioned or reside. In this way, the differences in personal software can be presented as differences that initially brought the couple together. The other important piece of this is wiling to learn the new software and engage in some of the opportunities presented. For example, there are often only certain apps allowed on Apple products and not available on Google and vice versa. In applying this metaphor to couples, the therapist can talk about the flexibility needed in relationships to adapt and allow for different uses of technology rather than to dictate how it should be used with family, friends, etc.

Emotional Maintenance. Of the strategies described, this one is of utmost priority for couples in bridging their cultural gaps with technology. Much of the literature on technology and relationships discusses the nature of how quickly and intimately relationships facilitated by online technology develop based on the increased level of self-disclosure (Lee et al., 2019). Part of how to emotionally maintain relationships when there are cultural differences between partners is to communicate emotions and insecurities (Seshadri & Knudson-Martin, 2013). In couple relationships where there are varying cultural origins, if and how emotional disclosures are made via technology may be dependent to some degree on one's cultural background. For example, some individuals may opt for social media as a place to self-disclose; others may believe that private text messages are more appropriate. In fact, some research suggests that disclosures made over social media in some contexts are less personal because they are offered instead to a large group, rendering the partner less special (Tokunga, 2016).

Positioning in Relation to Societal and Familial Context. The final strategy used by couples to negotiate difference noted by Seshadri and Knudson-Martin (2013) is how the couple establishes a boundary between themselves and those outside of their relationship. Generally, positioning oneself in societal and family contexts is grounded in Bronfenbrenner's ecological model and how each layer of our lives is recursively affected other contextual layers. Technology is pervasive in every area of our lives and therefore embedded in the levels described by Bronfenbrenner (Hertlein & Twist, 2019). For example, one study found that mass media has an impact on parent involvement with junior high students as well as the attitudes of the teachers toward Taiwanese youth regarding English language achievement (Kung & Lee, 2016). In addition, Lee et al. (2016) suggest expanding theoretical directions for problematic social networking use in teens can be achieved through further exploration of Bronfenbrenner's model. At the microsystem level, parenting style (authoritative, authoritarian, permissive, and rejecting-neglecting) is linked to self-regulation, which may in turn influence a teen's motivation for using social networking sites (SNSs). In addition, the support that parents offer may also influence whether their child looks for that support online. In short, the more support a parent offers, it is hypothesized that their teens will be less likely to rely on SNSs in problematic ways to ascertain that support (Lee et al., 2016).

Positioning one's self in broader contexts includes communicating boundaries to those outside of the relationship, managing (and limiting) reactivity to others, using humor, and asserting oneself in certain spaces. Communication boundaries outside of the relationship may include relying on cultural norms of announcing relationships via social media or establishing rules consistent with one's culture on with whom one communicates outside of their relationship. The couple can determine what platforms, if any, to announce their relationship in ways that are supportive by both cultural expectations. Couples should also be able to communicate why they selected certain sharing preferences if their selection to adopt a certain platform is divergent from their partner. In managing and limiting reactivity to others, members of the couple can consult and rely on their partner to learn another perspective to potentially reduce their reactivity to others' behaviors in online spaces. Couples can also look for ways to assert themselves in culturally appropriate ways online through joining certain sites together, assisting one another with writing posts that will be culturally consistent with and perhaps even combine elements from both of their cultures.

Conclusion

The interpretation of how technology is used in relationships is a function of many factors, including one's regional, national, or other cultural backgrounds. The differences that couples may experience are to be viewed as opportunities for connectedness and negotiation rather than opportunities for division. Using the approaches offered in the research for couple negotiation can be applied to couples who use technology differently and can serve as a further bonding experience.

References

Abbasi, I. S. (2019). Falling prey to online romantic alternatives: Evaluating social media alternative partners in committed versus dating relationships. *Social Science Computer Review*, *37*(6), 723–733. https://doi.org/10.1177/0894439318793947

Abel, S., Machin, T., & Brownlow, C. (2021). Social media, rituals, and long-distance family relationship maintenance: A mixed-methods systematic review. *New Media & Society*, *23*(3), 632–654. https://doi.org/10.1177/1461444820958717

Archambault, J. S. (2011). Breaking up 'because of the phone' and the transformative potential of information in southern Mozambique. *New Media & Society*, *13*(3), 444–456. doi:10.1177/1461444810393906

Bacigalupe, G., & Lambe, S. (2011). Virtualizing intimacy: Information communication technologies and transnational families in therapy. *Family Process*, *50*(1), 12–26.

Bacigalupe, G., & Cámara, M. (2012). Transnational families and social technologies: Reassessing immigration psychology. *Journal of Ethnic and Migration Studies, 38*(9), 1425–1438. https://doi.org/10.1080/1369183X.2012.698211

Bakardjieva, M. (2005). *Internet Society: The Internet in Everyday Life.* London: SAGE.

Barakji, F., Maguire, K. C., Reiss, H., Gaule, J., Smith, N., Pelliccio, L., Sellnow-Richmond, S., Jeon, J., & Oshagan, H. (2019). Cultural and transnational influences on the use of information communication technologies in adult long-distance family relationships: an extension of media multiplexity theory. *Journal of Family Communication, 19*(1), 30–46. https://doi.org/10.1080/15267431.2018.1530675

Barrantes Cáceres, R., & Cozzubo Chaparro, A. (2019). Age for learning, age for teaching: the role of inter-generational, intra-household learning in Internet use by older adults in Latin America. *Information, Communication & Society, 22*(2), 250–266. https://doi.org/10.1080/1369118X.2017.1371785

Beck, U., & Beck-Gernsheim, E. (2014). *Distant love: Personal life in the global age* (R. Livingstone, Trans.). Cambridge, England: Polity Press.

Belus, J. M., Pentel, K. Z., Cohen, M. J., Fischer, M. S., & Baucom, D. H. (2019). Staying connected: An examination of relationship maintenance behaviors in long-distance relationships. *Marriage & Family Review, 55*(1), 78–98. https://doi.org/10.1080/01494929.2018.1458004

Billedo, C. J., Kerkhof, P., & Finkenauer, C. (2015). The use of social networking sites for relationship maintenance in long-distance and geographically close romantic relationships. *Cyberpsychology, Behavior, and Social Networking, 18*(3), 152–157. https://doi.org/10.1089/cyber.2014.0469

Blank, G., & Lutz, C. (2018). Benefits and harms from Internet use: A differentiated analysis of Great Britain. *New Media & Society, 20*(2), 618–640. https://doi.org/10.1177/1461444816667135.

Calder-Dawe, O., & Gavey, N. (2016). Making sense of everyday sexism: Young people and the gendered contours of sexism. *Women's Studies International Forum, 55*, 1–9.

Campbell, E. C., & Murray, C. E. (2015). Measuring the Impact of Technology on Couple Relationships: The Development of the Technology and Intimate Relationship Assessment. *Journal of Couple & Relationship Therapy, 14*, 254–256. https://doi.org/ 10.1080/15332691.2014.953657

Canton, N. (2012). Cell phone culture: How cultural differences affect mobile use. Retrieved October 11, 2020, from: https://www.cnn.com/2012/09/27/tech/mobile-culture-usage/index.html

Cáceres, R. B., & Chaparro, A.C. (2017). Age for learning, age for teaching: the role of intergenerational, intra-household learning in Internet use by older adults in Latin America. *Information, Communication & Society.* https://doi.org/10.1080/1369118X.2017.1371785

Chen, B., & Marcus, J. (2012). Students' self-presentation on Facebook: An examination of personality and self-construal factors. *Computers in Human Behavior, 28*(6), 2091–2099. https://doi.org/10.1016/j.chb.2012.06.013

Chen L., & Nath, R. (2016). Understanding the underlying factors of Internet addiction across cultures: A comparison study. *Electronic Commerce Research and Applications, 17*, 38–48. https://doi.org/10.1016/j.elerap.2016.02.003.

Cheng, C., Lau, Y-C., Chan, L., & Luk, J. W. (2021). Prevalence of social media addiction across 32 nations: Meta-analysis with subgroup analysis of classification schemes and cultural values. *Addictive Behaviors, 117*, 106845–106845. https://doi.org/10.1016/j.addbeh.2021.106845

David, M. E., Roberts, J. A., & Christenson, B. (2018). Too much of a good thing: Investigating the association between actual smartphone use and individual well-being. *International Journal of Human-Computer Interaction, 34*(3), 265–275. https://doi.org/10.1080/10447318.2017.1349250

Dhir, A., Chen, S., & Nieminen, M. (2015). Psychometric Validation of the Chinese Compulsive Internet Use Scale (CIUS) with Taiwanese High School Adolescents. *Psychiatric Quarterly, 86*(4), 581–596. https://doi.org/10.1007/s11126-015-9351-9

Felton, E. (2014). A/Effective connections: Mobility, technology and well-being. *Emotion, Space and Society, 13*, 9–15. https://doi.org/10.1016/j.emospa.2014.09.001

Fernandes, B., Aydin, C., Uzun, B., Tan-Mansukhani, R., & Biswas, U. N. (2021). Psychometric properties of the compulsive internet use scale among adolescents in India, Philippines and Turkey. *Addictive Behaviors Reports, 13*, 100349. https://doi.org/10.1016/j.abrep.2021.100349

Fox, S., & Rainie, L. (2014). The Web at 25. PEW Research Center. Retrieved May 11, 2021 from: http://www.pewinternet.org/2014/02/25/the-web-at-25-in-the-u-s

Francisco, V. (2015). "The internet is magic": Technology intimacy and transnational families. *Critical Sociology, 41,* 173–190. https://doi.org/10.1177/0896920513484602

Gmel, G., Khazaal, Y., Studer, J., Baggio, S., & Marmet, S. (2019). Development of a short form of the compulsive internet use scale in Switzerland. *International Journal of Methods in Psychiatric Research, 28*(1), e1765–n/a. https://doi.org/10.1002/mpr.1765

Goodman-Deane, J., Mieczakowski, A., Johnson, D., Goldhaber, T., & Clarkson, P. J. (2016). The impact of communication technologies on life and relationship satisfaction. *Computers in Human Behavior, 57,* 219–229. https://doi.org/10.1016/j.chb.2015.11.053s

Hamill, L. (2011). Changing times: Home life and domestic habit. In *The connected home: The future of domestic life* (pp. 29–57). London: Springer London.

Hampton, A., Rawlings, J., Treger, S., & Sprecher, S. (2017). Channels of computer-mediated communication and satisfaction in long-distance relationships. *Interpersona, 11*(2), 171–187. https://doi.org/10.5964/ijpr.v11i2.273

Hertlein, K. M. (2012). Digital dwelling: Technology in couple and family relationships. *Family Relations, 61*(3), 374–387. doi:10.1111/j.1741-3729.2012.00702.x

Hertlein, K. M., & Ancheta, K. (2014). Advantages and disadvantages of technology in relationships: Findings from an open-ended survey. *The Qualitative Report, 19* (article 22), 1–11. Retrieved December 6, 2018, from https://nsuworks.nova.edu/tqr/vol19/iss11/2

Hertlein, K. M., & Blumer, M. L. (2013). *The couple and family technology framework: Intimate relationships in a digital age.* New York: Routledge.

Hertlein, K. M., & Chan, D. (2020). The rationale behind texting, videoconferencing, and mobile phones in couple relationships. *Marriage and Family Review, 56*(8), 739–763. https://doi.org/10.1080/01494929.2020.1737624

Hertlein, Twist, Twist, Markie L. C., & ProQuest. (2019). *The internet family: technology in couple and family relationships.* Routledge.

Hong, S., & Na, J. (2018). How Facebook is perceived and used by people across cultures: The implications of cultural differences in the use of Facebook. *Social Psychological and Personality Science, 9*(4), 435–443. https://doi.org/10.1177/1948550617711227

Janning, M., Gao, W., & Snyder, E. (2018). Constructing shared "space": Meaningfulness in long-distance romantic relationship communication formats. *Journal of Family Issues, 39*(5), 1281–1303. https://doi.org/10.1177/0192513X17698726

Kenaw, S. (2012). Cultural translation of mobile telephones: Mediation of strained communication among ethiopian married couples. *The Journal of Modern African Studies, 50*(1), 131–155. doi:10.1017/S0022278X11000632

Khazaal, Y., Chatton, A., Atwi, K., Zullino, D., Khan, R., & Billieux, J. (2011). Arabic validation of the Compulsive Internet Use Scale (CIUS). *Substance Abuse Treatment, Prevention and Policy, 6*(1), 32–32. https://doi.org/10.1186/1747-597X-6-32

Khazaal, Y., Chatton, A., Horn, A., Achab, S., Thorens, G., Zullino, D., & Billieux, J. (2012). French Validation of the Compulsive Internet Use Scale (CIUS). *Psychiatric Quarterly, 83*(4), 397–405. https://doi.org/10.1007/s11126-012-9210-x

Kim, D., Lee, Y., Lee, J., Nam, J. K., & Chung, Y. (2014). Development of Korean Smartphone addiction proneness scale for youth. *PloS One, 9*(5), e97920–e97920. https://doi.org/10.1371/journal.pone.0097920

Kim, Y., Sohn, D., Choi, S. M. (2011). Cultural difference in motivations for using social network sites: A comparative study of American and Korean college students. *Computers in Human Behavior, 27,* 365–372. https://doi.org/10.1016/j.chb.2010.08.015

Kolozsvari, O. (2015). "Physically we are apart, mentally we are not": Creating a shared space and a sense of belonging in long-distance relationships. *Qualitative Sociology Review, 11*(4), 102–115.

Kung, H., & Lee, C. (2016). Factors influencing junior high school students' English language achievement in Taiwan: a Bronfenbrenner's ecological system approach. *Journal of Educational Practice and Research, 29*(1), 35–66.

Laconi, S., Urbán, R., Kaliszewska-Czeremska, K., Kuss, D. J., Gnisci, A.,...& Király, O. (2019). Psychometric Evaluation of the Nine-Item Problematic Internet Use Questionnaire (PIUQ-9) in Nine European Samples of Internet Users. *Frontiers in Psychiatry, 10,* 136–136. https://doi.org/10.3389/fpsyt.2019.00136

Laconi, S., Rodgers, R. F., & Chabrol, H. (2014). The measurement of Internet addiction: A critical review of existing scales and their psychometric properties. *Computers in Human Behavior*. https://doi.org/10.1016/j. chb.2014.09.026.

Lee, J., Gillath, O., & Miller, A. (2019). Effects of self- and partner's online disclosure on relationship intimacy and satisfaction. *PloS One*, 14(3), e0212186–e0212186. https://doi.org/10.1371/journal. pone.0212186

Lee, E., Ho, S., & Lwin, M. (2016). Explicating problematic social network sites use: A review of concepts, theoretical frameworks, and future directions for communication theorizing. *New Media & Society*, 19(2), 308–326. https://doi.org/10.1177/1461444816671891

Lin, C. A., Atkin, D. J., Cappotto, C., Davis, C., Dean, J., Eisenbaum, J., …Vidican, S. (2015). Ethnicity, digital divides and uses of the internet for health information. *Computers in Human Behavior*, 51, 216–223. https://doi.org/10.1016/j.chb.2015.04.054

Lopez-Fernandez, O. (2015). Short version of the Smartphone Addiction Scale adapted to Spanish and French: Towards a cross-cultural research in problematic mobile phone use. *Addictive Behaviors*, 64, 275–280. https://doi.org/10.1016/j.addbeh.2015.11.013

Lortie, C. L., & Guitton, M. J. (2013). Internet addiction assessment tools: Dimensional structure and methodological status. *Addiction*, 108(7), 1207–1216. https://doi.org/10.1111/add.12202

Madianou, M., & Miller, D. (2011). Mobile phone parenting: reconfiguring relationships between Filipina migrant mothers and their left-behind children. *New Media and Society* 13(3), 457–470.

McDaniel, B. T., & Drouin, M. (2019). Daily technology interruptions and emotional and relational well-being. *Computers in Human Behavior*, 99, 1–8. https://doi.org/10.1016/j.chb.2019.04.027

Miller-Ott, A. E., Kelly, L., & Duran, R. L. (2012). The effects of cell phone usage rules on satisfaction in romantic relationships. *Communication Quarterly*, 60(1), 17–34. https://doi.org/10.1080/01463373.2012.64

Mok, D., Wellman, B., & Carrasco, J. (2010). Does distance matter in the age of the Internet? *Urban Studies*, 47(13), 2747–2783. https://doi.org/10.1177/0042098010377363

Monacis, L., Sinatra, M., Griffiths, M. D., & de Palo, V. (2018). Assessment of the Italian Version of the Internet Disorder Scale (IDS-15). *International Journal of Mental Health and Addiction*, 16(3), 680–691. https://doi.org/10.1007/s11469-017-9823-2

Morgan H. M., Entwistle V. A., Cribb A., Christmas S., Owens J., Skea Z. C., et al. (2017). We need to talk about purpose: a critical interpretive synthesis of health and social care professionals' approaches to self-management support for people with long-term conditions. *Health Expectations*, 20, 243–259. 10.1111/hex.12453

Morrissey, L., Wettersten, K. B., & Brionez, J. (2019). Qualitatively derived definitions of emotional infidelity among professional women in cross-gender relationships. *Psychology of Women Quarterly*, 43(1), 73–87. https://doi.org/10.1177/036168431880668

Murray, C. E., & Campbell, E. C. (2015). The pleasures and perils of technology in intimate relationships. *Journal of Couple & Relationship Therapy*, 14, 116–140.

Norton, A., Baptist, J., & Hogan, B. (2018). Computer-mediated communication in intimate relationships: Associations of boundary crossing, intrusion, relationship satisfaction, and partner responsiveness. *Journal of Marital and Family Therapy*, 44(1), 165–182.

Peters, C., & Allan, S. (2018). Everyday imagery. *Convergence: The International Journal of Research into New Media Technologies*, 24(4), 357–373. https://doi.org/10.1177/1354856516678395

Pontes, H. M., Caplan, S. E., & Griffiths, M. D. (2016). Psychometric validation of the Generalized Problematic Internet Use Scale 2 in a Portuguese sample. *Computers in Human Behavior*, 63, 823–833. https://doi.org/10.1016/j.chb.2016.06.015

Przybylski, A., & Weinstein, N. (2012). Can you connect with me now? How the presence of mobile communication technology influences face-to-face conversation quality. *Journal of Social and Personal Relationships*, 30, 237–246. https://doi.org/10.1177/0265407512453827

Sariyska, R., Reuter, M., Bey, K., Sha, P., Li, M., Chen, Y-F., Liu, W., Zhu, Y., Li, C-B., Suárez-Rivillas, A., Feldmann, M., Hellmann, M., Keiper, J., Markett, S., Young, K. S., & Montag, C. (2014). Self-esteem, personality and Internet Addiction: A cross-cultural comparison study. *Personality and Individual Differences*, 61-62, 28–33. https://doi.org/10.1016/j.paid.2014.01.001

Scheerder, A., van Deursen, A. J. A. ., & van Dijk, J. A. G. . (2019). Internet use in the home: Digital inequality from a domestication perspective. *New Media & Society*, 21(10), 2099–2118. https://doi.org/10.1177/1461444819844299

Seshadri, G., & Knudson-Martin, C. (2013). How couples manage interracial and intercultural differences: Implications for clinical practice. *Journal of Marital and Family Therapy*, 39(1), 43–58. https://doi.org/10.1111/j.1752-0606.2011.00262.x

Siibak, A., & Tamme, V. (2013). 'Who introduced granny to Facebook?': An exploration of everyday family interactions in web-based communication environments. *Northern Lights: Film & Media Studies Yearbook, 11*(1), 71–89.

Sullivan, K. T., Riedstra, J., Arellano, B., Cardillo, B., Kalach, V., & Ram, A. (2020). Online communication and dating relationships: Effects of decreasing online communication on feelings of closeness and relationship satisfaction. *Journal of Social and Personal Relationships*, 37(8–9), 2409–2418. https://doi.org/10.1177/0265407520924707

Taipale, S. (2019). *Intergenerational Connections in Digital Families.* Springer International Publishing AG.

Taipale, S. & Farinosi, M. (2018). The big meaning of small messages: The use of WhatsApp in intergenerational family communication. In J. Zhou & G. Salvendy (Eds.), *Human aspects of IT for the aged population 2018*, lecture notes in computer science (pp. 532–546). Cham: Springer.

Taipale, S., Petrovĉiĉ, A., & Dolniĉar, V. (2018). Intergenerational solidarity and ICT usage: Empirical insights from Finnish and Slovenian families. In S. Taipale, T.-A. Wilska, & C. Gilleard (Eds.), *Digital technologies and generational identity: ICT usage across the life course* (pp. 68–86). London & New York: Routledge.

Tokunaga, R. S. (2016). Interpersonal surveillance over social network sites. *Journal of Social and Personal Relationships, 33*(2), 171–190. https://doi.org/10.1177/0265407514568749

van Deursen, A. J. A. M., & Helsper, E. J. (2018). Collateral benefits of Internet use: Explaining the diverse outcomes of engaging with the Internet. *New Media & Society 20*(7), 2333–2351. https://doi.org/10.1177/1461444817715282.

van Deursen, A. J. A. M., & van Dijk, J. A.G.M. (2011). Internet skills and the digital divide. *New Media & Society, 13*(6), 893–911. https://doi.org/10.1177/1461444810386774

Yong, R. K. F., Inoue, A., & Kawakami, N. (2017). The validity and psychometric properties of the Japanese version of the Compulsive Internet Use Scale (CIUS). *BMC Psychiatry, 17*(1), 201–201. https://doi.org/10.1186/s12888-017-1364-5

22

CROSS-CULTURAL TECHNOLOGY USE IN MAINTAINING ROMANTIC AND FAMILIAL RELATIONSHIPS

Katherine M. Hertlein, Nicole Feno, Alysha Robinson, Norma Gomez, Jonathan Molina, and Teri Raven

Introduction

Increasing trends in globalization and migration have fueled the reliance on the use of electronic and web-based communication between family members and couples for connection and communication (Westjohn et al., 2009). In the United States alone, 81% of adults report using YouTube and 69% Facebook, with an overall proportion of social media users at 72.3% (Statista, 2021). In the United Arab Emirates, the proportion of the population using social media is 99%; South Korea follows at 89.3%, followed by Taiwan at 88.1% and the Netherlands at 88.0% (Statista, 2021). Technology is a major entity in personal relationships. Its dominance as a communication medium has dramatically altered the way people connect with partners, peers, and family members in a relatively short span of time (Bruess, 2019; Lomanowska & Guitton, 2016; McDaniel & Drouin, 2019; Taipale, 2019). Further, with the shift toward engagement in remote education, vocation, leisure, and other socialization due to the COVID-19 pandemic, Internet-based communications, and dependence on them as the primary way to connect with others, are infused into romantic and familial relationships more than ever (Garfin, 2020; Kluck et al., 2021).

Technology-informed or not, maintaining personal relationships is a complex process. In romantic relationships, it involves many elements including but not limited to communication processes, conflict management, attributions, attention to one's partner, social networks, dyadic coping, and forgiveness/response to partner transgressions (Lydon & Quinn, 2013; Sprecher et al., 2019; Stafford, 2019). Five maintenance behaviors have been identified as core predictors of positive, healthy relationships: positivity (e.g., kindness, refraining from criticism); openness (e.g., self-disclosure, and disclosure pertaining to the relationship); assurances (e.g., affirming commitment, faithfulness, and support); social networks (e.g., spending time with family and friends); and shared tasks (e.g., equitably

DOI: 10.4324/9781003297871-25

sharing responsibilities) (Stafford & Canary, 1991). Culturally, however, there may be some debate as to whether these factors contribute to a healthy relationship in every culture (Gaines & Ferenczi, 2019).

First, the aforementioned qualities of a healthy relationship cited from 1991 are 30 years old in their definition and contemporary relationships – in our more recent culture and in Western cultures in particular – highly value partner equality in healthy relationships, defined as equity fairness in which both partners are "equitably treated" (Stafford & Canary, 1991). In fact, social equity theory is one of the cornerstones of relational maintenance and places a heavy emphasis on reciprocity in relationships (Eastwick, 2013; Stafford, 2019). Second, different cultures vary in what they value. For example, partners in countries that identify as traditional/self-expression cultures report use of maintenance strategies to a greater extent than do their counterparts in the survival/modern values cultures (Yum & Canary, 2003). Third, the literature suggests that couples who are geographically (and, perhaps, surrounded by different cultures) are reliant on technology to moderate their relationships (Taylor & Bazarova, 2018). It is imperative that we better understand how technology use is informed by culture and contexts.

Given that technology usage is a worldwide phenomenon, little is known about the influence – if any – on how cultural norms affect technology use in personal relationships. To date, the published literature accomplishes two things: presenting a summation of how technology affects relationships (i.e., Caughlin & Wang, 2019), and a summation of cultural differences in relationships (i.e., Gaines, & Ferenczi, 2019). Few articles investigate the combination of technology use in different cultural contexts, a striking omission in the literature given the globalization of technology in our personal lives.

Maintaining Healthy Relationships

Behavioral relationship maintenance practices are central to the well-being of romantic and family relationships. Positivity, openness, and assurances are practiced as ongoing verbal interactions providing affirmation and promoting stability by reducing uncertainty. Shared tasks and networks promote interdependence within family members. Similar to romantic maintenance practices, family maintenance behaviors share commonalities cross-culturally, but also highlight different dynamics as centrally important depending on the family's culture. For example, reflective conversation orientation describes a family climate in which participation in communicative interactions about all topics is encouraged whereas conformity orientation represents a family climate in which uniformity of attitudes, values, and beliefs is expected (Aloia 2020). As these orientations are often reflective of cultural values, it follows that while the established five core maintenance behaviors can be consistent cross-culturally, there is variation on the relevance of specific behaviors in accordance with the family unit's culture.

Technology and Relationship Maintenance in U.S. Samples

The influence of smartphones on the processes of relationships includes how relationships are initiated, maintained, and end (Hertlein, 2012; Hertlein & Twist, 2019). For romantic couples, the Internet also inspires changes to the processes within personal romantic relationships (Coyne et al., 2011; Hertlein, 2012; Hertlein & Twist, 2019). Benefits include improved connection, access, and intimacy with one another (Billedo et al., 2015;

Currin et al., 2020; Hertlein & Ancheta, 2014; Hertlein & Chan, 2020; Hobbs et al., 2017; McCormack & Ogilvie, 2020). Drawbacks include the potential for hurt feelings from those who feel neglected by the individual using the phone and not attending to the relationship (Kushlev & Dunn, 2019; Latif et al., 2020; McDaniel & Radesky, 2018; Modecki et al., 2020). In studies using American samples, communication facilitated by technology has been associated with higher levels of relationship satisfaction (Roberts & David, 2016).

In families, technology enables new methods of communicating (e.g., Schofield-Clark, 2013) and allows parents to adapt their parenting practices (Johnson & Hertlein, 2019; Lanigan et al., 2009). Implications for technology use in the family may be that the accessibility and interference of smartphones may be conceptualized as technoference, or technology's interference with attentional processes to the tasks at hand (Braune-Krickau et al., 2021; Johnson & Hertlein, 2019; McDaniel & Coyne, 2016). Smartphones may upend the hierarchy in the family as those younger in the family may be more knowledgeable about technological systems (McDaniel & Coyne, 2016).

Technology and Relationship Maintenance in Multinational Samples

Globalization has influenced the trends in relationship maintenance (Sanri & Goodwin, 2014). Differences in how people communicate with one another are influenced by the norms and values of cultural groups (Canton, 2012; Na et al., 2015; Sanri & Goodwin, 2014; Yoshie & Sauter, 2020). Smartphones have the capacity to support and facilitate engagement in cultural customs but can also conflict with cultural or regional norms (Peters & Allan, 2018). One's use of technology and software choices reflects socioeconomic status, preferences in activities and communication patterns, and social status (Calder-Dawe & Gavey, 2016). For example, Facebook is perceived differently by varied cultures and may reinforce cultural differences (Hong & Na, 2018). Some of these differences relate to the construction of one's network depending on whether the user is associated with an individual versus a collectivistic culture (Na et al., 2015).

Madianou (2014) found smartphones are used in transnational families to maintain connections but, over time, do not find those interactions as necessarily satisfying. On the other hand, if parents can monitor how technology interferes with their day-to-day lives, they have higher levels of understanding of how it changes their practices. Those who do not allow as much interference may report feeling they are more effective in their parenting because they are not distracted (Modecki et al., 2020).

The challenges introduced to relationships according to a sample of participants based in the U.K., for example, included impaired trust, challenges in the interpretation of messages, and the intrusion from work life into one's home space (McCormack & Ogilvie, 2020). These findings, consistent with Hertlein's and Ancheta's (2014) and Hertlein's and Chan's (2020) findings, also present noticeable differences. In the McCormack and Ogilvie, 2020 sample from the U.K., participants noted technoference (McDaniel & Coyne, 2016) was the primary challenge to their relationship (McCormack & Ogilvie, 2020).

Outside of these studies, most of the remaining scholarship addressing technology use in different cultures is typically related to Internet addiction. Few articles examine differences between cultures and technology within personal relationships. One study identified differences in how Austrians and Americans use technology in their relationships. In a survey of 1,166 participants (half Austrian and half American), differences between the two populations included how acceptable technology was in relationships, how often they contacted their partner during the day, the presence of rules in their relationships, how affordable technology was in their relationships, the prevalence of sexting in their relationships, and the presence of using technology to spy on their partner (Hertlein, 2021). Specifically, Americans were more likely to spy on their partners, more likely to engage in sexting, were more likely to have rules in their relationship related to technology, reported that technology was more affordable for them than Australians, considered technology as more acceptable in their relationships, and contacted their partners more often using technology than Austrians.

Another study has looked specifically at the structure of relationships as defined by roles, rules, and boundaries in European couples. In a quantitative study of over 3,000 couples, Norton et al. (2018) found that electronic boundaries are a critical part of couple satisfaction and partner responsiveness. These findings suggest technology use in relationships might be tied to different behaviors and different levels of what is considered satisfying in a relationship (Hertlein, 2021). Still, there is little data about how technology is used to maintain relationships in multinational populations.

Purpose and Research Question

This study was part of a larger research project exploring how different cultures use technology in their relationships. Thus far, the research on technology in romantic and family relationships has predominately evaluated how electronic methods of communication such as email, text, and video influence (a) perceived intimacy and satisfaction in couple relationships and (b) the roles held by parents and children in family systems. As Sullivan et al. (2020) noted, "These mixed findings suggest a more nuanced view is necessary to understand the effects of online communication on intimate relationships" (p. 2410). The overarching purpose of this research was to understand how technology is used in personal relationships in a multinational sample. For the purposes of this study, personal relationships are defined as romantic couple relationships and family relationships.

Methods

Theoretical Perspective

This research was informed by a phenomenological perspective characterized by "the understanding of meaningful, concrete relations implicit in the original description of experience in the context of a particular situation and is the primary target of phenomenological knowledge" (Moustakas, 1994, p. 14). The purpose of this study was not to generate a theory about how people use their phones; rather, it was to understand how variations in culture affect how technology is used in personal relationships.

We aligned ourselves with an interpretive hermeneutic perspective as described by McCracken (1988). The value of this specific method is that it enables us to rely on what we already knew about how people process technology and through the Couple and Family Technology framework (Hertlein, 2012), but also allows for the generation of new knowledge and the emergence of detail and thick, rich description within what we know and our applied framework. One challenge of conducting cross-cultural research is ensuring that the scope of the research is broad enough to account for many of the different ways in which cultural issues may emerge in the topic (Norenzayan & Heine, 2005). Therefore, the interpretive hermeneutic approach would allow for this broad context. We wanted to understand how the intersection of technology use and one's nationality influenced both the structure and process of their relationships. That is, how are relationships maintained via technology in ways that are consistent with specific cultural norms? What are the influences of culture that are missed in the explanation of technology usage in relationships thus far?

Participants

The participants for the interviews were healthy adults aged 18 and over and who could speak conversational English. In total, we interviewed 31 participants. The contextual information for the participants can be found in Table 22.1.

Table 1 Demographics of Participants

Number	Gender	Age	Nationality	Living Arrangement
01	M	38	Irish	With spouse
02	F	21	Italian	With roommate
03	M	27	German	With fiancé
04	M	22	Mexican	With roommate
05	M	22	Romania	With roommate
06	F	26	Austrian	With partner and roommate
07	F	20	German	Living alone in a flat
08	M	22	German (Bavarian)	Living alone in a flat
09	F	20	Polish	Living alone in a flat
10	F	22	South Korea	Dormitory
11	F	32	Romanian	With spouse
12	F	34	Romanian	Living alone in a flat
13	F	30	Indian	With spouse
14	F	21	Mexican	With roommate
15	F	20	Mexican	With family (parents and brothers)
16	F	23	German (Bavarian)	With roommates
17	F	22	German	With partner
18	F	20	Japanese	With roommate
19	F	20	Japanese	Dormitory
20	M	29	Austrian	With fiancé
21	F	29	Austrian	With parents
22	M	25	Polish	Dormitory with sibling
23	M	25	Polish	With parents
24	F	22	Kazakhstan	Living alone in a flat
25	F	22	Austrian	With roommate
26	F	23	German	With roommate
27	F	40	UK	Living with young son
28	F	34	Austrian	With partner
29	F	24	Croatia	With partner
30	M	27	Romanian	With roommate
31	F	20	Mexican	With roommate

Procedures

Interviews were conducted by one faculty member and one student who spoke German. Subjects participated in a semi-structured interview lasting no longer than 60 minutes, ranging from 22 to 60 minutes. The interview schedule contained 17 questions assessing how technology influenced roles, rules, boundaries, and relational processes.

Analysis

The data was analyzed by open- and axial-coding and the constant comparative method alongside an a priori analysis (Strauss & Corbin, 1990). Given the number of interviews to be read, the first author numbered each interview, read each interview, and engaged at least two more analysts for each interview in a rotating fashion. For example, Interview #001 was read by the first, second, and third authors; Interview #002 was read by the first, third, and fourth author; Interview #003 was read by the first, fourth, and fifth authors and so on. The first author read all 31 interviews; the second read 15 interviews; the third and fourth read 18 interviews, and the last author read 19 interviews.

In the coding process, we used an a piori bracketing procedure (Patton, 2014). Because we were interested in the impact of technology on relationships following the areas of the Couple and Family Technology Framework, we organized the codes that emerged into the areas of how technology was used to express roles, rules, and boundaries. Each member of the research team looked for codes consistent with the areas in the Couple and Family Technology framework. The team met to review the codes, with each reviewer contributing their codes one at a time. Once we had the entire list of codes together, we referred to the research question and then composed themes based on the codes that answered the research question (Emerson et al., 1995).

Rigor

Our establishing rigor in this study was informed by the strategies identified by Anfara et al. (2002). Credibility, or the extent to which the analysis could be deemed credible, was achieved through engaging reviewers and coders who were separate from the research process and interviews. Dependability refers to how reliable the data is, and the primary strategy we used to demonstrate this was inclusion of codes that overlapped among the independent reviewers. Transferability, or how the data can be transferred to other populations, was accomplished by asking participants for examples of their comments to provide thick, rich descriptions. Confirmability, or the objectivity of the analysis, was identified through the findings aligning with previous findings on similar topics.

Findings

How Structure of Relationships Intersects with Cultural Technology Usage

Within the structure of the relationships, participants described relationship roles to be influenced by accessibility, knowledge of technology, and contextual issues such as privilege. Rules (either implicit or explicit) often were enacted regarding time spent with devices, developed out of comparison with peers, and established due to receiving unsolicited content. Finally, the boundaries in relationships were influenced by internal struggles of those using the technology, ambiguity of expectations, and accessibility of devices and software. Findings are presented by romantic relationships and then familial relationships.

Roles Change with Technology

Accessibility to Technology Affects Roles Taken in Relationships
Accessibility to technology influences what norms are adopted as appropriate behavior in relationships. On the positive end of accessibility, participants universally reported a great deal of accessibility because of Internet and smartphone technologies. Such technology allowed them to contact their significant other or family member independent of the time of day or night, and through a variety of mediums. For example, Participant 20 stated, "The possibility to give [my girlfriend] a call whenever I want to and whenever we've got time. It's more or less a 24-hour possibility to stay in contact." Another participant noted "It helps in creating an opportunity to talk." (P. 24) and still another stated "it helps you to meet random people, just encounter people you normally wouldn't be able to find." (P. 23).

Accessibility also meant more than just communication: it meant understanding physical access, as Participant 15 noted: "It was really good that I could share my location, my own location, so [my boyfriend] was in constant contact." Participant 17 supported this by saying:

> [My boyfriend and I] use text quite regularly. He doesn't go to Uni here but far...we don't see each other in the day very often and so we resulted, kind of, to texting to know about our lives and our day, and what we are doing, we're meeting, and what we're eating, and about the cat.

The access afforded by technologies benefitted both partner and familial relationships. One participant exemplified this by stating: "In terms of my family, or me in connection to my family, as I said I travel a lot, do a research project in India so without Internet or a smartphone I would not be able to stay in touch with them." (P. 29). Another participant noted: "the Internet connectivity, the ease of calling your parents anytime, anywhere, all you have to do is have an Internet connection, that's it." (P. 13). They opted to take a more active role in their personal relationships. The accessibility offered encouraged users to "update [family] about my daily life...and to solve my daily problems. (P. 07). Another participant stated: "I talk to [my parents] more now since they both started using the text messaging function. Before they would have the phone, but it was basically useless as they would not really answer the phone. Now with texting it's better." (P. 04).

Technological Acumen Shapes Relationship Roles. Technology knowledge shapes the roles and power in the relationship, perhaps in age-dependent ways. Participants either called or texted depending on who was more knowledgeable about technologies in the family system or in the romantic relationship. The difference in technological knowledge dictated who had more power in the relationship in many circumstances. One participant reported the difference in who had what knowledge in their romantic relationship:

My boyfriend knows my password from my mobile phone and I haven't got any problems at all that he can have a look at my pictures or, yeah. I don't want him to go through my messages but sometimes I say, "Just grab my phone and read what my sister has written or something like that." So, that's okay. He is keeping a [stricter alert]. I don't know his password and he would never tell it to me. So, when I need his cellphone I ask him and then he's entering the password and he's more like observing what I'm doing with his cellphone.

(P. 20)

The key in this passage is that she did not know her boyfriend's password and that he would not tell her; that suggests a power imbalance in the relationship that subjugates the female partner, which may imply cultural scripts related to gender being expressed in technological acumen.

Similar things occurred in families: those who were more familiar with phones (i.e., younger generations) often instituted rules in their families for the older generation. As one participant stated: "I think my grandma is more like, we set the rules and we tell her what not to do and what to avoid." (P. 06). Participant 02 also provided an example by saying:

Yeah, we have to teach my mom a lot, and my dad. My dad is actually really into technology, so he spends a lot of time figuring it out and he knows it, and he as well shows my mom. He is really into computers and stuff like that, everything, but my mom is not at all, so we have to show her like how to send a picture, and my dad helps her as well. (P. 02)

Rules about Technology in Personal Relationships

As mentioned above, rules pertaining to technology use in couple and family relationships were affected by time spent with devices, developed from comparison with peers, and influenced by the receipt of unsolicited content. Participants described the presence of both explicit and implicit rules. Implicit rules refer to rules made but not articulated, such as how to behave in a given context or situation. Such rules generally develop out of couples' time together and observations of each person's individual patterned behavior as well as the patterned behavior adopted as a couple (Meng et al., 2013). Explicit rules are discussed and agreed upon in an overt fashion (Steuber & Mclaren, 2015).

The presence of implicit rules was higher than explicit rules in both romantic and family relationships. Many participants used statements such as "no rules per se, but...," "this hasn't been stated," "not expressed," "not stated," or "it's understood" to describe the organization of technology use in their relationships. Thus, ambiguity surrounded many of the "rules" since most reported tended to be implicit.

In addition, most of the rules in personal relationships regarding technology tended to be regulative as opposed to constitutive (Roggensack & Sillars, 2014). For both familial and romantic relationships, rules governed time spent with one another in the presence of devices: in other words, when (and for how long) is it appropriate to be on one's phone while in a relational setting? Referring to her romantic relationship, Participant 25 stated: "It's not good for our relationship when we always check the emails and are on the phone and available." The rules governing time spent (present in both couple and family relationships) can be either implicit or explicit. Examples of implicit rules around time spent online within a romantic relationship included comments from Participant 13, who stated:

> He sits there for three hours and he can do that without noticing that you're out. He can really be hooked up to the computer and that is something I'm not okay with and we all fight all the time (P. 13).

Another participant supported this by saying: "So we don't have the official rules. But I don't know, when we are eating or if we're somewhere out having a drink, or dinner or whatever. We are trying not to stare at the phone the whole time." (P. 23). Another participant exemplified this by stating: "We don't use smartphones when we are like eating or in general, sharing quality time let's say watching a movie or so, usually like implicit rules not like stated explicit rule." (P. 08). Another participant stated their rules in their romantic relationship were not expressed but added: "we never use phones when we are together." (P. 04). Participant 12 stated: "My partner likes to play a game on his smartphone that in my opinion takes too much time. He keeps installing it and then deletes it when I am mad about it."

On several occurrences, participants noted explicit rules in their romantic relationship in the realm of using phones at bedtime, or even shared time together. One participant stated: "I've never had my phone at night for example in our bedroom." (P. 03). Another participant stated:

> We have a rule that we don't have it with us all the time and just checking the mails or the WhatsApp and messages, and no smartphone in the evening or in the night, I switch it off, I always switch it off. (P. 25).

Participants reported the presence of idiosyncratic rules related to the use of technology with one another. In one example, a participant discussed a rule in her romantic relationship about the length of messages:

> I have a rule to my boyfriend when we are communicating in mobile phone. It's like I don't like a short sentences so I just tell him "Hey, only short words." We have like this weird word it means yes. I mean I expect more longer sentences but he says only yes that I've gone mad and, "Why did you do? Talk like that, I don't like it." And I would upset him and he correct me, "Hey I didn't made these sentences." My automatically complete sentence, you know the iPhone. The phone makes my sentence sorry. (P. 12)

In another example, the rules in couples related to who reached out to who first: "No, you know, the rules are that I have to wait for him to contact me, because he said then he misses more, if I don't talk to him" (P. 26). The participant is implying that for her partner to miss her and want to talk to her he created the rule of her not being able to contact him first. Another participant supported this by discussing bedtime routines: "For [my boyfriend] it's like, okay, this phone is like disturbing our evening. Since he told me, I try to not do it when he is there." (P. 16)

As mentioned earlier, the presence of implicit and explicit rules was also observed within family relationships. An example of explicit rules in a family context came from Participant 02:

I don't think there [are] specific rules except that when we are eating or especially if we, if you are two people and you talk to someone, I don't like when the other person is on the phone, and vice versa. So we try not to use it too much, or we say, "Okay, now let's put away the phone and focus." Because why would we be together if we just use our phones. (P. 02).

The acknowledgement that families held few explicit rules except for mealtimes was supported by other participants. Participant 07 stated:

I think there are no explicit rules but like on the table when you're eating or having lunch or dinner, you can look at your phone but you have to limit this interaction with the phone because otherwise it would be rude and same goes with activities.

Another participant recalled the explicit rules set by their parents:

My parents set the rules out for us on which times we could use the cellphones. So, at night, I think around 9:00 PM they set, we came, we all collect all smartphones and all cellphones and put it in one spot so that we don't like browse all night. (P. 17)

Given the autonomy developmentally, however, the explicit rules set by parents may not be well-received. Participant 17 continued:

I always had problems with rules like that. I don't like being told that I can't use the cellphone. I think I can. I'm kind of addicted but that's not the problem. I would sneak out like five to seven days a week to just take it back after it was collected because it was collected in a public spot. (P. 17)

Other familial rules involve response time: "With my sister, the rule is just to respond to me within a week or a few days" (P. 16). One participant clarified that the rules regarding response time and checking phones might change based on the people involved:

That depends on the person you're with. If it's a close friend or if it's something formal like an interview or I know what the doctor or something like that I would never interrupt our conversations to check my phone but whenever I'm with my friends, or my mother right now. Also it depends on the importance I mean, if I wait and an email I applied for some jobs and I wait in response for the deadline then I will check my phone regularly but only with the person I can do that. I mean I wouldn't do that with someone like a doctor or like I said, when I'm interview wait a second I need to check my phone. (P. 13).

Participants in this study described giving more deference to parents and more conflict in couples than in family. Little pushback in families.

Boundaries about Technology Use in Relationships

Closely tied to explicit and implicit rules in personal relationships was the discussion of boundaries in technology within relationships. The rules described above concerned largely the way phones were used in in-person interactions. Boundaries refer to how you use technology outside of an immediate interaction with your partner or family, such as who you could access and who had access to you. A common boundary adopted by romantic couples concerns with whom one may communicate outside of the couple relationship. For example, Participant 17 offered:

> I think we don't have rules of who we can talk to. I think it's like unspoken rule that we are not on apps like Level ought to know or something like that where we could message people which romantically or sexually attracted to us, which is kind of the only rule. (P. 17).

In many cases, boundaries were explicitly stated to people outside of the relationship with varying degrees of success. Participant 18 recalled telling someone:

> 'You can't accept that I just want to be friends. I don't want to pursue a relationship. If you don't like acknowledge my boundaries then we just can't talk to each other anymore.' So, then I blocked him on every page that he could reach me.

This was a common occurrence supported by other participants, including Participant 8 who discussed boundaries around social media following: "I don't like it. For example my boyfriend...[has] followers...people really like pretty girls or something because [that's what on] the Instagram nowadays."

Other responses related to boundaries included unwanted or unsolicited contacts. Participant 08 noted:

> I did half a year of development aid in Nepal there were these earthquakes in 2014, I did some fundraising there and like constructing, collecting construction material and helping rebuild some broken villages, and some people there got my Facebook name and then months later like contacted me, I need money, can you provide some, certain stuff like that. (P. 08)

In other cases, participants noted boundary violations are when photos were shared with others without their authorized consent. Participant 09 noted: "I don't like who uploads my picture." This finding was true in both romantic and family relationships. Participant 02 stated:

> ...my brother posted a really embarrassing picture of my sister...He posted that picture in the big [group chat]. I think for him it was meant to be funny but my sister was like "Why are you doing this?" and "This is so mean and now everyone ...had to have it in their gallery" so it's really on everyone's phone now.

Another participant supported this by stating: "For me it would not be ok if my boyfriend would link me to pictures and to everything on Facebook." (P. 06).

Boundaries in families operated differently. Participants often described regulating their boundaries of who had access to them based on previous communications/interactions, and then a process of setting up chats that exclude the person who offended or upset them. In describing a parent, Participant 09 stated: "It became more and more clear that, uh, she was using the things I said or even when I responded to manipulate me. She was doing the same thing to my sister and brothers too, so we all just ended up creating another family chat that she isn't on." Participant 15 described a similar process in his family: "[My brother] just seemed to react badly to things and even was making screen shots of our conversations and sending them to other family members. I keep my distance and don't interact with him on text anymore."

Ambiguity. The ambiguity of who is in an individual's life can also create anxiety for boundary making. As Participant 03 described: "One of my girlfriend's favorite sentences is, "Who is she?" The thing is that it's very difficult I mean that this regards my phone and Facebook because I mean I'm not really hiding anything." In some cases, the internal struggle was a consequence of boundary violations in the past or the potential for perceived violations, making the waters on what constituted a boundary murky. For example, Participant 07 noted:

I have regularly contacted with my ex-boyfriend but it is not a problem for my boyfriend now because we talked about it, and it's okay for him and we trust each other. I wasn't so happy when he started following several models on Instagram but it's his life and there are other abstract concept because they are so far away and I do not see them as a danger. When I see I don't know girls in underwear also I asked him, "Why do you?" Oh, now I remember, I asked him but it's like his answer shows me that it is simply interesting that nothing that will disrupt our relationship. (P. 07).

Another example of a perceived boundary violation came from Participant 12 discussing how technology (phone interaction with her ex-partner and another female) ended the relationship: "I really couldn't continue, it wasn't the only reason but it was like a bomb that exploded everything. So, literally we ended up breaking up." (P. 31)

Accessibility. Other participants noted using accessibility features to establish those boundaries. For example, Participant 02 noted that: "You can choose how accessible you want to be because you can always, like on Instagram, you can have a private account so no one can contact you if you want or on Facebook as well. There is an option to hide your profile so only you can make friend requests for send messages." There was also a difference in the boundaries that participants put over their own information. Participant 06 noted:

For me it would not be okay if my boyfriend would link me to pictures and to everything on Facebook. Oh, look, baby look there and oh so sweet like you and I don't know. I don't think this would definitely not be okay for me, but obviously it's okay for others.

Accessibility also influenced what was appropriate in terms of boundaries around checking each other's phones. Participants in the study stated they used technology to maintain their relationship to see what others are doing and why their contacts are not responding to them. They want to maintain their own privacy, but by spying or looking in a way that hides their surveillance activities, their discoveries may hurt the relationship. We term this the "double-edged sword" of privacy: a balance of privacy for each person.

In discussing their checking of their partner's devices, Participant 10 stated: "One of my best friends told me like her boyfriend checks her phone. Like when they meet together, and they're like looking her SNS like, WhatsApp the Japanese version of WhatsApp. He asked, like, "Who is this boy?" Another participant supported this by stating: "Whenever he had like a Snapchat of her or like a text of her, he just hides the phone. So it was a problem for me because it will like why do you need to hide?" (P. 12). Another participant exemplified the secrecy surrounding breaking this boundary in his romantic relationship: "It's like he never usually gives his phone to me, I don't even know his password. So, it's like, very rarely, I do get his phone for some reason without he opened and that's when I really check his photos." (P. 13). Another described the utility of a phone for other tasks as one thing that compromises one's abilities supported this statement by saying:

> The problem is that it tends to fill up your phone and you have to remember to delete stuff check the things that are of no interest and they aren't wrong but the smartphone is when they get into your smartphone they also get into your yahoo account, they get into your Facebook account and then you start getting all that rubbish. (P. 16).

Participant 12 discussed it as an issue of trust in her romantic relationship: "We've never been the type of couple that checks each other too much or I don't know. We just trusted each other from the beginning and that went well. So, I never felt the need to check on him to his phone when he's sleeping."

Examples of the importance of privacy revealed anxiety tied toward someone checking the phone: "... it's good to have privacy, I don't have nothing to hide but I don't like anyone to take my phone and to check it." (P. 05) Another participant tried to clarify the reason why the boundary around their personal phone was so important:

> [There is] a lot of information there, it's your whole life there. Like in my relationship, I really try to keep that...it's your phone, it's your life; it's my phone, it's my life. If I want to show you something I'll show you, if you want to show me something open to see it...he knows and I know that we can trust each other 100%, so I don't expect anything on his cellphone that I wouldn't be allowed to see. (P. 14)

In family relationships, the accessibility factor was discussed in terms of who in the family had access to technology and how conversations were influenced based on the physical accessibility. For example, Participant 03 stated: "My mom doesn't use the phone too much, and even though she has one, it isn't the way she talks to us. I usually talk to my father and texting with him, and he sometimes passes things along to her."

Using Technology to Regulate Closeness and Distance

As mentioned, there are many ways in which smartphones can augment participants' sense of closeness and connection to one another. Some participants attributed this to the ability to speak to one another while at a distance or that it otherwise created a deep communication: "We met in person but of course the first context, the deeper context was initiated using the cellphone." (P. 20). In many cases, participants reported that accessibility was also a primary contributor to the challenges within their romantic relationships. One participant stated, "The problems we've had, it was because, actually a girl was texting him. And he also was like, whenever she texted her, he was like, hiding the phone. So, I was like, why do you hide?...whenever there was someone else, he was like, normal, but when I...didn't even read the messages, but I can see [them] in the phone" (P. 14). Other participants supported this by stating the Internet and smartphones create a "lack of attention towards the other, when you get absorbed into doing your own stuff. Also, because it's available, yeah, you can do this. And it makes it easier to ignore the other [partner]." (P. 23).

There is also an assumption that one's partner is accessible because the partner has the phone nearby. Participant 23 exemplified this by stating: "you're usually expected to be available if you have a smartphone. It's [a] default state." Another stated: "The problem is sometimes [my sister] texts me and I'm not in the mood to respond." (P. 16). The lack of accessibility was sometimes viewed as a hindrance because of the screen size. As one participant explained as it pertained to their romantic relationship:

Only one person has access to one smartphone. So we can't really share what we do on our smartphone. We can't send it to everyone easily. It's just one person with smartphone: interaction with everyone else is isolated. It isolates us from general conversation, point of connection. It just throws people out of the group, temporarily. I think it's more accepted nowadays, but it's still considered rude, especially in social meetings. (P. 24)

In family relationships, there seemed to be more impetus on those who are among younger generations to be reciprocal in their interactions with their family members. As one participant stated:

[My family] keep posting...[my siblings and I] would reply to the messages to just encourage the elders to keep using the phone but now it's like they are expecting too much like they want the reply, they want you to say something about which they posted and they don't really want to talk to you over the phone but they want replies and likes and comments for what they posted (P. 13).

Another participant stated: "They want to take pictures, or they want something interesting just because they want to post it online. It's not like it just happened, you are trying to generate the content." (P. 18). Other descriptions of connection with one's family was also dictated, in part, by the nature of the relationships. One participant stated:

I write my sister more because she uses her smartphone more than my parents do and I don't see her as much as I see my parents, so, it's more important to communicate with her via the smartphone. My parents are a little bit lazy with it, they don't respond very quickly, it takes a lot of time, so, it was much complicated, so, I don't prefer to communicate with them with the smartphone, I call them but I don't write them. (P. 16)

One participant summed it up by saying: "Let's say smartphones keep you connected whether you want it or not." (P. 08). The other characteristics that help improve connection are the various modalities in using technology and the increased description that goes along with it. Participant 31 stated:

> Because now it's like you have morning the panorama, like you have to see not just a text, but you can see what the other people is watching like. Also, I remembered like when I traveled, for example, I went to Mexico City and we were really worried about one night that we went out and it was a disaster. So it was really good that I could share my location.

Discussion

The purpose of this study was to better understand the way in which culture informs how technology is used in personal relationships. The general findings of this study revealed that the structure of relationships (as defined by roles, rules, and boundaries) is affected by how people use technology. Participants in the present study noted how the roles of family members change when children have more information about how to navigate technology than their parents, a finding consistent with previous literature (see, for example, Gee et al., 2018; Sun & McMillan, 2018). In addition, the accessibility affected the roles in romantic relationships by helping individuals transition into romantic roles in easier, quicker ways. This is consistent with research from Christopher et al. (2016), which discusses how texting and mobile communication helps young people shift more easily into relationship roles. The roles held can also be influenced by who is more knowledgeable in the way of technological acumen as the person who knows more about technology use may have more power and thus be more likely to surveille and take a role of more power in the relationship based on that knowledge.

The findings also revealed greater acknowledgement of implicit rules and boundaries governing technology use in relationships than explicit rules. When implicit rules are established in larger social groups such as family of origin or in the larger social network, and not specifically between the couple, complications can occur in each partner's understanding of what they are (Hertlein, 2012). Rules that are not discussed openly between partners can become problematic in that interpretations, assumptions, and prioritizations can vary widely between partners, potentially causing confusion and conflict. This is especially true when couples, for example, come from different cultures. Vandello and Cohen (2003) found that when rules are implicit in romantic relationships in cultures where honor is an organizing theme, the incidence of intimate partner violence is greater. In addition, technology has been referenced as that which perpetuates intimate partner violence (Hertlein, 2021; Lee & Anderson, 2016). Therefore, the implicit rules that are operating in these relationships may leave the couple subject to some challenging outcomes based on their culture.

Since technology use is a major means of communication, implementing healthy rules and boundaries becomes extremely useful to maintain relational health. Increasing clarity regarding privacy or personal time an individual needs would benefit the relationship in that the need for privacy or space at certain times would not be confused with negative behaviors such as avoidance. This is highly important because attachment behaviors (and the other side of the coin, avoidance) are affiliated with maintenance behaviors (Lee et al., 2019). Those who can exhibit more support, communication, and commitment will enjoy relationships that are characterized by higher levels of attachment (Lee, 2019). On the other hand, when individuals use their phone to avoid difficult conversations, this will detract from developing an attached relationship. What is universal in conversation is the exchange and turn-taking; what is culturally informed, however, is the response time (Stivers et al., 2009). The interpretation of one's partner taking longer to respond can affect how people interpret and make meaning of their partner's actions.

Cultural Differences/Universalities Using a Universal Tool

Technology as a universal tool may induce universal behaviors or differences. Norenzayan and Heine (2005) discussed how examining cultures in terms of universalities and differences can be accomplished with attention to three areas: differences in accessibility, function, and existence. Of these three, the first two were addressed in this study. Differences in accessibility refers to the differences in frequency of engaging in a behavior and/or similarity in attitude about something. In the present study, accessibility was an important factor in establishing and maintaining relationships, both couple and familial. The access encouraged relationships that were separated by geography but also set the stage for expectations of response time and interactions.

Examining differences in function describe whether some element has the same function in every culture or whether a component used can predict the same outcome in a different context. In the present study, the participants focused on technoference and how they must make judgment calls about whether to respond to the phone during interactions. Since phones have many functions both inside and outside of relationships, and the functions of when to use what modality can affect relationship tempo (Hertlein & Chan, 2020). Participants in the present study discussed more than the functions of when to use their phone. They also discussed the settings under which they felt it was appropriate to engage their phone while with a romantic partner or family member(s).

Implications for Practice

From a practice perspective, therapists can be instrumental in working with couples and families to make the implicit rules explicit. While this may seem like something that is naturally done within the therapeutic practice, it is not often that therapist go into detail about the rules specifically for phone use in couple relationships. Therapists may visit this in more detail as it pertains to children's use (see, for example, Fletcher & Blair, 2016), but again, the rules around timing and tempo of response may not be articulated. Another implication for therapists is to review and negotiate boundaries, including phone usage when in relational settings especially as it pertains to interdependence. This study explored how people used technology in their relationships but spent less time on the interaction and interdependence in relationships mediated by smartphones. Yet as Caughlin and Sharabi (2013) demonstrate, "communication that occurs via one mode can shape the very meaning of communication that happens via another mode." (p. 888). Examining interpretations and interdependence more specifically is an important direction for scholars.

Limitations

A primary limitation of this study was the sample. We relied on recruiting from a diverse sample; in so doing, we did not regulate the specific countries from which the participants originated. Some were from an exchange program offered at the local university and some were community members. Therefore, the lack of precision in the sampling may have made it difficult to make more meaningful interpretations. In addition, the fact that the interview questions were developed from a White, Western, middle-class person would naturally influence the language of the questions asked, which may impact this research on cultural understandings of technology.

Future Research

Because technology is used for regulating closeness and distance, further research may look at the stages of relationship building and how technology can be used adjunctively in this process (Eastwick, 2013). Another area of future research could be examining interdependence pattens of technology usage in personal relationships more closely. In the present study, participants described their interactions with technology to some degree as a response to their partner and the stimuli in front of them. For example, rules about who they communicated with were dependent on the person and situation in front of them. At the same time, interactions may result in outcome problems or coordination problems, which may have an impact on relationships (Caughlin & Sharabi, 2013; Machia et al., 2020). The extent to which phone use is coordinated and the outcomes such coordination creates is worthy of further study.

References

Anfara, V. A., Brown, K. M., & Mangione, T. L. (2002). Qualitative analysis on stage: Making the research process more public. *Educational Researcher, 31*(7), 28–38. https://doi.org/10.3102/0013189X031007028

Billedo, C. J., Kerkhof, P., & Finkenauer, C. (2015). The use of social networking sites for relationship maintenance in long-distance and geographically close romantic relationships. *Cyberpsychology, Behavior, and Social Networking, 18*(3), 152–157. http://doi.org/10.1089/cyber.2014.0469

Braune-Krickau, K., Schneebeli, L., Pehlke-Milde, J., Gemperle, M., Koch, R., & Wyl, A. (2021). Smartphones in the nursery: Parental smartphone use and parental sensitivity and responsiveness within parent–child interaction in early childhood (0–5 years): A scoping review. *Infant Mental Health Journal, 42*(2), 161–175. https://doi.org/10.1002/imhj.21908

Bruess, C. (2019). *Family communication in the age of digital and social media*. New York: Peter Lang, Inc.

Calder-Dawe, & Gavey, N. (2016). Making sense of everyday sexism: Young people and the gendered contours of sexism. *Women's Studies International Forum, 55*, 1–9. https://doi.org/10.1016/j.wsif.2015.11.004

Canton, N. (2012). Cell phone culture: How cultural differences affect mobile use. Retrieved October 11, 2020, from: www.cnn.com/2012/09/27/tech/mobile-culture-usage/index.html.

Caughlin, J., & Sharabi, L. L. (2013). A Communicative Interdependence Perspective of Close Relationships: The Connections Between Mediated and Unmediated Interactions Matter. *Journal of Communication, 63*(5), 873–893. https://doi.org/10.1111/jcom.12046

Caughlin, J., & Wang, N. (2019). Relationship Maintenance in the Age of Technology. In B. Ogolsky & J. Monk (Eds.), *Relationship Maintenance: Theory, Process, and Context* (Advances in Personal Relationships, pp. 304–322). Cambridge: Cambridge University Press. https://doi.org//10.1017/9781108304320.016

Christopher, F. S., Poulsen, F. O., & McKenney, S. J. (2016). Early adolescents and "going out" *Journal of Social and Personal Relationships, 33*(6), 814–834. https://doi.org/10.1177/0265407515599676

Coyne, S. M., Stockdale, L., Busby, D., Iverson, B., & Grant, D. M. (2011). "I luv u": A descriptive study of the media use of individuals in romantic relationships. *Family Relations, 60*(2), 150–162. https://doi.org/10.1111/j.1741-3729.2010.00639.x

Currin, J. M., Pascarella, L. A., & Hubach, R. D. (2020). "To feel close when miles apart": qualitative analysis of motivations to sext in a relationship. *Sexual and Relationship Therapy, 35*(2), 244–257. https://doi.org/10.1080/14681994.2020.1714024

Eastwick, P. R. (2013). Cultural influences on attraction. In J. Simpson and L. Campbell's (Eds.), *The Oxford Handbook of Close Relationships.* https://doi.org//10.1093/oxfordhb/9780195398694.013.0008

Emerson, R., Fretz, R., & Shaw, L. (1995). *Writing ethnographic fieldnotes.* Chicago: The University of Chicago Press.

Fletcher, A. C., & Blair, B. L. (2016). Implications of the family expert role for parental rules https://doi.org//10.1177/1461444814538922

Gaines, S., & Ferenczi, N. (2019). Relationship Maintenance across Cultural Groups. In B. Ogolsky & J. Monk (Eds.), *Relationship Maintenance: Theory, Process, and Context* (Advances in Personal Relationships, pp. 284–303). Cambridge: Cambridge University Press. doi:10.1017/9781108304320.015

Garfin, D. R. (2020). Technology as a coping tool during the coronavirus disease 2019 (COVID-19) pandemic: Implications and recommendations. *Stress and Health, 36*(4), 555–559. https://doi.org/10.1002/smi.2975

Gee, E., Takeuchi, L., & Wartella, E. (2018). *Children and families in the digital age: Learning together in a media saturated culture.* New York: Routledge.

Hertlein, K. M. (2012). Digital dwelling: Technology in couple and family relationships. *Family Relations, 61*(3), 374–387.

Hertlein, K. M. (2021). The weaponized web: Technology's enhancement and perpetuation of intimate partner violence. *International Journal of Systemic Therapy, 32*(3), 173–191.

Hertlein, K. M., & Ancheta, K. (2014). Advantages and disadvantages of technology in relationships: Findings from an open-ended survey. *The Qualitative Report, 19*(11), 1–11.

Hertlein, K. M., & Chan, D. (2020). The rationale behind texting, videoconferencing, and mobile phones in couple relationships. *Marriage and Family Review, 56*(8), 739–763.

Hertlein, K. M., & Twist, M. L. C. (2019). *The Internet family.* New York: Routledge.

Hobbs, M., Owen, S., & Gerber, L. (2017). Liquid love? Dating apps, sex, relationships, and the digital transformation of intimacy. *Journal of Sociology (Melbourne, Vic.), 53*(2), 271–284. https://doi.org/10.1177/1440783316662718

Hong, S., & Na, J. (2018). How Facebook is perceived and used by people across cultures: The implications of cultural differences in the use of Facebook. *Social Psychological and Personality Science, 9*(4), 435–443. https://doi.org/10.1177/1948550617711227

Johnson, D., & Hertlein, K. M. (2019). Parents' perceptions of smartphone use and parenting practices. *Qualitative Report, 24*(6), 14–23.

Kluck, J. P., Stoyanova, F., & Krämer, N. C. (2021). Putting the social back into physical distancing: The role of digital connections in a pandemic crisis. *International Journal of Psychology.* https://doi.org/10.1002/ijop.12746

Kushlev, K., & Dunn, E. W. (2019). Smartphones distract parents from cultivating feelings of connection when spending time with their children. *Journal of Social and Personal Relationships, 36*(6), 1619–1639. https://doi.org/10.1177/0265407518769387

Lanigan, J., Bold, M., & Chenoweth, L. (2009). Computers in the family context: Perceived impact on family time and relationships. *Family Science Review, 14*(1), 16–32.

Latif, H., Şimşek Kandemir, A., Uçkun, S., Karaman, E., Yüksel, A., & Onay, Ö. A. (2020). The presence of smartphones at dinnertime: A parental perspective. *The Family Journal, 28*(4), 432–440. https://doi.org/10.1177/1066480720906122

Lee, K., & Anderson, J. (2016). The internet and intimate partner violence: Technology changes, abuse doesn't. *Criminal Justice, 31*(2), 28–33.

Lee, J., Karantzas, G., Gillath, O., & Fraley, R. (2019). Relationship maintenance from an attachment perspective. In B. Ogolsky & J. Monk (Eds.), *Relationship Maintenance: Theory, Process, and Context* (Advances in Personal Relationships, pp. 47–68). Cambridge: Cambridge University Press. https://doi.org/10.1017/9781108304320.004

Lomanowska, A. M, & Guitton, M. J. (2016). Online intimacy and well-being in the digital age. *Internet Interventions: The Application of Information Technology in Mental and Behavioural Health, 4*(P2), 138–144. https://doi.org/10.1016/j.invent.2016.06.005

Lydon, J. E.., & Quinn, S. K. (2013). Relationship Maintenance Processes. In J. Simpson & S. Campbell (Eds.)., *The Oxford Handbook of Close Relationships* (pp. 1–30). Oxford University Press. https://doi.org/10.1093/oxfordhb/9780195398694.013.0026

Machia, L. V., Agnew, C. R., & Arriaga, X. B. (2020). *Interdependence, Interaction, and Close Relationships*. Cambridge University Press. https://doi.org/10.1017/9781108645836

Madianou, M. (2014). Smartphones as Polymedia. *Journal of Computer-Mediated Communication*, *19*(3), 667–680. https://doi.org/10.1111/jcc4.12069

McCormack, M., & Ogilvie, M. F. (2020). Keeping couples together when apart, and driving them apart when together: exploring the impact of smartphones on relationships in the UK. In A. Abela, S. Vella, & S. Piscopo (Eds.), *Couple Relationships in a Global Context* (pp. 245–259). Springer International Publishing. https://doi.org/10.1007/978-3-030-37712-0_15

McCracken, G. (1988). *Culture and Consumption: New Approaches to the Symbolic Character of Consumer Goods and Activities*. Bloomington: Indiana University Press.

McDaniel, B. T, & Coyne, S. M. (2016). Technology interference in the parenting of young children: Implications for mothers' perceptions of coparenting. *The Social Science Journal*, *53*(4), 435–443. https://doi.org/10.1016/j.soscij.2016.04.010

McDaniel, B. T., & Drouin, M. (2019). Daily technology interruptions and emotional and relational well-being. *Computers in Human Behavior*, *99*, 1–8. https://doi.org/10.1016/j.chb.2019.04.027

McDaniel, B. T., & Radesky, J. S. (2018). Technoference: Parent Distraction with Technology and Associations With Child Behavior Problems. *Child Development*, *89*(1), 100–109. https://doi.org/10.1111/cdev.12822

Meng, K., Harper, J. M., Coyne, S., Larson, J., Miller, R., & Sandberg, J. (2013). *Couple implicit rules for facilitating disclosure and relationship quality with romantic relational aggression as a mediator*. ProQuest Dissertations and Theses.

Modecki, K. L., Low-Choy, S., Uink, B. N., Vernon, L., Correia, H., & Andrews, K. (2020). Tuning into the real effect of smartphone use on parenting: a multiverse analysis. *Journal of Child Psychology and Psychiatry*, *61*(8), 855–865. https://doi.org/10.1111/jcpp.13282

Moustakas, C. (1994). *Phenomenological research methods*. Thousand Oaks, CA: Sage.

Na, J., Kosinski, M., & Stillwell, D. (2015). When a new tool is introduced in different cultural contexts. *Journal of Cross-Cultural Psychology*, *46*(3), 355–370. https://doi.org/10.1177/0022022114563932

Norenzayan, A., & Heine, S. J. (2005). Psychological universals. *Psychological Bulletin*, *131*(5), 763–784. https://doi.org//10.1037/0033-2909.131.5.763

Norton, A. M., Baptist, J., & Hogan, B. (2018). ComputerMediated communication in intimate relationships: associations of boundary crossing, intrusion, relationship satisfaction, and partner responsiveness. *Journal of Marital and Family Therapy*, *44*(1), 165–182. https://doi.org/10.1111/jmft.12246

Patton, M. Q. (2014). *Qualitative research and evaluation methods*. Thousand Oaks: Sage.

Peters, C., & Allan, S. (2018). Everyday imagery. *Convergence: The International Journal of Research into New Media Technologies*, *24*(4), 357–373. https://doi.org/10.1177/1354856516678395

Roberts, J. A., & David, M. E. (2016). My life has become a major distraction from my cell phone: Partner phubbing and relationship satisfaction among romantic partners. *Computers in Human Behavior*, *54*, 134–141. https://doi.org/10.1016/j.chb.2015.07.058

Roggensack, K., & Sillars, A. (2014). Agreement and understanding about honesty and deception rules in romantic relationships. *Journal of Social and Personal Relationships*, *31*(2), 178–199. https://doi.org/10.1177/0265407513489914

Sanri, Ç., & Goodwin, R. (2014). The influence of globalization and technological development on intimate relationships. In C. R. Agnew's (Ed.), *Social influences on romantic relationships: Beyond the dyad* (pp. 11–32). Cambridge, MA: Cambridge University Press.

Schofield-Clark, L. (2013). *The parent app*. New York: Oxford University Press.

Sprecher, S., Felmlee, D., Stokes, J., & McDaniel, B. (2019). Social Networks and Relationship Maintenance. In B. Ogolsky & J. Monk (Eds.), *Relationship Maintenance: Theory, Process, and Context* (Advances in Personal Relationships, pp. 152–177). Cambridge: Cambridge University Press. https://doi.org/10.1017/9781108304320.009

Stafford, L. (2019). Communication and Relationship Maintenance. In B. Ogolsky & J. Monk (Eds.), *Relationship Maintenance: Theory, Process, and Context* (Advances in Personal Relationships, pp. 109–133). Cambridge: Cambridge University Press. https://doi.org//10.1017/9781108304320.007

Stafford, L., & Canary, D. J. (1991). Maintenance strategies and romantic relationship type, gender and relational characteristics. *Journal of Social and Personal Relationships, 8*(2), 217–242. https://doi.org/10.1177/0265407591082004

Statista (2021). Active social network penetration in selected countries as of January 2021. Retrieved May 14, 2021, from: www.statista.com/statistics/282846/regular-social-networking-usage-penetration-worldwide-by-country/.

Steuber, K., & Mclaren, R. (2015). Privacy recalibration in Personal Relationships: Rule Usage Before and After an Incident of Privacy Turbulence. *Communication Quarterly, 63*(3), 345–364. doi:10.1080/01463373.2015.1039717

Strauss, A., & Corbin, J. M. (1990). *Basics of qualitative research: Grounded theory procedures and techniques.* Sage Publications, Inc.

Stivers, T., Enfield, N., Brown, P., Englert, C., Hayashi, M., Heinemann, T., Hoymann, G., Rossano, F., Ruijter, J. P. de, Yoon, K.-E., & Levinson, S. (2009). Universals and Cultural Variation in Turn-Taking in Conversation. *Proceedings of the National Academy of Sciences – PNAS, 106(26),* 10587–10592. https://doi.org/10.1073/pnas.0903616106

Sullivan, K. T., Riedstra, J., Arellano, B., Cardillo, B., Kalach, V., & Ram, A. (2020). Online communication and dating relationships: Effects of decreasing online communication on feelings of closeness and relationship satisfaction. *Journal of Social and Personal Relationships, 37*(8–9), 2409–2418. https://doi.org/10.1177/0265407520924707

Sun, X., & McMillan, C. (2018). Interplay between families and technology: future investigations. In J. Vandehook, S. M. McHale, and V. King's (Eds.), *Families and technology* (pp. 177–187). National Symposium on Family Issues (vol 9). New York: Springer. https://doi-org.ezproxy.library.unlv.edu/10.1007/978-3-319-95540-7_10

Taipale, S. (2019). *Intergenerational connections in digital families.* Springer International Publishing AG.

Taylor, S. H., & Bazarova, N. N (2018). Revisiting media multiplexity: A longitudinal analysis of media use in romantic relationships. *Journal of Communication, 68*(6), 1104–1126, https://doi-org.ezproxy.library.unlv.edu/10.1093/joc/jqy055

Vandello, J. A., & Cohen, D. (2003). Male honor and female fidelity. *Journal of Personality and Social Psychology, 84*(5), 997–1010. https://doi.org/10.1037/0022-3514.84.5.997

Westjohn, S. A., Arnold, M. J., Magnusson, P., Zdravkovic, S., & Zhou, J. X. (2009). Technology readiness and usage: A global-identity perspective. *Journal of the Academy of Marketing Science, 37*(3), 250–265. http://dx.doi.org.ezproxy.library.unlv.edu/10.1007/s11747-008-0130-0

Yoshie, M., & Sauter, D. A. (2020). Cultural norms influence nonverbal emotion communication: Japanese vocalizations of socially disengaging emotions. *Emotion 20*(3), 513–517. https://doi.org/10.1037/emo0000580

Yum, Y-O., & Canary, D. J. (2003). Maintaining relationships in the U.S. and Korea. In Canary, D. J. & Dainton, M. (Eds.), *Maintaining relationships through communication: Relational, contextual, and cultural variations* (pp. 277–296). Mahwah, NJ: Erlbaum.

23

EXPERIENTIALISM

Finding Unconditional Positive Regard in a World of Chaos

Tabitha N. Webster, Dumayi Gutierrez, and Reihaneh Mahdavishahri

Introduction

If you have ever picked up a Virginia Satir book, you immediately know who the author is; her unique voice is clear and resonates. You are enveloped and wrapped in her warm and unconditional positive cadence. Her voice is unmistakable and an immediate salve to the soul. Visions of being wrapped in a blanket by the fireplace, sipping a hot cup of chamomile tea always come to me when I read her works. There is comfort, authenticity, and safety in her voice.

If you have ever read anything from Carl Whittaker, you likely experienced a similar sensation of a clear, bright voice, full of sincerity and authentic humor, a bit of mischievous spirit – that unmistakable Whittaker style. For me, he conjures visions of camping, in the cool mountain air, staring up at the stars, pondering life's biggest questions. Sincerely laughing at the smallness we are. Whittaker creates an existential space of contradiction of both the importance and the irrelevance of life. There is honesty, sincerity, profound understanding, and mischievous joy in his voice.

Collectively we have taught marriage and family therapy (MFT) theories courses for over a decade, and it never ceases to amaze us that experiential therapy is often addressed as a "model" in textbooks, when in reality, it is a theoretical framework, like the way we teach modernism and postmodernism. Experiential therapy is not a model, but four models, under an umbrella of philosophical and theoretical assumptions that allow for each therapist to find ownership in the most congruent and authentic way. This is very much like the four models of postmodernism, and the way we teach it.

History and Theoretical Formation

The definition of experiential is relating to or derived from experience (Merriam-Webster, n.d.), and who are we today if not beings shaped by experiences of our past. Experiential therapy is rooted in humanistic and existential movements of 19th-century Europe, which prioritized subjective truth within human existence, lived experience, realization

DOI: 10.4324/9781003297871-26

of possibility, and relationship to the human world (Loeschen, 1994; Wong, 2006). Existentialism involves: 1) Unwelt or biological world (pleasure, warmth); 2) Mitwelt or social world (community and culture); and 3) Eigenwelt or psychological world (meaning making and understanding of experience) (Wong, 2006). In the United States, at a time when behaviorism and psychoanalysis were ruling the world of psychotherapy, humanistic therapists such as Rollo May, Abraham Maslow, Carl Rogers, and Carl Jung responded to their limitations and placed emphasis on the essential function of therapeutic relationships, shifting from symptomatic to positive human nature, self-actualization, self-expression in therapy, and freedom of existence (Elliot & Greenberg, 1997; Nichols & Davis, 2021; Price, 2011). These groundbreaking ideas in addition to influences from family systems therapy, Gestalt therapy, and psychodrama paved the way for experiential therapy. Centering client experience as it unfolds, communicating and processing them are among the fundamental goals of experiential therapy (Satir et al., 1991).

Experiential therapists play an essential role in facilitating the exploration and expression of clients' deepest emotional experiences and desires in safe therapeutic space. What truly stands out from humanistic perspective is honoring who we are and as social creatures the meaningful bonds that we foster. Emphasis on the therapist approach and presence includes "empathy, authenticity, and dedication to creating a bond with a client" (Price, 2011, p. 60). Socioculturally, experiential therapy works with, "Feelings produced through processes of marginalization and oppression, as well as those that emerge from growing awareness of power structures can mobilize us into action" (McDowell et al., 2023, p. 85). The main theoretical assumptions involve emotional expression exploration. Textbooks cite this as the condition for dysfunction in a family due to "emotional suppression." Experiential therapists as quoted from Nichols and Davis (2021) "tend to be fairly aggressive and attacking defenses to promote emotional expression." Experiential therapists rely on a fine-tuned unmasked use of self in the room as the mechanism of change (Roberts, 2005). Experientialism values creative spontaneity and emotional honesty as primary values to living a fully expressed life (Nichols & Davis, 2021). In the here and now, change occurs in session moments where we create novel emotional experiences with our clients. This highlights and emphasizes the key value of emotional experience for its own sake (Nichols & Davis, 2021). Through this dyadic approach, experiential therapy expanded from an individual and symptomatic perspective to internalized and externalized growth and empowerment of subjective truth.

In the framework of experientialism, social interactions shape experiences and relationships influence meaning creation (Greenberg et al., 1998). For example, a father might discuss with his son that "men can't express their emotions," thus, creating a relationship between father and son in which emotional expression from the males is "wrong." Yet, conformity causes increased distress and alignment of a reality which differs from the lived experience of the son. In this example, men clearly are emotional beings and increased stress is evident when feelings cannot be expressed in a healthy manner. Noting that what is considered "healthy" has many socially constructed discourses, defined by that specific society and culture. Eliciting third-order change from an attuned cultural lens "requires identifying, putting into words, sharing, and hearing felt experiences, of marginalization, oppression and privilege" (McDowell, Knudson-Martin, & Bermudez, 2023). Restriction in authenticity may occur in multiple intersecting factors such as gender, socioeconomic status, age, culture, religion and so on from societal conformities (Elliot & Greenberg,

1997; Haber, 2002). We later posit, while society's contextual definitions are inherently true to meaning-making of the human experience, experientialism's seemingly contradiction bypasses all social construction to find connection in the physiological underpinnings that make us all human beings.

One of the last consistent theoretical assumptions is unconditional positive regard, as I have heard other experiential therapists call it, love. Love, in this way, is an expression, obviously not in unethical romantic love, but as a fully actualized acceptance of SELF. This type of love holds no conditions. It expresses that nothing will limit the acceptance and affirmation of who you are, no matter what you have said or done. Clients are seen in a positive strength-filled and whole-person light. Everything the client needs is found inside themselves. Experiential therapists live in the "both/and." As such experiential therapists are actively engaged in both collaborative and directive roles, and are both supportive and challenging. The pure beauty and magic of experiential therapies is that these base assumptions are so humanly universal and can support change in almost any contextual situation, while at the same time "analyzing the power dynamics from the broadest global to the most intimate family relationships" (McDowell et al., 2023). To experience true unconditional positive regard and be fully SEEN is life changing both because of and regardless of positionality, cultural context, or country of origin.

Virginia Satir

Virginia Satir and Carl Whitaker are known as the pioneers of experiential therapy (Nicholas & Davis, 2021). We want to mention here, that while the EFT and IFS models are under the experiential framework umbrella, this chapter will focus mostly on Satir and Whitaker, as we hope others are writing full chapters on EFT and IFS in their own rights.

Virginia Satir (1916–1988) was born in the small town of Neillsville in rural Wisconsin and is often referred to as the *mother of family therapy*. Satir founded the Satir Model, sometimes called the Satir Growth Model, Satir Transformational Systemic Therapy, The Satir Change Model, or The Satir Communication Model. Satir's experiential family therapy invites family members to express their feelings, desires, and fears in the safety of the non-judgmental therapeutic environment that experiential therapists create (Loeschen, 1994; Satir et al., 1991). Helping individuals express their emotional experiences in the moment instead of suppressing them promotes a space in which open, honest, and congruent communication is encouraged and individuals are able to better understand themselves and their potentials for positive growth.

A teacher and a social worker, Satir began her clinical work in Chicago by seeing families in her private practice. In 1955 she joined the Illinois State Psychiatric Institute to train students in family therapy (Loeschen, 1994; Nichols & Davis, 2021). Her interest and groundbreaking work in family therapy led her to the Mental Research Institute (MRI) in Palo Alto in 1959 for the next 7 years of her professional life. In later years, Satir primarily focused on teaching and training new family therapists committed to promoting healthy communication patterns among family members by increasing clients' self-awareness and self-esteem (Andreas, 1991). In many ways Virginia Satir was ahead of her time in the history of family therapy development. Many of Satir's core beliefs in doing therapy resonate with social constructionism, postmodernism, and feminism, which later developed and hold much popularity today.

Satir identified as a strong existential humanist and went on the record to state,

"I am Me. In all the world, there is no one else exactly like me. Everything that comes out of me is authentically mine, because I alone chose it -- I own everything about me: my body, my feelings, my mouth, my voice, all my actions, whether they be to others or myself. I own my fantasies, my dreams, my hopes, my fears. I own my triumphs and successes, all my failures and mistakes. Because I own all of me, I can become intimately acquainted with me. By so doing, I can love me and be friendly with all my parts."

(Satir, 1988, p.28)

She emphasized processes of communication, potential, and complete engagement with families (McDowell et al., 2023). Scholars and therapists have noted Satir's work as "magic" – she promoted an atmosphere of attention to uniqueness of each individual in the room, connection and bonding within relationship, and upheld interaction of intrapersonal, interpersonal, and contextual factors (Haber, 2002). However, as one of the most influential women in the field of family therapy, Satir encountered several challenges throughout her career, including lack of recognition by the larger therapeutic community in the early stages of her work (Andreas, 1991; Loeschen, 1994). In 1972, a controversial duel of ideas was set up by the Family Process Advisory Editors titled "Is Virginia Satir dangerous for family therapy?" It was an attempt to evaluate and question the validity of Satir's ideas, pitting them against the work of Salvadore Minuchin. And so, she found herself being criticized and rejected by a predominantly male field at the time. Her undeniable warmth, authenticity, and vulnerability was generally seen as a weakness, and noted as dangerous, by many of her colleagues in the United States. Having enough of male-dominated discourse, Satir broke away from family therapy conferences in the United States and focused on continuing her work in Europe (McGoldrick & Hardy, 2019). The unfortunate consequences of this divisive and sexist challenge and Satir's then exit to Europe made her only a footnote in the history of family therapy in the United State. Fortunately, she was widely successful in the European and global context as a predominate thought leader in family therapy (Andreas, 1991).

Globally, Satir's works live on within organizations like the Virginia Satir Global Network and The Satir Institute of the Pacific. *The Satir International Journal*, which ceased publication in 2018, was a long-held empirical supporter of Satir's work, and was created by these two networks "to promote research, development, teaching and practice of the Satir Model in both the academic and practitioner community worldwide through the publication of material related to the Satir Model" (Satir International Journal, 2023). While the publication has ceased, the VSGN continues to hold annual conferences centered around the Stairs Model in the Global context. This year alone you can see presentations from Israel, Canada, Ireland, Turkey, France, China, Thailand, and the United States (Satirglobal.org, 2023). One presentation abstract by Sandy Novak posits that China now holds the largest number of Satir Practitioners, after Dr. John Banmen brought Satir's Model to China in 2003 (Satirglobal.org) or Lyla Harmon from Canada's work on Satir Applications with Indigenous Groups (Satirglobal.org).

While Satir continues to impact therapy in the global context, in the United States Satir's impact on family therapy remains significant primary as a historical footnote and mostly only lives in her publications including *"the peoplemaking"* and the revised *"the new peoplemaking"* edition, *"conjoint family therapy,"* and *"making contact"*. Satir's powerful work extended well beyond her therapy room as she made it her mission to "raise the consciousness of each individual regarding personal esteem and world peace" until her retirement through her workshops and advocacy work (Andreas, 1991; Loeschen, 1994; Satir et al., 1991).

Carl Whitaker

Carl Whitaker (1910–1991), an American physician and psychotherapist, is best known for his innovative, absurd, and directly confrontational approaches in family therapy and creating the Whitaker's Symbolic-Experiential Model (Nichols & Davis, 2021). Whitaker was an advocate for implementing family therapy in treatment of mental health issues and a pioneer in seeing beyond the individual symptoms and examining the relational context of human experience.

He was considered a charismatic and energetic person. He believed his confrontational and absurd tactics helped clients overcome their challenges and often pushed the boundaries of traditional psychotherapy practices of the time (Neill & Kniskern, 1989). Whitaker connected with his clients on a deep level and created an open and honest therapeutic space. He was known for his sense of humor, which he often used to diffuse emotionally tense scenarios and allowed for more flexibility to arise throughout the therapeutic process (Whitaker & Malone, 1981). Let's all be honest here, who can forget the ever-fated account of Whitaker wrestling on the floor with the kiddo in *The Family Crucible* (Napier & Whitaker, 1978). It was a clear demonstration of the Whitaker essence that created his lore in the pages of textbooks.

Amongst some of the few documented of Whitaker's innovative exercises were "the miracle of the onion" and the "wild party" (Keith, 2014). In the miracle of the onion exercise, each family member is asked to peel away a layer of an onion, which would facilitate the revelation of their true thoughts and feelings. This exercise was designed to help families move past any emotional barriers previously created and allow for more vulnerable and open expression of emotions (Keith, 2014). "The Wild party" exercise encourages family members to enact their true feelings in a playful and exaggerated manner to increase each member's awareness of their emotional experiences and facilitate the expression and communication of such emotions in the safety of the therapeutic space (Keith, 2014). Like all experiential modalities, for Whitaker, the key to desired change was hidden in the family's emotional system. Thus, raising the intensity of emotions in the family, facilitating the family's communication through experiential interaction, would lead to major shifts in the family (emotional) system (Whitaker & Malone, 1981).

Among other significant Whitaker's innovations is the practice of co-therapy, which started as an experiment in response to the demands of the job during World War 2 and soon became his standard for practice and focus of his teachings (Keith, 2014; Knapp, 1997). As the chairman of the department of psychiatry at Emory University in Atlanta, he wrote the *The Roots of Psychotherapy* with Dr. Thomas Malone in 1953. Before his retirement in 1982 at the University of Wisconsin, he spent ten years at the Atlanta Psychiatric Clinic providing family therapy to his psychiatric patients (Keith, 2014). Unlike his peer, Satir, he had significant success in the United States. However, that led to less of a spread of this methodology on the global scale during his lifetime.

On a relational level, Satir, Whitaker, and experiential therapists believed that relationships are a crucial aspect of clients' experiences and ultimately their lives. Satir's in-session interventions involved role playing, family sculpting, guided fantasy and contemplation, family patterns of relationship experience and reconstruction to intrapersonal and interpersonal actualization, and the use of healing touch (Satir, 1988). While Whitaker's techniques involved metaphor, humor, absurdity, disruption of feedback loops, and existential encounters (Nichols & Davis, 2021). Admittedly, Satir's and Whitaker's techniques are hard to teach. They exist in the intuitive and inherent gift of the person-of-the-therapist. Teaching these techniques, like in experiential therapy, is centered around challenging the defense systems of the trainee so these gifts can naturally shine through and be expressed fully and unconditionally.

In Symbolic Experiential, Whitaker emphasizes the importance of the person of therapist, stating "Theory and technique come alive and take form only when filtered through the personhood of a therapist" (Whitaker & Bumberry, 1988, p. 18; Bailey, 2022). He goes even further to state "My capacity to be real, to be alive during the session, to respond in a personal fashion is the essence of what I have to offer" (Whitaker & Bumberry, 1988, p. 18; Bailey, 2022). Whitaker was much more focused on what he was doing in session, stating "[the presumption is that] it is experience, not education that changes families (Whitaker & Keith, 1982). His main two main assumptions were around the idea of 1) creativity, spontaneity, humor, and play to "spur families toward the freedom of authentic communication" (Bailey, 2022). Play and spontaneity are a marker of a healthy and free system. The second assumption is 2) direct confrontation, challenging, and absurdity.

> *"[When clients] are then faced with the growth issues of choice, values and responsibility in an uncertain world. Again, I want to participate in an experience that shakes them. One that surprises them enough to break free of the family-of origin hypnosis we all are subject to. Confusion is, by itself, one of the most potent ways of symbolically opening up the infrastructure of the family.*
> Whitaker & Bumberry, 1988, p. 18; Bailey, 2022.

In order for this process to occur, experiential therapists must know that the client is the expert of their own lives and internal systems. However, experiential therapists often take an active and directive role to perturb the system so it can naturally reorganize itself rather than using forceful control, structure, or psychoeducation. This allows for clients' systems to be then able to reorganize in a naturally adaptive and responsive way that is unique to each client system. This ultimately shapes maladaptive emotion into new adaptive emotion and a new perspective, leading to "not only understanding but responding in ways that prioritize connection" (McDowell et al., 2023). To do this, experiential therapists must know that the client is the expert in their lives and that this stance is primary in session. With all these factors integrated together, the capacity for client growth increases, creating change within the system (Greenberg & Goldman, 1988; Paivio & Bahr, 1998).

In the late 1960s and early 1970s, psychotherapy moved towards evidence-based modalities like cognitive behavioral approaches and postmodern approaches like solution-focused ones. With Satir's leaving the United States and Whitaker's style being considered hard to teach and with ever-growing legal implications, experientialism in the United States became untrendy. However, even though experiential family therapy started losing momentum, it inspired influential figures like Drs. Sue Johnson and Richard Schwartz (Nichols & Davis, 2021).

Intersectional and Cross-Cultural Adaptability

Experiential therapy naturally builds warmth, safety, and belonging in diverse communities. As congruence and authenticity are centered, our ability to live our lives is fostered. As an entity, experiential therapy centers on self-actualization and growth regarding sociocultural context, yet Satir's Growth Model has specifically been utilized with culturally diverse and international communities. Although critiqued for a large focus on gender and power outside of feminist family therapy techniques, it also recognized social context, binary and gendered societal messages, and empowerment through equality within relationships (Maxey, 2021). A few empirical studies have shown adaptability within Hispanic and Asian cultures. Bermudez (2008) provides a thorough application with Hispanic families through the value of family or *familismo,* immigration status, language, acculturation, and culturally responsive work that is internally intertwined. Thus, emphasizing family bonds as strengths that have transcended over hundreds of generations. Cheung and Chan (2002) bring the cultural sensitivity of Satir's model outside of Western, individualistic binds and into collectivistic, Chinese culture. They describe Satir's communication stances and focus on congruence. One of Satir's descriptions of unhealthy coping mechanisms take form in survival stances: placator (people pleasers), blamer (blame others), super-reasonable (logic and rules emphasis), irrelevant (no consistent ground for self, other or context), and congruent (balance of self, others, and context) (Satir, 1991). Embedded within the model, congruence takes shape through cultural empowerment to reconnect with ancestorial resources; meaning the client's ability to heal is already embedded deep within them (Cheung & Chan, 2002). Satir's model is uniquely built to honor the collectivistic values and individual self. Growth is interpersonally connected. As an individual family member centers their inner strengths and healing, the entire family can benefit from and express their own strengths (Epstein et al., 2012). Regarding cultural influence, ingredients of interaction and softening family rules (Satir, 1991) come to play important factors when creating change in my sessions. For example, a self-identified African American lesbian client came in stating that her parents viewed her sexual orientation as "wrong" because her culture values heterosexual relationships. The rigidity of reflexivity with her sexual orientation caused her extreme distress. I used this assumption to navigate conflict with their values and increase awareness of how each moment of reality is constructed and how each specific individual gives unique meaning to their own unique experience. This increase in awareness promoted healthy functioning, which in turn decreased the distress of not conforming to their culture but being aware of their own experience of being authentically themselves.

In the continued spirit of Satir and in my own adaptation of Satir and Latinx couples, survival stances were very helpful in recognizing various intersecting processes for Latinx LGBTQ communities. In Gutierrez (2019), I share an example of Latinx lesbian experiences through an experiential lens:

> "She may face expectations of rejection because her family may be highly religious (i.e., social environment) and lives in a country where lesbians are outwardly discriminated against. She describes experiencing internalized heterosexism. Part of

the therapist's assessment of the problem is that she developed a placating stance to survive her family system. She pleases her family by continuing to adhere to gender, sexuality, and traditional norms by putting her authentic self and desires second, to avoid conflict, tension and possible abandonment from her family and possible danger when she is out in public. She continues this stance at school within her interpersonal relationships to continuously avoid conflict and potential danger. This specific stance she has taken may exacerbate feelings of shame, guilt and distress from internalized heterosexism; ultimately influencing and diminishing her intrapersonal processes of self-worth and self-esteem. Through experiential theory, change occurs when families and clients remove defense mechanism and can fully express their feelings. Fighting emotional suppression begins with processing from inside (i.e., emotions) moving to external expression (i.e., behavior) (Hale-Hanif, 2012). So, for this example, it would be beneficial for her to express feelings of internalized heterosexism with her family, friends and community. Lastly, one possible intervention here would be role-playing and practicing responses of a coming-out conversation with the safest person in her circle."

Gutierrez, 2019, p. 40–41

Neuroscience of Experiential Therapy

More recently, neuroscience research is giving Satir and Whitaker's experiential therapy a chance to regain its momentum and re-establish itself once again as an exciting approach to family therapy. The magic of what Satir and Whittaker tapped into during the 60s we now have supportive neuroscience that explains the power of their theoretical assumptions of their experiential therapies.

Exciting research coming from interpersonal neurobiology (IPNB), founded originally by Dr. Daniel Siegel, is a consilient, multidisciplinary framework that seeks to examine the connection between the brain and mind (Bailey, 2022). IPNB looks at the ways in which our experiences, particularly our relationship with others, shapes neurobiological connections (Bailey, 2022). IPNB and its now over 85 published books, in the *Norton Interpersonal Neurobiology Series*, have laid the foundation for finding strong support for experiential therapy's legitimacy in creating long-lasting, physiological change (WWNorton.com, 2023; Bailey, 2022). Under the interpersonal neurobiology framework other important neuroscience has emerged including Stephen Porges' Polyvagal Theory, Pat Ogden's Sensorimotor Psychotherapy, Daniel Hill's Affect Regulation Theory, Louis Conzolino's Neuroscience of the Human Relationship, and so many more. As an aside, two of my personal favorites from the Series is *Healing the Traumatized Self* by Paul Frewen and fellow neurofeedback practitioner Ruth Lanius and *Art Therapy and Neuroscience of Relationship, Creativity and Resiliency*, by our dear colleague Noah Hass-Cohen and her writing partner Joanna Clyde Findlay. As one can imagine from the title it has many intersections with experientialism.

IPNB argues that experiential therapy has the capacity to promote multilevel change across the family system as well as the individuals' neural system. The significant shifts in individuals' experiences through the expression of their deep emotions and desires, facilitated by the safe presence of the experiential therapist, leads to interpsychic and intrapsychic changes that move individuals toward growth (Bailey, 2022).

The IPNB conceptualizations reflects what Satir and Whitaker already knew, that a healthy, integrated, and regulated nervous system is formulated through relationship, or as Dan Siegel says, the exchange of information and energy flow (Siegel, 2012).

The energy flow we are talking about is the actual electrical signatures that each human produces from the electrical pathways of neurons found in the physical brain and heart and other innervated locations in our physical bodies. As well as the acknowledgement that we communicate via sound waves and other felt sensory information.

The development of a healthy, integrated nervous system is formulated by a nurturing and regulated relationship with our caregivers in infancy (Siegel, Schore & Cozolino, 2021). The immense work of attachment theory and developmental trauma describes what physiologically can go awry if we do not have healthy, co-regulating caregivers in those developmental years (Siegel, Schore & Cozolino, 2021). Most if not all the concerned clients that come to therapy have some foundation in these developmental areas. As such, it becomes an incredibly important and often unidentified task for the therapist to be the co-Regulator for the clients' nervous systems, until the point where clients can begin to self-regulate (Siegel, Schore & Cozolino, 2021). Often in therapy we term this attunement, presence, and therapeutic alliance. All key elements of person-of-the-therapist as the mechanisms of change in experiential therapy.

Bailey's article (2022) is a brilliant review that describes how these new understandings support Whittaker and Satir in neuroscience. One example Bailey states is regarding the brain's resonant circuitry, which is where clients feel seen by their therapist. This resonant circuity is both intra- and interpersonal attunement: "this requires therapists to develop presence to pay attention to their own experience and be attuned to their clients. Whittaker consistently brought here and now of himself to his therapeutic process, in addition to the reflections on his experiences with his clients" (Bailey, 2022).

The theoretical assumption of spontaneity, creativity, play, and emotional honesty is demonstrated again by Satir and Whitaker (Nichols & Davis, 2023). We now understand that individuals that struggle with play, creativity, spontaneity, and emotional honesty in their personal lives have lower levels of connection in the corpus callosum. The corpus callosum is the neuronal connection between the brain's two hemispheres (Bailey, 2022). The active, creative, and spontaneous nature of experiential therapies begins to build more of these pathways and connections. There are many positive associations with increased hemispheric connectivity (Bailey, 2022).

Virginia Satir was not very concerned with teaching techniques but with engaging her students and trainees in fine-tuning their instruments (Bailey, 2022). More explicitly, this is person-of-the-therapist work, meaning having them work on and learn self-regulation and explore of their own defense mechanisms and emotional suppressions (Bailey, 2022). The concept of resonance, which the field of neurofeedback talks about frequently, and can also be seen in Dan Siegel's work, is the idea that we need another safe, connected, nervous system to develop our own safe, connected nervous system (Fisher, 2014; Seigel, 2012). Again, we see this resonance/attunement/presence concept described in Alan Shore's work describing right brain to right brain nonverbal communication and synchronization in mothers and infants (Schore, 2019). This is to say further that these nonverbal, energetically based connections are key to all health determinates (Bailey, 2022) and are key mechanisms for change in these experiential approaches. As demonstrated and taught by Satir and Whitaker, the use of self in session is tapping into the power of that resonance, connection, and co-regulation (Baily, 2022).

The last tenant of experiential therapies being supported by neuroscience that I want to mention here is our every growing understanding of neuroplasticity. We now understand that new and novel experiences are the primary mechanism for how the brain develops new neuronal connections (e.g., new pathways) (Fisher, 2014). As those experiences are repeated over time, with an ongoing relationship with the therapist, we see these connections become the new default pathways (Fisher, 2014). The Bailey article (2022) continues to describe a multitude of other experiential assumptions that can now be supported by neuroscience. We cannot recommend enough that you check out that article, as a full articulation of these connections (Bailey, 2022).

The last statement I want to make here is that when we initiate something so fudamentally human, hacking into physiological underpinning, something that society and social constructs cannot permeate, such an action methodically holds global possibilities. Experientialism is concerned with process over content. It focuses on the unique but consistent needs of being a human, wired with this physiology. Of course, it can be highly utilize in China and resonate with Indigenous communities in Canada, (satirglobal.org), because it bypasses the content to initiate true second-order change processes in human physiology. Culture may dictate what expression looks like, but it cannot change the inherent human fact of physiology that we all do express, every day. We cannot change the fact that we all need human connections to develop. We cannot change the fact that we all process the world through relationships and an exchange of energetic information flow (Seigel, 2012). Experiential, both theoretically and functional, is an expression of being human.

Case Study: A Snapshot

I fell in love with Satir's experiential therapy early on as a master's student. Having some understanding of neuroscience coming into marriage and family therapy training, having an undergraduate degree, and time spent in a neuroscience doctoral program, her work intuitively resonated with what I believed about the world, but on a different note, I felt like I hadn't experienced much of it in my own childhood. Her ideas of unconditional positive regard, warmth, and authenticity resonated with the type of therapist I wanted it to be and knew I would have to work towards. It was during these earlier years of my training that I had a family come into therapy. I know the countries of origin for these clients but will speak broadly for confidentiality.

The parents had recently adopted elementary-aged siblings from an Eastern European country. The children had been in limited-resourced orphanages most of their lives and had suffered many developmental and childhood traumas. The eldest child had essentially been the younger siblings' caretakers for most of their lives. One parent was Canadian and had only been living in the states for a few years. They reported that their Canadian upbringing bent them towards more progressive ideals about parenting and desires to connect to their new children. They generally had a warm demeanor but expressed feeling very disconnected from their partner and their struggles with the new children in their life. The second parent was an immigrant from East Asia and reported having more traditional ideologies around parenting and children's role in a family system. They expressed a strong meaning of the word respect and what it meant in the parent-child relationship.

The couple met in East Asia and lived there for several years prior to moving to Canada, where they lived for a few more years, and then moved to the United States for a job opportunity. They had been married for over a decade when they adopted the children. The stated goals for the family were around children's behaviors, primarily the eldest child, and creating connections in this newly formed family structure.

In the early sessions with the parents, I tried very hard to understand the seemingly opposing perspectives on parenting, one being considered relatively progressive and the other relatively traditional. There seemed to be several "stuck points" where each parent was not able to do things differently based on opposing positions.

The children were recently adopted from Eastern Europe, and English was not their primary language; they struggled to express themselves in English. The family spoke mostly French at home, as it was the language they all had the most fluency in. As such, it was the primary language the family was communicating in at home. Both parents also spoke the Eastern Asian language and were trying to teach their children it, as well as English. I only know English, and vocabulary level understanding of Spanish and ASL. So, as you all can imagine communicating through verbal speech was a unique challenge in this case.

For a variety of reasons, we had been doing sessions for several months with little movement in the places where both the parents and children have been stuck in their new relationships. Always looking for low-speaking interventions when I had the whole family, I decided to engage them in a sculping activity that Satir is well known for. I gave the oldest child the prompt to create a scene about their new family using their family as the characters as they would see on TV or in a movie.

As the child built this picture in the room, they placed the more traditional parent standing on a chair and made the parent have "mad" eyebrows and a "yelling" mouth. This parent also was sculpted to have their finger pointing at the ground in a "you're in trouble gesture." They placed their youngest sibling in the corner, crouched in a ball and facing the corner of the room. They placed the second parent in the doorway halfway in and out of the room with their hands covering their ears. They placed the middle sibling lying face up in the middle of the room, spreading their limbs like a starfish. I asked them to place themselves in the picture and they placed themselves lying under the chair with the first parent standing on, creating the image that this parent was quite literally standing over them in an aggressive-looking manner. They had also reached out to the middle sibling on the floor and were just barely touching their fingertip to fingertip. And this was the scene.

Outside of giving the prompt, there was very little to no speaking communication. Yet it created a very powerful visual to the internal emotional experience and suppression of this child's fear in their new home. It was immediately clear to the parent on the chair who was very hurt and saddened that they were being experienced in this way. Even though we had tried many times to verbalize this concern, they were now experiencing it in a new way.

The parent halfway out the door began to get tearful, and without prompting or encouragement, gathered each family member up and out of their sculpted positions onto the couch. The parent literally wrapped their arms around everybody and all of them began to cry. I later discovered this was the first time they had done a "family hug."

While part of these dynamics had been clear to me for some time, I had not successfully translated the concerns or created disruption in the system. It very clearly took such a powerful intervention for it to be communicated and resonate with the parents the level of distress, fear, and mistrust the children had been experiencing. From that session forward the parents were better aligned and very engaged in working on co-regulation with each of the children and with each other. It quite literally was the disruptor we needed.

I hope that this example demonstrates how powerful a relatively simple non-speaking, new experience for this family was. It allowed them to put down many of the defense mechanisms that other talk strategies had not been able to access. It demonstrates that while many cultural factors are important to who we are and to how we live, if we can hack into primal physiological supported interventions that are uniquely human and therefore universal to humanity, these experiential practices can be beneficial, powerful, even seemingly magic, in the intersection of most cultural and societal structures.

It also demonstrates that all societies and cultures have different values, beliefs, expectations, and language expression for emotional experiences; basic non-speaking, expressive techniques can bypass those differences. We can only encourage you to try a sculpting activity with any family cases you have. It can also be done with individuals by recruiting dolls, stuffed animals, pillows, figurines, etc. We have found this helpful when working with individuals or if other family members are unavailable in sessions.

Research Agenda

Although there was, and still is, a critique of the ability to translate and teach experiential techniques, the heart of experiential is to believe in clients and families unconditionally, a subjective outcome that can be explored. Studies collectively have a pattern of using therapeutic alliance, empathy, mood disorder inventories, a certain number of sessions, and the use of certain experiential interventions (Elliott et al., 2004). The best way to measure and assess this therapy seems to be from the client's experience in the session. In a session, we work to heighten emotion, challenge defenses, create lived experiences, and actively engage in this work. If measures were taken at any other time, other than in session, we would posit, true experiential results could not be assessed.

One area of significant controversy within this research involves the assumption that experiential therapies are inferior to evidence-based theories like CBT or DBT. However, Elliott, Greenberg, and Lietaer (2004) in metanalysis of 74 comparison studies found experiential therapies' outcomes were demonstrated to be statistically equivalent to cognitive behavioral therapies. Investigations have found that experiential therapies are effective for the treatment of depression, anxiety, and trauma, as well as having possible physical health benefits and applicability to clients with schizophrenia. For example, Carryer and Greenberg (2010) conducted a study on the expression of aroused emotion and therapeutic outcome when working with clients diagnosed with depression. This study found that even a moderate level of heightened emotional arousal was helpful and improved therapeutic outcome. Another study discussed by Greenberg (2013) examined changes in expressing anger for participants who are more inclined to becoming perpetrators of domestic violence. Results showed that after going through experiential treatments, the participants' experience and expression of anger declined significantly and they were within the normal range. Even through a sociocultural attuned quantitative lens, centering emotional experiences is completely viable (Gold et al., 2007; Gold et al., 2011), and can be utilized through an experiential framework moving forward.

Three Key Takeaways

- The experientialist voice has transcended over time and been adapted into culturally responsive frameworks across the globe.

- The intuitive and holistic person-centered theory underlying experientialism is now being supported by modern-day neuroscience.
- In a time of unrelenting global turmoil and unrest affecting humanity, understanding experientialism as a contemporary theoretical framework, not an irrelevant historical model, allows us to foster self-growth, connection, and support the inherent universality of being human.

Resources and Further Reading

Brothers B. J. (2011). Virginia Satir: foundational ideas. Routledge. Retrieved November 7 2022 from http://site.ebrary.com/id/10647693.

Satir V. (1978). Your many faces. Celestial Arts.

Satir V. (1988). The new peoplemaking. Science and Behavior Books.

Satir V. Banmen J. Gerber J. & Gomori M. (1991). The Satir model: Family therapy and beyond. Science and Behavior Books.

Satir V. & Banmen J. (2008). In her own words ... Virginia Satir: selected papers 1963–1983. Zeig Tucker & Theisen.

Satir International Journal (ceased publishing 2018) https://journals.uvic.ca/index.php/satir

Satir Institute of the Pacific https://satirpacific.org/

The Virginia Satir Global Network https://satirglobal.org/

We recommend reading the references too!

References

Andreas, S. (1991). *Virginia Satir: The patterns of her magic.* Science & Behavior Books.

Bailey, M. (2022). Science catching up: Experiential family Therapy and neuroscience. *Journal of Marital and Family Therapy, 48,* 1095–1110. DOI: 10.1111/jmft.12582

Bermudez, D. (2008). Adapting Virginia Satir techniques to Hispanic families. *The Family Journal, 16*(1), 51–57. https://doi.org/10.1177/1066480707309543

Carryer, J. R., & Greenberg, L. S. (2010). Optimal levels of emotional arousal in experiential therapy of depression. *Journal of Consulting and Clinical Psychology, 78*(2), 190–199. https://doi.org/10.1037/a0018401

Cheung, G., & Chan, C. (2002). The Satir model and cultural sensitivity: A Hong Kong reflection. *Contemporary Family Therapy, 24*(1), 199–215.

Elliott, R., & Greenberg, L. S. (1997). Multiple voices in process-experiential therapy: Dialogues between aspects of the self. *Journal of Psychotherapy Integration, 7*(3), 225–239.

Elliott, R. K., Greenberg, L. S., & Lietaer, G. (2004). *Research on experiential psychotherapies.* In M.J. Lambert (Ed.), *Bergin and Garfield's handbook of psychotherapy and behavior change* (5th ed.). (pp. 493–539). John Wiley & Sons Inc.

Epstein, N. B., Berger, A. T., Fang, J. J., Messina, L. A., Smith, J. R., Lloyd, T. D., Fang, X. & Liu, Q. X. (2012). Applying western-developed family therapy models in China. *Journal of Family Psychotherapy, 23*(3), 217–237. https://doi.org/10.1080/08975353.2012.705661

Fisher, S. F. (2014). *Neurofeedback in the treatment of developmental trauma: Calming the fear-driven brain.* W W Norton & Co.

Gold, S. D., Feinstein, B. A., Skidmore, W. C., & Marx, B. P. (2011). Childhood physical abuse, internalized homophobia, and experiential avoidance among lesbians and gay men. *Psychological Trauma: Theory, Research, Practice, and Policy, 3*(1), 50–60. https://doi.org/10.1037/a0020487

Gold, S. D., Marx, B.P., & Lexington, J.M. (2007). Gay male sexual assault survivors: The relations among internalized homophobia, experiential avoidance, and psychological symptom severity. *Behavior Research and Therapy, 45*(3), 549–562. https://doi.org/10.1016/j.brat.2006.05.006.

Gold, S. D., Feinstein, B. A., Skidmore, W. C., & Marx, B. P. (2011). Childhood physical abuse, internalized homophobia, and experiential avoidance among lesbians and gay men. *Psychological Trauma: Theory, Research, Practice, and Policy, 3*(1), 50–60.

Greenberg, L. S., & Goldman, R. L. (1988). Training in experiential therapy. *Journal of Consulting and Clinical Psychology, 56*(5), 696–702.

Greenberg, L. S. (2013). Anchoring the therapeutic spiral model into research on experiential psychotherapies. In K. Hudgins & F. Toscani (Eds.), *Healing world trauma with the therapeutic spiral model. Psychodramatic stories from the frontlines* (pp. 132–148). Jessica Kingsley Publishing.

Greenberg, L. S., Watson, J. C., & Lietaer, G. (1998). *Handbook of experiential psychotherapy.* Guilford Press.

Gutierrez, D. M. (2019). *Adapting and utilizing the minority stress model: adding sexually marginalized Latinx voices and cultural factors.* [Doctoral dissertation, The University of Iowa]. ProQuest Dissertations Publishing.

Haber, R. (2002). Virginia Satir: An integrated, humanistic approach. *Contemporary Family Therapy, 24*(1), 23–34.

Hale-Haniff, M. (2012). Virgina Satir's Growth Model. Family Therapy Review: Contrasting contemporary models. *Contemporary Family Therapy, 24,* 7–22.

Johnson, S. M. (2019). *Attachment theory in practice: Emotionally focused therapy (Eft) with individuals, couples, and families.* The Guilford Press.

Keith, D. (2014). *Continuing the Experiential Approach of Carl Whitaker.* Zeig, Tucker & Theisen.

Knapp, J. V. (1997). Family Systems Psychotherapy, Literary Character, and Literature: An Introduction. *Style, 31*(2), 223–254. www.jstor.org/stable/45063758

Loeschen, S. M. (1994). *Magic of Satir: Practical Skills for Therapists* (3rd ed.). Halcyon Publishing Design.

Luepnitz, D. A. (1989). Virginia Satir: The limitations of humanism. *Journal of Feminist Family Therapy, 1*(3), 73–83. https://doi.org/10.1300/J086v01n03_05.

Maxey, V. A. (2021). The intersectional growth model: The Satir growth model informed by intersectional feminism. *Contemporary Family Therapy, 43*(1), 54–68. https://doi.org/10.1007/s10591-020-09553-7

McDowell, T., Knudson-Martin, C., & Bermudez, J. M. (2023). Socioculturally attuned family therapy: guidelines for equitable theory and practice (Second Edition). Taylor and Francis.

McGoldrick, M., & Hardy, K. V. (2019). *Re-visioning family therapy: Addressing diversity in clinical practice* (3rd ed.). Guildford Press.

Merriam-Webster. (n.d.). Experiential. In *Merriam-Webster.com dictionary.* Retrieved February 15, 2022, from www.merriam-webster.com/dictionary/experiential

Napier, A. Y., & Whitaker, C. A. (1978). *The family crucible* (1st ed.). Harper and Raw.

Neill, J. R., & Kniskern, D. P. (1989). *From Psyche to System: The Evolving Therapy of Carl Whitaker.* Guilford Press.

Nichols, M. P. & Davis, S. D. (2021). The essentials of family therapy (12th ed.). Pearson Education.

Paivio, S., & Bahr, L. (1998). Interpersonal problems, working alliance, and outcome in short-term experiential therapy. *Psychotherapy Research, 8*(4), 392–407.

Price, M. (2011). Existential-humanistic psychologists hope to promote the idea that therapy can change not only minds but lives. *American Psychological Association, 42*(10), 58.

Roberts, J. (2005). Transparency and self-disclosure in family therapy: Dangers and possibilities. *Family Process, 44,* 45–63.

Satir V. (1988). *The new peoplemaking.* Science and Behavior Books.

Satir, V., Banmen, J., Gerber, J., & Gomori, M. (1991). *The Satir Model: Family Therapy and beyond.* Science and Behavior Books.

Schore, A. (2019) Right Brain Psychotherapy. Norton Professional Books. ISBN: 978-0-393-71285-8

Siegel, D. J. (2012). *The developing mind: How relationships and the brain interact to shape who we are* (2nd ed.). The Guilford Press.

Siegel, D.J., Shore, A.N. & Cozolino, L. (2021). *Interpersonal Neurobiology and Clinical Practice.* Norton, W. W. & Company, Inc. ISBN:9780393714579

The Virginia Satir Global Network. *The Voices of Satir: Online Conference 2023.* Retrieved February 18th, 2023 from https://satirglobal.org/virginia-satir-global-network-2023-online-conference/

Whitaker, C. A., & Bumberry, W. M. (1988). *Dancing with the family: A symbolic-experiential approach.* New York: Brunner/Mazel.

Whitaker, C. A., & Keith, D. V. (1982). Symbolic-experiential family therapy. In J. R. Neill & D. P. Kniskern (Eds.), *From psyche to system: The evolving therapy of Carl Whitaker* (pp. 330–363). Guilford Press.

Whitaker, C.A., & Malone, T.P. (1981). *Roots Of Psychotherapy* (1st ed.). Routledge. https://doi.org/10.4324/9781315799155

Wong, P. T. P. (2006). Existential and humanistic theories. In J. C. Thomas & D. L. Segal (Eds.), *Comprehensive handbook of personality and psychopathology*. Wiley.

24

IMMIGRANT AND REFUGEE FAMILIES

Theory and Practice

Zamzam Dini, Marwa W. Ibrahim, and Connor Callahan

The Immigrant Experience

Immigrants choose or are forced to migrate for a multitude of reasons ranging from increasing financial stability through employment to reuniting with family members or war. Whatever the purpose of migration, post-resettlement, individuals and families go through the process of acculturation. Acculturation is the process of social, psychological, and cultural change that immigrants experience, which stems from balancing two cultures while adapting to the prevailing culture of the host society (Silva et al., 2017). Race, gender, socioeconomic status (SES), and community acceptance are all factors that impact the acculturation process and resettlement experience for immigrant families and individuals. In this chapter, we introduce some possible presenting problems or lived experiences immigrant and refugee families might desire to discuss in addition to common mental health-related issues addressed in therapy. A common misconception when working with immigrants of any generation, a first-generation (1G) recent immigrant or a second-generation (2G) immigrant, is the goal of assimilation. To clearly understand what assimilation is, we discuss the different types of acculturation developed by Berry (1997).

Acculturation

Historically, acculturation was conceptualized as a linear process where a family moves from holding the culture of origin to assimilating with the host culture. Figure 24.1 illustrates this relationship. While this linear process might have accurately reflected how some European immigrants assimilated into American society, this process produces increasing acculturative stress for individuals and families with identities that do not match the dominant American culture.

Due to the limitations of conceptualizing acculturation as a linear process, Berry (1992) developed a bidirectional acculturation process that identifies a feedback loop between the host culture and the emigrating individual or family. Essentially, acculturation is measured on a two-dimensional process to the degree to which a family a) desires to maintain their

DOI: 10.4324/9781003297871-27

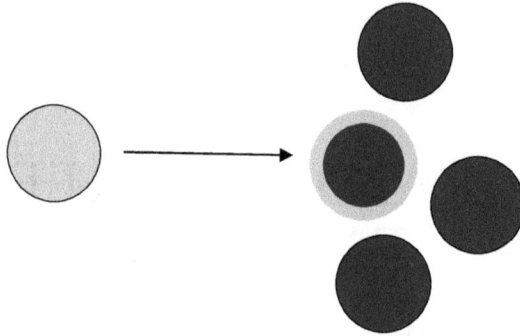

Figure 24.1 The linear process of acculturation misunderstood with assimilation.

culture of origin and b) desires to interact with individuals outside their culture of origin (Berry, 1992). Using these two dimensions, four types of acculturation emerge: assimilation, marginalization, separation (or segregation), and integration. Assimilation occurs when the emigrating family has no desire to hold on to any aspect of their culture of origin and ultimately adapts to the dominant culture. Separation or segregation occurs when the emigrating family only desires to hold on to their culture of origin without intending to interact with the dominant culture. Marginalization occurs when the emigrating family has no interest in either holding on to culture of origin or interacting with the dominant culture. Lastly, integration is when the emigrating family desires not only to hold on to components of their culture of origin but also seeks out interactions with the dominant culture (Berry, 1992). Figure 24.2 illustrates the types of acculturation on a multidimensional scale.

Society often expects immigrants to "assimilate" into the dominant culture. Individuals and families attempting to maintain some part of their culture of origin are seen as rejecting the dominant culture. This assumption is harmful and xenophobic. As we see in the types of acculturation identified by Berry (1992), assimilation means letting go of one's culture of origin and ultimately adopting the dominant culture. To expect communities who escaped war, persecution, and violence to let go of the only thing they have left, which is their culture, is a cruel expectation. Berry (1992) explains that integration is the only healthy way to acculturate; anything outside of that can produce acculturative stress (Berry, 1997). This point is crucial for clinicians working with immigrants and refugees. The desire for the immigrant family to interact with the dominant culture should be welcomed, and the desire to hold onto some culture of origin practices should also be respected. Figure 24.2 illustrates what healthy acculturation can look like through the integration process. We have added the generational component to Berry's (1992) idea of integration to show that acculturation happens internally and externally. The circles without borders illustrate first-generation immigrants, while the circles with the rings show how second-generation immigrants may acculturate. There is also an internal process of cultural exchange where values, ideologies, and thoughts are influenced by the host society and vice versa, represented by the dots in the circles (Figure 24.2). Acculturative stress is heightened for immigrants considered People of Color (POC) because we live in a racialized society that centers Whiteness or the White experience. However, the answer to that acculturative stress is not always assimilation.

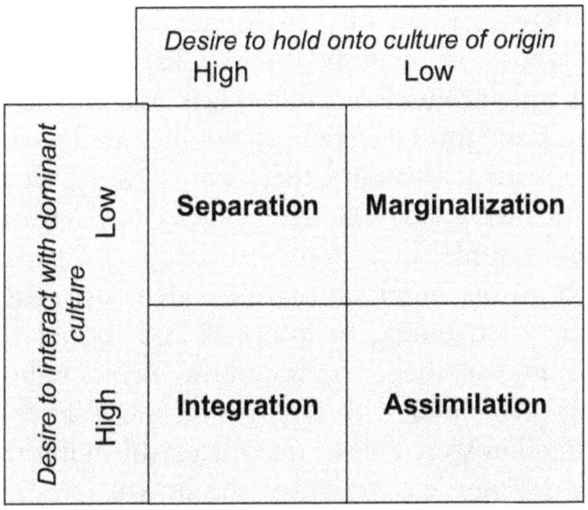

Figure 24.2 The Four Types of Acculturation according to Berry (1992).

The Refugee Experience

Refugees are a subset of immigrants with traumatic experiences attached to their immigration stories. Since 2001, the world has witnessed some of the worst humanitarian crises in history. The crises, such as the war in the Middle East, famine linked to climate change-induced drought, and extreme financial difficulties, have displaced millions of people. Refugees often experience hardships like political/religious persecution, oppressive regimes, and even torture before they are forced to leave for their safety (Perera et al., 2013; Hecker et al., 2017; Porter & Haslam, 2005). After the decision to leave, they are forced to endure the act of migration, which can be extremely dangerous and even deadly. Upon arrival to a new country, refugees must navigate grueling immigration systems. Depending on the country, refugee families must simultaneously move forward from the trauma they experienced before migration and endure the stress of learning a new language, acculturating, and navigating a new way of life (Halcón et al., 2004; Weine et al., 2011; O'Donnell et al., 2020). This phenomenon is encapsulated in two concepts called pre-emigration trauma and post-migration stress (Hecker et al., 2017; Porter & Haslam, 2005; Steel et al., 2017).

There is strong evidence that rather than ending refugee families' stress and trauma, resettling in a host country exponentially increases the stress and trauma due to continued exposure to post-migration stresses (Bentley et al., 2019; Phipps & Degges-White, 2014). Dealing with the psychological distress of the previously discussed traumatic experiences can negatively affect parents' and grandparents' ability to perform effective and healthy caregiving. This increases the possibility that offspring in these families may suffer the consequences of the impact of trauma (e.g., secondary traumatic stress). Recently, this phenomenon has been identified as intergenerational trauma. A minimum requirement for clinicians working to support refugee families is to be trauma-informed in their practice. We will provide resources and examples of trauma treatment modalities in the Resources section.

Strength and Resilience in Immigrant and Refugee Families

Strength and resilience are essential attributes of immigrants and refugees. It takes immense courage and logistical planning to support your family as you navigate the complex immigration process and create a new life in a foreign land. Without firsthand experience or insider knowledge of what it is like to be forcibly displaced from your home and create a new life elsewhere, it is tough to understand or even imagine the overlapping experiences that go into immigration. Immigrant and refugee families are incredibly skilled in adaption and assessing the situation to understand their status (Juang et al., 2018). The experience immigrant families possess gives them the resilience to navigate future family stressors with some wisdom. For example, most families struggled during the initial COVID-19 government shutdown; however, immigrant families demonstrated collective resilience by supporting each other by contributing to informal and formal community food banks, opening their doors to family members who found themselves unhoused after being unable to pay rent, and helping each other with daycare responsibilities (Solheim et al., 2022). Immigrant and refugee families were able to quickly establish informal social supports that were no longer available during the government shutdown.

Culturally Sensitive Approaches to Therapy Are Critical

We have established that immigrants and refugees are not monolithic. Many experiences grounded in race, gender, SES, and the intersectionality of those identities are not commonly shared. Considering this, cultural expertise is impossible, as no person can become an "expert" in any given culture. Culturally sensitive and attuned approaches represent a better understanding that even if a family has origins in a specific culture, the family may not ascribe to all the norms and values of the culture of origin. This highlights the need for cultural humility when working with immigrant families and remaining curious. When we stay curious, we empower families to define their culture, decreasing our likelihood of imposing our assumptions on the family. These assumptions are often rooted in stereotypes, possibly perpetuating racist and xenophobic ideas about immigrant and refugee families. Immigrants and refugees are among the more vulnerable populations. Because of the often underrepresentation of mental health providers with shared backgrounds and experiences, our ethical responsibility is to incorporate cultural humility into our work to reduce the structural oppression rooted in mental health treatment. In the next section, we discuss why not incorporating culturally sensitive approaches can result in imposing Western family practices and structures on immigrant and refugee families and individuals.

The Mismatch with Current Clinical Approaches in the Field

Historically, the mental health field has actively harmed, ignored the needs of, and pathologized the lives of historically marginalized communities and POC, especially the African American community in the United States. (You can read a historical chronology of the American Psychological Association's (APA, 2021b) contributions to the perpetuation of inequality in the United States and APA's apology (APA, 2021a) for racism in the field of psychology in the resources section.) When we focus on MFT specifically, the theories that guide us and helped establish the field were grounded in the assessment and evaluation of heteronormative WEIRD (Western, educated, industrialized, rich, and democratic) families (Henrich et al., 2010). Due to the origins of the foundational theories in MFT (Bowen Family Systems Theory, Structural Family Therapy, etc.) centering on WEIRD standards, there needs to be a level of intentionality and awareness of these biases when working with

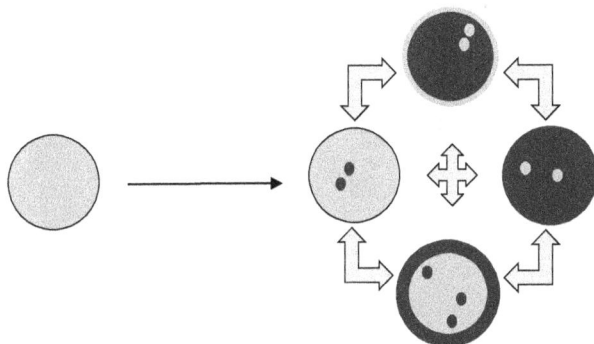

Figure 24.3 Integration as a feedback loop where the host culture and immigrant family influence each other at different generational time points.

non-WEIRD families. For example, Duvall's (1957) Family Development Theory assumes that couples will have children as they move through various relationship stages.

While some immigrants and refugees may have shared experiences that result from building a new life in a foreign country or growing up bicultural (or multicultural) as a child of immigrants, we must emphasize that there will always be nuanced differences in immigrant and refugee experiences. Families with similar cultural backgrounds and/or ethnicities may function differently depending on factors like acculturation, racial identity, religion, etc. Understanding the intersectionality of identities and lived experiences is necessary when working with such a diverse population.

Kimberlé Crenshaw coined the term *intersectionality* to describe the unique ways Black women's identities were oppressed within systems (i.e., law, healthcare) in the United States and how they were unique compared to other intersectional identities (e.g., white women, Black men) (Crenshaw, 1991). Crenshaw (1991) argued that all aspects of one's identity needed to be understood as simultaneously interacting with each other and influencing one's worldview in society. Bešić's (2020) work visualizes how identities intersect, creating the intersection onion represented in Figure 24.3.

One of the central ethical values held in many fields is to *"do no harm."* Therefore, we have an ethical responsibility to be knowledgeable enough to do no harm when working with immigrants and refugees. Imposing Western family functioning on immigrants and refugees and then labeling their behavior pathological causes harm. For example, ask yourself if this family is *really* enmeshed/codependent or do they have a family structure beyond the nuclear family, allowing other adults in the family system to take on a parental role. When a 25-year-old college student who lives at home comes to therapy for family issues, is your first thought *why is a 25-year-old living with their parents?* I've had clients who have told me horror stories of therapists saying culturally incongruent things to them. A client thinking about whether she should keep on her hijab informed me of a previous therapist who told her to prioritize her happiness and leave Islam altogether. My client was so shocked at the suggestion that she left that therapist and didn't go to therapy again for years, finally explicitly seeking a Muslim therapist. In a chapter on values-sensitive therapy, Doherty (2001) explained how current therapy often imposes Western values on clients and provides insights into how we can be aware of this in our practice. (See Resources section.)

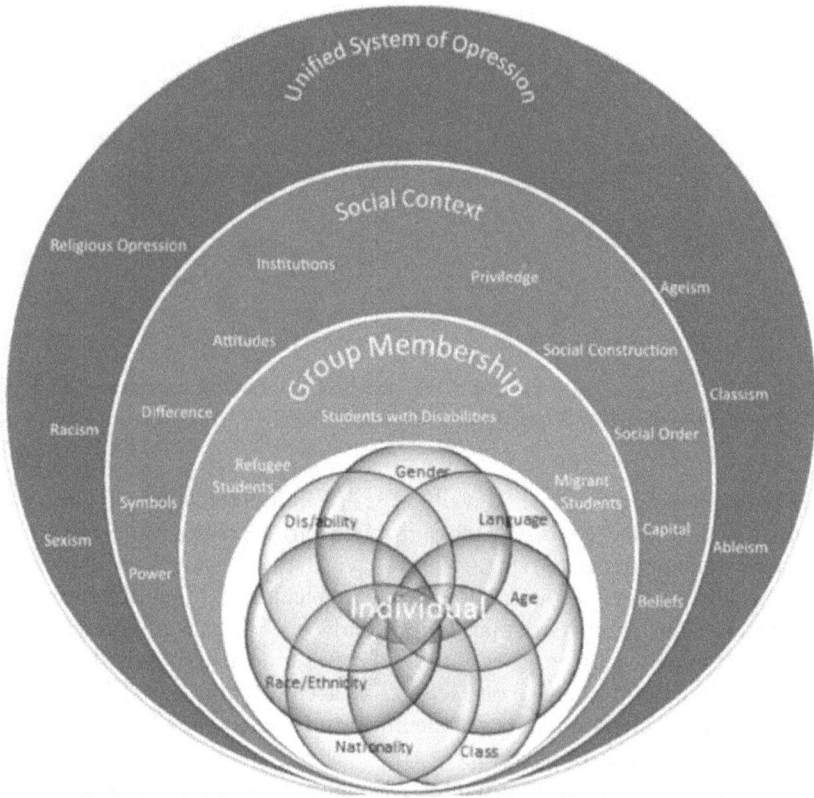

Figure 24.4 The intersection onion represents how identities and systems of oppression intersect and overlap. (Bešić, 2020).

Working with Immigrants and Refugees

Due to their unique experiences, we want to provide guidance for addressing concerns immigrant and refugee families bring to therapy, as illustrated by case examples. We hope these case examples highlight the nuances of this work often missed by Western approaches. We will also provide guidance about addressing identified barriers from a systemic lens through discussions about the role of the therapist role and the system.

Addressing Trauma: Research and Practice

While immigrant (and specifically refugee) populations have a higher prevalence of trauma exposure, there is little guidance in the literature on how to address this specific trauma in therapy. Clients who want to work with these populations often must specialize in trauma treatment, necessitating additional training after graduation. The lack of familiarity or understanding of trauma, its symptoms, and how it might show up directly impacts the confidence, comfortability, and appropriate assessment capabilities of new therapists and those unfamiliar, leading to various knee-jerk reactions. This can look like referring out too quickly, immediately trying to ground the client by shutting down any emotional reactivity, premature feelings of unsafety, and/or institutionalization.

Subsequently, this also perpetuates systems of oppression built into our institutions that continually disenfranchise Black, Indigenous, People of Color (BIPOC), minoritized, and often underrepresented communities in treating mental health concerns. Essentially, we fear what we do not know. Working with clients with trauma history goes beyond learning a specific intervention and requires intentional learning and understanding on a theoretical level. How we conceptualize health and dysfunction, understand and assess change, and define the role of the therapist, all impact the effectiveness of addressing trauma properly. This is even more important when working with immigrant and refugee populations with multiple intersecting marginalized identities and adverse experiences.

Trauma is a Relational Experience

We experience trauma through a relational lens. The grief we experience after losing our loved one, the violence committed against each another, witnessing others commit violence against another, etc. In response, orienting trauma treatment through a relational lens only makes sense. Trauma is multidimensional, contextual, spatial, physiological, and emotional (Yehuda, 2002). Untreated trauma can also be (and usually is) passed down through intergenerational transmission to the offspring (Heberle et al., 2020). It is essential to understand and acknowledge that trauma experienced directly and trauma that is transmitted generationally may not present in the same way. People who have experienced trauma have a heightened nervous system that can easily activate through interactions and environmental triggers (Ursin & Erikson, 2010). For example, when a client shares their experience of rape, and the clinician feels discomfort, the communication of our comfort level occurs on a physiological level.

Interpersonal Neurobiology of Therapy

Interpersonal neurobiology (IPNB) posits that our nervous systems constantly communicate (Siegel, 2012). Creating safety is of great importance when working with clients who have experienced trauma, and those with a history of oppression. When we say, "creating a safe space," this can include physical safety, emotional safety, and unconditional positive regard. Emotional safety looks like allowing the expression of emotion, being comfortable with tears and pain, and acknowledging feelings in general. Unconditional positive regard, popularized by humanistic psychologist Carl Rogers, involves meeting the client where they are at, allowing clients to show up how they need to, and believing the experiences they share. In this section, I want to emphasize physical safety. Safety, not just in the physical space, like where the exit is situated in the room or what type of images and artwork is presented. We will introduce and discuss trauma-sensitive office space later. The physical safety here could be defined more as physiological safety. Is the clinician's nervous system communicating a sense of safety to the client's nervous system?

Part of understanding how to work with clients with a history of trauma is learning to ground yourself and relax your nervous system. This is essential to communicating safety to your clients. Immigrants, particularly refugees, have experienced atrocious traumas that might include torture, war, and sexual violence. By their nature, these topics are not comfortable for anyone to discuss. However, for those working with immigrants, and refugees in particular, it is imperative that you face these stories head-on to provide one of the few spaces of healing available for these communities. You do not have to be a trauma therapist to support clients with a history of trauma. Providing safety and being a compassionate witness is enough to stimulate the healing process. (See the Resources Section for trauma-specific models that offer therapists additional resources.)

Addressing Acculturative Disparities

Acculturative stress theory characterizes acculturative stress, a byproduct of acculturation, as the adverse behavioral and emotional reactions attributed to the process and experiences of adjusting to a new cultural environment (Berry, 1997). Often, family members acculturate at different rates for various reasons, creating acculturation disparities (Meschke & Juang, 2014). Second-generation (2G) refugees, who tend to have more accelerated acculturation, might view their first-generation (1G) refugee parents' slow pace of acculturation as closemindedness or rigidity, whereas 1G refugees may view their more acculturated children as rejecting the culture of origin. Meschke and Juang (2014) explained that acculturation disparities impact meaning-making, often resulting in misaligned communicative expressions and leading to further communication challenges. In the following case example, we illustrate what acculturative disparities can look like in the therapy room.

The Yusuf Family

I once worked with a refugee family from East Africa. The family comprised two 1G parents and five 2G children (between approximately 15 and 4) born in the United States. The parents were in the middle of divorce proceedings, and the court ordered family therapy for the children and the father due to parent estrangement. The advantage of being trained in Marriage and Family Therapy was that I could see many variations of family constellations in this family system. With a co-therapist, I worked with the father individually, the three older children individually, the father with the two youngest children, and the father with the three older children. I even met with the mother as a resource to the therapeutic system.

The first author is a second-generation East African refugee and had some cultural insight to support this family. My co-therapist was an African-American woman whose age aligned more with the father and therefore had some insight that I also lacked; we made a great team. The father's main concern was wanting his children to like him again after a history of intermittent involvement in their lives. The children reported they could not trust their father after leaving without warning. We initially had family therapy with the three older children and their father. Whenever we asked the father to express his desire to be with his children, his answer always was, "because they are my children." After hearing that, the children would immediately shut down, feeling that they needed an "apology" from dad and some "proof" that he was willing to change.

I remember sitting in a session with the family, and one of the children said that dad only cared about her grades and not her. I paused the teen and asked the father to respond to her statement. The father explained that education was his only means of survival when growing up in his country of origin. He felt the same urgency and importance when considering his children's education. I could see the frustration on the children's faces and had to pause the father. I explained to the father that his children did not have to worry about survival, shelter, safety, etc., as he did growing up. This anxiety and worry drove the father to have his children study every evening after school from a textbook he bought, continuing their learning until bedtime. The children explained that they wanted their father to care about things besides their grades, like how they were feeling or what they did for fun, and the session fell silent.

At this point, we realized we had to have separate sessions with the older children to provide context for their father's behavior. I explained that their father did not have first-hand experience with what it's like to grow up in this country. We also spent some time with the father to explain that his children had their basic needs met, introducing Maslow's hierarchy of needs (Maslow, 1969) and describing his children's importance of emotional connectedness. In all honesty, it took more than one discussion with both parties to move toward a place of understanding; however, our continual talks about the experiences of everyone in the room provided ample context to produce empathy. As I continued working with this family, I felt like a cultural translator between the two generations, constantly providing context and interpreting perceived differences in values and attitudes. Although being a cultural insider may have played a part in joining with the clients, I am confident that if a therapist approached this family with patience, cultural sensitivity, and open-mindedness, they would be able to build a bridge between the perceived cultural/generational gap in this family system.

Language Barriers

One byproduct of acculturation is immigrant families' generational differences in language skills (Cox et al., 2021). As children of immigrant parents enroll in schools and engage with the dominant culture, the natural result is an advanced acquisition of the host language. As 1G parents maintain their language of origin as their primary method of communication, children born in a host country switch their primary language (English in the United States, for example) from the language of origin to the host language as they grow. As we know, language is deeply connected to identity and the self. Communication limitations due to a lack of knowledge of the host language make it more challenging to integrate into a community. Now, imagine a family where chronic language restrictions are getting in the way of meaningful dialogue between parents and children. How connected will the family members feel? How will they discuss abstract, difficult-to-explain experiences like biculturalness, discrimination, or depression/anxiety? Cox and colleagues (2021) describe this phenomenon of family systems with differing language skills as Shared Language Erosion (SLE). Their phenomenal work describes how SLE plays a role in parent-child conflicts, attachment development, peer influence/selection, and parental competence (Cox et al., 2021). The following example illustrates how this might occur in multilingual families experiencing acculturation.

The Gutierrez Family. *I received a referral from an ER for an older pre-adolescent client. The presenting problem for this client was suicidality and depressive symptoms. As with all minor clients during intake, I briefly met with the parents separately, then individually met with the young client, and concluded with everyone in the room. Due to the client's young age, I suggested having family and individual sessions to understand the family system better. I noticed an interesting dynamic in the room during the first family session. Since the parents were divorced, the client was living with her mother. However, the client was closer to her father, who was heavily involved in her treatment* and highly supportive and understanding. The mother's primary language was Spanish, and the second language was English. The father was fluent in both Spanish and English. The young client spoke both languages but not at the same level of fluency and felt more comfortable having therapy in English. I asked the parents if they wanted a Spanish interpreter to support me during family sessions, and they both kindly declined. As a therapist who does not speak Spanish, I realized that the space would become imbalanced if I were not careful and intentional.

Due to language limitations, the young client often described having more open and honest conversations with her father than with her mother. The client explained that she couldn't find the right words in Spanish to describe her intrusive thoughts when feeling depressed. There was a moment during a family session when I asked the mom to express the feelings she experienced when she saw her daughter want to describe something to her but couldn't due to the language. The mom started crying and explained her experience while the dad interpreted it for me. Structural Family Therapists would describe the young client and father as forming a coalition against the mother in this family system. Mom and dad had many points of conflict, some being parenting styles but other issues more related to their relationship. Dad was able to be the fun and lenient parent, highly influencing the young client's perception of her mother. As someone who doesn't speak Spanish, I had to rely on the father to interpret our discussions that entire session. This lack of shared language created an unavoidable power imbalance at that time. Luckily, I had a rudimentary knowledge of Spanish from school, so I tried and listened for some vocabulary I could identify.

I remember one session where I asked the mom about emotional reactivity, and the father asked the question in a way that might come off as rude and even called her "the devil." I then realized the father was not a neutral party in this situation who could be objective when playing this different role as an interpreter. After that instance, I rearranged our family sessions by separating the young client and the parents for portions of the session. The young client had great difficulty in watching her parents constantly fight and often blamed herself for the state of her family, but she couldn't have those discussions with her mother and often got one side of the story due to that.

Racialization of Identity

When refugees acculturate within a racialized society, the acculturation process differs, depending on their ethnicity. The process by which people become racialized is contingent on various factors. The particulars of history, geography, the need for capital, and the attributes of various populations all contribute to it (Yarbough, 2010). This means education level, foreign policy, SES, and country of origin should all be considered in the racialization process. In many cases, processes and experiences of racialization depend upon the "cultural distance" between a specific group and the dominant racial/ethnic group, such that racialization remains intimately connected to acceptance into and by the nation (Yarbough, 2010). Two immigrants who are labeled "White" on the census and have accented English could be treated differently simply because one is from Sweden and the other from Lebanon. Living in a racialized society means one's experience with racism varies based on where a person's humanity is placed on the racial spectrum of social hierarchy (from Whiteness to Blackness), the ability to assimilate into the dominant culture, and acceptability (from the host culture).

Medford (2019) found that working-class, second-generation, Black immigrants believed that their ethnic background provided them little to no advantages, so they identified as African Americans. But the middle-class, second-generation, Black immigrants attributed their success to their ethnicity and so-identified as "West Indian" (Medford, 2019). This process of ethnic self-selection is partially responsible for the misperception that Black immigrants are blanketly more successful than African Americans. This racialization of immigrant groups embeds them into the social hierarchy perpetuated by racism embedded in American culture. Often, immigrants and refugees hail from ethnically homogenous societies and do not identify with the racialization that occurs when they resettle in countries like the United States, Canada, the UK, etc.

Due to this nuance, 1G refugees might not be as aware of being racialized compared to 1.5G and 2G refugees and focus solely on discrimination due to immigrant status. However, racial trauma and/or stress is one component of continuous traumatic stress (CTS) (Hecker et al., 2017) that impacts the lives of POC daily. Unlike post-traumatic stress (PTS), which identifies an initial incident responsible for the trauma response, CTS results from traumatic incidents that frequently happen every day (Hecker et al., 2017). Therefore, it is vital to ask about racially motivated stressors separate from immigrant-related stress when assessing immigrants and refugees that we work with.

Transnational Characteristic

Due to the migration history of immigrants and refugees, their families are often structurally transnational. Multiple branches of family members live in various countries throughout the world. Some family members may remain in the country of origin, while others emigrated to host countries as immigrants or refugees, often not in the same country. Take my family, for example; most of my family remained in Somalia. Still, I also have family members that emigrated to Kenya, Uganda, the UAE, Sweden, the UK, Canada, China, Turkey, and Australia, while I live in the United States with my immediate family. Although technological advances (e.g., online messaging and video calls) have made it easier to stay connected to family members across the globe, there is still a sense of loss when your family members live far away from you. This phenomenon is best explained through the lens of Ambiguous Loss Theory.

Ambiguous Loss. Ambiguous loss is the most challenging type of loss because there is no apparent resolution (i.e., closure), and it creates confusion about who is in or outside the family (i.e., boundary ambiguity) (Boss, 2004). These types of loss are frozen because they have an element of uncertainty and ambiguity. Boss (2004) described two types of ambiguous loss: a) psychologically present but physically absent, and b) physically present but psychologically absent. Immigrant and refugee families can experience either category depending on which branch of the family we focus on. However, families that live in the diaspora are more likely to experience ambiguous loss within the context of family members being psychologically present and physically absent.

Although family members might not be together physically, they are aware of what family members are experiencing; they might be responsible for financially sustaining family members overseas and/or closely following political strife or natural disasters in the country of origin. Families living in the diaspora might go years without being able to visit family back home. During that absence, family members might get sick, pass away, move away, etc. Acknowledging the ambiguous loss in immigrant families is crucial as this frozen grief can become a barrier to a healthy resettlement or acculturation experience. For example, traditions may end, roles become hard to define (role ambiguity), attachments may become less secure, caretaking stressors might create resentments, identity shifts can result in self-doubt, etc. (Boss, 2004).

Role of the Clinician

A clinician working with immigrants and refugees is a unique witness to the complexity of the immigration experience and its interplay with mental, physical, and social health. This unique position comes with the great responsibility of using what we bear witness to to deepen our understanding of our clients, bridge the gaps in our knowledge regarding their immigration experience, and cultivate the foundational skills necessary to intervene in a culturally sensitive and competent manner. A clinician working with immigrant clients holds the roles of a witness, a multiculturally competent professional, and an advocate. To better demonstrate the integration of these roles, I introduce the case of Fatima. Fatima is a pseudonym for a client I worked with in an outpatient counseling setting. I slightly altered the details of this case to protect the client's confidentiality but retained the core elements relating to her immigration experience.

Fatima is a 45-year-old who identifies as an Arab Muslim female. She immigrated to the United States from Iraq when she was 30. Fatima speaks Arabic as a primary language. Fatima reported frequently struggling in her relationship with her children. In particular, she expressed difficulty communicating and understanding her 12-year-old son, who speaks primarily in English, which places the responsibility of communication and oversight on her 25-year-old daughter, who speaks English and Arabic fluently. Fatima tried learning English in the past but reported difficulty in remembering the information she acquired. Fatima's difficulty in learning English adversely impacts her self-efficacy and self-esteem. Fatima's relationship with her daughter is also somewhat turbulent due to acculturative differences. Fatima expects her daughter to attend to matters that involve speaking English, such as communicating with medical doctors or setting up services through their county's human services office. When her daughter does not respond to her requests promptly or if she declines to take responsibility for some tasks, Fatima is left feeling disappointed and further internalizes the belief that everyone around her is failing her. Fatima reached out to me because I am an Arabic-speaking clinician and expressed comfort in knowing she can express herself to me without involving an interpreter. Fatima's stated goal for therapy includes reducing feelings of depression and navigating family difficulties. I, the second author of this chapter, identify as a North African Arab female who immigrated to the United States from Egypt when I was 11 years old and experienced/continue to experience variations of acculturative stress on individual and family levels.

Challenging Homogeneous Assumptions

The cultural homogeneity myth refers to the belief that those holding similar cultural identities share similar experiences. Although this is sometimes true, it should not be a generalized assumption when working with clients. When I met Fatima for the first time, I realized the similarities in our ethnicity, cultural backgrounds, and immigration histories. We learned Arabic as a first language, immigrated from Muslim and Arab countries, and navigated similar systems in our acculturation processes. However, despite the similarities in our backgrounds, we each hold unique, distinct experiences that differentiate the frameworks through which we see and interpret struggles and triumphs. For example, my family and Fatima's family experienced drastic changes in familial dynamics due to the immigration experience. Fatima and I experience and interpret these changes quite differently, as will be described later.

Often, clients seek clinicians who identify similarly due to the belief that these clinicians will be more competent in tackling their concerns. Likewise, many clinicians assume that holding similar identities as their clients makes them more effective at their work. Although having similar identities, especially marginalized aspects, can be an informative and powerful experience, we must be careful not to conform to the homogeneity myth. My immigration experience and ethnocultural background aided my work with Fatima in multiple ways. First, it helped me ask better questions to deepen my understanding of her experiences. My immigration experience as an Arab Muslim woman strengthened the questions I asked, not the assumptions I made. For example, instead of telling Fatima, "Moving to a new country can significantly change the relationship between parents and their children," it is more appropriate to ask, "In what ways do you think the move to the United States impacted your relationship with your children?".

A Witness of Experience

Maya Angelou wrote, "There is no greater agony than bearing an untold story inside of you." One of the most critical roles a clinician can embody when working with immigrant clients is the role of a witness: someone who patiently sits with the client as they tell their stories resisting any temptation to center on anything other than the client's narrative. When working with immigrant and refugee clients, you are working with a population that holds told and untold stories of loss, victory, trauma, resilience, coping, and resistance. As a bearer of witnesses, you listen and allow your five senses and the space around you to be a welcoming canvas for the client's story. As a bearer of witness, you can empathetically join the client in their tears, laughter, hope, and sorrow while staying grounded in your self and experience. You are aware of your own cognitive, physical, and emotional reactions to the client's story and effectively regulate them without interrupting the client's therapeutic process. As a bearer of witness, you consider the untold story of the client alongside the told story. With Fatima, the told story is the story of her immigration, her difficulty in learning English, and her family's difficulties. The untold stories I had to inquire about sensitively were her trauma history before immigration, the stress associated with the immigration process, and the post-immigration acculturative stress. Witnessing Fatima's experience involves intentional observation and inquiry to capture a nuanced picture closer to her reality.

A Multiculturally Competent Professional

Your role of bearing witness to Fatima's experiences is essential but insufficient without multicultural competence. Being a multiculturally competent clinician allows you to integrate and utilize what you bear witness to deepen your understanding and intervene effectively. As a multiculturally competent clinician, you pay attention to the nuances in your client's story. For example, in learning about Fatima's difficulty with her daughter, one could assume that the parentification of Fatima's daughter is a primary concern. However, upon working with Fatima, you realize that her expectation of her daughter may stem from more than role reversal of parent-child roles due to the immigration process. For example, you look more into Fatima's Islamic and Iraqi cultures and note the significant emphasis on children being righteous towards their parents. For Fatima, her daughter's resistance to a parental role could mean that she is not doing her part as a child of caring for and being righteous towards her mother.

An Advocate

One of the most unique and challenging aspects of working with Fatima as an immigrant client is the level of advocacy I had to take on as a clinician. To assess Fatima's need for advocacy, I needed to be aware of systems and how they advantage and disadvantage specific populations. Fatima experienced considerable difficulty navigating healthcare, governmental, or social support systems due to language barriers and a lack of familiarity with such systems. It became evident that this difficulty in navigating such complex systems exacerbated Fatima's symptoms through helplessness, feelings of stagnation, and self-blame. My responsibility as a clinician was to help Fatima contextualize her symptoms and externalize what needed to be externalized, such as her guilt. I witnessed the shame and helplessness on Fatima's face ameliorate with the mere acknowledgment of the flaws inherent in the systems she is working very hard to navigate. I did so by acknowledging how difficult it is for me to navigate these systems sometimes as an English-speaking professional. In addition to recognizing the systemic barriers, my responsibility as a counselor was to advocate for Fatima to address them to aid her therapeutic progress.

It is essential to realize that advocacy can take on different shapes and forms in the therapeutic space. Before engaging in advocacy work, assessing the client's need and readiness for advocacy is crucial. The client may want their therapeutic space to be an action-free space of reflection and processing while reserving their work with their caseworker to pursue these resources. Your role as an advocate will vary significantly based on the client's needs and readiness for a change and your professional limits of competence. With Fatima, our advocacy work mostly involved the identification of her needs in a given situation and pulling together different resources inside and outside the therapeutic space to help address her needs. My advocacy with her ranged from simply offering the phone number for a housing service that utilizes interpreters to reaching out on her behalf to set up services such as medication management. It is also essential to identify the goal for advocacy in each situation where advocacy efforts are relevant. With Fatima, reducing feelings of overwhelm, improving self-efficacy, and tackling helplessness drove our advocacy work.

Ethical Considerations

In working with immigrant and refugee clients, clinicians sometimes feel that the client's needs are outside of their scope of practice. This pressure can often lead to feelings of helplessness. The clinician must recognize that many of the issues immigrant/refugee clients face are systemic and cannot be addressed fully in the therapy room. Clinicians must be aware of their limitations as advocates to ensure ethical practice and uphold nonmaleficence. For example, Fatima had requested that I translate legal paperwork and other mail correspondence during some of our sessions, which I politely declined. Although I am Fatima's Arabic-speaking clinician, I am not an interpreter or a legal professional and could cause harm by completing non-therapy-related paperwork on behalf of Fatima. To balance adherence to my ethical guidelines with continued advocacy, I spent a portion of these sessions assisting Fatima in identifying and brainstorming available resources to translate the documents and helping her set small, realistic goals to make self-advocacy more manageable. Whenever there was a lack of resources, I verbalized my genuine concern and labeled the systemic barriers to externalizing Fatima's feelings of helplessness. Additionally, I helped Fatima identify alternative resources and develop ways of coping with the situation without appropriate resources.

Lastly, a clinician working with immigrant and refugee clients must secure adequate supervision and consultation experiences. Supervisors and colleagues often need more training or experience to assist you. Finding or creating these spaces for yourself is a sound idea, which sometimes means extending beyond the organizations of which you are a part. Finding these spaces could mean connecting with a colleague who works with immigrant or refugee clients and is willing to partake in the journey of being a witness, competent professional, and an advocate with you.

Future Steps for Research

Immigrants and refugees are becoming more visible in our societies as the world becomes more virtually connected. Representation is becoming increasingly important, and people are more intentional about inclusivity. Research has shed light on the experiences of pre-migration trauma in refugee families (Perera et al., 2013; Hecker et al., 2017; Porter & Haslam, 2005) and described the acculturation process for immigrant families at large (Berry, 1997; Meschke & Juang, 2014; Silva et al., 2017). It is now essential for us to understand the experiences of immigrant and refugee families as they continue to build their lives in a new society. Questions about how refugee families are coping with the legacy of trauma, how generations born outside of the country of origin are developing their identities, and what resilience factors are being passed down from generation to generation should be pursued.

Takeaways

- *The acculturation process immigrants and refugees face is more complex than initially conceptualized in the literature and involves an interactive exchange between the individuals, families, and the host society.*
- *In working with immigrants and refugees, a clinician must be aware of the interlocking systems of oppression and trauma that clients oftentimes experience and navigate before and after immigration.*
- *A clinician working with immigrants and refugees is uniquely positioned to uphold the essential roles of a witness, a multiculturally competent professional, and an advocate.*

Resources Section

APA. (2021a). *Apology to people of color for APA's role in promoting, perpetuating, and failing to challenge racism, racial discrimination, and human hierarchy in U.S.* www.Apa.Org. www.apa.org/about/policy/racism-apology

APA. (2021b). *Historical chronology.* www.Apa.Org. www.apa.org/about/apa/addressing-racism/historical-chronology

Boss, P. (2007). Ambiguous loss theory: Challenges for scholars and practitioners. *Family Relations*, *56*(2), 105–110.

Doherty, W. J. (2001) Values-Sensitive Therapy. In Jon Carlson and Diane Kjos (Eds.), *Theories and Strategies of Family Therapy*. (pp 1–48). Boston, MA: Allyn & Bacon.

Falicov, C. J. (2017). Multidimensional Ecosystemic Comparative Approach (MECA). In J. Lebow, A. Chambers, & D. C. Breunlin (Eds.), *Encyclopedia of Couple and Family Therapy* (pp 1–5). Springer International Publishing. https://doi.org/10.1007/978-3-319-15877-8_848-1

Grand, D. (2013). *Brainspotting: The Revolutionary New Therapy for Rapid and Effective Change*. Sounds True.

Hart, S. (2019). *Brain, Attachment, Personality: An Introduction to Neuroaffective Development*. Routledge. https://doi.org/10.4324/9780429472541

Levine, P., & Kline, M. (2012). Use of Somatic Experiencing Principles as a PTSD Prevention Tool for Children and Teens during the Acute Stress Phase Following an Overwhelming Event. *Post-Traumatic Syndromes in Childhood and Adolescence: A Handbook of Research and Practice*, 273–295. https://doi.org/10.1002/9780470669280.ch15

Macaluso, N. (2015). *Toward an integrative somatic depth psychotherapeutic model for relational trauma: Exploring the psychotherapy client's lived embodied experience – ProQuest*. www.proquest.com/openview/f32469179ecbca653aab2d8d58e4aef9/1?pq-origsite=gscholar&cbl=18750

Robjant, K., & Fazel, M. (2010). The emerging evidence for Narrative Exposure Therapy: A review. *Clinical Psychology Review*, *30*(8), 1030–1039. https://doi.org/10.1016/j.cpr.2010.07.004

References

Bentley, J. A., Dolezal, M. L., & Alsubaie, M. K. (2019). Does duration of residency in the United States influence psychological symptoms and postmigration stressors among refugees? Potential implications of populism for refugee mental health. *International Perspectives in Psychology: Research, Practice, Consultation*, *8*(3), 161–176. http://dx.doi.org.ezp3.lib.umn.edu/10.1037/ipp0000109

Bešić, E. (2020). Intersectionality: A pathway towards inclusive education? *Prospects*, *49*(3), 111–122. https://doi.org/10.1007/s11125-020-09461-6

Berry, J. W. (1992). Acculturation and adaptation in a new society. *International Migration*, *30*(s1), 69–85. https://doi.org/10.1111/j.1468-2435.1992.tb00776.x

Berry, J. W. (1997). Immigration, acculturation, and adaptation. *Applied Psychology*, *46*(1), 5–34. https://doi.org/10.1111/j.1464-0597.1997.tb01087.x

Boss, P. (2004). Ambiguous loss research, theory, and practice: Reflections after 9/11. *Journal of Marriage and Family*, *66*(3), 551–566. https://doi.org/10.1111/j.0022-2445.2004.00037.x

Cox, R. B., Desouza, D. K., Bao, J., Lin, H., Sahbaz, S., Greder, K. A., Larzelere, R. E., Washburn, I. J., Leon-Cartagena, M., & Arredondo-Lopez, A. (2021). Shared language erosion: Rethinking immigrant family communication and impacts on youth development. *Children (Basel)*, *8*(4), 256. https://doi.org/10.3390/children8040256

Crenshaw, K. (1991). Mapping the margins: Intersectionality, identity politics, and violence against women of color. *Stanford Law Review*, *43*(6), 1241–1299.

Duvall, E. M. (1957). *Family development*. Philadelphia: Lippincott.

Halcón, L. L., Robertson, C. L., Savik, K., Johnson, D. R., Spring, M. A., Butcher, J. N., Westermeyer, J. J., & Jaranson, J. M. (2004). Trauma and coping in Somali and Oromo refugee youth. *Journal of Adolescent Health*, *35*(1), 17–25. https://doi.org/10.1016/j.jadohealth.2003.08.005

Heberle, A. E., Obus, E. A., & Gray, S. A. O. (2020). An intersectional perspective on the intergenerational transmission of trauma and state-perpetrated violence. *Journal of Social Issues*, josi.12404. https://doi.org/10.1111/josi.12404

Hecker, T., Ainamani, H. E., Hermenau, K., Haefele, E., & Elbert, T. (2017). Exploring the potential distinction between Continuous Traumatic Stress and Posttraumatic Stress in an East African refugee sample. *Clinical Psychological Science*, *5*(6), 964–973. https://doi.org/10.1177/2167702617717023

Henrich, J., Heine, S. J., & Norenzayan, A. (2010). The weirdest people in the world? *Behavioral and Brain Sciences*, *33*(2–3), 61–83. https://doi.org/10.1017/S0140525X0999152X

Juang, L. P., Simpson, J. A., Lee, R. M., Rothman, A. J., Titzmann, P. F., Schachner, M. K., Korn, L., Heinemeier, D., & Betsch, C. (2018). Using attachment and relational perspectives to understand adaptation and resilience among immigrant and refugee youth. *American Psychologist, 73*(6), 797. https://doi.org/10.1037/amp0000286

Maslow A. H. (1969). The farther reaches of human nature. *Journal of Transpersonal Psychology, 1*(1), 1–9.

Medford, M. M. (2019). Racialization and Black multiplicity: Generative paradigms for understanding Black immigrants. *Sociology Compass, 13*(7). https://doi.org/10.1111/soc4.12717

Meschke, L. L., & Juang, L. P. (2014). Obstacles to parent–adolescent communication in Hmong American families: Exploring pathways to adolescent mental health promotion. *Ethnicity & Health, 19*(2), 144–159. https://doi.org/10.1080/13557858.2013.814765

O'Donnell, A. W., Stuart, J., & O'Donnell, K. J. (2020). The long-term financial and psychological resettlement outcomes of pre-migration trauma and post-settlement difficulties in resettled refugees. *Social Science & Medicine, 262*, 113246. https://doi.org/10.1016/j.socscimed.2020.113246

Perera, S., Gavian, M., Frazier, P., Johnson, D., Spring, M., Westermeyer, J., Butcher, J., Halcon, L., Robertson, C., Savik, K., & Jaranson, J. (2013). A longitudinal study of demographic factors associated with stressors and symptoms in African refugees. *American Journal of Orthopsychiatry, 83*(4), 472–482. https://doi.org/10.1111/ajop.12047

Phipps, R. M., & Degges-White, S. (2014). A new look at transgenerational trauma transmission: Second-Generation Latino immigrant youth. *Journal of Multicultural Counseling and Development, 42*(3), 174–187. https://doi.org/10.1002/j.2161-1912.2014.00053.x

Porter, M., & Haslam, N. (2005). Predisplacement and postdisplacement factors associated with mental health of refugees and internally displaced persons: A meta-analysis. *JAMA, 294*(5), 602. https://doi.org/10.1001/jama.294.5.602

Siegel, D. J. (2012). *The developing mind* (2nd Ed.). New York, NY: The Guilford Press.

Silva, N. D., Dillon, F. R., Verdejo, T. R., Sanchez, M., & De La Rosa, M. (2017). Acculturative stress, psychological distress, and religious coping among Latina young adult immigrants. *The Counseling Psychologist, 45*(2), 213–236. https://doi.org/10.1177/0011000017692111

Solheim, C. A., Ballard, J., Fatiha, N., Dini, Z., Buchanan, G., & Song, S. (2022). Immigrant family financial and relationship stress from the COVID-19 pandemic. *Journal of Family and Economic Issues, 43*(2), 282–295. https://doi.org/10.1007/s10834-022-09819-2

Steel, J. L., Dunlavy, A. C., Harding, C. E., & Theorell, T. (2017). The psychological consequences of Pre-Emigration Trauma and Post-Migration Stress in refugees and immigrants from Africa. *Journal of Immigrant and Minority Health, 19*(3), 523–532. https://doi.org/10.1007/s10903-016-0478-z

Ursin, H., & Eriksen, H. R. (2010). Cognitive activation theory of stress (CATS). *Neuroscience & Biobehavioral Reviews, 34*(6), 877–881. https://doi.org/10.1016/j.neubiorev.2009.03.001

Weine, S. M., Hoffman, Y., Ware, N., Tugenberg, T., Hakizimana, L., Dahnweigh, G., Currie, M., & Wagner, M. (2011). Secondary migration and relocation among African refugee families in the United States. *Family Process, 50*(1), 27–46. https://doi.org/10.1111/j.1545-5300.2010.01344.x

Yarbrough, R. A. (2010). Becoming "Hispanic" in the "New South": Central American immigrants' racialization experiences in Atlanta, GA, USA. *GeoJournal, 75*(3), 249–260. https://doi.org/10.1007/s10708-009-9304-7

Yehuda, R. (2002). Post-Traumatic stress disorder. *New England Journal of Medicine, 346*(2), 108–114. https://doi.org/10.1056/NEJMra012941

25

SYSTEMIC THERAPY IN CENTRAL AND SOUTH AMERICA

Past, Present, and Future

Ruth Casabianca

Introduction

Systemic Therapy (ST), whose baselines were founded the United States, towards the mid 20th century, had a brief dissemination history almost parallel in different nations in Europe, such as Italy, Germany, the United Kingdom, and Belgium – as examples of being pioneer countries – then expanding rapidly to different Western European and South and Central American areas.

In the late 1970s, and especially in the 1980s, ST development gained more popularity in the aforementioned countries of Central and South America, including, a little bit later, some Caribbean Islands. In fact, not all the countries in this location of the American continent present neither the same interest nor the grade of development of the models settled in the circular epistemology described like "Systemic Psychotherapy," nor is the case as it happens in the world, if we incorporate a global wide vision (Casabianca, 2022).

Nonetheless, it is highly significant to rescue F. Kaslow's opinion. She noted the American families' impact – and also European and Asian ones – suffered the effect of much wider contexts. This includes the wars, most flourishing economies or those with scarce resources, to name as an example. And, indeed, this was a **shared rule,** beyond the local particularities of the impact (Kaslow, 2001). This similitude in suffering beyond their particular development, the different countries here analyzed started incorporating a particular form of understanding. Their approach to dealing with bonding behaviors exclusively centered on the person that were the rule in the field of mental health.

One might well ask why to include in an *International Handbook of Couple and Family Therapy* a chapter about this topic. Beyond the editor's personal motivation, to whom I deeply express my gratitude for inviting me to participate, I understand it is highly important to emphasize the notable influence ST has achieved as years go by within the wide variety of psychotherapies implemented in the mental health field, especially in the familial and community-social areas influencing in some Central and South American countries. A significant proportion of such countries are exposed to sudden changes in governance and have high vulnerability in their social and economic conditions. It is important

DOI: 10.4324/9781003297871-28

to highlight that some of these countries have achieved the inclusion of ST in establishing policies and laws that today rule their social organization and, consequently, improve conditions for the wellbeing of their populations.

As S. Campos González, from Chile (2023) expressed: "it is of primary importance to incorporate Systemic Therapy in public policies, health, education and community work" …"Its importance has raised awareness as long as the symptoms diminish, the perception of the existence improves and quality of life scales improve too."

As was mentioned before, not all the developing countries in Central, South America, and the Caribbean Islands, neither introduced nor spread ST with the same intensity and in the same working fields.

These differences may be due, for example, to dominant local traditions leading the field of mental health and psychotherapies in particular that had accepted or rejected relational visions from the different Systemic Models; proximity or distance to the information centers or "the teachers" during a time when (virtual communication) being neither widespread nor popularized as it is today; local material and cognitive resources, facilitating or restricting the foreign scientific information; local culture in different populations presenting features more or less tending to value closer social bonding or wider community links (that makes up the heart of the systemic vision), and, without any doubt, the presence of therapists and professors determined to introduce and disseminate the latest news – especially in the context of universities and private institutes that train therapists – even at the risk of being criticized or rejected.

It is impossible to give a detailed description of the developments that have taken place in all the countries in Central and South American territories (more than 30), but it should be noted that certain similarities are shared by many of the countries likely due to the "Latin-American culture" in the macro sense. Most of Central and South American regions shared the colonization that handed down a language derived from Latin and Latin traditions and values, especially those from Spain, Italy, Portugal, and France that helped faciliate the growth of relational therapies, based on their worldviews and derived interactional close style life. Some Caribbean islands do not belong to this cultural group but were considered here because they are defined by most geographers to belong to Central America (Wikipedia, 2022).

Representing Latin American countries mentioned above, the data about Argentina, Brazil, Chile, Colombia, Costa Rica, the Cayman Islands, Peru and Mexico are specifically included. Some of them come from cultural manifestos and demographic studies, others from information spread on-line and, most of them, from prestigious systemic therapists from the above mentioned countries: Lic. H. Hirsch from Argentina, Dra. Rosa María Macedo, from Brazil, Mag. Natalia APU from Costa Rica, Mg. Sylvia Campos González from Chile, Dra. Katherine Wittaker from Cayman Islands, Eduardo Villar MD from Colombia, Mg. Paulina Medina Mora from México, and Mg. Roxana Zeballos from Perú.

Brief Description of the Cultural Contexts of the Involved Countries

Latin American countries – except Brazil which was under a Portuguese colonization- share the Spanish language with idiomatic expressions and colloquialisms that characterize each one of the countries (Guyana and Belize were colonized by France are not part of the Latin countries because they do speak English). Likewise, different social classes and diverse age groups have rooted their own terms and expressions that need to be known and considered in therapeutic interventions.

In most of the Caribbean Islands with a Latin colonization, the same thing happens, though they present a different racial cross-breeding and multiple cultures that are originated basic-ally by migrations coming from some of the continental American and European countries.

In particular, the Cayman Islands, with a British colonization, speak English and pre-sent characteristics that differ from Latin American countries. The same happens with other Caribbean Islands – colonized by Saxon countries – that do not share with the rest of Central or South America the Latin cultural influence, the language, or local lifestyle customs (e.g., Aruba, Saint Martin, the Bahamas, to name a few). Nevertheless, they are also considered by most of the experts in geography part of Central American territory (Wikipedia, 2020).

Despite the diversity in different cultural aspects arriving in postmodernity, Latin coun-tries share in common the prevalence of values regarding **the importance of the family as the context of human development,** and also transcendence as a facilitator of models of coexistence and ethics. Beyond these facts that – especially in this century – in most of them, the traditional structures and modes of coexistence have changed as well as a significant proportion in the number of divorces that has also increased (currently between 30% to 65% of the registered marriages in the different societies). It is difficult to present precise statistics regarding this topic because many families agree to not formalize the relationship via official records; consequently, it is not possible to know the exact number of either the unions or separations.

As in the rest of the world, each country in Central and South America has "traditional" groups that describe most families in the area: families with heterosexual parents and two or more children. These traditional families trend strongly toward the conservation of couples and extended families and adherance to religious values (primarily values con-sistent with Catholic, Jewish or Christian/Protestant traditions). These groups co-live with other families that are more "progressive": such families are characterized as being: single-parent families (generally the mother), LGTB couples (with a legalized marriage in some of the countries, like in Argentina), with one child or no children, with more liberal life values and customs. (Casabianca, 2007). This trend in changes in family structure and dynamics is seen in most Latin American countries. Nevertheless, **the values of social con-gregation** – whether within couples or families or in neighborhoods or communities **is the most common in Latin-American societies.**

An example of family types mentioned above is expressed by Roxana Zeballos from Perú: "families are very solidary in our society and, it is the place where we all go like a first resource"…It is also important to have into account how important grandparents' education on children is"… "In the field of community problems, ST is, nowadays, almost a requirement to enter as a professional (psychologist, medical doctor, social worker), in health and social welfare institutions" (Casabianca & Zevallos, 2022). Consequently, sys-temic professionals are in high demand to work in those organizations.

In relation to other aspects in Latin Americans, the co-living in diversity may be present in a lesser or lower degree of conflict among them, a phenomenon that also happens among the different social classes and racial groups: the white supremacy of white *mestizos*, local native groups, and a minor population from African or Asian origin wen relating to the number of people with the other groups. Conflicts currently appear more related to the differences in economic income (poverty indexes have raised in most of the Latin-American countries, thus, class division), or political convictions that have been outlining themselves like more dichotomous than previously, mainly among democratic and autocratic tenden-cies. All of this happens in the majority of Latin American countries, with some differences of course, depending basically on the governments and their own policies (La Nación+, 2022, 2023).

Especially researched in this chapter among the Caribbean Islands, the Cayman Islands present a different cultural influence coming from the British In the Cayman Islands, almost half of the population is comprised of ex-patriots (a total of 71.105 inhabitants in 2021). The rest of the population was born or naturalized there, representing 130 nationalities. The population in the Cayman Islands does not support ST; as a result, it is difficult to empathize and build rapport at the therapeutic sessions. Nevertheless, ST has developed in different workplaces beyond the clinic, and as time goes by the use of technologies for virtual family therapies have become necessary for treatment as well as the need of systemic confidentiality (Casabianca & Wittacker, 2023).

The importance of considering the characteristics of the social contexts of the countries evaluated in this chapter is related to both the understanding of how much ST is included as an alternative therapy and, "how to make therapy" in these societies. In other words, consider the social guidelines and cultural values that need to be respected in each of the cultures.

How Did Systemic Therapy Begin and Become Rooted in Central and South American Countries?

In most of the countries, ST began in the 1980s due to the efforts of some "daring therapists" most of whom went abroad to North America or Western Europe to study. Thus, ST in South and Central America has been deeply influenced by the systemic developments in such foreign countries. None of the existing models of therapies before ST considered the basic assumptions of systems theory or cybernetics. In fact, the Central and South American pioneers described the beginnings of implementing the new approach ST in mental health as difficult, delayed or directly rejected where therapists worked. Different traditions of individual substantiation based in lineal logics – both in the psychotherapeutic field and traditional psychiatry – strongly resisted the so-called new epistemology. As noted by R. M. Macedo from Brazil, "the strong influence of psychoanalysis, and lately the wide acceptance of Cognitive-Behavioral Therapies – especially by psychiatrists that emphasizes therapies based on evidence – are very popular in teams working in those hospitals with an international projection"… "private institutions, universities and professional associations with a family or systemic profile – like ABRATEF (Associação Brasileira de Terapia Familiar) – helped to the systemic formation and its development" (Macedo, 2021).

In Argentina, despite the fact that there already existed an Association of Family Therapy in the 1970s, at those times wrongly, the therapies under a psychoanalytical approach ascribed their theoretical and technical concepts to the therapies implemented in families, couples. or groups (the word "concepts" describes and transfers the principles that base psychoanalysis to the family therapy field). The great influence of psychoanalysis happened in most of the Central and South American countries, and that is why it took years for ST to be accepted in the family of "respected" psychotherapies. The fact that those professionals who studied and were trained in foreign countries decided not only to work in their offices using this new ST approach but also to teach other curious colleagues who started to evaluate the beneficial results in treated patients with ST. The relationship "colleagues-students" multiply progressively, and, consequently, patients began to demand ST.

At the beginning of the 21st century, countries like Colombia had not made any important progress in including ST, since historically, the models for treatment focused on medical models and cognitive behavioral therapies (Terjesen & Doyle, 2022). Nevertheless, in the last years ST acceptance kept growing as the benefits started to be perceived in fields like children and adolescent therapy and in social networks and communities (Villar, 2023).

The Associations of Systemic Therapy are undoubtedly the institutions that principally gathered the different fields (psychology, medicine, social work and psycho-pedagogy) together and inspired the acceptance of ST epistemology at the universities. The adoption grew progressively to the graduate and post graduate studies in psychology and psychiatry. Indeed, they were factors not only facilitating ST acceptance but also stimulating formal education of therapists with a systemic orientation. In almost all the countries included and mentioned in this chapter, both situations have been produced as is seen in the opinions given by the professionals who were interviewed for this opportunity. Today also ST is taught at other universities in places like Equator and Uruguay.

Another important phenomenon to mention is that over time ST started to be developed in its conceptual aspects. Its interventions to solve problems expanded into other areas besides clinical cases: working organizations (enterprises); schools and their problems of teacher-student relationships; in the juridical field: adoption, divorce, and mediation especially; in jails; at work with different community problems, like migration.

An additional factor believed to influence ST's rooting in different Central and South American countries – beyond the evidence is treats bonding problems were its quality of being a brief type of therapy and problem-resolution centered. When compared with long individual treatments focusing on personal development, ST allows to save money, time, and energy, in countries where these types of resources are progressively reduced (e.g., Argentina).

What is Currently Happening with Systemic Therapy in Central and South American Countries?

In present times, ST has seen diverse acceptance in Central and South American countries. Nevertheless, in most of the continental countries as well as in some Islands, have incorporated ST especially for working in the clinical field with family and couples cases. In the Caribbean Islands, the different grades of acceptance has to do with cultural diversity present in most of most of them due to a high level of migrations among American countries as well as inter-continental migration.

ST development and implementation have been earlier and more intense in the countries mentioned especially in this chapter. The numerous fields of implementation in the present times showed how ST has spread to areas of work in some unthinkable ways in the beginning stages.

According to what N. Apu (2023), "Costa Rica is a melting pot"... "We live the migration from close countries, principally from Nicaragua, Venezuela and Colombia"... "The fundamental contributions of ST have been [able] to improve communication among family members, to reduce the levels of violence, and to strengthen affective bonding among groups. To develop a better living based in understanding, establishing clear limits, parents (men) are involved in raising their children, boys and girls. Families succeed in solving those problems [from which] they suffered, look for and strengthen support networks in the community, looking together to find solutions the benefit them." (Apu, 2023).

Moreover, the ST fields of implementation have widened in present times. In several countries, ST has extended to areas of work which were previously thought of as unthinkable. In part, this phenomenon has to do, probably, with the global vision of the ecological thinking (countries like Brazil, Chile and Mexico have been in the most affected countries due to their geophysics catastrophes). Presently, in Costa Rica there are governmental offices that are opening to the systemic therapy consultation in cases of addiction, child violence, abandonment and in certain areas of health. This is especially the case in countries in the south of Latin America (Argentina, Brazil, Chile, and Peru) and in the north (Mexico).

Some countries, like Chile and Peru, for example, advanced with the gender inclusion approach in their public health and education policies, while in other countries this matter is taken care of at the clinics and private institutions exclusively. In countries like Brazil, Chile, and Peru – also Equador to a lesser degree – have ST offerings have multiplied especially to address community problems. For individual concerns, individual treatments tend to be offered (see, for example, Aravena et al., 2022; Hutz et al., 2013). The trend to gender inclusion in therapies based in the neurosciences and cognitive-behavioral approaches in dealing with individual problems appears in almost all the countries in Central and South America.

Nevertheless, there may not be a conflict between individual and relational approaches in every country. In Argentina, for example, though in psychiatry there is a strong tendency to observe the neurosciences knowledge, it is very common to consider also the focus on the influence of the family over the problems coming to the consultation, especially when working with children or adolescents. Generally, they present a binocular vision in the field of mental health, especially when working with minors.

According to Paulina Medina Mora from Mexico (Casabianca et al., 2021) the systemic areas of work have been extended from clinical consultations at the office to the different social institutions, including "multiple voices" in possible dialogues within the relationships among nations. In present times, therapists are dealing with challenges such as problems with gender inequity, social inequality and injustice, discrimination, immigration, and violence.

In Chile, the emphasis is in indicating ST "for problems related with family communication, transitions of the vital cycle and untimely events, and social intervention in mental health related to situations of socio economical vulnerability (Campos Gonzalez, 2023). Chile presents a long tradition of psychosocial work with vulnerable families (including "people of the streets" (homeless) in different regions of the country (Bernales, 2010). Narrative-based therapies have been gaining ground, especially in the field of communities psychosocial therapy. Nevertheless, the mixture of models is not conflicting when selecting therapies between more prescriptive or narrative, all **in accordance with the types of problems and the style of consultants and therapists.** This also happens clinically where couple and family problems are prioritized, observing that global research have shown around 75% of effectiveness for different types of problems. (Davis, Lebow & Fraenkel 2012).

It is important to note in Northern South America, a systemic approach has been implemented when working with networks and socio-economic vulnerable neighborhoods with significant poverty and its consequences. In some cases, systemic programs have been included that have been sponsored and supervised by both foreign organizations and professionals with experience in the mental health field (Falicov, 2013).

In Argentina – from H. Hirsh´s perspective (2020) – presently, it is difficult to get families together for therapy due to economic or other concerns. This phenomenon is more frequent in big cities. Likewise, in this country, a significative development has been perceived in new interventions in couple therapy, implementing the inclusion of advanced technological devices therapy (cellular, computers), and centered in focusing over the resources of the consulting population (Hirsch, 2020).

In the same way, systems therapists also work with families with chronic illness, with judicial issues, and with problems with divorces, abuse, false memories, and other populations considered beyond more traditional problems (Hirsch, 2020; Fernández Moya, 2007). One such positive example is from the work of C. Rausch Herzcovici in schools in Buenos Aires Province, with a program to change healthy eating habits at a primary level (Kowalski, 2017).

Central and South American countries where ST grew did so when ST in different relational models were included in the present university curricula. They were also included in formal grade or post-grade courses and scholarships in psychology and medicine or in private training institutions that acquired support for their programs from institutions of international prestige. They may have also been included in educational programs with agreements of exchange teaching programs with foreign universities. These actions favored research and scientific debate with the world, and, with it, further development and scientific acknowledgement of the systemic approach in those countries.

It should be noted that the development of ST in these countries can also be attributed to access to knowledge online around the world, especially for those professionals involved in family and couple therapy, from universities around the world.

Future Outlook

As noted by M. Ceberio, "psychotherapists' role is like catalysts of the crisis", and consequently, we can not abandon our vision and field of action referring to indispensable relations (Ceberio, 2016).

Thus, we do not know yet for sure how the future of ST will look in its various relations with its aims of resolving human problems, focusing on the mutual interactions and influences among living human beings and their context. As noted here, Central and South American countries, in most cases, have specific difficulties yet at the same time are cultures with profound roots and social bonds that should be to take advantage of and increase ST development.

As noted by N. Apu from Costa Rica (2023), "For the challenges we have as a society, I believe that Systemic Therapy has a great future. Systemic therapies will contribute to the improvement of Costa Ricas´s society unquestionably. I believe that it is highly important."

In this regard, those of us who have shared the practices of ST know that it will be our responsibility to investigate the different fields of human interaction, to communicate our knowledge beyond our own walls of our working place, to be creative and ethical to face the problems that do not have yet built solutions, without losing our focus. This will require a compromise between science, collaboration "with and from" the other sciences, accepting the complexity, mutuality, and the uncertainty of the evolution of our countries and our neighbors.

Acknowledgements

I want to thank the International Family Therapy Association (IFTA) for the stimulus they have always given me to investigate the topic within its context. Likewise, I want to pay tribute to the multiple professionals and friendly relationships established in many meetings organized by the IFTA, which gave me much of the material for this text. And, last but not least, I would like to thank to all the colleagues from different countries that contributed with their information to this chapter: Natalia Apu from Costa Rica; Silvia Campos Gonzáles from Chile; Hugo Hirsch from Argentina; Rosa María Macedo from Brazil; Paulina Mora Medina from Mexico; Katheryne Whittacker from Cayman Islands; Eduardo Villar from Colombia; Roxana Zeballos from Peru.

References

Aravena, J., Gajardo, J., Saguez, R., Hinton, L., & Gitlin, L. N. (2022). Nonpharmacologic Interventions for Family Caregivers of People Living With Dementia in Latin-America: A Scoping Review. *The American Journal of Geriatric Psychiatry, 30*(8), 859–877. https://doi.org/10.1016/j.jagp.2021.10.013

Bernales, S. (2010). *Ethical dilemmas in psychosocial interactions from a contextual relational perspective.* Presentation al 2010 Congress of the International Family Therapy Association. Buenos Aires. Argentina

Casabianca, R. (2007). The heterosexual couples' therapy in current postmodernist Argentine culture: a challenge to creativity and an ethical issue for therapists. In *Sistemas familiares de la Asociación de Psicoterapia Sistémica de Buenos Aires. 23*(2), 19–28.

Casabianca, R. (2022). The Systemic Therapy across the world: a global view from the past to the future. In Jorge Fernandez Moya y Federico Richard, Comp.: "*El pensamiento sistémico en Mendoza, 1975–2021*". Mendoza. Universidad del Aconcagua.

Casabianca, R., & Apu, N. (2023). Interview to Mag. Natalia Apu, from Costa Rica. Retrieved

Casabianca, R., & Campos González, S. (2023). *Interview to Mag. Sylvia Campos González, from Chile.* Online

Casabianca, R., & Hirsch, H., (2020). Interview to *Lic. Hugo Hirsch from Argentina.* Online

Casabianca, R., Macedo, R. M. (2021, 2023). *Interview to Dr Rosa M. Macedo from Brazil.* Online

Casabianca, R., & Zevallos, R. (2020, 2023). *Interview to Roxana Zevallos from Peru.* Online

Casabianca, R., Mora Medina, P., & Villar, E., & Wittacker, K. (2021). *What takes place with Family Therapy in those countries that are in development in Central and South America: difficulties and hope facing the future.* Presentation to the 2021 International Family Therapy Association Congress. Online

Ceberio, M. (2016). Latin American systemic therapy: Is it only an illusion? *Interactions, 2*(1), 97–106.

Davis, S., Lebow, J., & Sprenkle, D. (2012). Common factors of change in Couple Therapy. *Behavior Therapy, 43*(1), 36–48.

Falicov, C. (2013). Supervisión en el Instituto Chileno de Terapia Familiar.

Fernández Moya, J. (2007). *Eslabones: una propuesta sistémica para abordar la discapacidad múltiple.* Mendoza. Universidad del Aconcagua.

Fernández Moya, J. Richard, F. (2022). *El pensamiento sistemico en Mendoza, 1975–2021. De la psicología a las ciencias sociales: historia, presente y perspectivas futuras.* Universidad del Aconcagua, Argentina.

Herscovici, P. (2020). https://www.youtube.com/watch?v=xXl8r_t2g3o

Hirsch, H. (2020). Recursos. Personal questionnaire on line.

Hutz, C. S., & Gomes, W. B. (2013). Counseling and psychotherapy in Brazil: From private practice to community services. In R. Moodley, U. Gielen, & R. Wu (Eds.), *Handbook of counseling and psychotherapy in an international context* (pp. 95–105). Routledge.

Instituto Nacional de Estadísticas y Censos INDEC (2010). Buenos Aires, Argentina

*Instituto Nacional de Estadística e Informática de Perú (*INEI) (2022). Lima, Perú https://es.wikipedia.org

Kaslow, F. (2001). *Families and Family Psychology at the Millenium: Intersecting crossroads. 56*(1), 37–46.htpss//doi.org/10.1037/0003-066X.56.1.37

Kovalsky, I., Rausch-Herscovici, C., Indart Rougieri, P., De Gregorio, M.J. Zonis, Orellana, L., (2017). MNC Public Health, 17, 401, https://doi.org/10.1186/s12899-017.4327-3

La Nación + (2022, 2023). *Programas periodísticos v*arios. Canal Privado de TV. Argentina.

Terjesen, M., & Doyle, K. A. (2022). *Cognitive behavioral therapy in a global context.* Springer.

26

RISKS AND SIDE-EFFECTS IN SYSTEMIC FAMILY THERAPY

Matthias Ochs, Jakub Caha, and Tomáš Řiháček

Introduction

In a recent overview concerning Family-Based Psychological Interventions (FBPI)[1] Carr (2022, p. 69) stated: "Gurman and Kniskern (1978b) concluded that deterioration in family therapy did not occur at a higher rate than in individual therapy. However, no current systematic reviews or meta-analyses have been published on negative effects, deterioration, or adverse events associated with FBPIs."

Many reasons for negligence...

Indeed, for a long time, risks, negative side effects, and harms were rarely mentioned in the professional discourses of all psychotherapy approaches, not only in family and systemic therapies; there were no in the scientific community general accepted definitions, categories or concepts – that only changed recently (e.g., Linden & Strauss, 2018, 2022). The reason, why it went that way, seems to be a mixed bag. Some of the possible reasons for this include according Märtens & Petzold (2002, p. 11–30):

- The few existing studies on the side-effects of therapy don't attract interest; in addition Schermuly-Haupt et al. (2018) e.g. revealed only a dozen hits in Pubmed/PsychInfo research 1964–2011.
- Danger of discussion: more "school bickering," political power games and mutual devaluations; defended and marginalized issue for the profession, no open/transparent discourse.
- Reasons on the part of the therapists: persuasion, that PT harm is not possible, "self-serving bias," legal consequences (Hermes & Lindel, 2020). (Busch & Lemme (1992): 70% of therapists reject the idea of negative events/adverse effects; Walfish et al. (2012): 50% of therapists state, that deteriorations are not existent in their therapies.)
- Difficulties of determining adverse effects because of unclear standards, insufficient conceptualization and definitions (Klatte et al., 2022).
- Often comparison of arithmetic means: deteriorations remain undetected (e.g., Bergin, 1971; Barlow, 2010)

DOI: 10.4324/9781003297871-29

- Negative therapy courses seem underrepresented because of dropouts or premature termination.
- Multifactorial: deteriorations are not easy to trace back to therapy
- Course of disease is in mental illnesses not foreseeable.
- Clients' belief: deteriorations are normal part of psychotherapy (by the way, this is also therapists' belief, as we are showing later. Actually, clients' beliefs might be instilled by therapists' comments).
- Given psychotherapist optimism about their ability to help (...) there are not surprising that therapists have been overlooking worsening and deterioration of their clients in the course of treatment (Hannan et al., 2005; Hatfield et al., 2010; Barkham et al., 2017)
- Clients tend to defer to their therapists and withhold their negative reactions (Farber, 2020; Hill et al., 1993; Rennie, 1994)

... especially in Systemic Family Therapy

In addition to the above, there may be in the context of systemic family therapy some epistemological issues (constructivism, systems theory (Ochs, 2020) that have to be considered, discussed as follows.

Constructivism

The epistemology of constructivism considers human knowledge as a constructed process that develops on neurobiological, psychological, and socio-cultural levels, and postulates, that no single human being has an objective access to reality; the epistemological opposite of constructivism is the idea that human knowledge is some kind of copy of reality (naïve realism) (Ochs & Kriz, 2022a).

So, if – according to epistemological constructivism – everything mankind can think of is a construction, then also adverse side-effects/negative events can be "only" a construction, so it doesn't make sense to investigate them and to reify and "objectify" them in that way. In addition, social constructionism-inspired systemic therapy approaches argue that therapy is ("only") conversation (e.g., Boscolo & Betrando, 1996) – but conversation/communication is an everyday social event, where the concepts of adverse side-effects/negative events are not meaningful (because every day social events are not professional medical discourses). Moreover, the systemic intervention technique of reframing, which is theoretically rooted in constructivism, operates with the "calculus" that everything (also every phenomena that is labeled as side-effects/negative events) can be put into a "positive" frame (e.g., loss of job can be framed as a restart, anxiety symptoms can be framed as a gain in liveliness, depression can be viewed as an opportunity to recalibrate one's meaning of life, etc.).

Systems theory

Dynamical systems theories (Kriz & Ochs, 2022) try to conceptualize pattern formation, change, and stabilization in living complex systems (such as the society, organizations, families, workplace teams, human beings, brains, interactions such as psychotherapy sessions) in terms of circular non-linear feedback process between system components, system levels, and between system and environments.

But if – according to dynamical systems theories – everything is circular, no causal attribution is possible between phenomena that could be labelled as harms and negative events and therapy. Above all, complexity sciences postulate that living complex systems need "order and disorder" for developing, growing, and differentiating (Morin 2008, S. 63): distortion, irritation, and "mistakes" are necessary to stimulate the reciprocal feedback process between system components and system levels.[2] This is because this is the only possible way for a living complex system to adapt and accommodate its structures and dynamics in the contexts of environment impulses and systems inherent antagonistic tensions (Kriz & Ochs, 2022). Telfener (2022, p. 82f) described this issue in the following way:

> Within the systemic framework, it is a mistake to fear mistakes, since the possibility of a miscalculation is not separate from the possibility of understanding. Errors are important, and there is no logical way to avoid them in psychotherapy. Errors are signals that can help professionals to correct their process (they are usually within a behavioral domain). Keeney (1983) thinks that trying to avoid mistakes is a mistake since the basis for the self-correction emerges from the same possibility of generating errors and differences, which allow us to change our behaviour and the process.

The medical vs. the contextual model of psychotherapy

The concept of risks and side-effects of treatments is more or less borrowed from the medical model – it even reminds of instruction leaflets of pharmaceutical products. So it could be argued, that the implementation of the concept of risks and side-effects into systemic family therapy contributes to the medicalization of the field. Medicalization means the extensive and vast conceptualization and explanation of phenomena in the context of illness and health from a natural science and somatic-focused perspective. If you do this, a massive reduction of the complex interdependencies between somatic, intra- and interpsychic such as socio-cultural aspects is happening (Ochs & Kriz, 2022b, S. 337 f.). Because of this, the contextual model of psychotherapy (e.g., Wampold, 2001; Elkins, 2009) (which e.g. does not use medical concepts such as risks and side-effects) is preferred in psychotherapy in general. In systemic therapy this medical model is especially problematic, because 1.) it implies an expert position (someone defines which phenomena should be considered as risks and side-effects – and which not) – that position contradicts the social constructionism non-expert position (Bertando & Lini, 2021), and 2.) it implies a linear causality between treatment and (to minimize) negative side-effects, risks and harms, that does not make sense in the systems theory concept of complex, non-linear, multilevel, circular feedback processes.

... and also many reasons for (a new) interest in the topic

The reasons for the growing interest in the topic in the psychotherapeutic profession and psychotherapy research are also multifaceted. Recent evidence (e.g. Leichsenring et al., 2022) reveals that the huge psychotherapy effect sizes that were reported in the last decades (0.8, sometimes even up to 1.2[3]) are probably artefacts of overestimations (e.g., due to publication bias, researcher allegiance, weak comparators, or other shortcomings in study design). More realistic effect-sizes are about 0.30 or below in comparison with TAU or placebo, especially if effect-sizes are adjusted for biases. Large effect sizes ($\geqslant 0.80$) were only achieved with weak comparators (e.g., waiting list control group, no treatment). The difference in response rates in comparison to placebo is between 10% and 15%, indicating small effect sizes in terms of success rate differences (0.20–0.30) (Leichsenring et al., 2019). Moreover, on average 8% of adult clients in routine practice settings deteriorated (the estimates ranged from 3% to 14% depending on the particular study) (Lambert, 2013). In studies on clients with depression, the deterioration rates ranged from 0% to 25% (median 4%) (Cuijpers et al., 2018).

For the systemic field in Germany there was another incidence that directed our focus to the topic of side-effects, risks, and harms of psychotherapy. In 2017 the IQWiG (Institut für Qualität und Wirtschaftlichkeit Gesundheitswesen, translated: Institute for Quality and Economy in Public Health) published a review regarding the benefit and medical necessity of systemic therapy for adults as a psychotherapy approach (IQWiG, 2017)[4]. In a press release (24.07.2017) concerning the publishing of that review the IQWiG stated: "In the systemic therapy studies, that IQWIG analysed, no negative events/adverse effects were reported[5], because of that, we cannot make any statements about that, and it is not possible for us to weight the benefits against the possible harms." This "calculation" made by the IQWiG is of course not only applicable to systemic family therapy but to all psychotherapy approaches (e.g., behavioral and psychodynamic ones) (Ioannidis et al., 2004).

What are the Risks and Side-Effects of Psychotherapy?

The area of risks and side-effects is a broad and conceptually complicated area. Linden (2013) suggested that side-effects should be distinguished from other similar concepts such as treatment non-response (i.e., clients reporting no progress in treatment) and treatment-unrelated illness deterioration. He proposed using the etiologically neutral concept of "unwanted events" as an umbrella term that covers all kinds of undesired reactions clients may have in the course of treatment. Schermuly-Haupt et al. (2018) further elaborated on this classification and distinguished between events unrelated to the treatment (i.e., those attributable to the natural course of an illness and those caused by external factors) and events associated with the treatment. They termed the latter group "adverse treatment reactions" and divided them into side-effects (i.e., clients responding adversely to a correctly indicated and properly conducted treatment) and malpractice (i.e., reactions caused by incorrect treatment).

One of the most challenging problems in studying unwanted events is finding their cause. While we agree that it is essential to conceptually distinguish events caused by the treatment from those based on other factors, it is seldom possible in practice. In their rational-empirical model, Curran et al. (2019) demonstrated that adverse effects can be caused by many factors, including those pertaining to the client, therapist, treatment process, and client-therapist relationship. Therefore, both unwanted events in general and adverse effects specifically should be treated as multifactorial. In empirical studies, this problem is typically simplified to asking clients whether *they* attribute the event to the treatment, external factors, or both (e.g., Rozental et al., 2016). However, clients' opinions can hardly be considered "unbiased" evidence of causality. Reporting adverse events is related to clients' personality traits (Chvála et al., 2022) and may be influenced by other client-related factors such as treatment expectations, preferences, and previous treatment experience (Curran et al., 2019). Therefore, we argue that this phenomenon must be studied from diverse perspectives, including that of therapists and clients.

Proceeding from the psychotherapy experts' perspective, Ladwig et al. (2014) identified six domains of adverse effects. The first domain, *intrapersonal changes caused by psychotherapy*, included, for instance, feeling more guilty, shameful, lonely, anxious, sad, and unworthy, having worse symptoms, less self-accepting, and having suicidal thoughts or intentions. The second domain, *therapeutic malpractice*, described experiences such as being hurt by the therapist's statements, feeling ridiculed, harassed, attacked, and forced to unwanted treatment activities. The third domain, *intimate relationship*, comprised deterioration in a client's relationship with their partner, but also partner noticing negative changes in the client. The fourth domain, *family and friends*, included worsening of a client's relationships with their family, friends, and other people. The fifth domain, *work*, comprised diverse work-related difficulties such as worse concentration, absenteeism, conflicts with colleagues and superiors, and increased carelessness. Finally, the sixth domain, *stigma*, covered feeling stigmatized by psychotherapy, having financial worries and problems with insurance, and decreased career opportunities.

While the experts in Ladwig et al.'s (2014) study identified tangible and often severe unwanted effects potentially connected with psychotherapy, clients may add other aspects they experience as uncomfortable or hindering. Indeed, Vybíral et al. (2023) conducted a qualitative meta-analysis of client-reported negative experiences and found some categories not mentioned by Ladwig et al. (2014). One of the main clusters in Vybíral et al.'s (2023) study focused on clients' perception of the therapeutic relationship. Some clients complained about their therapist being too distant, non-empathetic, and untrustworthy. Others felt confused and uncertain in the relationship or experienced "lack of chemistry" between themselves and their therapist. Another cluster dealt with a perceived lack of fit between the clients' needs, expectations, and preferences on the one hand, and the therapeutic approach, interventions, and various practical aspects of therapy, on the other. Special attention was drawn to termination that could be experienced as mishandled or premature by the client and could leave the client feeling abandoned or resentful. Although Ladwig et al. (2014) identified many adverse impacts of psychotherapy, clients in Vybíral et al.'s (2023) meta-analysis described other, more subtle reactions, such as fearing the therapeutic process, experiencing high in-session arousal that led to no resolution, and losing motivation and hope. These experiences are easy for a therapist to dismiss as fleeting and unimportant, on the one hand, or expectable and inevitable, on the other. From the clients' perspective, however, these may become legitimate reasons for dropping out from the treatment and coming to hate psychotherapy.

What do we know about the Prevalence of Risks and Side-effects?

As we have already mentioned, a non-negligible proportion of clients tends to deteriorate in psychotherapy. However, deterioration (i.e., an increase of symptoms and/or a decrease in well-being) is just one of the possible risks and side-effects clients may encounter during their treatment. If we consider unwanted events more broadly, we get a different picture. Linden et al. (2018) concluded that "[d]epending on data gathering method, sample and therapy form, incidences of side-effects between 3% and 100% of all psychotherapy cases were reported" (p. 378). Looking at different types of negative experiences, experiences that were most frequently reported across studies, included the resurfacing of unpleasant memories, experiencing unpleasant feelings, and feeling more stress (Pourová et al., 2022; Rozental et al., 2016; Strauss et al., 2021). Other reactions, such as feeling stigmatized or dependent on therapy, occurred less often. However, even reactions that occur relatively rarely may be alarming given their severity. For instance, 1% to 12% of clients reported suicidal thoughts that they explicitly attributed to the treatment (Pourová et al., 2022; Strauss et al., 2021).

What Possibilities do we have to Measure Risks and Side-Effects and Collect Data Regarding those Phenomena?

Several questionnaires have been developed to assess the occurrence and/or severity of unwanted events. These include, for instance, the Vanderbilt Negative Indicators Scale (VNIS; Suh et al., 1986), Experiences of Therapy Questionnaire (ETQ; Parker et al., 2014), Unwanted Effects–Adverse Treatment Reaction checklist (UE-ATR; Linden, 2013), Inventory for the Assessment of Negative Effects of Psychotherapy (INEP; Ladwig et al., 2014), Negative Effects Questionnaire (NEQ; Rozental et al., 2016), Positive and Negative Effects of Psychotherapy Scale (PANEPS; Moritz et al., 2019), and Psychotherapy Side Effects Scale (PSES; Chen et al., 2023). Despite the profusion of these questionnaires, none of them covers all aspects of unwanted events (Herzog et al., 2019) and researchers must carefully select a measure depending on what they intend to study.

Using standardized scales allows researchers to collect data on large samples, estimate the prevalence of different types of unwanted events in the population, and make comparisons across samples. To understand the nature and context of these experiences, however, qualitative methods may be necessary. Some of these methods have been specifically developed to capture the process and outcomes of psychotherapy, including open-ended post-session questionnaires, such as the Helpful Aspects of Therapy form (HAT; Llewelyn, 1988) and the Important Events Questionnaire (IEQ; Cummings et al., 1992), and post-treatment interview schedules, such as the Client Change Interview (CCI; Elliott & Rodgers, 2008) and Change After Psychotherapy (CHAP; Sandell, 2015). These methods can help us elucidate the complex role of these events in the therapeutic process.

Are there Specific Risks and Side-effects of Systemic and Family Therapies?

Märtens (2002, p. 225 ff.) explored the following aspects of systemic therapy in terms of risks and side-effects: the setting as risk-factor, couple therapy, short-term nature of treatment, pressure to participate (in multiple person settings), treatment without direct contact with therapist (e.g., in the case of non-participation of a family member in family therapy), one-way mirror, shame and publicity (in multiple-person settings), and conjoint therapy. Also, Märtens (2002) explored under the headline "dangerous interventions?" genogram work, family constellation work and circular questioning; he mainly criticized insufficient criteria for indication and contra-indication of those systemic interventions. In the case of instance genogram work, for example, there is the question of whether the (uncovering) exploration of intergenerational patterns could produce malign effects (e.g., in the case of family violence and abuse experiences or in the case of family secrets). Regarding family constellation work there are well-known risk and harm-associated case reports (e.g., a family constellation work-associated suicide). In addition, Strauß (2018, S. 916 f.) broached the issue of non-reflected partisanship of the systemic family therapist as a potential risk factor and lacking motivation of the index-patient to participate in family therapy. Furthermore, Sydow (2015, S. 109 ff.) noted additional issues in family therapy if family members are also in individual therapy.

Pfautsch & Ochs (2023) reported on a qualitative/exploratory online study among systemic counsellors/therapists (180 responses, including 50 usable data sets). The results show that in the systemic field this topic is considered to be significant. Examples of side-effects cited were symptom deterioration and destabilization of the social environment. Among the various causes adduced were inadequate fixation to resources plus deficient appreciation of problems and suffering, confusing questioning techniques, and lack of competence in connection with intrapsychic phenomena. Supervision, intervision, and further training are referred to as important spaces of resonance that should be drawn upon to reflect regularly and proactively on the relevant topics and to develop competencies and routines for dealing with them in the therapeutic/counselling process.

Results of an exploratory focus-group investigation

We conducted and facilitated four focus group discussions regarding the question: How do family and systemic therapists conceptualize risks and side-effects of family and systemic therapy? The participants of the focus groups were family and systemic psychotherapists. Data were analyzed using the method of reflexive thematic analysis (Braun & Clarke 2006; Caha, 2023): besides focusing on emerging themes, issues, and contents, the interaction and communication process of conceptualization of risks and side-effects by the participating family and systemic therapists was taken into account. Two of the focus groups were online in the Czech language: the participants were systemic family therapy trainers in a Czech systemic therapy training institute. Two focus groups were realized in the context of research workshops at European conferences 2022, one in the English language (in September 2022 at the European Family Therapy Association (EFTA) conference in Ljubljana, Slovenia, which was attended by therapists of various nationalities) and one in the German language (in September 2022 at the Deutsche Gesellschaft für Systemische Therapie, Beratung und Familientherapie (DGSF) conference in Dresden, Germany, which was attended by German systemic therapists).

1. 1.   Dynamic dialogue process

1. 1. 1.   UNCERTAINTY, UNCLARITY, AMBIVALENCE

The themes of uncertainty, unclarity, and ambivalence regarding the topic of risks and side-effects are situated beyond all that is happening in the focus group discussion. The therapists do not know in advance what is going to happen in the therapy. The topic of side-effects cannot be grasped easily, and there is always some ambivalence in the interpretation of specific events.

Therapist[6] 1: And how about this, is it a negative side-effect? I don't know. I really don't. Perhaps that's just life, right?
T2: I don't know either.

1. 1. 2.   DYNAMICS OF THREE STRATEGIES

Within this background, the dynamics of three discourse streams – three strategies – is taking place. These strategies give the therapists directions of thinking about the topic of side-effects, conceptualizing it, understanding their causes, and dealing with them. Rather than being separate, virtual "pure forms" these three strategies exist in lively blending. Occasionally, we can even detect more strategies within one utterance.

1. 1. 2. 1. DENIAL STRATEGY

This is a protective discourse direction that expresses the **need to believe in flawlessness of the therapy** – if it turned out that the therapy is not without its flaws, the speaker would not be able to carry on with it.

T2: *You know, I find it terribly irritating, and I don't know why...*
T1: *Because we need to believe in it.*
T2: *Well, yes, otherwise we couldn't do it.*

In accordance with this strategy, the concept of side-effects is not appropriate for the context of the therapy; **the therapy has no side-effects at all.** On the contrary, what could be habitually considered a side-effect is in fact a part of a healthy therapeutical process: **there can be disruptions that make it possible for the system to develop its structures.**

T1: *(...) the family therapy is set in a certain way where working with those negative side-effects is actually a part of it. Like mending those disruptions in relationships is in fact sort of groundwork of what we do there. So, basically all those negative side-effects are immediately integrated back again, and they become an important part of this work. It is actually a therapeutical process.*

This strategy is distinguished by a **heavy emotional charge,** which can be manifested as anger towards this topic or those who present it. In other cases, it can be expressed with emotions of panic, consternation, or irritation.

T1: *It made me angry, as I said before.*
T2: *We already mentioned that we find this topic a bit annoying.*
T1: *Perhaps the researcher has nothing to do, so he comes up with stuff like this...*
T2: *He was looking for something to tinker with, and this is what he found (laughter).*
T1: *Exactly, that was the first thing that occurred to me.*

1. 1. 2. 2. ACKNOWLEDGEMENT STRATEGY

The heart of this strategy is **the acknowledgement of the fact that the therapy has side-effects,** which is inevitable and needs to be borne in mind. The therapist is expected to feel responsibility for the clients not leaving therapy in a worse state than they had been in before.

T1: *When you said a while ago that it's about working with disruptions or that it's a part of the process itself in fact, I've been thinking about it. Why do we call it negative side-effects? They are simply side-effects and like you said, they keep coming back, and for me, it's important to be aware of it. To realize that there are some side-effects or that there can be some things going on, different from what we think it is about.*

According to this discourse, side-effects are inevitable because of the very fact that therapy is essentially an intervention, a certain "penetrative touch," to a system that works in a certain way. It is necessary to try and work responsibly and **strive to minimize harms** instead of doubting or undermining one's self and one's work.

T1: *(…) the therapy is by definition some kind of stimulation, as we said. We can't avoid affecting those people, but we try to do it in a reasonable way.*
T2: *Yes, in a beneficial way, if possible.*
T1: *But we can't be sure what will happen. If we believe Maturana[7] and Ludewig[8], it's impossible not to affect them. We actually want to do that, but in an adequate way.*

This narrative provides relief. One does not have to be so afraid of side-effect as clients are largely doing the therapy so to speak by themselves while the therapist's task is more or less to "hold the power."

T1: *I've got this feeling (…) that it's OK. It's not like there's something wrong with me if the therapy has some negative side-effects because it is somehow important, even liberating. It doesn't mean that I am doing something wrong, there are also simply some limits of the therapy.*

1. 1. 2. 3. UNPREDICTABILITY STRATEGY

According to the unpredictability, **therapy is an uncertain experiment, and we cannot guarantee the results to be achieved.** We never know for sure which therapy really turns out to be helpful, to whom it helps, and whether the client will evaluate it subjectively as beneficial or not. Uncertainty is something the therapist should be able to cope with.

T1: *So, you know, it's these kinds of things that make you come back into the room and see, "ok, maybe one layer is visible to me, maybe two or three layers, but there are many other layers that we can't see." So that kind of is what I think about side-effects and all of that. That's where they lie and where they live, they live in the unforesaid and in the unforeseen.*

1. 2. Side-effects

The domain of side-effects is an emerging typology of what side-effects or risks systemic and family therapists see with psychotherapy focused on the family and systemic level. Side-effects are categorized as follows:

- Those that have an impact on the entire system. Their subtheme includes life crises as a result of the therapy.
- Side-effects as experiences of the individuals in the therapy.
- Separation of the client from psychological care as a side-effect.

1. 2. 1. THE THERAPY HARMS THE SYSTEM

In the discussions, there were often examples of side-effects that relate to the client's whole family or system. At a general level, **uncovering of compensation mechanisms can break**

Table 1 The classification of themes proposed by the thematic analysis

Side effects	Effects on the entire system
	Side effects as individual experience
	Separation of the client from psychological care
Sources of side-effects	Non-consensuality
	Setting
	Authoritative and directive approach
	Process-related risks
	The client is the cause
	It's the therapist's fault
Mitigation of side-effects/best practice	Good communication
	Sensitivity, reflexivity and listening
	Treating the system well

something that worked and thus potentially result in undesirable events. For example, family therapy can result in the feeling of humiliation as there are always "witnesses" who can see and hear what happens in the therapy session/in the system, for an individual with "more serious problems," the therapy in the family setting can result in the labelling/pillory effect. There is also the risk of overburdening of the "healthy part of the system," according to therapists.

T1: Or there's the other extreme. We might overburden those who are already...
T2: Those who are struggling to keep things working.
T1: Yes, those who are working hard to keep things working. Like when the kids express they want more from the father, we may burden the mother who is already overstrained. And because she feels guilty for marrying a nutcase and for her children suffering, she feels like she should work twice as hard.

1. 2. 1. 1. LIFE CRISES

This is a subtheme of the theme "The therapy harms the system." A **family therapy can result in events that have a significant impact on clients' lives and that can be described as ethically problematic.**[9] These often include a divorce, a break-up, and escalation of family conflicts. On the other hand, there can also be a situation when partners find out they are not happy together, but they do not want to or they are not able to separate for a serious reason.

T1: There can be people who start the therapy, for example, because of some psycho-somatic issues, and it is during the therapy when they discover how poorly they are doing, in fact. (...) but sometimes they also reach this moment when they actually don't want to change it and they just continue living, knowing they are doing so bad.

1. 2. 2. SIDE-EFFECTS AS INDIVIDUAL EXPERIENCES

Besides the whole systems, the family and systemic therapy may also impact participating individuals, according to therapists. **The central theme here is deterioration, i.e. the state**

when the therapy client's experiencing of symptoms intensifies. An example would be the repetition of hurtful patterns from the client's everyday life in the therapy situation.

T1: *If there is a woman who has attachment issues, (...) it's not easy for her to confide in others. Then she comes to a therapy session and this thing happens. It could be something that brings her back to a traumatizing experience, perhaps something in childhood with her parents when she felt like... You know, when she felt like that. This could be retraumatizing for this patient or client. She might never be able to come to a therapist again because she will remember these painful feelings.*

1. 2. 3. SIDE-EFFECTS AS SEPARATION FROM PSYCHOLOGICAL CARE

The client's **discontinuation of the therapy is considered a negative impact per se.** In some cases, the danger related to the drop-out is the fact the client reached stronger awareness of their problems without having developed capacities to deal with them.

T1: *(...) the therapy (can be) ineffective and people can say: "In our case, therapy won't help. We tried a therapy, and it didn't work out." Or "Those therapists also think that I'm just a nutcase."*

1. 3. Sources of side-effects

Regarding the causes of side-effects, we can observe splitting on the attribution axis ("The client is the cause" vs. "It is the therapist's fault"), and furthermore, there is a specific type of approach that can lead to side-effects (authoritative and directive). Some causes of side-effects seem to form an integral part of the therapy process (whether in general or in the family therapy). Moreover, there are two other phenomena that can result in side-effects according to some opinions expressed in the discussion: requirements on the setting[10] and non-consensual participation in the therapy.

1. 3. 1. NON-CONSENSUALITY

The theme of non-consensuality refers to situations when **it is unclear whether all participants are willing to engage,** or when someone was forced to join the therapy and only participates with repulsion.

T1: *Well, talking about the family therapy, the family also consists of those who didn't come there, but they were sort of dragged to be there. Typically, it's the kids.*

Children are frequently mentioned in this case. They may not realize what they are taking part in, and they can be exposed to witnessing something in the therapy that they would usually be protected from by their family.

T1: *(...) perhaps those children don't show it, but later they can feel like that and unconsciously they can experience some bad feelings – because they were present in a situation where they shouldn't have been. I think this might be more common in family therapy than we realize.*

1. 3. 2. SETTING

The issue of the setting was heard in the discussion as something demanding, unclear, and difficult. **The basic position is that the failure in maintaining the setting may lead to side-effects.**

T3: For example, in family therapy, I place great emphasis on the requirement of the setting. Like if we want it to be somehow useful, we can't do that without the Dad. (...) And that we can't really have this approach like "we'll have Grandma today, and next time we'll have Mum." This is something that must be clear (that the setting, e.g., who is partici-pating in the respective session, is not arbitrary or random).

Another source of danger is **some level of automaticity** in the therapist's work (i.e., their selection of a certain setting without considering alternatives based on the clients' needs).

T1: (...) I noticed that I often like to invite people, I mean even more participants, and I tend to see them as a system. But perhaps sometimes it might be more useful if there's only one person. (...) I wonder if it's some kind of habit, some routine of mine when I want to have them all there.

1. 3. 3. AUTHORITATIVE AND DIRECTIVE APPROACH

Authoritative and directive approaches to work were repeatedly mentioned in the discussion as potentially harmful for the client. An example is labeling an individual as defective – this relates to an imperative of change.

T1: I see a huge risk here if I were the one who says: "Listen, you have a problem, and you'd better do something about it." As an authority, the therapist can produce a nega-tive effect like shaming someone or overloading the weakest link (...).

At the family/systemic level, this approach is often manifested as **"pushing the system to change,"** which is not necessarily based on the system's needs and decisions, but rather the therapist's orientation.

1. 3. 4. PROCESS-RELATED RISKS

The risks related to the nature of the therapeutic process are not often clear and visible for the clients in advance. **Clients rarely have – unlike therapists – the same and sufficient understanding of what the therapy process is, and what kind of uncertainty and risks it conveys.** Although therapists can try to explain the risk right from the start, clients may find it incomprehensible.

T1: And what is important, this person probably orients themselves more based on how they feel around me than based on what I tell them. So when I tell them nicely, in a close contact, "We're setting out for a journey," they reply "Hooray" because they hear me, not because they perceive the contents. They feel they are coming with me, but not... So in a way, I promise them my presence, but not the result. So, this person accepts being with me, not results.

1. 3. 4. 1.   CAUSES SPECIFIC FOR THE FAMILY THERAPY PROCESS.

Because there are always multiple actors present, **the safety of the therapeutic space can be limited** for the clients.

T1: *Well, there is also another side-effect with family therapies when you create such a strong feeling of closeness and safety, and those people really say things they wouldn't even mention under normal circumstances. And then they can use it against each other. They can get access to some sensitive feelings, and then perhaps the husband uses that against his wife, or a parent against the child.*

In family therapy, sometimes **there is not enough space for sharing and taking care of sensitive feelings and topics.** Family therapy can generally deal better with the interpersonal than with the intrapsychic. A personality disorder, for example, was considered unsolvable in the discussion, and in such cases, the therapy is only expected to focus on better adaptation of the other members in the system.

1. 3. 5.   THE CLIENT IS THE CAUSE

In one discussion string of the focus groups, responsibility for side-effects was attributed to clients. For example, it can be clients whose psychopathology prevents the therapist from effective work.

T1: *Me and my co-therapist sometimes we can achieve very few, very small (effects). Not because we are not good psychotherapists, but because the psychopathology, it's enormous. Sometimes, with multi-problematic families, the person to trust and to cooperate you don't find. Father – a psychopath. Mother – high borderline. Adolescent daughter – just came from the hospital with a suicide attempt. Young children of eight is the healthiest of all, but you can not rely on her, as a co-therapist, let's say, because you are overburdening her with that… .*

Some clients in the therapy process are not able to view certain things in time or communicate sufficiently (e.g., the client is going through a certain discomfort, suffering due to something in the therapy). There can also be incompatibility in needs and expectations of individual clients within the system in family therapy.

1. 3. 6.   IT IS THE THERAPIST'S FAULT

The sources of side-effects that are localized as the therapist's responsibility are probably the most extensive theme of this domain. They can be categorized as three subthemes – methodical errors, issues related to the therapist's experiencing, and errors due to insensitivity.

1. 3. 6. 1.   METHODICAL ERRORS

This theme covers situations when the therapist makes a certain intervention too early or too late, when they stick to the techniques and methods too rigidly while losing contact with the clients, when they do not intervene sufficiently into the events in the therapy process or, on the contrary, when they are drowning in details.

T1: So I came up with an intervention, I wanted to give him a prod with a confrontation. And I did so sort of clumsily – I asked him whether he ever heard the saying "If you wanna fuck, you have to be friendly." But it appeared to be such a no-go for him; it took us three more sessions to mitigate the impact of this sentence.

1. 3. 6. 2. ISSUES RELATED TO THE THERAPIST'S EXPERIENCING

These can be situations when the therapist falls in love with the client (and consequently concludes the therapy or starts a sexual relationship with the client) or when the **therapist's behaviour is directed according to their own motives.**

1. 3. 6. 3. ERRORS DUE TO INSENSITIVITY

"There is something going on with the process, negative feelings are surfacing, and it depends on how they get detected and addressed whether they will turn into side-effects or not." **Errors caused by insensitivity or carelessness occur when the process of "detection" fails.** This includes overlooking certain family dynamics; for example, when some members of the system are non-consensual participants in the therapy or when they are experiencing something that may harm them.

T1: When I come across these repeated topics with my clients, for example, three break-ups in a row, then I feel like… You know, somehow it looks like the same thing, and I feel my work quality drops off. I tell myself: "OK, let's hear this once again" and my empathy is fading out.

1. 4. Mitigation of side-effects/best practices

The last of the three themes discussed are best practices. The discourse around this domain focuses on prevention or mitigation of side-effects by means of following the best practice principles of psychotherapy work, which are discussed here.

1. 4. 1. GOOD COMMUNICATION

It is crucial for the client to be able to open and share their lived experience in therapy. **The therapist's task is to encourage clients to share, and to give them appreciation when this process is successful.** The therapist also needs to be able to sense what is going on in the therapy and be able to bring up and thematize such things.

T1: Negative side-effects occur at that moment when one doesn't bring "the stuff" to therapy and doesn't address it. I remember one couple. The guy said that at the previous session, he didn't feel taken care of. That we didn't protect him from his wife. The fact that he was able to express it, that's something we appreciated so much, but then we were like… how to deal with it? He was really worried to deal with it somehow, the client himself. But later it proved somehow beneficial.

1. 4. 2.   SENSITIVITY, REFLEXIVITY, AND LISTENING

A therapist needs to monitor the therapy progress and the clients' experiences. This can also be expanded by working with things that were "left unsaid" by clients.

T1: But I guess, there are also things that I haven't been told and I can... well... unless it makes me too anxious on that day, I can also think about the things I didn't learn about. (...) If they say "This was great and that was great," I can realize later we only talked about those great things. But then I can also say: "Look, last time you mentioned things that were great, but perhaps you didn't mention what wasn't great, so how about we try to talk about such things too?"

The therapist should sensitively work with their own internal dialogue.

1. 4. 3.   TREATING THE SYSTEM WELL

While dealing with families, the therapist needs to balance modeling and non-competing while working with the family.

T1: (...) Very often we actually relate to those children in front of their parents, and at that moment, it can be difficult for the parents. You see, they are in this situation when we treat the child in a different way, we ask different questions, or the child responds differently. Even if we don't want to become their competitors, in a way that's what happens... .
T2: On the other hand, this is the way for them to learn that things can be done differently. Through us, they learn a different way of communication with the children.
T1: So it's actually a balance between modeling and non-competing.

The therapist needs to work sensitively with the setting and its changes if they are necessary. The therapist needs to minimize the risk of labeling one member of the system and overburdening another one via active encouragement of the system members to explicitly take over shared responsibility for solving their shared situation. Moreover, it is desirable for the therapist to help the system to become more adaptive in dealing with various situations, and the therapist also needs to be able to favour every participant equally.

Concluding Annotations

As stated, in recent years the topic of risks and side-effects has become an important perspective in psychotherapy practice and research (e.g., Linden & Strauss, 2018) – mainly for two reasons:

1. As we know, we cannot avoid risks and side-effects since they are a vital part of any expert-working, effective psychotherapy (Linden, 2013). Therefore, we have to develop a practice and research perspective on the prevention of them to imporove psychotherapies – especially in the context of our developing understanding, that the once reported relative high effects-sizes of psychotherapy (0.8, sometimes up to 1.2 (BPtK, 2013)) were merely overestimations due to methodological flaws of studies.

2. For ethical reasons we must take the topic of risks and side-effects into account, because one important part of the Hippocratic Oath is as we know: "Primum non nocere" ("First do no harm").

Ochs & Pfautsch (2022; see also Ochs & Borcsa, in prep.) recommend regarding prevention and managing of risks and side-effects by:

- the use of respective questionnaires (see above); some of the already established questionnaires include items that focus on "systemic" aspects. For example, the Inventory for the Assessment of Negative Effects of Psychotherapy (INEP; Ladwig et al., 2014) includes the items (also a version of INEP is available that allows to assess negative effects not only after termination but also in the course of the therapy):
  o "Since the termination of therapy, I experience my relationship with my partner in comparison to the period before the start of the therapy… less/more conflicted."
  o "My relationship to my family since termination of therapy compared to before the start of the therapy is… better/worse."
  o "The relationship to my friends since termination of therapy compared to before the start of the therapy is… better/worse."
- use of Routine Outcome Monitoring (ROM) (e.g., Lambert & Harmon, 2018) or Systematic Client Feedback (SCF) (for systemic therapy see Tilden, 2020; Rober, van Tricht & Sundet, 2021). There are reliable and valid systemic questionnaires available that can be used for ROM including EVOS (Evaluation of Systems, Aguilar-Raab et al., 2015, 2018) or SCORE-15 (Systemic Clinical Outcome and Routine Evaluation Stratton et al., 2020).
- use of conventional quality control formats, such as inter- and supervision, further training and education on the topic.
- In some countries, because of professional legal regulations, you have to educate and inform every patient at the beginning of psychotherapy about possible risks and side-effects. Besides this, from time to time a proactive realizing of the issue into the psychotherapeutic discourse by the therapist is strongly recommended, for example, by asking questions such as:
  o "I want to invite you to think about whether you are experiencing any kind of negative outcomes or uncomfortable processes that possibly could be associated with the psychotherapy that we are undergoing."
- use of reflexive questions regarding the therapeutic relationship is advised (Schlippe & Schweitzer, 2012, S. 275). For example:
  • How do you feel regarding our collaboration? Are you having the impression that we are succeeding? Are we talking about the issues that are important to you? Are we communicating in a way that is helpful and useful for you?
  • Which of the aspects we were talking about could become important for you? Supposed the session would end now – for which of your concerns you would already have a solution, and on which issues we should have had elaborated more?

Telfener (2022) puts the reflexive moment of the therapeutic relationship in the centra of a successful handling of psychotherapeutic risks and side-effects. "The helping professional relationship asks for a high degree of reflexivity, otherwise the relationship becomes one of friendship. The risk of undesired outcomes emerges from this failure to consider therapy as a second-order process. The aim in therapy is not to fight the other's ideas and propositions, nor to arm wrestle, but rather to create a synergy."

The perspective of psychotherapy approach specific risks and side-effects besides a perspective of risk ans side-effects, that occur in all kind of psychotherapy approaches, is still under debate – also there are hints, that such a perspective could be useful should be further elaborated (for the psychodynamic approaches, see, e.g., Fäh, 2002; Kächele & Hilgers, 2018: for behavioral approaches see Jacobi, 2002; Nestoriuc & Rief, 2018; for Gestalt psychotherapy approaches see Fuhr & Gremmler-Fuhr, 2002). But what seems to be clear is that the belief of many psychotherapists that they are doing no harm and producing no side-effects (Busch & Lemme, 1992) – e.g., because they think that they are way above average regarding their therapeutic competencies (Lake Wobegon-effect of psychotherapists (Walfish et al., 2009), Ochs & Pfautsch, 2022) – is a stance that needs to be challenged!

Notes

1   We refer to systemic therapy as a psychotherapeutic approach, that developed from the Fifties in the last century until now in different developmental phases (from the Palo Alto informed strategic perspectives to structural family therapy, development-oriented family therapy approaches such as proposed by Virginia Satir or Walter Kempler, to systemic-constructionist approaches, solution focused and narrative therapy, such as systemic-dialogical approaches or family constellations work (z.B. Schweitzer & Ochs, 2020; Hunger-Schoppe, 2021)). Also, the so called "trademark-therapies" (Sydow et al., 2018, S. 944). could be subsumed under the umbrella of systemic therapy (Hanswille, 2022): Attachment-Based Family Therapy (ABFT), Multidimensional Family Therapy (MDFT), Multisystemic Therapies (MST), Mentalization Based Family Therapy (MBFT or MBT-F), Family-Based Treatment for Adolescent Eating Disorders (FBT) Functional Family Therapy (FFT) Behavioral Couple Therapy for Alcohol and Drug Abuse (BCT) Emotion focused Therapy and Couple- und Family Therapy (EFT und EFFT) Internal Family Systems (IFS), Ego-State-Therapy (EST).

2   The generic principles that are derived from the synergetic systems theory (Haken, 1983) are a heuristic for understanding and managing self-organized change processes (Schiepek et al., 2015). One premise of that principle is that change sensible periods in living complex systems are associated with instabilities. Accordingly, the fifth generic principle is called "destabilization" – development is proceeded by distortion, without order-order-passages there is no development. In which way destabilization and distortion could or should be a result of therapeutic interventions is unclear against the background of recent results from psychotherapy research on risks and side-effects. Moritz et al. (2019, S. 579) refer to "anecdotal reports that some destabilization may be a prerequisite for improvement" (by the way also psychoanalytic reports) – but infer on the base of their own empirical results: "no evidence was found for this 'no pain, no gain' hypothesis" (see Moritz et al., 2015) – a negative correlative association was found between positive effects and side-effects in psychotherapy. Taking this empirical situation into account the question of how many systems theoretical-derived destabilization and distortion is necessary may need to be discussed again… .

3   www.bptk.de/wp-content/uploads/2019/01/20130412_BPtK_Standpunkt_10_Tatsachen_Psychot herapie.pdf

4   From 2014 to 2017 12 experts over a period of 3 years worked on that review: 3,133 potentially relevant sources were identified, 2,837 of these were excluded after full-text inspection; an additional 231 sources were systematic reviews, screened to identify relevant primary studies. The remaining 65 publications for 28 studies fulfilled the pre-defined inclusion criteria for the report. Further search of study registers/other resources resulted in 28 additional documents from 14 additional studies. A total of 42 RCT studies from all possible sources were included as relevant to the aim of the report. Of these 42 studies, only 33 studies had data that could be utilized; 33 studies over 9 mental disorders areas were considered. (www.iqwig.de/download/n14-02_abschlussberi cht_systemische-therapie-bei-erwachsenen_v1-0.pdf)

5 Not "reported" does not mean "not present"…
6 Hereinafter referred to as "T" (therapist) with a number identifying various speakers in the focus groups. The numbers of the therapist "T" are relevant for each quotation only, not throughout the text, i.e., "T1" is not an actual therapist, it's just the first speaker in a specific quotation out of the focus groups.
7 Umberto Maturana
8 Kurt Ludewig
9 The concepts of "moral controversy," "ethical problems," or something "negative" occurred repeatedly in the discussion and were not clearly anchored with any explicit value system or a specific perspective. In this chapter, these (and similar) terms are always used as a reference to utterance in the discussion without a clearly specified anchoring unless stated otherwise in the text.
10 The setting in this context refers to "which people participate in the therapy process," and it is understood as a category that should be more or less constant in the therapy.

References

Aguilar-Raab C., Grevenstein D., Schweitzer J. (2015) Measuring social relationships in different social systems: The construction and validation of the Evaluation of Social Systems (EVOS) Scale. *PLoS ONE*, 10(7): e0133442. doi:10.1371/journal.pone.0133442

Aguilar-Raab, C., Grevenstein, D., Gotthardt, L., Jarczok, M. N., Hunger, C., Ditzen, B. & Schweitzer, J. (2018). Changing me, changing us: Relationship quality and collective efficacy as major outcomes in systemic couple therapy. *Family Process*, 57(2), 342–358.

Barkham, M., Lutz, W., Lambert, M. J., & Saxon, D. (2017). Therapist effects, effective therapists, and the law of variability. In L. G. Castonguay & C. E. Hill (Eds.), *How and why are some therapists better than others?: Understanding therapist effects*. American Psychological Association, pp. 13–36. https://doi.org/10.1037/0000034-002

Barlow D. H. (2010) Negative effects from psychological treatments: a perspective. American Psychologist, 2010 Jan; 65(1):13–20. doi: 10.1037/a0015643. PMID: 20063906

Bergin, A. E. (1971). The evaluation of therapeutic outcomes. In A. E. Bergin & S. L. Garfield (Eds.), *Handbook of Psychotherapy and Behavior Change*. John Wiley, pp. 217–270.

Bertrando, P., & Lini, C. (2021). Towards a systemic-dialogical model of therapy. *Human Systems*, 1(1), 15–28. https://doi.org/10.1177/26344041211003853.

Boscolo, L., & Bertrando, P. (1996). Systemic therapy with individuals. London: Karnac.

BPtK Bundespsychotherapeutenkammer (Hrsg.) (2013). 10 Tatsachen zur Psychotherapie BPtK-Standpunkt. Berlin: BPtK.

Braun, V., & Clarke, V. (2006). Using thematic analysis in psychology. *Qualitative Research in Psychology*, 3(2), 77–101

Busch, I., & Lemme, R. (1992). Schulenspezifische Unterschiede hinsichtlich der Einstellung der Therapeuten zur Wirkung von Psychotherapie? Diplomarbeit. Berlin: Technische Universität

Carr, A. (2022). Psychological treatment in the family format. In G. J. G. Asmundson (Ed.), *Comprehensive clinical psychology*. 6 (pp. 58–74) Amsterdam: Elsevier.

Caha, J. (2023). "They come with the hope that something will improve… but let's define 'improve' first.": Side effects of family and systemic therapy from the perspective of therapists [Master's thesis, Masaryk University]. https://is.muni.cz/th/eho5n/Jakub_Caha_-_Diplomova_prace_-_FINAL.pdf

Chen, F., Liu, L., Zhao, X., Feng, Q., Ge, C., & Zhao, Y. (2023). The preliminary development and psychometric properties of the Psychotherapy Side Effects Scale. *Brain Behaviour*, e2885. https://doi.org/10.1002/brb3.2885

Chvála, Ľ., Řiháček, T., & Vybíral, Z. (2022). A pilot study of HEXACO dimensions and therapeutic change as potential predictors of negative effects of psychotherapy. *Československá Psychologie*, 66(5), 532–542. https://doi.org/10.51561/cspsych.66.5.532

Cuijpers, P., Reijnders, M., Karyotaki, E., de Wit, L., & Ebert, D. D. (2018). Negative effects of psychotherapies for adult depression: A meta-analysis of deterioration rates. *Journal of Affective Disorders*, 239, 138–145.

Cummings, A. L., Martin, J., Hallberg, E., & Slemon, A. (1992). Memory for therapeutic events, session effectiveness, and working alliance in short-term counseling. *Journal of Counseling Psychology*, 39(3), 306–312. https://doi.org/10.1037/0022-0167.39.3.306

Curran, J., Parry, G. D., Hardy, G. E., Darling, J., Mason, A. M., & Chambers, E. (2019). How does therapy harm? A model of adverse process using task analysis in the meta-synthesis of service users' experience. *Frontiers in Psychology*, 10, 347. https://doi.org/10.3389/fpsyg.2019.00347

Elkins, D. N. (2009). The medical model in psychotherapy. Its limitations and failures. *Journal of Humanistic Psychology*, 49, 66–84. DOI 10.1177/0022167807307901

Elliott, R., & Rodgers, B. (2008). Client Change Interview. Retrieved from www.drbrianrodgers.com/research/client-change-interview

Fäh, M. (2002). Wenn Analyse krank macht. Methoden-spezifische Nebenwirkungen psychoanalytischer Therapien. In Märtens M, Petzold H (Hrsg.), *Therapieschäden. Risiken und Nebenwirkungen von Psychotherapie*. Grünewald, Mainz, S 109–147

Farber, B. A. (2020). Disclosure, concealment, and dishonesty in psychotherapy: A clinically focused review. *Journal of Clinical Psychology*, 76(2), 251–257. https://doi.org/10.1002/jclp.22891

Fuhr, R., & Gremmler-Fuhr, M. (2002). Therapieschulenspezifische Nebenwirkungen von Gestalttherapie. Märtens, M. (2002) Nebenwirkungen und Risiken in der Systemischen Therapie. In M. Märtens & H. Petzold, (Hrsg.), *Therapieschäden* (S. 148–180) Mainz: Matthias Grünewald.

Hannan, C., Lambert, M. J., Harmon, C., Nielsen, S. L., Smart, D. W., Shimokawa, K., & Sutton, S. W. (2005). A lab test and algorithms for identifying clients at risk for treatment failure. *Journal of Clinical Psychology*, 61(2), 155–163.

Hanswille, R. (2022). Varianten der Systemischen Therapie und manualisierte/integrative Therapien. In R. Hanswille (Hrsg.), *Basiswissen Systemische Therapie: Gut vorbereitet in die Prüfung* (Kapitel 9) (267–302). Vandenhoeck & Ruprecht, Göttingen.

Haken, H. (1983). Synergetics. Heidelberg: Springer.

Hatfield, D., McCullough, L., Frantz, S. H. B., Krieger, K., Hatfi, D., McCullough, L., Frantz, S. H. B., & Krieger, K. (2010). Do we know when our clients get worse? An investigation of therapists' ability to detect negative client change. *Clinical Psychology and Psychotherapy*, 17(1), 25–32.

Hermes, M., & Lindel, B. (2020). Haftungsfragen in der Psychotherapie. *Psychotherapeut*, 65, 32–35. https://doi.org/10.1007/s00278-019-00394-w

Herzog P, Lauff S, Rief W, Brakemeier EL. (2019). Assessing the unwanted: A systematic review of instruments used to assess negative effects of psychotherapy. *Brain and Behaviour*, e01447. https://doi.org/10.1002/brb3.1447

Hill, C. E., Thompson, B. J., Cogar, M. C., & Denman, D. W. (1993). Beneath the surface of long-term therapy: Therapist and client report of their own and each other's covert processes. *Journal of Counseling Psychology*, 40(3), 278–287. https://doi.org/10.1037/0022-0167.40.3.278

Hunger-Schoppe, C. (2021). Systemische Therapie. Stuttgart: Kohlhammer.

Ioannidis, J. P., Evans, S. J., Gøtzsche, P. C., O'Neill, R. T., Altman, D. G., Schulz, K., & Moher, D. (2004). Better reporting of harms in randomized trials: an extension of the CONSORT statement. *Annals of Internal Medicine*, 141, 781–788.

IQWiG – Institut für Qualität und Wirtschaftlichkeit im Gesundheitswesen (2017). Systemische Therapie bei Erwachsenen als Psychotherapieverfahren. Köln: IQWIG.

Jacobi, F. (2002). Risiken und Nebenwirkungen verhaltenstherapeutischer Behandlung. In Märtens, M., Petzold, H. (Hrsg.), *Therapieschäden. Risiken und Nebenwirkungen von Psychotherapie*. Grünewald, Mainz, S. 89–108

Kächele, H., & Hilgers, M. (2018). SpezifischeNebenwirkungen von psychodynamischer Psychotherapie. In M. Linden & B. Strauß (Hrsg.), *Risiken und Nebenwirkungen von Psychotherapie* (S. 41–58) Berlin: Medizinisch Wissenschaftliche Verlagsgesellschaft

Klatte, R., Strauss, B., Flückiger, C., Färber, F., & Rosendahl, J. (2022). Defining and assessing adverse events and harmful effects in psychotherapy study protocols: A systematic review. *Psychotherapy*. Advance online publication. http://doi.org/10.1037/pst0000359

Kriz, J. & Ochs, M. (2022). Erkenntnis- und wissenschaftstheoretische Grundlagen II: Systemtheorien. In R. Hanswille (Hrsg.), *Basiswissen Systemische Therapie* (Kapitel 3) (S. 51–75). Vandenhoeck & Ruprecht, Göttingen.

Ladwig, I., Rief, W., & Nestoriuc, Y. (2014). Welche Risiken und Nebenwirkungen hat Psychotherapie? – Entwicklung des Inventars zur Erfassung Negativer Effekte von Psychotherapie (INEP). *Verhaltenstherapie, 24*, 252–263. https://doi.org/10.1159/000367928

Lambert, M. (2013). The efficacy and effectiveness of psychotherapy. In M. Lambert (Ed.), *Bergin and Garfield's Handbook of Psychotherapy and Behavior Change*. John Wiley & Sons, pp. 169–218.

Lambert, M., & Harmon, K. (2018). The merits of implementing routine outcome monitoring in clinical practice. *Clinical Psychology: Science and Practice, 25*. e12268. DOI 10.1111/cpsp.12268

Leichsenring, F., Steinert, C., & Ioannidis, J. P. A. (2019). Toward a paradigm shift in treatment and research of mental disorders. *Psychological Medicine, 49*, 2111–2117.

Linden, M. (2013). How to define, find and classify side effects in psychotherapy: From unwanted events to adverse treatment reactions. *Clinical Psychology and Psychotherapy, 20*(4), 286–296. https://doi.org/10.1002/cpp.1765

Linden, M., & Strauß, B. (2018) (Hrsg.). Risiken und Nebenwirkungen von Psychotherapie. Erfassung, Bewältigung, Risikovermeidung. Berlin: Medizinisch Wissenschaftliche Verlagsgesellschaft.

Linden, M., & Strauß, B. (2022) (Hrsg.). Erfassung von Psychotherapie-Nebenwirkungen. Berlin: Medizinisch Wissenschaftliche Verlagsgesellschaft.

Linden, M., Strauß, B., Scholten, S., Nestoriuc, Y., Brakemeier, E.-L., & Wasilewski, J. (2018). Definition und Entscheidungsschritte in der Bestimmung und Erfassung von Nebenwirkungen von Psychotherapie. *Psychotherapie, Psychosomatik, Medizinische Psychologie, 68*, 377–382.

Llewelyn, S. (1988). Psychological therapy as viewed by clients and therapists. *British Journal of Clinical Psychology, 27*(3) pp 223–237. https://doi.org/10.1111/j.2044-8260.1988.tb00779.x

Märtens, M. (2002) Nebenwirkungen und Risiken in der Systemischen Therapie. In M. Märtens & H. Petzold, (Hrsg.), *Therapieschäden* (S. 216–244) Mainz: Matthias Grünewald.

Märtens, M., & Petzold, H. (2002) (Hrsg.), Therapieschäden .Mainz: Matthias Grünewald.

Morin, Edgar (2008): On Complexity (Advances in Systems Theory, Complexity, and the Human Sciences). New York: Hampton Press.

Moritz, S., Fieker, M., Hottenrott, B., Seeralan, T., Cludius, B., Kolbeck, K., et al. (2015). No pain, no gain? Adverse effects of psychotherapy in obsessive-compulsive disorder and its relationship to treatment gains. *Journal of Obsessive-Compulsive and Related Disorders, 5*, 61–66.

Moritz, S., Nestoriuc, Y., Rief, W., Klein, J. P., Jelinek, L., & Peth, J. (2019). It can't hurt, right? Adverse effects of psychotherapy in patients with depression. *European Archives of Psychiatry and Clinical Neuroscience, 269*(5), 577–586. https://doi.org/10.1007/s00406-018-0931-1

Nestoriuc, Y., & Rief, W. (2018). Risiken und Nebenwirkungen von Verhaltenstherapie. In M. Linden & B. Strauß (Hrsg.), *Risiken und Nebenwirkungen von Psychotherapie* (S. 59–74) Berlin: Medizinisch Wissenschaftliche Verlagsgesellschaft.

Ochs, M. (2020) Die erkenntnistheoretischen Säulen und praxeologischen Grundorientierungen systemischen Arbeitens. In P. Bauer & M. Weinhardt (Eds.), *Systemische Kompetenzen entwickeln: Grundlagen, Lernprozesse und Didaktik*. Vandenhoeck & Ruprecht, Göttingen, pp 134–157.

Ochs, M., & Kriz, J. (2022a). Erkenntnis- und wissenschaftstheoretische Grundlagen I: Konstruktivismus. In R. Hanswille (Hrsg.), *Basiswissen Systemische Therapie* (S. 31–48). Vandenhoeck & Ruprecht, Göttingen.

Ochs, M., & Kriz, J. (2022b). Systemische (Psychotherapie-)Forschung. In R. Hanswille (Hrsg.), *Basiswissen Systemische Therapie* (S. 337–351) Göttingen: Vandenhoeck & Ruprecht.

Ochs, M., & Pfautsch, B. (2022). Kommen Systemiker:innen (auch) aus Lake Wobegon? Teil 1: Risiken und Nebenwirkungen systemischer Therapie und Beratung. *Familiendynamik, 47*(4), 284–293.

Parker, G., Paterson, A., Fletcher, K., McClure, G., & Berk, M. (2014). Construct validity of the Experiences of Therapy Questionnaire (ETQ). *BMC Psychiatry, 14*(1), 369. https://doi.org/10.1186/s12888-014-0369-6

Pfautsch, B., & Ochs, M.(2023): Antizipation von Nebenwirkungen – Ausdruck von Professionalität? Teil 2: Empirische Befunde zu Risiken und Nebenwirkungensystemischer Therapie und Beratung: Ergebnisse einer qualitativ-explorativen Online-Befragung. *Familiendynamik, 48*(2).

Pourová, M., Řiháček, T., Chvála, Ľ., Vybíral, Z., & Boehnke, J. R. (2022). Negative effects during multicomponent group-based treatment: A multisite study. *Psychotherapy Research*. Advance online publication. https://doi.org/10.1080/10503307.2022.2095237

Rennie, D. L. (1994). Clients' deference in psychotherapy. *Journal of Counseling Psychology, 41*(4), 427–437. https://doi.org/10.1037/0022-0167.41.4.427

Rober, P., Van Tricht, K., & Sundet, R. (2021). 'One step up, but not there yet': Using client feedback to optimise the therapeutic alliance in family therapy. *Journal of Family Therapy, 43*(1), 46–63.

Rozental, A., Kottorp, A., Boettcher, J., Andersson, G., & Carlbring, P. (2016). Negative effects of psychological treatments: An exploratory factor analysis of the negative effects questionnaire for monitoring and reporting adverse and unwanted events. *PLoS ONE, 11*(6), 1–22. https://doi.org/10.1371/journal.pone.0157503

Sandell, R. (2015). Rating the outcomes of psychotherapy using the Change After Psychotherapy (CHAP) scales: Manual and commentary. *Research in Psychotherapy: Psychopathology, Process and Outcome, 18*(2), 32–49. https://doi.org/10.7411/RP.2015.111

Schermuly-Haupt, M.-L., Linden, M., & Rush, A. J. (2018). Unwanted events and side effects in cognitive behavior therapy. *Cognitive Therapy and Research, 42*(3), 219–229. https://doi.org/10.1007/s10608-018-9904-y

Schiepek, G., Eckert, H., Aas, B., Wallot, S., & Wallot, A. (2015). Integrative psychotherapy: A feedback-driven dynamic systems approach. Hogrefe Publishing. https://doi.org/10.1027/00472-000

Schlippe, A. von, Schweitzer, J. (2012). Lehrbuch der Systemischen Therapie und Beratung I: Das Grundlagenwissen. Göttingen: Vandenhoeck & Ruprecht.

Schweitzer, J. & Ochs, M. (2020). The Heidelberg Systemic Research Conferences: Their History, Goals and Outcomes. In M. Ochs, M. Borcsa, & J. Schweitzer (Eds.), *Systemic Research in Individual, Couple, and Family Therapy and Counseling.* Cham: Springer International, pp 1–10.

Stratton, P., Carr, A., & Schepisi, L. (2020). The SCORE in Europe: Measuring effectiveness, assisting therapy. In M. Ochs, M. Borcsa & J. Schweitzer (Eds.), *Systemic Research in Individual, Couple, and Family Therapy and Counseling.* Cham: Springer International, pp. 367–384.

Strauß, B. (2018). Risiken und Nebenwirkungen. In K. v. Sydow & U. Borst. (Hrsg.), *Systemische Therapie in der Praxis* (S. 912–919) Weinheim: Beltz.

Strauss, B., Gawlytta, R., Schleu, A., & Frenzl, D. (2021). Negative effects of psychotherapy: Estimating the prevalence in a random national sample. *The British Journal of Psychiatry Open, 7*(6), e186. https://doi.org/10.1192/bjo.2021.1025

Suh, C. S., Strupp, H. H., & O'Malley, S. S. (1986). The Vanderbilt process measures: The psychotherapy process scale (VPPS) and the negative indicators scale (VNIS). In L. S. Greenberg & W. M. Pinsof (Eds.), *The Psychotherapeutic Process: A Research Handbook.* Guilford Press, pp 285–323.

Sydow, K. v. (2015). Systemische Therapie. München: Ernst Reinhardt.

Sydow, K. von, Borst, U., & Geyerhofer, S. (2018). Aus- und Weiterbildung in Systemischer Therapie an Hochschulen und privaten Instituten. In K. von Sydow & U. Borst (Hrsg.), *Systemische Therapie in der Praxis* (S. 944–962). Weinheim: Beltz.

Telfener, U. (2022). Getting Sick from Psychotherapy. Our Co-Responsibility in Unintended and Undesired Outcomes. In P. Barbetta, M.E. Cavagnis, I.-B. Krause, U. Telfener (Eds.), *Ethical and Aesthetic Explorations of Systemic Practice.* New Critical Reflections, pp. 75–95.

Tilden, T. (2020). The Idiographic Voice in a Nomothetic World: Why Client Feedback Is Essential in Our Professional Knowledge. In Ochs, M., Borcsa, M., Schweitzer, J. (Eds.), *Systemic Research in Individual, Couple, and Family Therapy and Counseling.* European Family Therapy Association Series. Springer, Cham. https://doi.org/10.1007/978-3-030-36560-8_21

Vybíral, Z., Ogles, B. M., Řiháček, T., Urbancová, B., & Gocieková, V. (2023). Negative experiences in psychotherapy from clients' perspective: A qualitative meta-analysis. Psychotherapy Research. https://doi.org/10.1080/10503307.2023.2226813

Walfish, S., McAlister, B., O'Donnell, P. & Lambert, M. J. (2009). Are all psychotherapists from Lake Wobegon? An investigation of self-assessment bias in mental health providers. Unveröffentlichtes Manuskript

Walfish, S., McAlister, B., O'Donnell, P., & Lambert, M. J. (2012). An investigation of self-assessment bias in mental health providers. *Psychological Reports, 110*(2), 639–644.

Wampold, B. E. (2001). Contextualizing psychotherapy as a healing practice: Culture, history, and methods. *Applied & PreventivePsychology, 10,* 69–86.

27

INTERRACIAL COUPLES

Clinical Considerations for a Contemporary World

Maxine R. Notice

A Modern Experience

Wendell and Sherry had been dating for two years before the lock down of March 2020. Though they had initial concerns about losing privileged freedoms, they quickly decided to make the best of the situation by following a strict safety protocol, and spending lots of connective time together. Wendell, a first-generation Black Caribbean-American male in his early 30s, found himself excited to spend uninterrupted time sharing some of his Trinidadian culture with his girlfriend. As the restaurant he worked at was temporarily closed, he had hopes to develop new recipes at home to share with his partner. Sherry, a Korean-American female in her late 20s, was ecstatic to work from home as a junior para-legal. As she prepared to enter law school in the fall semester, she was grateful for as much rest and relaxation as she could get before an uptick in her educational commitments. As their time in close proximity began Wendell and Sherry came to grow a deeper fondness for one another's ability to make the best of a difficult situation. They worked earnestly at deepening their relationship by having in-depth conversations, sharing in the care of their shared space, and engaging in personal projects to keep their moods elevated.

As the days at home turned into weeks Wendell and Sherry both began to struggle with understanding the rapidly changing world. Feeling confined and cut off from the world quickly gave way to trepidation. In April, Sherry was made aware that her younger cousin was verbally berated at a local grocery store for being Asian. Sherry's concern for her family was overwhelming as she grappled with the influx of Asian hate assaults taking place across the country. In May, the killing of a Black man in Minneapolis, George Floyd, by local law enforcement ignited a global outcry not yet witnessed in the 21st century. For Wendall, the repetitive playing of the video footage across media outlets depicting the killing led to immediate feelings of rage, despair, and hopelessness.

As global citizens began to rally together in local cities to protest racial injustice, police brutality, and systemic racism, Sherry and Wendell came to an impasse about their involvement with supporting the movement of the time. The couple argued about their concerns of remaining safe, avoiding illness and physical harm. Yet as their contention grew, they remained silent about their personal worries about being supported, understood, and seen

DOI: 10.4324/9781003297871-30

by one another during this difficult time. Moments of laughter were now filled with silence, as each person contemplated the state of their relationship. When violence made its way to their local city, as a young Black man James Scurlock was killed during a local protest by a White business owner, Wendell began to sink into a deeper state of despondency. It was this catalyst that caused Sherry to find a local couples therapist to help them deal with all that was taking place.

Introduction

This chapter is deliberate in presenting the contemporary experiences of interracial couples, and how they impact their current clinical needs in relational therapy. In recent years, it has become commonplace for therapists to have many couples that share the same predicament of Wendell and Sherry. While these couples may have a deep desire to thrive in their relationships, a plethora of historical and contemporary issues threaten to widen the gap in their ability to be fully seen and cared for, within their relationships, and within the therapeutic environment. To begin, a review of the historic narratives surrounding interracial couples will be presented. This is followed by a brief exploration of the current state of concerns facing interracial couples. This is done to provide insight, and present parallels that highlight the evolution of systemic interactions surrounding interracial couples across time. Finally, we conclude with addressing the role of relational therapists in effectively supporting interracial couples through their clinical and research practices. This chapter intends to paint a picture of the need for further research on interventions, theories, and best practices for relational therapy with interracial couples. It also expresses the need for interracial couples' voices to be sought out and elevated as they identify their needs in relational therapy. This chapter primarily focuses on the research done on heterosexual, interracial relationships within the United States. Definitions have been operationalized for a clear understanding of the language and concepts used throughout the chapter. At the conclusion of this chapter, readers will leave with the understanding of the following notions:

1. It is essential for clinicians to have a contextual understanding of the systemic history of anti-miscegenation within the United States.
2. There is a connective thread that binds our country's past to the relevancy of contemporary issues clinicians must be prepared to support interracial couples in addressing.
3. Clinicians must develop contextual awareness and cultural attunement to effectively support interracial couples clinically in creating shared meaning.

The Past is Not Dead

The choice to enter into an interracial relationship has for a long time been frowned upon within the United States. Historically, the choice to racially intermix romantically has been proposed as a cause of mental illness and seen as hate for one's own race. Societal norms, laws, and scare tactics have attempted to discourage the intermixing of different racial groups and have been somewhat effective in keeping people of different races apart. Through experiences of lynching, segregation, media-driven scare tactics, and government-enforced laws on race mixing, interracial couples have been exposed to multiple levels of risk to their physical, mental, and developmental well-being.

As many researchers of interracial couples have echoed (Bacigalupe, 2003; Ham, 2003; Killian, 2001a; McDowell et al., 2005), it is useless to attempt to understand the current experiences of interracial couples in the United States without first acknowledging the racially charged histories that have transgenerationally shaped the way these couples are viewed and treated in this country. DeFrancisco and Palczewski (2007) describe race as "the social identification attached to physical traits such as skin and hair color, despite huge variations among people that are considered a part of a racial group" (p. 22). Dating back to the times of slavery, racial minorities have found themselves at the whims of those identifying as racially dominant in society. "Race as a socially constructed variable, and as a social stimulus, fall into the category of social environment causal conditions" (Leslie & Young, 2015, p. 792). Since the inception of our country, Whites have dominated Blacks solely based on the construct of racial identity. Our history of interracial coupling has been based on one of ownership. It is well documented that White slave owners frequently forced Black women into cohabitation and pregnancy (Franklin, 1966). This process, though frequently occurring, was taboo to speak of, and became all the more so as bloodlines became intermixed across time. With this history of exploiting and demeaning minority populations, the involvement of Whites and Blacks in romantic relationships continues to be a source of anger for many in the Black community. Long (2003) notes that the lasting effects of negative treatment of Blacks by Whites is seen especially in the anger Black women hold for Black men involved with White women.

Between 1661 and 1967, approximately 30 states had anti-miscegenation in their state laws; the first of which were observed in Virginia (Wehrly et al.,1999). One law, implemented in 1662 Virginia, doubled a fine for those engaging in interracial fornication (Kennedy, 2004). Interestingly, the state of Virginia would also go on to be the proverbial tipping point in our nation's history for the deconstruction of these laws. The 1967 Supreme Court ruling of Loving v. Virginia determined that interracial couples of all races were allowed to date, marry, and live in a land that acknowledged the legitimacy of their union. However, this newfound freedom did not come with the respect and social acceptance that interracial couples desired. The picture of interracial love had changed from one of lawlessness to that of pervasive experiences of systemic racial discrimination.

"Racial discrimination may be defined as concrete actions which adversely affect the personal safety, security, or social and economic opportunities of persons whose skin color or ethnic heritage differs from that of the perpetrator" (Killian, 2003, p. 6). Although Loving v. Virginia was the country's best attempt to move toward a narrative of inclusion, the dominant discourse was intolerance. A tone of discrimination continued to be seen through the harsh observance of "formal and informal racial caste rules, meant to... reinforce the lesson of white supremacy, and black subordination" (Kennedy, 2004, p. 221). The common discourse "a system of statements, practices, and institutional structures that share common values" (Hare-Mustin, 1994, p. 19), was intolerance and discrimination against interracial couples and families. As time advanced, clear markers of our nation's undertone regarding interracial couples continued to be felt. In 1983, intolerance toward interracial couples was recognized nationally, when the Texas Civil Liberties Union called for the removal of three justices of the peace who refused to perform interracial marriages (Ho, 1990). This blatant disrespect by multiple members of a larger societal power structure continued to sustain the view of interracial couples as unnatural.

Traditionally interracial couples in the United States have lived in hiding. Laws regarding anti-miscegenation have been noted within the American colonies, as early as

1705 (Cumminos, 1963). From the times of slavery, where Black and Brown people were counted as three-fifths of a White person, oppressors have used ideals of intermixing of the races as a sexual conquest or trivial event of sport. Blacks historically had no control of how they were used intimately for the desires of Whites. As whispers of interracial mixing continued after slavery among lower class Whites and Blacks, societal powers did all they could to keep people of different races from loving one another. Not until the Supreme Court verdict of 1967, which ended all race-based legal restrictions on marriage, were interracial couples allowed to legally live their lives in plain view (Loving v. Virginia, 1967). This victory was a small one in the United States, as interracial relationships continued to be outlawed throughout other countries, such as in South Africa with the Prohibition of Mixed Marriages Act (Union of South Africa, 1949).

Although strides are continuously being made on behalf of interracial and multiracial couples and families, the hurts of their past in this country is not easily forgotten or erased, especially as larger systems continue to inflict pain. In Alabama, anti-miscegenation laws remained on the state books until they were finally overturned in the year 2000, 33 years after the Supreme Court ruling (Hartill, 2001). Alabama, the last state to overturn this law, is simply another demonstration of the power that larger society wields over those in inter-racial couples. By failing to unify their state legislation to the national law for over 30 years, a message was sent by those in power that discrimination was lawful, socially acceptable, and a state norm. In addition, it is important to remember that changes in laws may not change people's beliefs and attitudes and discriminatory attitudes and discourse may persist long after laws have changed.

In conjunction with experiences of being ostracized, interracial couples have frequently been barred from living and raising families in certain areas. There is a long history of mixed-race families being labeled as their minority identifying race while looking for housing, being denied housing based on racial discrimination, and only being able to find housing among accepting minority communities (Villazor, 2018). Stemming from a set of prejudiced beliefs, racism is continually manifested in both overt hostile actions, and subtle acts directed against people of color (Rains, 1998). These experiences have plagued inter-racial couples across our country as systems have historically pushed back against the cul-tural shifts toward interracial coupling.

Since that time of transition in the United States, people have speculated about the impact interracial couples would leave on the fabric of American life. Many feared the influence these couples would have on the status quo of the White dominant social order in America. These fears included the potential influence mixed race couples would have on changing historically upheld laws to the developmental fears of raising a generation of biracial children (Danko et. al., 1997). Despite their ability to be recognized legally as legitimate partnerships, interracial couples continued to be discredited by larger factions of society.

Though interracial couples have continuously been met with push back from larger society, there have always been allies attending to the needs of interracial couples. These allies have been cited in the literature as being present as early as the 1800s, with the movement to support multiracial couples. In Chicago, the Manassah Society for Black-White couples supported this movement of intercoupling from 1830 to 1932 (Poe, 1993). After the Civil Rights movement, the multicultural movement began to make a signifi-cant impact with the creation of Interracial Intercultural Pride Inc., in San Francisco in 1978. The creation of multiple organizations that outwardly supported the unique needs of interracial couples and families were necessary to stake their claim in society, among a mass of the population that continued to attempt to silence them (Poe, 1993). As time has passed, we have come to see the necessity of these external supports, as interracial couples continue to encounter modern-day threats to their existence within our society.

It is Not Even Past

Interracial couples continue to grow as a demographic in this country. There has been an exponential increase in the number of interracial marriages in the decades following the end of the miscegenation laws. Kenney and Kenney (2012) noted from 2010 U.S. Census data that 2.4 million of a total 60 million marriages were interracial. "In 2015, 17% of all U.S. newlyweds had a spouse of a different race or ethnicity, marking more than a fivefold increase since 1967" (Livingston & Brown, 2017, para. 1). The latest projections show "all states experienced an increase in the percent of interracial and interethnic married coupled households from 2000 to 2012–2016" (Rico et al., 2018). This growth shows the need for continued insight into the factors that make these couples unique.

Despite exponential growth, interracial relationships are still commonly viewed as inherently dysfunctional, unnatural, and doomed (Perry & Sutton, 2008). These old narratives threaten our ability to seek out and acknowledge the value that interracial couple configurations bring to our communities as well as our clinical practices. Research literature and writings on interracial couples within the field of marriage and family therapy continues to be a smaller subset of information. The limited information and attention paid to the uniqueness of interracial couples, along with a lack of incorporation of the clients' voice, may affect the efficiency in which relational therapists are able to identify important client factors, and work with these couples in relational therapy.

According to the U.S. Census Bureau, interracial couples make up from 7.4 to 10.2 % of all married-couple households (Rico et al., 2018). Additionally, in recent years there has been an increase in positive approval of interracial couples within the United States, with a current historic high of 94% (McCarthy, 2022). Like most couples, relational distress may lead interracial couples to seek therapy. However, given the diversity in racial, ethnic, and cultural background experiences, interracial couples are likely to face more challenges than same-race couples (MacNeil & Adamsons, 2014). To manage the relational nuances influenced by racial differences and societal messages, therapists must understand the unique systemic circumstances that affect interracial relationships and how these factors influence clinical treatment.

The impact of suffering through an extended history of segregation and fear has influenced many interracial couples today to seek a lifestyle of invisibility. Fusco (2010) found that couples in interracial relationships are more likely than couples in same-race relationships to hide their relationships due to fear of rejection. Having to make substantial decisions regarding their visibility to the outside world, interracial couples have gone on to experience subsequent difficulties within the safety of their relationship. Feeling unsafe to connect to other portions of society, interracial couples may express frustrations solely with one another (Solsberry, 1994). Feelings of being unsafe have been palpable in recent years, as the overturning of laws legalizing abortion (Roe v. Wade, 1973), and the impending challenge of affirmative action (Fisher v. University of Texas, 2016), initially led many Americans to believe there could be a discernible threat to the laws upholding interracial marriages in the United States (Loving v Virginia, 1967; Ciesmeier & Goodwin, 2022).

Some research suggests that people in interracial relationships experience more conflicts than same-race couples, thus creating a risk of partners feeling unsafe with their relationship (Porter and Thomas, 2012). Brownridge (2016) found indications "that interracial couples in the U.S. have higher rates of intimate partner violence than same-race relationships" (p. 865). It is plausible that this is due to the lack of visibility and connection interracial couples find in our society. If these external and internal constraints are experienced on a regular basis, interracial couples are sure to suffer a negative impact in their lives.

Leslie and Young (2015) noted that racial differences did not just touch on the difference in skin color, but to the history of social interactions and experiences tied to one's race (p. 792). The ways in which interracial couples have historically come to their own personal understanding of race goes on to shape their interactions within their relationship, as well as with the larger society. Circumstances of this nature are currently making situations harder as partners may struggle to speak with their partner about their personal experiences regarding race. As these concepts are heavily charged in our daily observations within our country, couples may not have a history discussing issues such as race, policing tactics, and politics in racially mixed settings. This can lead to an overwhelming avoidance of these discussion topics within the relationship. In connection, Zebroski (1999) found that Black and White interracial couples have come to expect negative reactions from members of their own racial groups, as well as from individuals of other racial groups. Adjustment toward the expectation to be treated in demeaning ways from one's own ethnic group may partially account for an increase in the vigilance of these individuals to remain safe as a couple unit.

Therapists should recognize the ways in which varying systems have colluded to sequester interracial couples into a realm of invisibility and silence. It has been noted that at multiple levels of our society, interracial and multiracial units have historically been stricken from our collective memories. This has been a common issue in the past, with interracial couples and families rarely being visible in mainstream images throughout society. Bell and Hastings (2015) noted that interracial couples and families must become "normalized in our visual landscapes" (p. 768). These researchers believed that without the push for the inclusion of interracial couples and families in our advertising, programming, and books, there will continue to be a failure of our society to align with the actual trends of our changing population (Bell & Hastings, 2015). With global move toward diversity, equity, and inclusion movements in recent years there has been an uptick in interracial couples in advertising campaigns. Yet researchers still find "ads depicting Black and White couples elicited more negative emotions and attitudes toward a brand than comparable ads showing same-race couples" (Bhat et al., 2018). This reality indicates that as the world takes a step in the right direction, our work with interracial couples will still be laced with the nuance of society confronting its discriminatory leanings on a regular basis.

In addition to the old adages that have plagued the circumstances of interracial couples in the United States, they are continually threatened by a barrage of new factors impacting our entire society. During the COVID-19 pandemic, African Americans and Latinx Americans experienced a rate of hospitalization approximately two times greater than White Americans (Center for Disease Control and Prevention, 2022). The disparity in infection, hospitalization, and death rate is one that is connected to social determinants of health that continually remain overlooked in minoritized populations in the United States. The threat of financial ruin, prolonged symptoms, and death is a concern for interracial couples living through the time period of COVID-19.

While the entire nation has dealt with the experiences of the post-pandemic world, people of color, specifically those in interracial couples, may be charged with making more specific decisions regarding their connection to specific socio-political movements. Members of interracial couples are in a unique position to determine their engagement and support of causes such as The Black Lives Matter movement, and the Stop AAPI Hate community. Whether in solidarity with a partner, or in respect to their own ethnic background, couple members must take extra care with deciding and making known their stance on these issues. While lending support may account for a deeper connection within their relationship, there is still a risk of the couple losing support from surrounding family and friends that do not share the same connection to the cause.

To fully grasp the extent to which interracial couples are affected daily by their racially mixed relationship status, it is important to look at areas that are viewed as clinically unique to these couples. Many of the unique clinical challenges identified by the literature on interracial couples can be categorized within the realm of support. Many researchers ascertain support as a key intervention area for interracial couples seeking relational treatment (Debrosse et al, 2022). Support is defined as the act or process of receiving practical and emotional assistance from a network of people or entities in which the subject is regularly involved. The prevalence of the presentation of clinical issues related to social support and community acceptance have been explored by many researchers in the field of marital and family therapy (Csizmadia et al., 2015; Estrada, 2005; Killian, 2003; Leslie & Young, 2015; Poulsen, 2003). Although these two issues are repetitively explored in the literature, this does not imply that these are the only unique or relevant issues to interracial couples. Challenges such as managing societal disapproval, navigating the effects of racial privilege, and discrimination are additional stress factors added to the relationships of interracial couples.

The current concerns faced by interracial couples are at risk of becoming compounded by the historical threats these relationships are commonly exposed to. This includes the threat of intimate partner violence (Brownridge, 2016), lack of social and familial support (Brummett & Afifi, 2019; Grether & Jones 2021), conflict management, and relationship instability (MacNeil & Adamsons, 2014). These issues in conjunction with the socio-political concerns of the time create an increase in needs of interracial couples as they seek clinical services. The growing needs of these clients call for an expansive outlook to be maintained by relational therapists working to serve this population.

An Ode to The Future

As we prepare to face the current and future needs of interracial couples, it is imperative that therapists explore ways to grow their skills to support this population. As systemic therapists, we believe in the importance of people having access to therapy with competently trained therapists. Systemic therapists strive to effectively serve couples and families of all varieties; thus it is imperative for them to be educationally versed in the unique life issues that might bring interracial couples into therapy and the barriers that might hinder their engagement in therapy. As interracial couples are at risk for being stigmatized, marginalized, and overlooked in our country, it is essential that therapists understand the influence of supportive relationships and connections on the relationship patterns of interracial couples and how that can influence their engagement in couples therapy.

Therapists must recognize the ongoing relevance of the social environment in which couples interact with one another. It is undeniable that interracial couples face distinct challenges that shape the course and quality of their relationship. The experiences that impact these couples in their daily lives do not disappear as they enter the therapy room. In fact, the therapeutic environment is another social space in which couples can find themselves feeling supported or scrutinized. It is for that reason that relational therapists must become proactive in their actions to learn and understand the needs of interracial couples. A formative step to accomplish this comes with considering continuing education around this subject area. Therapists should seek out training, continuing education credits, conference curriculum, and current literature on doing effective therapeutic work with interracial couples.

Implications for Clinical Practice

Acknowledging the current contextual difficulties interracial couples face as a threat to their mental health, physical safety, and relationship well-being, many may not deem the therapy room as a safe place to bring the problems of their relationship. There may be a desire to minimize contention and downplay difficult experiences tied to overlapping contemporary issues. Therapists do well to remember that given the past societal hurts, many interracial couples could benefit from a combination of therapeutic support, and support from other external outlets. This may come through the form of support groups, psychoeducational materials, and interventions for coping with stressors (Negy & Snyder, 2000). These resources can also be found through their engagement with and practice of religious or spiritual traditions (Vazquez & Goodlow, 2019). Modern-day outlets that may be of assistance in connecting interracial couples to support include use of social media, multicultural magazines, and readings, as well as video media addressing real-life issues of interracial couples and multiracial families. To support relational therapists in starting this journey, a resource list is included within this chapter.

As therapists consider the societal levels of stress and anxiety accumulated within the last decade, we must be sure to not overlook the unique presentation of interracial couples in connection to these happenings. To do so would be to situate oneself within the dominant discourse, denying the influence of privilege and power that shapes our experiences of the world. It is important that as a field of systemic practitioners, there is forward movement with intent set on creating space for identifying the clinical needs of all interracial couple configurations. This implies accounting for diversity in the racial, ethnic, sexual, gender, and ability of these couples. This can be introduced to one's therapeutic practice by allowing more space for interracial couples to identify themselves. By creating space for more inclusive gathering of demographic information from clients, therapists will be able to identify the unique intricacies of their identity. It is unrealistic to box clients into five categories of race in a very colorful society. Creating more inclusive methods for collecting this information can assist in identifying clients more accurately within our practice records. These are a few of the ways that relational therapists can begin to shift the dominant culture to one that better values our interracial couple clients.

Therapists can also assist interracial couples in their clinical practice by keeping an eye on the expression of common couple problems, such as communication issues, parenting, financial issues, and life adjustments (Leslie & Young, 2015). As most interracial couples will present in therapy for these issues, therapists must be aware of the ways in which the couple's connections to larger systems may be shaping their experiences of common problems. The experience of interracial couples having similar clinical issues as same-race couples, such as communication issues, may be ripe with added complexity due to differences in racial, cultural, or ethnic backgrounds (Motoyoshi, 1990). These added complexities are factors that go on to affect the course of a relationship for interracial couples. Multiple studies looking at marital satisfaction, stability, and longevity suggest that interracial couples experience lower levels across all areas compared to same-race couples (Bratter & King, 2008; Debrosse et al., 2022; Fu & Wolfinger, 2011).

Smith and Trimble's (2016) meta-analysis of client experiences in treatment found that "diverse clients tend to see therapist's multicultural competence as highly related to, yet distinct from, other positive counselor attributes" (p. 64). A therapist's ability to join well with interracial couple clients does not indicate that their minority clients feel comfortable addressing issues of racism, privilege, or discrimination freely within the therapy room. This may also be amplified, given the visible racial, ethnic, or cultural background of the therapist. In addition, researchers found that culturally diverse clients are "more likely to prematurely discontinue treatment when their therapist does not demonstrate multicultural competence" (Smith & Trimble, 2016, p. 64).

As relational therapists, it is our duty to find ways to better acknowledge and demonstrate competence in addressing the needs of interracial couples. Literature historically notes that the first step for therapists to build knowledge and efficiency when working with these populations is to identify and understand one's own beliefs about interracial relationships (Estrada, 2005; Kenney & Kenney, 2012). Therapists must acknowledge the power we hold, and how it is wielded in the therapy room with not one, but two clients with varying needs and lived realities.

It is recognized that only one piece of literature can be found that examines the perspective of relational therapists on working with interracial couples in therapy. Poulsen's (2003) research noted that out of 140 members of the American Association for Marriage and Family Therapy (AAMFT) selected to participate in interviews about working with interracial couples, 41 returned letters noting they had insufficient experience working with interracial couples, or because they were currently no longer in clinical practice" (p.167). Seven participants were asked questions about their initial response to interracial couples, common client issues and concerns, and experiences of providing relational therapy. Their responses indicated the use of a non-expert stance to provide space for clients' narratives, concerns about therapeutic techniques being sufficient enough to deal with issues related to race, and the maintenance of curiosity to learn about the experiences of each individual (Poulsen, 2003).

Coupled with these attempts of inclusiveness, Poulsen (2003) also highlights therapists continued internal struggle with their thoughts and beliefs of interracial relationships. It is important to note that without substantial examination of our knowledge and practices of relational therapy with interracial couples as a field, we are at risk of allowing our personal beliefs to color our clinical conceptualizations and work with these couples. Clinicians who provide therapy to interracial couples need to assist dyads with managing both family, and larger societal disapproval, while also navigating the effects of racial privilege (Leslie & Young, 2015). This charge is a large one to lead if relational therapists are not conscious about their personal beliefs about interracial couples and power exhibited by larger systems in which they are situated.

An increase in the world's population and globalization have created a steady incline of interracial coupling. Working with differences in cultures between interracial couples of two minority groups may lead to instances of detachment from each individuals' personal culture and the dominant culture. It is noted that language barriers may contribute to difficulties in drawing on a shared social-support system including friends, faith-based institutions, or other community groups (Negy & Snyder, 2000). Versatility in helping interracial couples find supportive ways to connect and develop personal meaning may call for the use of more diverse clinical techniques and tools. Creating meaning and connection through shared tasks such as community cooking, gardening, or learning a new skill such as dancing could work as outlets for interracial couples to create new experiences together while building community.

A key factor that assists with helping therapists prepare for such detailed work is the use of relevant educational materials. In recent years the clinical literature on interracial couples has slowly grown, denoting further reference to clinically focused writings, books, and theoretical tools to assist therapists specifically in learning about therapeutic work with interracial couples. Robinson (2017) also suggested that "therapists working with interracial couples must develop the skills of using the research literature to inform their work with clients. This also includes matching clinical theory with pertinent clinical problems, thus creating the highest possibility for success" (p. 282).

Theoretical-based literature includes examples of working with interracial couples using narrative therapy (Kim et al, 2012), emotionally focused therapy (Dansby Olufowote et al., 2022), and medical family therapy (Samman et al., 2022). Recent literature focusing on interracial couples also addresses a variety of clinical issues including parenting (Roy et al., 2020), same-sex relationships (Rosenthal et al., 2019; Sully et al., 2022), and relationship satisfaction (Brooks, 2021). This information creates a starting point for clinicians as they assist these couples with addressing contemporary issues and concerns.

Along with the use of relevant clinical materials to guide relational therapy practices, it is imperative for therapists to break the code of silence in clinical supervision about their self-of-the-therapist issues related to race, privilege, and power (Estrada, 2005). Coming to a comprehensive understanding of these issues can assist therapists and supervisors with identifying how personal locations and identities impress upon their work with interracial couples. The process of being curious can help therapists remain open to the shifting needs of treating interracial relationships in connection to their socio-political context.

Implications for Research

As we sharpen our clinical minds to address the contemporary issues of interracial couples in the therapy room, we must recognize that best practices will be formulated based on growing research. It is important to note that much of the systemic research literature about interracial couples focuses on clinical areas of treatment and clinical growth areas for clinicians, and also tends to be less empirical and more practice-oriented (Leslie & Young, 2015). There is a dearth of clinical writings that use interracial couples as a direct source of information on their personal experiences, hopes, and desires for using relational forms of therapy. If we consider the increased demographic growth, lack of systematic literature, and the absence of the clients' voice in research, it is imperative for researchers to start at ground level as they begin to design research agenda that promote efficiency in addressing the needs relevant to the experiences of interracial couples. An increase in qualitative research studies will be sure to speak to the lived reality of interracial couples.

Kilian's (2001b) qualitative research reflected couples' hopes that helping professionals would act as strong advocates when they worked with interracial couples experiencing difficulties, as opposed to pointing to racially based differences as a reason for interracial couples to give up on their union. This research gave voice to interracial couples by asking them candidly what would be useful from professionals during their engagement with couples therapy. This inquiry sought to gather information on interracial couples' perceptions of relational therapy, and the unique needs they may bring to the therapeutic setting. These qualitative questions gave members of interracial couples the ability to state what they believed marriage and family therapists should know when working with this population. These questions were asked with the intention of getting direct user feedback to offer insight to current practitioners on culturally competent care.

As researchers it is important to be vigilant in the way we are exploring the full realities of interracial couples. Measurement constructs may not take into account the full depth of daily adaptations needed to live as interracial couples. The scarcity of research on interracial couples' mirrors society's fixation on racial segregation. This essentially impedes upon the research of marriage and family therapists and has left us with a shortage of information pertaining to the experience of interracial and interethnic couples identifying outside of Black and White racial categories.

In reality, the limited writings about these couples usually entail information pertaining to marital satisfaction, communication, and differences in language (Bacigalupe, 2003; Negy & Snyder, 2000; Schueths, 2015; Song, Bergen, & Schumm, 1995). Some of these writings focus on the cultural intersections experienced within these couples, given the specific influence that cultural background may play in interracial couples with partners presenting from one or more ethnically different locations.

Researchers can assist in developing a more concise subset of literature but attending to the proper use of terminology. The term *interracial* is often used interchangeably with intercultural and interethnic, and is sometimes referred to as *inter-married*, *intermixing*, or *heterogamy* by researchers and in popular culture (Henderson, 2000; Reiter & Gee, 2008). This practice can muddle the attention paid to the uniqueness of these couples and their presence within systemic literature. Additionally, in the United States, most systemic literature focuses on Black-White couplings and no other racial coupling constellations.

Researchers should realize that any combination of racial, ethnic, and cultural mixing is sure to add to the variation of stories that comprise the lives of interracial couples. Wang (2012) reported that 9% of Whites marry out of their race compared to 17% of Blacks, 26% of Hispanics, and 28% of Asians. With other racial and ethnic populations intermarrying, there is sure to be an intersection of cultural, ethnic, and racial experiences as these couples operate within the dominant American culture of Whiteness. With the varying rates of intermarriage, it is important for clinicians to not overlook the needs of interracial couple combinations where neither partner is White (Jacobs & Labov, 2002).

Conclusion

With over five decades since the legalization of intermarriage, numbers across the country continue to steadily climb. Though there are new challenges that present themselves, our current place in history may be seen as formative for interracial couples in the United States. Being more visible than ever, interracial couples have the opportunity to find connective community and support through the difficulties they face. Visibility has effectively translated to interracial couples gaining continued national support. This is demonstrated by improved racial and ethnic measures on our most recent national census (Jones et al., 2021), and also as demonstrated in the passing of the Respect for Marriage Act (2022), which requires all states to federally recognize interracial marriages. These shifts in governmental recognition and protection are a step in the right direction of changing the contextual experience of interracial couples in our country. Remaining aware of contextual factors impacting these couples at the local, national, and global level is just one effective measure therapists can take. Therapists must continue to build upon this step by improving the efficiency of their work by demonstrating cultural humility, attunement, and advocacy for the needs of their interracial couples. Engagement with current literature, resource cites, and continuing education will help therapists to be prepared for the charge of creating safe and supportive spaces to provide resources and care to interracial couples.

References

Bacigalupe, G. (2003). Intercultural therapy with Latino immigrants and white partners: Crossing borders coupling. *Journal of Couple & Relationship Therapy, 2*(2/3), 131–149. https://doi.org/10.1300/j398v02n02

Bell, G. C., & Hastings, S. O. (2015). Exploring parental approval and disapproval for Black and White interracial couples. *Journal of Social Issues, 71*, 755–771. https://doi.org/10.1111/josi.12147

Bhat, S., Myers, S., & Royne, M. (2018). Interracial couples in ads: Do consumers' gender and racial differences affect their reactions? *Journal of Current Issues & Research in Advertising, 39*(2), 160–177. https://doi.org/10.1080/10641734.2018.1428249

Bratter, J. L., & King, R. B. (2008). "But will it last?": Marital instability among interracial and same-race couples. *Family Relations: An Interdisciplinary Journal of Applied Family Studies, 57*(2), 160–171. https://doi.org/10.1111/j.1741-3729.2008.00491.x

Brooks, J. E. (2021). Differences in satisfaction? A meta-analytic review of interracial and intraracial relationships. *Marriage & Family Review.* https://doi.org/10.1080/01494929.2021.1937443

Brownridge, D. A. (2016). Intimate partner violence in interracial relationships. *Journal of Family Violence, 31*, 865–875. https://doi.org/10.1007/s10896-016-9809-z

Brummett, E. A., & Afifi, T. D. (2019). A grounded theory of interracial romantic partners' expectations for support and strain with family members. *Journal of Family Communication, 19*(3), 191–212. https://doi.org/10.1080/15267431.2019.1623220

Centers for Disease Control and Prevention. (2022, December 28). Risk for COVID-19 infection, hospitalization, and death by Race/Ethnicity. *Centers for Disease Control and Prevention.* Retrieved February 28, 2023, from www.cdc.gov/coronavirus/2019-ncov/covid-data/investigations-discovery/hospitalization-death-by-race-ethnicity.html

Ciesemier, K., & Goodwin, M (2022, June, 12). *How Dismantling Roe Puts Interracial Marriage at Risk* [Audio Podcast]. www.aclu.org/podcast/how-dismantling-roe-puts-interracial-marriage-at-risk

Csizmadia, A., Leslie, L. A., & Nazarian, R. (2015). Understanding and treating interracial families. In S. Browing & K. Palsley (Eds.), *Understanding and treating the contemporary family: Translating research into practice* (pp. 89–107). New York, NY: Routledge.

Cumminos, P. (1963, December 17). The Harvard Crimson. Retrieved from www.thecrimson.com/article/1963/12/17/race-marriage-and-law-pamerican-racism/

Danko, G. P., Miyamoto, R. H., Foster, J. E., Johnson, R. C., Andrade, N. N., Yates, A., & Edman, J. L. (1997). Psychiatric symptoms in offspring of within vs across racial/ethnic marriages. *Cultural Diversity and Mentadl Health, 3*, 273–277. https://doi.org/10.1037/1099-9809.3.4.273

Dansby Olufowote, R. A., Samman, S. K., & Frick, H. (2022). Medical family therapy with diverse populations part II: Understanding & treating interracial & international couples with chronic illness using emotionally focused MedFT. *International Journal of Systemic Therapy, 33*(4), 250–275. https://doi.org/10.1080/2692398X.2022.2125264

Debrosse, R., Thai, S., & Brieva, T. (2022). When skinfolk are kinfolk: Higher perceived support and acceptance characterize close samerace (vs Interracial) relationships for people of color. *Journal of Social Issues*. https://doi.org/10.1111/josi.12534

DeFrancisco, V. P. & Palczewski, C. H. (2007). Communicating gender diversity: A critical approach. Los Angeles, CA: Sage Publications.

Estrada, D. (2005). Supervision of cross-cultural couples therapy: Giving voice to the code of silence in the supervision and therapy room. *Journal of Family Psychotherapy*, 16(4), 17–30. https://doi.org/10.1300/J085v16n04_02

Fisher v. University of Texas at Austin, 579 U.S. (2016)

Franklin, J. H. (1966). *From slavery to freedom*. New York, NY: Knopf.

Fu, V. K. & Wolfinger, N.H. (2011). Broken boundaries or broken marriages? Racial intermarriage and divorce in the United States. *Social Science Quarterly*, 92, 1096–1117. https://doi.org/10.1111/j.1540-6237.2011.00809.x

Fusco, R.A. (2010). Intimate partner violence in interracial couples: A comparison to white and ethnic minority monoracial couples. *Journal of Interpersonal Violence*, 25, 1785–1800. https://doi.org/10.1177/0886260509354510

Grether, S. T., & Jones, A. (2021). Examining the relationship between social support and interracial divorce in Louisiana. *Journal of Family Issues*, 42(8), 1831–1851. https://doi.org/10.1177/0192513X20957363

Ham, M. D. (2003). Asian American intermarriage: A socio-political construction and a treatment dilemma. *Journal of Couple & Relationship Therapy*, 2(2/3), 151–162. https://doi.org/10.1300/J398v02n02_11

Hare-Mustin, R. T. (1994). Discourses in the mirrored room: A postmodern analysis of therapy. *Family Process*, 33(1), 19–35. https://doi.org/10.1111/j.1545-5300.1994.00019.x

Hartill, L. (2001). A brief history of interracial marriage, *Christian Science Monitor*, 93, 15. Retrieved from www.csmonitor.com/2001/0725/p15s1.html

Henderson, D. (2000). Racial/ethnic intermarried couples and marital interaction: Marital issues and problem solving. *Sociological Focus*, 33, 421–438. https://doi.org/10.1080/00380237.2000.10571178

Ho, M.K. (1990). *Intermarried couples in therapy*. Springfield, IL: Charles C. Thomas.

Jacobs, J. A., & Labov, T. G. (2002). Gender differentials in intermarriage among sixteen race and ethnic groups. *Sociological Forum*, 17, 621–646. https://doi.org/10.1023/A:1021029507937

Jones, N., Marks, R., Ramirez, R., & Rios-Vargas, M. (2021, August 12). 2020 Census illuminates racial and ethnic composition of the country. Census.gov. Retrieved March 2, 2023, from www.census.gov/library/stories/2021/08/improved-race-ethnicity-measures-reveal-united-states-population-much-more-multiracial.html

Kennedy, R. (2004). *Interracial intimacies: Sex, marriage, identity, and adoption*. New York, NY: Vintage.

Kenney, K. R., & Kenney, M. E. (2012). Contemporary US multiple heritage couples, individuals, and families: Issues, concerns, and counseling implications. *Counselling Psychology Quarterly*, 25(2), 99–112. https://doi.org/10.1080/09515070.2012.674682

Killian, K. D. (2001a). Crossing borders: Race, gender, and their intersections in interracial couples. *Journal of Feminist Family Therapy: An International Forum*, 13(1), 1–31. https://doi.org/10.1300/J086v13n01_01

Killian, K. D. (2001b). Reconstituting racial histories and identities: The narratives of interracial couples. *Journal of Marital and Family Therapy*, 27(1), 27–42. https://doi.org/10.1111/j.1752-0606.2001.tb01137.x

Killian, K. D. (2003). Homogamy outlaws: Interracial couples' strategic responses to racism and to partner differences. *Journal of Couple & Relationship Therapy*, 2(2/3), 3–21. https://doi.org/10.1300/J398v02n02_02

Killian, K. D. (2012). Resisting and complying with homogamy: Interracial couples' narratives about partner differences. *Counselling Psychology Quarterly*, 25(2), 125–135. https://doi.org/10.1080/09515070.2012.680692

Killian, K. D. (2013). *Interracial couples, intimacy, & therapy: Crossing racial borders*. New York, NY: Columbia University Press.

Kim, H., Prouty, A. M., & Robertson, P. E. (2012). Narrative therapy with intercultural couples: A case study. *Journal of Family Psychotherapy*, 23, 273–286. https://doi.org/10.1080/08975353.2012.735591

Leslie, L. A., & Young, J. L. (2015). Interracial couples in therapy: Common themes and issues. *Journal of Social Issues, 71,* 788–803. https://doi.org/10.1111/josi.12149

Livingston, G., & Brown, A. (2017, September 08). Intermarriage in the U.S. 50 years after Loving v. Virginia. Retrieved from www.pewsocialtrends.org/2017/05/18/intermarriage-in-the-u-s-50-years-after-loving-v-virginia/

Long, J. (2003). Interracial and intercultural lesbian couples: The incredibly true adventures of two women in love. *Journal of Couple & Relationship Therapy, 2(2/3),* 85–101. https://doi.org/10.1300/J398v02n02_07

Loving v. Virginia, 388 U.S. (1967).

MacNeil, T. A., & Adamsons, K. (2014). A bioecological view of interracial/same-race couple conflict. *International Journal of Conflict Management, 25,* 243–260. doi:10.1108/IJCMA-08-2012-0063

McCarthy, J. (2022, February 21). U.S. approval of interracial marriage at new high of 94%. Gallup.com. Retrieved February 28, 2023, from https://news.gallup.com/poll/354638/approval-interracial-marriage-new-high.aspx

McDowell, T., Ingoglia, L., Serizawa, T., Holland, C., Dashiell, J. J., & Stevens, C. (2005). Raising multiracial awareness in family therapy through critical conversations. *Journal of Marital and Family Therapy, 31,* 399–411. https://doi.org/10.1111/j.1752-0606.2005.tb01579.x

Motoyoshi, M.M. (1990). The experience of mixed-race people: Some thoughts and theories. The *Journal of Ethnic Studies, 18,* 77–89. Retrieved from https://eric.ed.gov/?id=EJ419413

Negy, C., & Snyder, D. K. (2000). Relationship satisfaction of Mexican American and non-Hispanic White American interethnic couples: Issues of acculturation and clinical intervention. *Journal of Marital and Family Therapy, 26,* 293–304. https://doi.org/10.1111/j.1752-0606.2000.tb00299.x

Perry, B.C., & Sutton, M. (2008). Policing the colour line: Violence against those in intimate interracial relationships. *Race, Gender and Class, 15(3/4),* 240–261. Retrieved from www.jstor.org/stable/41674663?seq=1#metadata_info_tab_contents

Poe, J. (1993, May 03). Multiracial people want a single name that fits. Retrieved from www.chicagotribune.com/news/ct-xpm-1993-05-03-9305030077-story.html

Porter, H., & Thomas, D.T. (2012). "We told you that's how they are": responses to White women in abusive intimate relationships with men of color. *Deviant Behavior, 33,* 469–491. https://doi.org/10.1080/01639625.2011.636661

Poulsen, S. S. (2003). Therapists' perspectives on working with interracial couples. *Journal of Couple & Relationship Therapy, 2(2/3),* 163–177. doi:10.1300/J398v02n02_12

Rains, F. V. (1998). Is the benign really harmless? Deconstructing some "benign" manifestations of operationalized white privilege. In J. L. Kincheloe, S. R. Steinberg, N. M. Rodrfuez, & R. E. Chennault (Eds.), *White reign: Deploying whiteness in America* (pp. 77–102). New York, NY: St. Martin's Griffin.

Reiter, M. J., & Gee, C. B. (2008). Open communication and partner support in intercultural and interfaith romantic relationships: A relational maintenance approach. *Journal of Social and Personal Relationships, 25(4),* 539–559. https://doi.org/10.1177/0265407508090872

Respect for Marriage Act, H.R.8404, 117th Cong. (2022) www.congress.gov/bill/117th-congress/house-bill/8404

Rico, B., Kreider, R., & Anderson, L. (2018, July 09). Growth in interracial and interethnic married-couple households. Retrieved from www.census.gov/library/stories/2018/07/interracial-marriages.html

Roe v Wade, 410 U.S. 113 (1973)

Rosenthal, L., Deosaran, A., Young, D. L., & Starks, T. J. (2019). Relationship stigma and well-being among adults in interracial and same-sex relationships. *Journal of Social and Personal Relationships, 36(11–12),* 3408–3428. https://doi.org/10.1177/0265407518822785

Robinson, M. C. (2017). Black and White biracial marriage in the United States. *The Family Journal, 25,* 278–282. https://doi.org/10.1177/1066480717711117

Roy, R. N., James, A., Brown, T. L., Craft, A., & Mitchell, Y. (2020). Relationship satisfaction across the transition to parenthood among interracial couples: An integrative model. *Journal of Family Theory & Review, 12(1),* 41–53. https://doi.org/10.1111/jftr.12365

Samman, S. K., Frick, H. A., & Dansby Olufowote, R. A. (2022). Medical family therapy with diverse populations part I: Interracial couples navigating infertility, racialized pregnancy, and pregnancy loss. *International Journal of Systemic Therapy*, *33*(4), 227–249. https://doi.org/10.1080/26923 98X.2022.2128623

Schueths, A. M. (2015). Barriers to interracial marriage? Examining policy issues concerning sueU.S. Citizens married to undocumented Latino/a immigrants. *Journal of Social Issues*, *71*, 804–820. doi:10.1111/josi.12150

Smith, T. B., & Trimble, J. E. (2016). Therapist multicultural competence: A meta-analysis of client experiences in treatment. In Smith, T. B., & Trimble, J. E (Eds.), *Foundations of multicultural psychology: Research to inform effective practice* (pp. 49–64). Washington, DC: American Psychological Association. doi:10.1037/14733-003

Solsberry, P. W. (1994). Interracial couples in the United States of America: Implications for mental health counseling. *Journal of Mental Health Counseling, 16*, 304–317. Retrieved from https://psyc net.apa.org/record/1995-10522-001

Song, J. A., Bergen, M. B., & Schumm, W. R. (1995). Sexual satisfaction among Korean-American couples in the midwestern United States. *Journal Of Sex & Marital Therapy, 21*(3), 147–158. doi:10.1080/00926239508404395

Sully, H., Perrone, K., Barrera, S., & Simon-Dack, S. (2022). Preconscious categorization impacts how interracial same-sex couples are perceived by others: Implications for counseling and super-vision. *Journal of Gay & Lesbian Mental Health, 26*(4), 403–425. https://doi.org/10.1080/19359 705.2021.2012732

Union of South Africa. (1949). Prohibition of mixed marriages act, Act No. 55 of 1949.

Vazquez, V., Otero, I., & Goodlow, J. (2019). Relationship stigma and Black-White interracial marital satisfaction: The mediating role of religious/spiritual well-being. *Mental Health, Religion & Culture*, *22*(3), 305–318. https://doi.org/10.1080/13674676.2019.1620189

Villazor, R. C. (2018). Residential segregation and interracial marriages. *Fordham Law Review*, *86*(6), 7th ser., 2716–2726. Retrieved from https://ir.lawnet.fordham.edu/cgi/viewcontent.cgi?arti cle=5516&context=flr

Wang, W. (2012). The rise of interracial marriage: Rates, characteristic vary by race and gender. Washington D.C.: *Pew Research Center Publications*. Retrieved from www.pewsocialtrends.org/ 2012/02/16/the-rise-of-intermarriage/

Wehrly, B., Kenney, K. R., & Kenney, M. E. (1999). *Counseling multiracial families*. Thousand Oaks, CA: Sage.

Zebroski, S. A. (1999). Black-white intermarriages: The racial and gender dynamics of support and opposition. *Journal of Black Studies. 30*, 123–132. Retrieved from www.jstor.org/stable/2645 896?seq=1#metadata_info_tab_contents

Resources

Resource Guides

1. Ackerman Institute for the Family: The Multiracial Family and Couples Project – www.ackerman. org/research/the-multiracial-family-project/
2. Loving Day Campaign – https://lovingday.org/resources/
3. University of Michigan: Interracial Resources – https://guides.lib.umich.edu/c.php?g=282906&p= 1885158

Books

4. Karis, T. A., & Killian, K. D. (2011). *Intercultural couples: Exploring diversity in intimate relationships*. Taylor and Francis.
5. Killian, K. D. (2013). *Interracial couples, intimacy, and therapy: Crossing racial borders*. Columbia University Press.
6. Roy, R. N., & Rollins, A. (2019). Biracial families: Crossing boundaries, blending cultures, and challenging racial ideologies. Springer .
7. Thomas, V., Wetchler, J. L., & Karis, T. A. (2003). *Clinical issues with interracial couples: Theories and research*. Haworth Press.

Readings

8. Berkley, C. (2021, February 21). *The difficulty finding a therapist as an interracial couple.* Medium. Retrieved March 2, 2023, from https://zora.medium.com/the-difficulty-finding-a-therapist-as-an-interracial-couple-9c2d765a6c46
9. Dansby Olufowote, R. A., Seshadri, G., & Samman, S. K. (2022, August 16). *Why your interracial/multinational couples might be dropping out: A self-of-the-therapist exploration of critical factors.* Family Therapy Magazine. Retrieved March 2, 2023, from https://ftm.aamft.org/why-your-interracial-multinational-couples-might-be-dropping-out-a-self-of-the-therapist-exploration-of-critical-factors/
10. Stritof, S. (2020, June 20). *How to overcome the different challenges of an interracial marriage.* Verywell Mind. Retrieved March 2, 2023, from www.verywellmind.com/interracial-marriage-challenges-2303129

Academic Articles

11. Brown, C. C., Williams, Z., & Durtschi, J. A. (2019). Trajectories of interracial heterosexual couples: A longitudinal analysis of relationship quality and separation. *Journal of Marital and Family Therapy, 45*(4), 650–667. https://doi.org/10.1111/jmft.12363
12. Brownridge, D. A., Taillieu, T., Chan, K. L., & Piotrowski, C. (2021). Understanding the elevated prevalence of intimate partner violence in interracial relationships. *Journal of Interpersonal Violence, 36*(7–8), NP3844-NP3868. https://doi.org/10.1177/0886260518781803
13. Calderon, P. S. P., Wong, J. D., & Hodgdon, B. T. (2022). A scoping review of the physical health and psychological wellbeing of individuals in interracial romantic relationships. *Family Relations: An Interdisciplinary Journal of Applied Family Studies.* https://doi.org/10.1111/fare.12765
14. Fall, S. L., & Wittenberg, B. M. (2022). Experiences of white partners in black–white romantic relationships in the united states: A qualitative study. *Family Relations: An Interdisciplinary Journal of Applied Family Studies.* https://doi.org/10.1111/fare.12778
15. Feustel, I. D. B. (2022). It all started at a post office: Interracial love and its complexities. *Journal of Child and Family Studies.* https://doi.org/10.1007/s10826-022-02248-7
16. Genç, E., & Su, Y. (2021). Black and white couples: Exploring the role of religiosity on perceived racial discrimination and relationship satisfaction. *American Journal of Family Therapy.* https://doi.org/10.1080/01926187.2021.1958269
17. Han, B. (2021). Race, gender, and power in Asian American interracial marriages. *Social Science Research, 96.* https://doi.org/10.1016/j.ssresearch.2021.102542
18. Hart, J. S. (2022). Changing eyes and ears: Using racial lifemaps to address microaggressions with interracial couples. *Journal of Couple & Relationship Therapy.* https://doi.org/10.1080/15332691.2022.2053261
19. Lemay, E. P., Jr., & Teneva, N. (2020). Accuracy and bias in perceptions of racial attitudes: Implications for interracial relationships. *Journal of Personality and Social Psychology, 119*(6), 1380–1402. https://doi.org/10.1037/pspi0000236.supp
20. Lengyell, M., Weststrate, N. M., & Moodley, R. (2022). Interracial couples' experiences with coparenting school-aged mixed-race children. *Cultural Diversity and Ethnic Minority Psychology.* https://doi.org/10.1037/cdp0000556
21. Ngcongo, M. (2021). Re-imagining the surveillance power of the close social network on interracial couples. *Journal of Family Studies.* https://doi.org/10.1080/13229400.2021.1908158
22. Stillwell, A., & Lowery, B. S. (2021). Gendered racial boundary maintenance: Social penalties for White women in interracial relationships. *Journal of Personality and Social Psychology, 121*(3), 548–572. https://doi.org/10.1037/pspi0000332

28

SINO-AMERICAN FAMILY THERAPY

A Chinese Perspective on Traditional Western Family Therapy Methods

John K. Miller, Hu Yaorui, and Dai Xing

The History of Sino-American Family Therapy

In 2005 the lead author participated in a special delegation of Western family therapy scholars who traveled to China to meet with Chinese family therapists for an intercultural exchange of ideas. At the time family therapy was becoming popular in China, as the culture opened up to Western modes of mental health treatment. Of all the Western mental health methods available to them, family therapy seemed to be the best fit for the Chinese culture given the history of filial piety and collectivistic social organization. The delegation was one of the first of its kind, and led to many future collaborations between Chinese and Western family therapy experts. Later that year the lead author, in collaboration with Western and Chinese scholars, founded the ***Sino-American Family Therapy Institute*** (SAFTI). The Institute was established to further the development of research and the practice of couples and family therapy in China and throughout Asia in association with western scholars and therapists. The Institute strives to foster relationships between scholars, clinicians, and students in the United States and Asia through education, research, and exchange programs. One of the main activities of the Institute is the delivery of rigorous, high-quality, competency-based clinical trainings for students and scholars learning the practice of marriage, couples, and family therapy. The faculty is comprised of Western, Chinese, and Southeast Asian experts. The Institute also fosters opportunities for faculty and students to engage in academic writing, research, and scholarly collaborations. Additionally, students from the United States, China and Southeast Asia are eligible to pursue professional intercultural experiences that include cross-cultural scholarly exchanges in family therapy in Asia. These exchanges have been carried out annually by faculty members since 2005. To date the Institute has hosted over 200 Western family therapy scholars and students to China and Southeast Asia for intercultural exchanges, and several Chinese family therapy scholars for academic and scholarly exchange trips to North America. The SAFTI is accredited by the *International Accreditation Commission for Systemic Therapy Education* (IACSTE) and most students become members of the *International Family Therapy Association* (IFTA)

DOI: 10.4324/9781003297871-31

during their training. Early in the development of the Institute the faculty and students began conducting couples and family therapy sessions using an amalgama of Western and Eastern methods. Students training at the Institute needed direct client contact experiences as well as live supervision opportunities. Previous research about Chinese peoples' preference for various treatment methods revealed that those surveyed would prefer an expert-based, family-focused, structured, brief, directive, intervention-rich, and team-based service (with several therapists observing and offering feedback). Over the years the Institute's students and faculty refined their way of conducting therapy using a seven-step team family therapy protocol. Each of the 20 therapists take turns bringing a case for the Seven-Step Team Family Therapy (SSTFT) sessions, with the other therapists serving as the observing/reflecting team. Team members generally practice various systemically informed models of treatment, but the team members are not required to follow one therapy model. We have found that this diversity of perspectives contributes greatly to both the treatment and the supervision process. The Institute faculty supervise all cases. A translator is present for all sessions to assist with clear communication when needed. The group has been conducting SSTFT consultations continuously since 2016. We designed our SSTFT with three fundamental goals in mind. Firstly, we designed the service to provide a high-quality therapy consultation service that was tailored to fit with the Chinese culture. Secondly, we designed the service to simultaneously provide SAFTI students with the chance to receive high-quality supervision experiences with live case consultations. Finally, we created the service to foster cross-cultural opportunities for participating Western and Chinese supervisors, clients, and training therapists. To date, all clients that have utilized the service reported that it was useful and helpful in addressing their problems.

The Seven-Step Team Family Therapy Protocol (SSTFT)

Step 1: The Pre-Session Briefing with the Team

During the first 30 minutes of the service the lead therapist for the case provides a standardized briefing for the team before the family arrives. The briefing details the people involved with the case and the nature of the problem, treatment history, attempted solutions, a genogram, supervision goals, and what the therapist is seeking from the consultation for the family. If this is the first session, this information will be gleaned from the initial phone contacts and intake paperwork. Each team member receives a paper copy of the pre-session briefing prepared by the lead therapist. Each team member takes notes on the briefing report throughout the session and returns it to the therapist at the end of the consultation to facilitate as much feedback as possible from the team to the therapist. The team and supervisor use the remaining time to ask follow-up questions about the case until the clients arrive.

Step 2: The Family Session

For the next 45 minutes the lead therapist conducts the first part of the session with the family. Generally speaking, the therapist's job during this part of the session is simply to get the family to describe as completely as possible their thinking about the areas of inquiry listed below. The therapist usually speaks less than 20% of the time during this part of the session, while the clients talk about 80% of the time. The therapist resists any attempt at intervention at this stage, but instead guides each member of the family to respond to the questions. The therapist maintains a "here and now" focus during the interview by limiting historical discussions and asking typical brief and single consultation questions (Miller & Slive, 2004). For example;

- "How would each of you describe the problem today and what would you like to get out of the session?"
- "How would we know that this session had been useful to you?"
- "What have you tried in the past that helped?" What are some things you haven't yet tried, but that you think might help?"
- "Can you think of any other available resources?"
- "If the problem disappeared tomorrow, what other problems might you have?"
- "Can you think of any times when the problem would usually occur, but for some reason it did not (exceptions)?"

The team's task during this part of the session is to generate as many ideas as possible in four areas of inquiry. These include:

1. Compliments, commendations, and validations for the client or family
2. Other questions to ask the family to give further detail or sponsor creative thinking
3. Alternative stories (reframes) that could be used to describe the situation
4. Interventions to be delivered to the family either in session, and/or to take home at the conclusion of the session

The supervisor's job is to keep things on time, organize the team's feedback, keep the supervision questions in mind, and occasionally call into the session to ask follow-up questions or make suggestions to the therapist.

Step 3: Team Break and Construction of a Team Message

During this step the family takes a break in another room while the lead therapist meets with the team and supervisor for about 30 minutes. The family is sometimes given a task to do among themselves during this step. In the observation room each member of the team shares their thoughts with the therapist regarding the four areas of inquiry described previously. After the entire team has express their ideas, the lead therapist selects five team members to take into meet with the family to share their feedback. During step 3 the lead therapist may alter a team member's message to best fit with what they think the family needs (we have termed this "tailoring the message"). Additionally, the lead therapist may suggest a team member come up with a suggestion that they think would be useful (we have termed this a "plant"). The supervisor also provides supervisory advice about the case to the team and therapist during step 3, and always serves as a member of the team that goes into the therapy room to meet the family during step 4.

Step 4: Team Metalogue in the Presence of the Family or Client System

At the beginning of step 4 the family is brought back into the therapy room and introduced to the five team members who have been selected by the therapist to give feedback to the family. The supervisor also always participates as a reflecting team member. The supervisor and the therapists offer their reflections on the four areas of inquiry described previously. The family sits at one side of the room, while the team, supervisor, and lead therapist sit at another. After introductions, the supervisor usually gives the following message directly to the family. "We have talked with your therapist about ideas we have for you to take home tonight. We tried to think of as many things as we could. These five team members represent the entire team that was observing. I'm the supervisor. We have no secrets from you, and we want you to know everything we are thinking. To help facilitate this, we want to have a condensed version of the conversation we just had with your therapist in front of you and have you overhear us. It will perhaps sound odd, but we will talk about you as if you are not in the room to preserve the tone of the original conversation. We ask you to pretend there is an invisible wall between you and us. We will pretend that you can see and hear us, but that we cannot see or hear you. We had to take our best guess about what is happening based on what we heard tonight. We ask that you lower your expectations about our feedback, as all we know is what we heard in the last 45 minutes. Hopefully, some things will be useful, but some things might be off target. If so, please feel free to let your therapist know after we leave. We will talk for about 30 minutes and then leave. We advise you to take notes on what stood out for you and talk about it with the therapist after we leave. Do you have any questions about this idea? Is it ok with you for us to proceed?" Each member of the family is provided with a pad and pen to take notes, and the supervisor waves his hand to indicate the wall is up once the family is ready to begin. Each team member takes turns talking to the therapist about their feedback in the four areas of inquiry. The lead therapist listens and takes notes. The last feedback message is given by the supervisor. The aim of the supervisor's feedback is usually to "wrap up" the feedback that was provided in one take-home message and to emphasize possible interventions. The team's focus is on the process (metalogue), instead of merely the content of the family situation. This step usually takes about 30 minutes. Our hope is that team metalogue guides the family to "second-order thinking" (thinking that is up one level of abstraction, getting at the process of how things happen instead of simply the "what is happening," or content). The idea of a metalogue was introduced by Gregory Bateson, relating to a discussion of a problem in such a way that the structure of the conversation matches elements of the problem (Bateson, 1972). The development of the use of the team in this way was also influenced by the work of Tom Anderson with reflecting teams (1987). This "invisible wall" strategy was modified from a technique developed by Dr. Wendel Ray at the Mental Research Institute (MRI), (Ray, Keeney, Parker & Pascal, 1992). Dr. Ray has served as a co-supervisor during several SSTFT consultations in China and Cambodia, as have several other visiting Western family therapists.

Step 5: Post-Team Family Reaction and Intervention Construction

During this step the supervisor lowers the imaginary "invisible wall," thanks the family for coming in, and the team and supervisor leave the therapy room. The team and supervisor return to the observation room, and the lead therapist asks each family member what they noticed from the team's comments. The therapist uses the information from the family about what they observed to help construct a final message to the family and one or more interventions to take home. Once complete, the therapist leaves the family in the therapy room and returns to the observation room. This step usually takes about 15 minutes.

Step 6: Appreciative Inquiry Interview with Family

At the beginning of step 6 the supervisor returns to the therapy room to ask the family a few questions about their experience with the therapist. In many situations the family has worked with the therapist in family therapy in the past. But even if this is the client's first experience with the therapist, we have found it useful also to conduct step 6, and the family usually has some productive feedback to provide. The following is a typical explanation provided by the supervisor to the family: "If you don't mind, I would like to take a few minutes to ask you a few questions about your experience with your therapist. These questions don't have anything to do with your case, but are focused on feedback you have for your therapist. I am your therapist's supervisor, and we are always working on improving things so we can provide our clients the best service possible. With this in mind, your feedback is very important to us. Your therapist is observing our conversation from the observation room, and I'm sure will be very interested in your thoughts. Is it ok with you that I begin?" The three questions asked of the family focus on what they appreciate, and include:

1. What are characteristics of your therapist that you appreciate?
2. What are the things that your therapist did that helped with your problem?
3. What advice would you give your therapist?

At the conclusion of the interview the clients are thanked for their feedback and depart the therapy offices. This approach is modified from Cooperrider & Srivastva's 1987 work on "appreciative inquiry" (AI), instead of criticism and problem solving, as a strengths-based and positively focused way to gather feedback and promote meaningful change. This focus on the positive instead of negative feedback is also in keeping with Paul Watzlawick's fundamental tenant of avoiding negation when talking with clients (Miller & Ray, 2021). He felt that negative criticism of people will do little to promote meaningful change. We find that this step is also a strategy to help the family think about things in a different way. This part of the interview helps the family see themselves not only as people with a problem seeking help from "experts," but also as people who are experts themselves in helping the therapist and the team become better in their work. We have found without exception that the family is happy and honored to be asked these questions and eager to provide feedback. At the end of this part of the interview the family is thanked and departs from the therapy offices.

Step 7: Post-Session Supervisory Discussion with the Lead Therapist and the Team

During this final step the supervisor returns to the observation room to discuss the client's feedback about the lead therapist, the lead therapist's thoughts about the session, and any final supervisory feedback to the lead therapist and the team. Interestingly, the lead therapist is almost always surprised to hear what the family had to say about all the things they appreciated about them as a person, and what they did to help in therapy. The advice the family provides to the therapist is usually productive as well, and often involves encouragement from the family for the therapist to push them more or take more direct action in their interventions. This step usually takes about 15 minutes.

Case Examples

The following are three case examples describing Chinese families seen using this 7-step protocol. The case descriptions are amalgamated from many cases and all identifying information has been changed or removed. The purpose of these case descriptions is to show how the therapy teams work, and to demonstrate some common problems that therapists work with that are unique to the Chinese context.

Case Example 1: Family Therapy for School Refusal of 16-Year-Old Daughter

During steps 1–3 the team learned about a family with a daughter that was refusing to go to school. A middle-aged mother and father attended the consultation with their only child, a 16-year-old daughter. The parents explained that the daughter was previously a good student in junior high but when she entered high school, she began to miss classes with greater frequency until eventually she stopped going altogether. She had missed school for over a month now, and both parents expressed their great concern for the situation. The daughter explained that she felt the problem was that the pressure was too much for her. She felt pressure to perform academically, and also generally in life as the only child in the family. The parents' response to the situation was to further pressure the daughter about the importance of high achievement in school for her future happiness, get good test scores on the Gaokao (高考) (national college entrance exams), to get into a good college, find a good husband, and to fulfill the hopes of the extended family. The parents lectured the daughter about all the sacrifices the family had made for her to have this chance. The mother talked about how she had given up her career to stay home and attend to the daughter full-time. The father talked about how hard he was working to provide for the family, spending most of the month out of town on business trips. The conversation slowly shifted from the daughter's school refusal to the family communication patterns and problems.

Next the team proceeded with step 4 where the metalogue discussion of the team occurs in the presence of the family utilizing the invisible wall technique. During the metalogue the team discussed how it would make sense that the parents would be anxious about the situation given their tremendous devotion to the daughter and how much the family had invested in her doing well. The team also appreciated the difficult situation the daughter was in as she faced the tremendous expectations of both parents and four grandparents. The team wondered if perhaps one good part of the school refusal problem was that it promoted a sort of "family reunion," as dad returned home more when the problem became worse to help the mother deal with the daughter's problem. The parents were complimented by the team in that while they had different ideas about how to deal with their daughter, they were able to come together to work on it. The team wondered if the daughter was showing her loyalty to her parents by helping bring them together. The team offered several interventions to consider. If the daughter was able to return to school, it would be important for the parents to have some hobbies and activities they could do together once she was away. They could start to develop these hobbies and activities even now to start getting ready, and as a sort of demonstration to the daughter that they would be alright after she launched. The team also discussed how the parents seemed to disagree about how to handle the problem, which had led to several fights. They suggested that the parents experiment with changing roles for a few days a week, with the mother taking the father's disciplinarian role, and the father taking mom's support and nurturing role. This way they might gain some empathy for the difficulty of each of the roles.

During step 5 after the team left the room the family discussed with the therapist their reaction to the team feedback. The mother expressed interest in the exchange of roles idea, and they talked about how to carry it out in the following week. The daughter talked about how she appreciated that the feedback from the team had helped take the focus off of her. The father talked about how the team discussion prompted him to think about how much time he was away, and that he wanted to spend more time home with the family in the future. The therapist ended the session with recommendations and suggestions that fit with the family reaction to the team metalogue discussion.

During step 6 the therapist left the room and went to the observation room to observe the appreciative inquiry interview of the family by the supervisor. The supervisor entered the therapy room and proceeded to interview the family about their experience with their therapist. The family was very happy to be asked about their experiences. The parents both expressed that they appreciated it when the therapist gave them direct advice and suggestions about things they might do differently. They also appreciated that the therapist asked thought-provoking questions that made them think differently about their situation. Both the parents and the daughter agreed that one of the main advantages of the therapy was that during the sessions they could have conversations with each other that they could never have at home because at home it would quickly turn into an argument. When asked about characteristics of the therapist that they appreciated, the family discussed the therapist's patient, caring, and calm approach during the sessions. When asked what advice they would give to the therapist, they suggested that the therapist feel free to challenge them more and feel free to give more direct interventions.

The family was thanked for their valuable feedback and they departed the therapy offices while the team and the supervisor conducted the post-session discussion (step 7). The therapist shared her reaction to the appreciative inquiry. She was surprised to hear that they had so many positive things to say about her as a therapist and that they wanted her to be more directive. She discussed how difficult this was for her as a new therapist to challenge and be directive to clients as she worried it would come across as rude behavior. The team discussed how this is a common value in Chinese culture (non-directiveness), but that this is not always what clients want or need. The supervisor suggested that each therapist in the team consider the feedback from the case and how they each utilize directiveness and challenge in their own clinical practices.

The therapist followed up with the family 3 months after the consultation and the family reported that they were doing much better. The family felt the greatest help from the session was that they could express themselves in the session without it turning into a fight, which is what usually happened at home before. They had followed the team's suggestion that the father spend more time at home, and the parents had begun going out once or twice a week on dates. The daughter returned to school shortly after the SSTFT session.

Case Example 2: Po Xi Wen Ti (The Mother-in-Law Problem)

During steps 1–3 the team learned about a family with intergenerational struggles. A couple in their 30s presented for the SSTFT consultation complaining of family conflict, especially between the husband's mother and his wife. The couple had married 3 years before. The husband's mother had recently divorced from his father, and she moved in with the young couple to help them take care of their 2-year-old son. This living arrangement is common in China, as is the conflict that sometimes emerges between the mother-in-law and the wife. In China this is commonly called the "po xi wen ti," or "mother-in-law problem." The husband reported that the conflict usually emerged when he returned home from work. He often felt "pounced on" by both his wife and his mother, who were upset with each other over some disagreement that had occurred between them during the day. Their conflict usually involved something related to the care of the 2-year-old son, like what to feed him that day. The husband felt he was in the role of the "judge" and this was a no-win situation for him. He was afraid that if he said anything to support his wife, his mother would be upset, and vice versa. To avoid conflict at home he had begun staying at work late, which only exacerbated the conflict at home. The unresolved conflict between his wife and his mother had also caused conflict in his marriage. In fact, they both reported that it had gotten so bad that they had considered divorce. They both reported that they didn't really want to divorce, but they also could not keep living in this situation. The therapist asked what the husband's mother would say was the problem if she was in the session, and the husband reported that she would probably say that she was upset that the wife "did not accept her influence and knowledge" about how to take care of the infant son. She might also talk about how she felt she did not have a place in the family anymore since her divorce, and her growing sense that she was irrelevant. The therapist asked the couple to rate how willing they were to work on improving the relationship on a scale of 1–10, with 10 being the most committed. Both reported a 10.

During Step 4 (the metalogue) the team used the invisible wall technique and discussed in front of the family about how they were not surprised that the couple was having difficulty in their marriage given all that was happening for them recently. They discussed how couples with young children often experience their lowest level of marital satisfaction at this stage, even if there are no other problems. In addition to this, the birth of their son coincided with the divorce of the husband's parents and his mother's subsequent move into the couple's small apartment. The couple had only recently married, and were dealing with the stressors of having their first child and the husband's increasing workload at the office. Another team member talked about the idea of the "crucible of intimacy" in relationships, and that the family conflict was perhaps this young couple's "relationship test" that may eventually make them stronger. They explained the idea that most significant relationships have struggles (a crucible) that tests the strength of the relationship. If they pass through the crucible without destroying the relationship, they usually have a more intimate and stronger bond (Schnarch, 1991). The team members discussed how it may seem that this current challenge will never end, but that it would one day. In the future if they can look back at this situation with the feeling that it was hard, but that they had worked together to solve it, they would likely be much stronger as a couple.

Another team member discussed the importance of working on the couple relationship, given that they were both at a "10" regarding their willingness to work on the problem. They suggested that the couple talk together privately to come up with a plan about how to talk to the mother-in-law about the conflict at home. The couple should mutually agree on a message that the husband gives to his mother. The trick would be coming up with a message that recognizes the mother-in-law's influence, since the team guessed that it would be important to her. The team encouraged the husband to get more involved in the relationship between his mother and his wife, even though it would likely be difficult at first. The team predicted that there would be many invitations in this situation for the couple to argue, but that they should do their best to maintain a sense of togetherness. One way to promote this would be to regularly have a time together that was just for the two of them. The team wondered aloud what it would take to help the young couple to create this opportunity. Finally, one team member talked about what they thought the 2-year-old son would advise the couple to do if he was able to talk. This may sound strange, but the infant has perhaps the greatest stake in the couple improving the relationship, so he might have some valuable advice if he could speak.

Next the therapist moved to step 5, the team departed, and the couple talked about the idea of the "crucible of intimacy." The couple agreed with each other that they very much wanted to pass this test. Responding to one question from a team member, the couple talked about getting a maid (called an "Ayi" in China, or 阿姨) to relieve some of the pressure in the home and give the couple a chance to spend more time together. The husband agreed to get involved more between his mother and his wife, and asked that the wife try to help him by not "pouncing" on him when he returned from work each day. The wife committed herself to trying to minimize the conflict with the mother-in-law, and asked that her husband help her in this by committing to spend more time together as a couple.

During step 6 the therapist left the therapy room and observed the supervisor conduct the appreciative inquiry interview with the family. The couple reported that they greatly appreciated the therapist's neutral stance toward the family situation. They also discussed how her calm and relaxed presence had helped them to think more clearly about the situation. They felt one of the main things about the therapy that had helped them was that it was one of the only opportunities they had during the week to talk together as a couple and that this alone had been a major contributor to their positive change in treatment.

During the post-session supervisory meeting during step 7 the supervisor discussed with the team the general dilemma of the "po xi wen ti" issue in China. The supervisor prompted the team to consider why it was called a "mother-in-law" problem, when it seemed systemically that all family members contributed something to the maintenance of the family conflict. We discussed how it might be more appropriately called a "mother-in-law, father-in-law, son, wife, daughter-in-law problem." Other members of the team talked about families they had seen in China that had managed this family situation well, and we talked about our views of the dynamics of these families. Several team members discussed the importance of the husband allowing himself to be triangulated into the conflict between his mother and his wife. Likewise, the team discussed the importance of the husband's father's involvement. The supervisor suggested that each team member continue to look out for these family dynamics in their clinical work and continue the discussion into the future so that we can all benefit from the ideas.

The lead therapist followed up with the couple 3 months after the SSTFT session. The couple reported that after the session they went out to a restaurant, had a glass of wine, and came up with a plan for how to improve the situation. The husband would find a time to talk with his mother privately about the environment in the home and ways to improve it. He reported that the conversation went well, and they talked about a balanced plan for his mother to develop some activities outside the home while still maintaining connection with her grandson. They also reported that they had hired a maid, and that the addition of this extra person in the home had helped de-escalate things. The wife reported that when the husband came home each day, she tried to make a special effort to welcome him with a warm and relaxed manner, which they both agreed helped a great deal.

Case Example #3: Child School Behavior Problem

During steps 1–3 the team learned about a single mother family with an 8-year-old son. After the mother's divorce from the father 2 years previously, she and son moved into a small apartment with the mother's mother. The father separated from the family soon after the son was born and had recently remarried. The therapist reported that he was completely cut-off from the mother and son. The mother and son had presented for therapy initially with concerns about the son's school behavior after receiving several complaints from his teacher. The teacher complained that the son was more and more distracted in class and that his performance had begun to fall. The mother reported that she was increasingly anxious about the situation, which prompted her to scold the son more and more. But she conceded that this did not seem to help the situation and apparently just contributed to a growing sense of anxiety in the home. Early during the family interview (step 2) the therapist asked what they thought the goal of the session was for each of them. The mother said that her goal was to get some ideas about how to separate the sleeping quarters for the mother and son. As is common in Chinese culture, the mother and son shared a bed since the child's early years. The mother felt this arrangement had gone on too long to be healthy for everyone, but she felt she had failed in her efforts to move the son to his own bed. Each time they tried to have him sleep in his own bed he would wake with anxiety and go to the mother's bed to calm down. Other times the mother would awake to find that she was anxious about her son and would compulsively check on him, which also disrupted her sleep. The son stated that he was not worried about the sleeping situation, but instead thought that the goal of the session should be to help his mother feel more happy and less anxious. He talked about how he worried about his mother and felt that she was sad and lonely. He worried about her feelings when she was on her own, and thought that she did not do enough things to take care of herself. He was worried she had no friends or social life. The mother stated that she was not averse to more self care and even creating more of a social life for herself, but that she felt her life was not so important and that her main concern was for her son and his school grades. The theme of "mutual concern" repeated throughout the family interview.

During step 4 the team utilized the invisible wall technique to share their impressions of the family situation. One team member talked about how impressed they were with the son and his apparent maturity. The team member stated that while the son was reported to be only 8 years old, he acted and appeared as a 28-year-old. Another team member talked about their feeling that the apparent maturity and mutual concern expressed in the home was evidence that the mother had done a fine job raising the boy despite the obvious difficulties they faced. Still, they wondered whether since the mother had focused almost exclusively on her role as a mother that she may have neglected her role as a woman and an individual. They wondered if this lack of self care might have unintentionally and subconsciously brought some pressure to the son. The team member wondered aloud what it would take for the mother to expand her own life as an individual and a woman. They shared a general reflection they had that in most love relationships it is about "connection," but that uniquely in parent-child relationships love is also about "separation." At first mothers and children are close, but as they develop together it is time to separate a little to begin school. Yet this will often raise anxiety for both the mother and the child, but this is normal and usually fades in time. There is a sacrifice that a mother has to make in the early stages where love is about connection, but also a sacrifice that a mother must make when it comes time to separate. The team member talked about the mother's attempt to separate the sleeping quarters, and perhaps this situation was part of that sacrifice of "separation" in loving parental relationships. Other team members asked if the son had any friends or hobbies of his own and suggested that it would be equally important for the son to develop himself in this way in parallel with the mother's efforts.

During step 5 the mother expressed that the team discussion encouraging her to develop her multiple roles and to engage in more self care was powerful for her. She admitted that she had all but given up on herself as a person and could see now that this might not be helpful. She agreed with the idea that of parental sacrifice and committed to work harder in the sacrifice of parental separation. She committed to working more on self-care, exercise, getting her hair done, joining a dance class she had been considering, and building her friendship group. The son reported that he was especially struck by the statement that he acted more like he was 28, instead of 8 years old. He agreed with this idea and stated that he would like to go back to being 8 years old again if he could. The therapist asked how he thought he could accomplish going back to 8, and he said that he thought is would help if he could play football, and spend more time with his friends. The therapist ended with asking each of them to try out the ideas they had developed during the session and report back later on the outcome of their efforts.

During the appreciative inquiry (step 6) the mother and son reported to the supervisor that they really appreciated the therapy time in that it helped lower anxiety in their home between sessions. The mother felt that she was better able to compartmentalize her moments of heightened anxiety with the knowledge that she would be meeting with the therapist each week to process things.

After the family departed the therapy offices the team discussed with the supervisor the idea of avoiding negation, distinguishing between indicative versus injunctive language, and speaking the clients' language (Miller & Ray, 2021). These are three central tenants from the work of Paul Watzlawick from the Mental Research Institute (MRI) that were demonstrated in this case. Instead of focusing on what the family was doing wrong (negation), the team had successfully focused attention on what they were doing well (positive connotation). As the old Chinese proverb goes, "It is better to light a candle than curse the darkness." The team had given attention to providing descriptive and behavioral suggestions (injunctive) instead of solely focusing on ideas and concepts (indicative). Finally, the team had worked to craft a message that fit the family's apparent language of "mutual sacrifice," which seemed to strike a chord with them. While each therapist on the team is free to practice and relate to various family therapy models, we generally find these three tenets are useful organizers across all models of treatment.

Six months later the mother and son returned for another team consultation. The mood was elevated, and they reported that they were doing much better and mainly wanted to return to show us all the changes they had made. The mother looked notably different, in that she had lost weight, was smartly dressed, and generally happier in her expressions. She reported that the son had transitioned to his own bed and that he was doing much better in school. The son seemed more care-free, and reported that he had joined the school football team and made some new friends. When the therapist asked how he had managed to do all this, he proudly raised his arms in the air and proclaimed "I'm no longer 28! I'm 8 years old again!"

Conclusion

These three case examples provide a glimpse of the unique problems facing Chinese families, and how this SSTFT protocol may be useful for other global supervisors and the therapists they supervise. We have found one advantage of this method lies in the ability of the team to help capitalize on the "wisdom of the crowd," a concept proposed by the English social scientist Sir Francis Galton in 1907 that demonstrated the group as a whole is often wiser than any one individual in the group. This idea is very consistent with Chinese culture's focus on communal collaboration and collectivism as an ancient core value. In our experience, this method of team consultation matches the Chinese tendency to "gather around" a problem in an effort to solve it as a group.

The diversity of the team feedback also serves as a sort of projective opportunity for the family. We have had visiting international supervisors and team members from around the world participate on the team. The fact that the consultant was from a different culture was rarely a disadvantage in our view. Conversely, the family usually found their feedback especially profound precisely because the feedback was coming from the perspective of someone from another culture. We believe this is because there is a special utility and weight a team member from another culture can offer to the family. Their feedback is novel, unique, and often from a completely different worldview. Many seminal international (non-US) family therapy leaders who have had a large impact on the development of family therapy in the United Stats match this idea (Paul Watzlawick, Salvador Minuchin, Insoo Berg, Michal White, Ivan Bozomony Nagy, the Milan Group, etc.).

It is almost always illuminating which of the team's feedback messages stands out most profoundly for the family during step 5. This information becomes an important clue for the therapist about how best to intervene with the family. Finally, the "appreciative inquiry" in step 6 conducted at the conclusion of the session provides a valuable opportunity for the family to express what they feel is most helpful about the therapist, and the therapist's interventions. It also provides important feedback for the therapist about how the family perceives them in therapy and where their next learning edge might be.

References

Anderson, R. (1987). The reflecting team: Dialogues and metadialogue in clinical work. *Family Process. 26*, 415–528.

Bateson, B. (1972). *Steps to an Ecology of Mind: Collected Essays in Anthropology, Psychiatry, Evolution, and Epistemology*. University of Chicago Press. ISBN 0-226-03905-6.

Cooperrider, D. L. & Srivastva, S. (1987). Appreciative inquiry in organizational life. In Woodman, R. W. & Pasmore, W.A. (Eds.), *Research in Organizational Change and Development*. (pp. 129–169). Vol. 1. Stamford, CT: JAI Press.

Miller, J. K., & Slive, A. (2004). Breaking down the barriers to clinical service delivery: Walk-in family therapy. *Journal of Marital and Family Therapy, 30*(1), 95–103.

Miller, J. K. & Ray, W. (2021). Three central concepts in teaching and learning with Paul Watzlawick: The importance of avoiding negation, distinguishing between indicative and injunctive language, and speaking the client's language. *International Journal of Systemic Therapy* 32(3), 219–228. https://doi.org/10.1080/2692398X.2021.1942750.

Ray, W., Keeney, B., Parker, K., & Pascal, D. (1992). The invisible wall: A method for breaking a relational impasse. *Louisiana Journal of Counseling & Development*, 3(1), Spring, 32–34.

Schnarch, D., (1991). Constructing the sexual crucible: An integration of sexual and marital therapy. New York: Norton.

29

AN ADAPTIVE APPLICATION OF EMOTIONALLY FOCUSED THERAPY (EFT) WITH IRANIAN IMMIGRANT COUPLES

Reihaneh Mahdavishahri

Theory Introduction

Formulated in the early 1980s by Les Greenberg and Sue Johnson, emotionally focused therapy (EFT) was born out of the need for more humanistic, validated, clearly defined, and less behavioral approaches to couple therapy (Johnson, 2019b). EFT is an evidence-based model grounded in humanistic experiential therapy and systems theory, as well as attachment theory and theory of adult love. As an integrative approach, EFT examines the individuals' intrapsychic emotional experiences and processes and integrates such understandings with the interpersonal experiences and interactions between the partners (Johnson, 2019b).

Attachment Theory

Attachment theory, originally developed by Bowlby (1969) and later extended by Hazan and Shaver (1994), is an interpersonal theory of human development and adult romantic love, which seeks to examine and explain the dynamics of interpersonal relationships and attachment to selected others. According to Bowlby (1969), we are all wired to operate from an attachment system, a complex psychological system that drives us to seek support from others in times of distress. Bonding, which is at the core of this system, is not only a social behavior but a survival strategy we engage in with emotion and emotion regulation as the primary elements of this engagement. This attachment system is shaped by the quality and the intensity of our relationships with key others leading to an interplay of (cognitive) working models of self and others and their associated emotion regulation strategies (Bowlby, 1969; Hazan & Shaver, 1994).

Seeking physical and emotional proximity to key others is among the fundamental tenets of attachment theory (Bowlby, 1969). It is through this connection and the responsiveness

DOI: 10.4324/9781003297871-32

of these key figures that a sense of safe haven develops that leaves an imprint on our nervous system. With comfort and reassurance reliably obtained from our attachment figures, we start to build a grounded, autonomous, and positive sense of self and feel confident in our abilities to explore the world around us (Hazan & Shaver, 1994). The more *responsive, accessible,* and *engaged* our attachment figures are the stronger and more resilient we are in adapting to the world around us. However, if key others are unresponsive, inaccessible, and/or hostile when we seek their support, we adopt insecure working models that include either patterns of anxious engagement with others, deactivated avoidant strategies, or wavering between fearful and longing strategies (Johnson, 2019b).

In summary, attachment theory seeks to explain how early caregiving experiences shape individuals and their internal working models of self and others and impact their perceptions, emotional experiences, and behavioral patterns (Hazan & Shaver, 1994). Grounded in such tenets, EFT then seeks to explain the model of relationships by privileging emotion and bonding and identifies *responsiveness* as the means through which we achieve relationship satisfaction and a sense of stability (Johnson, 2019b). While physical proximity may be less prominent in adult attachments and relationships, *the need for accessibility, responsiveness, and engagements in adult emotional bonding remains the same* (Johnson, 2019b).

EFT as a Culturally Informed Model

EFT's grounding in humanistic approaches lies in its non-pathologizing and empathic understanding of individuals' experiences, particularly their immediate emotional experiences (Johnson, 2020). The collaborative therapeutic relationship allows for a safe space in which clients' find comfort in the therapists' validation and empathy to explore and create new experiences. EFT therapists pay significant attention to the internal processes and interactional patterns that create crucial feedback loops between the partners without imposing judgment or prescribing the couple *"the right way of interacting"* with one another (Johnson, 2020). These crucial elements make EFT an appropriate fit for working with multicultural couples. As experiential therapists, EFT therapists privilege emotions and corrective emotional experiences in the here and now, which may lead to long-lasting change for the couple, holding space for the corrective emotional experience to be shaped and informed by the couples' unique cultural background.

The art of therapy is the ability to see beyond what is being presented and delve into the intricate workings of a relationship. EFT therapists are well equipped with a systemic lens that allows them to explore the context of the distressed couples' interactions and support them in breaking these rigid cycles. This lens offers a deep understanding of the couple's dynamic and how it plays out in their daily lives and allows the therapist to identify the underlying emotional experiences that drive these rigid interactional patterns (Johnson, 2020). Immigration and the family's immigration story is among those contextual factors that EFT therapists' systemic lens allows them to consider and explore to better support their immigrant clients (Karakurt & Keiley, 2009).

Immigration brings about significant changes and challenges that can impact the developmental life stages of individuals and families. As immigrants adapt to a new environment and culture, they must navigate the tension between maintaining their individual growth and the systemic growth of their family unit. This tension arises from the opposing forces of *morphostasis*, the need to maintain stability and continuity, and *morphogenesis*, the drive for change and adaptation. The immigrant family unit is then faced with the task of finding a delicate balance between these opposing forces. On one hand, they work on maintaining a sense of stability and continuity by preserving their cultural traditions, values, and beliefs, and on the other hand, they have to adapt to the new environment and culture by embracing new experiences, learning new skills, and developing new relationships (Liu & Wittenborn, 2011).

The stress that immigration brings to normal developmental life stages can manifest in different ways, such as cultural identity confusion, family conflict, social isolation, and mental health challenges that all may manifest in the rigidity of the couples' negative interactional patterns. By acknowledging the tension that the couple has been dealing with, including generational tension passed down from first-generation immigrants to their children, EFT therapists can work with immigrant families to name and identify their unique challenges and promote resiliency and a new way of responding to the stress of immigration (Liu & Wittenborn, 2011).

In addition, EFT therapists recognize the importance of examining each partner's attachment history. This exploration enables the couple to gain a greater awareness of how their past experiences may have influenced their current experiences and the ways in which they seek support and respond to the needs of those around them. This process of exploration and reflection allows the couple to make sense of their present struggles and work towards developing more secure attachment styles (Liu & Wittenborn, 2011).

Theory Approach to Functional and Dysfunctional Relationships

As an integrative approach that incorporates experiential, systemic, and attachment-oriented models of therapy, EFT invites couples to experience their emotions rather than merely describe them throughout the therapeutic process (Johnson, 2020). Emotion is then perceived to be the key agent of change in EFT. Problems are perceived to be the result of negative patterns of interactions among the partners, maintaining the systemic concept of circular causality (Johnson, 2020).

In EFT, healthy relationships are defined by a pattern of a secure attachment bond between partners, characterized by reciprocated (emotional) accessibility and responsiveness. This secure attachment bond enables partners to find a sense of security and safety in their relationship and navigate the world around them by engaging in strategies such as regulating their emotions, resolving conflict, and communicating in effective ways (Johnson, 2020). This effective dependency, as Johnson (2020) calls it, allows the partners to be independent and connected simultaneously. The internal working models of those with secure attachments entails a positive and competent sense of self (Johnson, 2020).

When the attachment bond between the partners is threatened or lost, it leads to relationship distress (Johnson, 2020). The attachment strategies partners engage in in such times of relationship distress determines the wellbeing of their relationship. Those with anxious attachment patterns are likely to be more sensitive and to perceive distance in the relationship as inherently negative and threatening. They seek to find reassurance from their partners by engaging in fight responses that aim to dispute such distance. They are often preoccupied with their internal distress and anxiety, which keeps them from properly reaching out to their partners or hearing about their needs in the relationship (Johnson, 2019b).

On the other hand, those with avoidance attachment strategies tend to engage in flight responses designed to dissolve such distress by increasing (physical and emotional) distance in the relationship (Johnson, 2019a). They often minimize or ignore their attachment needs and have difficulty in trusting others to meet such needs. Their view of others is casted by a shadow of unreliability and untrustworthiness while suppressing the negative views they may hold about themselves. There are also those that engage in fearful avoidant attachment strategies, which are marked by their desire for connection and their fear of it. They tend to have negative views of self and others, have difficult time finding safety within themselves and with others, and often have a history of traumatized or disorganized attachment with their primary caregivers (Johnson, 2019b).

When there is distress in the relationship, partners may then engage in any of such attachment strategies and get caught up in negative cycles of interactions that further threaten their emotional connection and security (Johnson, 2019b). If partners perceive that there is a persistent lack of responsiveness, emotional accessibility, and engagement in the relationship, the security of their bond is further threatened, and they may continue to utilize the secondary and insecure strategies to cope with such distress (Johnson, 2019b).

Therapy Goals and Applications

The three primary tasks of EFT include creating a safe therapeutic alliance to support the couple engage in the process of change; to use an attachment-oriented lens in supporting each partner in accessing, experiencing, and expanding their emotional experiences; and to create a space in which couples can restructure their interactive patterns (Johnson, 2019b; Johnson, 2020). The ultimate goal that these tasks seek to achieve is helping the partners to expand and reorganize their emotional experiences with one another and form new interactional patterns (Johnson, 2020).

The goal of stage one in Emotion Focused Couple Therapy (EFCT) is to identify the negative cycle of interaction and to support the couple in achieving a degree of de-escalation when it comes to getting caught up in this cycle. The four steps of stage one allows the therapist to help each partner identify forgotten or unaddressed attachment needs and reframe the key issues of the relationship in terms of the cycle and the underlying primary emotions and attachment needs fueling the cycle (Johnson, 2019a; Johnson, 2020).

The goal of stage two in EFT is to break the negative cycle of interaction. The three steps of stage two are formulated to help the couple hold a compassionate and accepting space to share their primary emotional experiences and unmet attachment needs with each other. The couple becomes more aware of their negative cycle of interaction and finds more ways to break this cycle by learning how to identify and share about their vulnerable emotions when facing a conflict. Stage three sets the stage for a new and positive cycle of interaction in which the couple integrates the new ways of connecting with each other, sharing their vulnerabilities with each other, and together finding new and effective solutions for challenges that may come their way (Johnson, 2019b; Johnson, 2020).

Stigma

The stigma of mental health issues and emotional distress is compounded by social, familial, and cultural expectations and pressures around being the *perfect couple* and thus keeps many partners from reaching out for help (Laveist & Isaac, 2012). Research indicates that stigma surrounding marital and relationship problems is prevalent in many immigrant communities. These studies have found that immigrants are less likely to seek professional help for relationship problems than non-immigrants due to such cultural factors (Laveist & Isaac, 2012).

In some cultures, there is a strong emphasis on preserving *the family honor and reputation* and seeking help for relationship problems may be viewed as a sign of weakness or failure. Others may view relationship problems as *private matters* not to be shared with outsiders or discussed openly with strangers. Additionally, some cultures may view relationship problems as spiritual issues rather than psychological ones, which can further discourage help-seeking behavior (Abbott et al., 2012).

Help-seeking Barriers

Help-seeking barriers refer to specific challenges immigrant couples often face when accessing mental health care services, preventing them from seeking and receiving much needed mental health care (Laveist & Isaac, 2012). As discussed, stigma associated with mental health conditions and marital discord significantly impacts immigrant couples' help-seeking behavior (Laveist & Isaac, 2012; Taylor, 2020). In addition, limited services available in languages other than English, lack of culturally informed care, cultural incompetency of care providers as well costs are among other barriers that immigrant couples face when experiencing emotional distress and relationship discord.

While these factors prevent many immigrant couples from seeking out help, few studies have examined the factors that lead to the high dropout rates of this population from mental health care. This gap within the literature prevents mental health professionals from providing effective and informed care and implementing the concerns of this population within their practices.

Challenges Faced by Iranian Immigrant Couples

Infidelity

As a relationship therapist, I have found that the majority of my couples seek my help to recover from the emotional trauma of infidelity. A significant breach of trust and a violation of the emotional bond between partners, infidelity can stem from a variety of underlying issues, including emotional disconnection, unmet needs, or a lack of emotional safety in the relationship (Johnson, 2019a). When working with Iranian immigrant couples, I have found a noticeable link between their immigration story and their story of seeking comfort and support outside their relationship. Immigration adds a new intersection to our identity. This complex layer is a new experience to navigate and comprehend. For many immigrants, the emotional turmoil of navigating life in a foreign country, away from the help of their support system, can leave them feeling frightened, vulnerable, and uncertain.

Immigration can result in a significant transformation of one's sense of self, altering their understanding of themselves and their relationships with others. Thus, the immigration process can have a profound impact on the individual identities of each partner within an immigrant couple, ultimately affecting their dynamic as a unit. The couple must confront a multitude of challenges as they navigate the complexities of adapting to a new culture, creating a shared sense of meaning and purpose, and re-establishing their emotional bond. This vulnerable moment can often lead to a deep sense of disconnection from one's sense of self, their relationship, and the role they used take in this partnership. Seeking comfort and support elsewhere then becomes an illusory safe haven for the partner that may have lost their access to the comfort their relationship once brought. This alternative comfort, though it may be fleeting and inadequate, provides a temporary respite from the pain of losing a meaningful connection (Karakurt & Keiley, 2009).

Birth

The birth of a child represents a major life cycle transition for mothers, their partners, as well as their families (Milgrom & Gemmill, 2015). Welcoming a new baby signifies three significant life-altering changes at once including pregnancy, birth, and becoming a parent (Milgrom & Gemmill, 2015). According to the Centers for Disease Control (CDC), one in seven women with a recent birth report experiences symptoms of peripartum depression (Bauman et al., 2020). Women of Color (WOC) and immigrant women are three times more likely than White and native-born women to experience perinatal depression.

Pregnancy and birth embody unique moments in the couple's relationship with expected and unexpected challenges and demands (Pilkington et al., 2016). Given the vulnerability that pregnancy and birth invite into relationships, couples are at increased risk of experiencing relationship distress and potentially attachment bond injury (Akhtar, 2011; Don & Mickelson, 2012). Attachment bond between partners can either be a protective factor or a risk factor for onset and severity of perinatal depression for many women during their pregnancy and after birth of their child (Bifulco & Thomas, 2013). However, little is known about the experiences of immigrant women and ways in which their attachment bond with their romantic partners may impact their pregnancy and postpartum experiences (Bifulco & Thomas, 2013; Laveist & Isaac, 2012.

Idealized cultural messages and images of pregnancy and motherhood are often incompatible with the reality of perinatal depression and thus lead many women to suffer in silence due to the shame and guilt of not living up to expectations (Milgrom & Gemmill, 2015; Stone & Menken, 2008). Immigrant women are more likely to report experiencing shame and blame from healthcare providers following post-delivery services and visits (Jones et al., 2007; Sanchez, 2022; Taylor, 2020). Fear of being reported for neglect and losing their children are also among important contributing factors to low utilization of mental health services by immigrant mothers (Jones et al., 2007; Taylor, 2020). Negative cultural beliefs concerning mental health issues also contribute to the experiences of immigrant mothers' postpartum, including minimizing their emotional distress to avoid facing stigma (Jones et al., 2007; Sanchez, 2022; Taylor, 2020).

Unfair division of childcare and domestic responsibilities has been identified as among the risk factors for relationship dissatisfaction following birth (Van Gelderen et al., 2020). Unequal division of childcare and domestic responsibilities is rooted in patriarchal gender-based social and cultural norms, which have left women responsible for the majority of childcare and household responsibilities (Laveist & Isaac, 2012). Perceived unfairness and unequal division of childcare have been reported to increase psychological distress in mothers and decrease relationship satisfaction. Particularly among employed mothers, lack of participation from their partners in childcare has been associated with more distress (Goldberg & Perry-Jenkins, 2004).

In a collectivist culture such as Iran, there exists a beautiful and powerful tradition of coming together to support and uplift new mothers during their postpartum journey. This deep-rooted emphasis on communal care and support demonstrates that the well-being of the mother is the foundation for the well-being of the entire family and community. The outpouring of practical assistance, emotional support, and guidance given to new mothers not only aids in their physical and mental recovery, but also empowers them to take on their new role with confidence and grace. By upholding these collectivist values, Iranian families ensure that new mothers feel seen, heard, and supported, allowing them to thrive and fully contribute to the flourishing of the family and community as a whole. The act of supporting new mothers in collectivist cultures serves as a powerful reminder of the strength and interconnectedness that can be found in social connections and the beauty of interdependence.

Immigration can then have a significant impact on the support that new immigrant mothers receive, particularly since many of these women had to leave behind their primary sources of support such their families, their friends, and communities. These mothers are then left isolated and alone in navigating the complex challenges that pregnancy and birth invites to their lives. This unique and vulnerable moment is bound to bring about feelings of uncertainty, sadness, and loss of the community that once embraced them.

Infertility

In cultures where motherhood is highly valued, infertility can have more severe consequences such as relationship distress, divorce, family conflict, and isolation. Studies have shown that women experiencing infertility in such cultures are more likely to struggle with depression, anxiety, chronic health conditions, and emotional dysregulation (Soltani et al., 2014). Stigma of infertility can further isolate these women and keep them from seeking and receiving emotional and mental health support. The journey of infertility can be an incredibly challenging and emotionally taxing experience for immigrant Iranian couples, often leading to disconnection and heartbreak. As they navigate the complex and unpredictable road ahead, these couples may struggle with feelings of resentment, hopelessness, and despair, as the emotional burden of infertility takes a toll on their relationship. The emotional stress of infertility can feel overwhelming, and it is not uncommon for these couples to feel lost and unsure of how to move forward (Soltani et al., 2014).

Through my work with immigrant Iranian couples, I have had the privilege of witnessing the transformative power of Emotionally Focused Therapy (EFT) when applied in a culturally sensitive and informed way. These three case examples serve as a testament to the efficacy of this approach, offering a window into the unique challenges that immigrant Iranian couples face and the ways in which EFT can help them overcome these obstacles. By placing cultural context and understanding at the forefront of my work, I have been able to create a safe and supportive environment for these couples to explore their emotions, deepen their connections, and work towards a more fulfilling and satisfying relationship. Through these case examples, I hope to illustrate the immense value of culturally sensitive therapy and the positive impact it can have on the lives of immigrant couples, paving the way for greater healing, growth, and transformation.

Case Example: Infidelity

Sarah and Amir have been together for over 7 years now. They met through mutual friends in Tehran and after dating for about two months they decided to get married. Less than three years into the marriage, Amir and Sarah were awarded the diversity visa program, also known as the *green card lottery,* and shortly after moved to southern California. Their immigration story was a story of joy, excitement, as well as grief and separation from friends, family, and their community. Sarah was able to start her graduate studies shortly after settling in southern California and within two years, found herself in a highly successful world of finance. On the other hand, Amir has been struggling to *find his place in society* as he puts it. He was in medical school in Tehran with less than two years left of his program when they moved, and he hasn't been able to pursue medicine due to barriers related to cost and language. When I first meet with them, they seem defeated and reluctant to speak of any hope for their marriage, yet a glimmer of optimism persisted, a small flame flickering in the face of doubt and uncertainty.

Amir described himself as a *"proud* Iranian man" whose *"dignity"* was shattered when Sarah disclosed a three-month affair to him. *"I don't even know why I'm here. It should be over; I should walk away...this is the worst thing that can happen to a man...but she is all I've got here, and I hate that."* While acknowledging that the affair was a mistake, Sarah expressed that she had her *reasons* and that she had grown weary of the persistent feeling of loneliness that she has been living with since their move to the States. *"He is always angry and resentful; he just shuts down and shuts me out and walks away...what was I supposed to do? I was tired of it all... ."* Sarah says as she wipes away her tears. It soon becomes clear what their cycle looks like; Sarah tends to blame him for shutting her out and Amir grows more and more resentful of their disconnection. But there is much more that fuels the engine of this never-ending cycle... .

Our work began to look like grief counseling at first; grieving the loss of the relationship as it was, grieving the loss of the parts of themselves left in Tehran and grieving the loss of their love as it was. When I first named the affair as an attachment injury, *a significant moment in the relationship when trust is violated and partner(s) is left abandoned,* Amir started to cry. *"I have never allowed myself to feel that I was abandoned; how can a strong man be abandoned."* In every session I would gently explore what it means to him to be a *strong* and *proud* Iranian man and validate the grief he feels at the loss of these parts of his identity. Over time, I started to explore if this *"strong"* part has been limiting for him and perhaps has kept him from embracing the more vulnerable parts of himself. Sarah was able to share about her longing for these vulnerable parts and the deep pain she has felt over the years when these parts became more and more inaccessible. *"I felt abandoned too! I felt ashamed for making it here while he was home depressed and lost!."* The affair started to look less like a cruel malicious act intended to strip Amir of his pride and more as a signal of distress in search of renewed connection, a plea that carried the weight of loneliness and the urgency of a desperate need to be loved again.

With each step of the EFT dance in the first two stages of our work, we uncovered the buried longings for love, connection, and support that lay hidden within them. As they moved more in sync, the emotions began to flow freely, and the unspoken desires were brought to the surface, allowing us to explore their deepest needs further. At the end of stage two, we started our work on the attachment injury of the three-month long affair using the attachment injury resolution model. Sarah was able to learn about Amir's internalized cultural messages around the *pride and dignity of an Iranian man* that has kept him from acknowledging and supporting Sarah in her endeavors after their move to the States. Sarah was able to learn about Amir's fears of losing himself and the man Sarah fell in love with when they first met. In the safety of our validating and non-judgmental therapeutic space, Amir began to explore what it would be like for him to acknowledge and embrace these more vulnerable parts. The parts that would allow him to be excited for Sarah without taking Sarah's success to mean that he has somehow failed her. Sarah was able to remain soft and responsive as Amir's most vulnerable parts were showing themselves and embraced these parts alongside him.

Amir's vulnerability invited Sarah to talk more about her grief over the past few years. *"I lost everyone that has ever loved me or supported me when we moved here...they became these faces on my WhatsApp calls that I couldn't touch or embrace...and Amir was so lost in figuring out what he wanted to do that didn't even realize how deeply I was longing for that kind of support... ."* Amir began to see the hurt and the sadness that Sarah had been carrying with herself all these years. *"I didn't see it...I thought surely you were doing fine since you had your job and your friends, everything that I wanted for myself too but were not good enough to get it...I didn't even see it... ."* Amir and Sarah were able to bond over their shared grief and the losses they each experienced when they left Tehran. They began to imagine a new beginning in the relationship, a new way for them to be together and remain engaged while letting go of these limiting cultural messages they continued to carry within themselves. Amir was able to explore and pursue a new career path for himself and with Sarah's ongoing support was able to reimagine success in a new way. *"I wanted to be a musician when I was much younger, but I was told in order to be a worthy son I needed to pursue medicine, so I did...but now I play guitar at these weddings and birthday parties and even though there is not a lot of money it, I come home a happy man!."* This newfound perspective allowed him to genuinely celebrate Sarah's achievements without feeling threatened or diminished by them, paving the way for a more authentic and fulfilling cycle of interaction between them.

At the end of our work together, Sarah and Amir were no longer defeated by their negative interactive cycle but instead found new ways of acknowledging, embracing, and validating each other's experiences without judgment or resentment.

Case Example: Infertility

Ali and Mojdeh have been together for over 10 years now. *"We were young when we got together maybe too young, but I wouldn't change a thing!"* Ali says as he sighs heavily looking down. Second generation Iranian-Americans, they met when they were 19 and freshmen in college. They moved in together about two years ago and have been trying to have a child since then. Mojdeh has been told she may not be able to get pregnant and has been in IVF treatment for the past 6 months. *"I feel like I'm in this alone; every appointment, every procedure, every injection even scheduling to have sex with him...it's all been me! I need to know if I'm wasting my time with him because I can't keep doing this by myself"* Mojdeh says as she fights back her tears. They seem to be caught up in a persistent cycle of craving connection but encountering rejection, missing each other's' signals for love and togetherness every time.

But the story runs a bit deeper than this... . After the couple seem to be de-escalated and are no longer *fighting relentlessly almost every night*, Mojdeh begins to share about the *shame* she feels for her difficulty getting pregnant. *"I see it in his mom's face when she visits, every time she comes over, she asks if I'm pregnant yet and tells me it's such a bad sign that I'm not...just last week she told me how she became pregnant after her first try... what am I supposed to say to that? And he just sits there and watches her say all these nasty things...,"* Mojdeh says as she starts crying. *"And what keeps you from saying something* to your mom Ali?" I ask him. *"She's my mom what can I tell her...she is sensitive, and I don't want to get caught up in the middle of these two."* Ali's response to his mother or lack thereof is rooted in his position in the family, the only son of a proud first-generation Iranian family that has installed in him a strong sense of responsibility and family loyalty. This strong sense of family loyalty has kept Ali from acknowledging and validating Mojdeh's pain of disconnection as it brings about his fears of losing his mother's love and support if he were to take any actions.

In stage two, we spent some time exploring what it would look like for Ali to remain loyal to his parents while supporting Mojdeh in ways that she wants to be supported. Ali begins to allow himself to hear more about the loneliness Mojdeh has been feeling while accessing his sense of responsibility and loyalty to the bond he shares with her. Receiving Ali's validation, Mojdeh begins to share about her experiences without blaming or judging his mother. This space allows the couple the opportunity to remain engaged and responsive to each other's needs without crowding it with other people's expectations or judgments. Over time, Mojdeh and Ali are able to find new ways of asking for support and privacy from his mother without jeopardizing Ali's bond with his family and Ali begins to see Mojdeh as an ally on his side not against him or his family.

While Mojdeh continues to navigate the emotional challenges related to her fertility, she no longer feels alone in this, as Ali has been able to join her on her doctor's appointments and has been a consistent support by her side. At the end of stage three, the couple has been able to talk more openly about their experiences without blaming or judging each other and instead have been able to hold a validating space where they each explore new ways of connecting with each other. Mojdeh no longer fears rejection for her difficulty conceiving as Ali continues to reassure her of his unwavering support for her. As we end our work together, the couple discloses exploring adoption as a new possibility for expanding their family.

Case Example: Postpartum Depression

Rosie and Dave welcomed a baby girl named Ava about seven months ago. While Rosie describes her pregnancy as smooth and uneventful, things took an unexpected turn when she had to do an emergency C-section after spending 12 hours at the hospital thinking she was going to give birth naturally as she had previously planned. Three days later they went home with their daughter, but Rosie was not feeling excited. After a week of paternity leave, Dave went back to work leaving Rosie to care for Ava on her own for the majority of the day. "I can't keep doing this, I am tired all the time, I haven't been able to sleep properly since Ava was born and I just can't do this anymore...I can't... ." Rosie says as she cries. *"I know it's been hard for you, but I can't just leave work right now, I have to support our family, I have to pay the mortgage, pay for groceries...staying home is not an option for me right now I'm sorry,"* Dave says while his desperation is palpable. Ever since their move to the States three years ago, Dave has been working to support his family financially while the couple decided that Rosie would stay home and manage their household.

Birth is a collective experience for many Iranians as families often get together to support the mother and help raise the newborn baby for at least a couple of months. Maternal grandparents are often the caretakers that take an active role in supporting the family in different ways. Rosie's parents live in Iran and have not been able to secure a visa to come and visit the couple. *"I never thought I'd be doing this by myself...my sisters had my mom when they had their babies, I never thought I wouldn't be able to have that kind of support, no one prepares you for that...And he is just not here, and I feel like I just can't rely on him anymore,"* Rosie says.

As we dive deeper into their fears, Rosie talks about her sense of abandonment and the *heavy* weight of motherhood that she has been carrying on her shoulders while feeling so lost in her new role. Dave talks about growing up with a father that was always working and never really there and not knowing that he had to do *fatherhood* any differently; he talks about his fear of ending up like him. *"When we found out that my dad had only days to live, I was relieved that I didn't have to travel all this way to see him and say goodbye to him... I felt guilty as hell for thinking it, but he was a stranger to me...,"* Dave says as he wipes away his tears.

In stage two, we delve deeper into their inner world and bring to light the parts of themselves that have been hidden away beneath layers of fear, mistrust, and uncertainty. This process requires a great deal of vulnerability, as we explore the perceptions, emotions, and desires that they each hold about themselves and about each other. This work cannot come to fruition if we are not able to assist Dave in finding new ways of providing Rosie with tangible support. Exploring his fears around fatherhood has allowed Dave to reimagine himself in this new role and give room to the possibility that he will not *fail* Ava if he is present with her. In the reassurance and validity that Rosie is able to offer him, Dave begins to take on a more active role in caring for Ava and starts to share the weight of parenthood with Rosie.

Rosie and Dave soon stop coming to therapy as they have been able to navigate the challenges of parenthood on their own.

Future Research

EFT has been established as a popular approach to couple therapy in Iran and there has been more recent research demonstrating its effective application with Iranian couples. However, such findings remain limited and there has been a huge gap in the literature when it comes to an adaptive application of EFT in which specific steps and stages are enhanced to better meet the unique needs of multicultural couples. Integrating the research findings coming out of Iran where EFT therapists are working with diverse dynamics in their unique cultural context can help bridge this current gap and inform a more sensitive application of this approach with Iranian immigrants.

Three Takeaways

- EFT therapists pay significant attention to the internal processes and interactional patterns that create crucial feedback loops between the partners without imposing judgment or prescribing the couple *"the right way of interacting"* with one another.
- EFT therapists possess a systemic perspective that enables them to delve into the context surrounding the problematic interactions of distressed couples and help them break free from these rigid cycles.
- The experience of immigration can bring about a profound shift in an individual's self-perception and their interactions with others. As a result, the immigration journey can deeply influence the personal identities of each partner in an immigrant couple, ultimately reshaping their collective dynamic.

Resources and Additional Reading

- The International Centre for Excellence in Emotionally Focused Therapy (ICEEFT) **https://iceeft. com/what-is-eft/**
- Spengler, P. M., Lee, N. A., Wiebe, S. A., & Wittenborn, A. K. (2022). "A comprehensive meta-analysis on the efficacy of emotionally focused couple therapy." *Couple and Family Psychology: Research and Practice*, advance online publication.
- **Becoming an Emotionally Focused Therapist: The Workbook** (2nd edition, 2022) by James L. Furrow, Susan M. Johnson, Brent Bradley, Lorrie Brubacher, T. Leanne Campbell, Veronica Kallos-Lily, Gail Palmer, Kathryn Rheem & Scott Woolley. New York, NY: Routledge.
- **An Emotionally Focused Workbook for Couples: The Two of Us** (2014) by Veronica Kallos-Lily and Jennifer Fitzgerald. New York, NY: Routledge.
  This book is in press in Hungarian and has been translated into:
  Dutch (2016) Stichting EFT Nederland. **LINK: Click here.**
  German (2016) Junfermann Verlag. **LINK: Click here.**
  Japanese (2021) **LINK: Click here.**
  Korean (2016) **LINK: Click here.**
  Polish (2019) Wydawnictwo Uniwersytetu Jagiellonskiego. **LINK: Click here.**
- **Attachment Theory in Practice — Emotionally Focused Therapy (EFT) with Individuals, Couples and Families** (2019) by Sue M. Johnson. New York, NY: Guilford Press.
  This book is now available in a full-accessible audio book format (e-pub).
  This book is also in press in Chinese (simplified), Finnish, Greek, Russian, Serbian, Spanish, and Turkish, and has been translated into:
  Chinese (Complex) (2022) **LINK: Click here.**
  Danish (2019) Forlaget Mindspace. **LINK: Click here.**
  Dutch (2020) Stichting EFT Nederland. **LINK: Click here.**
  Farsi (2022) **LINK: Click here.**

References

Abbott, D. A., Springer, P. R., & Hollist, C. S. (2012) Therapy with immigrant muslim couples: Applying culturally appropriate interventions and strategies. *Journal of Couple & Relationship Therapy*, 11(3), 254–266, DOI: 10.1080/15332691.2012.692946

Akhtar, S. (2011). *The mother and her child: Clinical aspects of attachment, separation, and loss.* Jason Aronson.

Bauman, B. L., Ko, J. Y., Cox, S., D'Angelo, D. V., Warner, L., Folger, S., Tevendale, H. D., Coy, K. C., Harrison, L., & Barfield, W. D. (2020). *Vital Signs:* postpartum depressive symptoms and provider discussions about perinatal depression — United States, 2018. *MMWR. Morbidity and Mortality Weekly Report*, 69(19), 575–581. https://doi.org/10.15585/mmwr.mm6919a2

Bifulco, A., & Thomas, G. (2013). *Understanding adult attachment in family relationships: Research, assessment, and intervention.* Routledge.

Bowlby, J. (1969). *Attachment and loss.* Basic Books.

Don, B. P., & Mickelson, K. D. (2012). Paternal postpartum depression: The role of maternal postpartum depression, spousal support, and relationship satisfaction. *Couple and Family Psychology: Research and Practice*, 1(4), 323–334. https://doi.org/10.1037/a0029148

Goldberg, A. E., & Perry-Jenkins, M. (2004). Division of labor and working-class women's well-being across the transition to parenthood. *Journal of Family Psychology*, 18(1), 225–236. https://doi.org/10.1037/0893-3200.18.1.225

Hazan, C., & Shaver, P. (1994). Attachment as an organizational framework for research on close relationships. *Psychology Inquiry*, 5(1), 1–22. https://doi.org/10.1207/s15327965pli0501_1

Johnson, S. M. (2019a). Attachment in action — changing the face of 21st century couple therapy. *Current Opinion in Psychology*, 25, 101–104. https://doi.org/10.1016/j.copsyc.2018.03.007

Johnson, S. M. (2019b). *Attachment theory in practice: Emotionally focused therapy (Eft) with individuals, couples, and families.* The Guilford Press.

Johnson, S. M. (2020). *The practice of emotionally focused couple therapy: Creating connection.* Routledge, Taylor & Francis Group.

Jones, H. L., Cross, W. E., & DeFour, D. C. (2007). Race-related stress, racial identity attitudes, and mental health among Black women. *Journal of Black Psychology, 33*(2), 208–231. https://doi.org/10.1177/0095798407299517

Karaku, G., & Keiley, M. (2009). Integration of a cultural lens with Emotionally Focused Therapy. *Journal of Couple & Relationship Therapy, 4*(1), 1–14. 10.1080/15332690802626684.

Laveist, T. A., & Isaac, L. A. (2012). *Race, ethnicity, and health: A public health reader.* John Wiley & Sons.

Liu, T., Wittenborn, A. (2011). Emotionally Focused Therapy with culturally diversed couples. In J. L. Furrow, S. M. Johnson, & B. A. Bradley (Eds.), *The Emotionally Focused casebook* (pp. 295–316). Routledge

Milgrom, J., & Gemmill, A. W. (2015), *Identifying perinatal depression and anxiety: Evidence-based practice in screening, psychosocial assessment, and management.* Wiley Blackwell.

Pilkington, P., Milne, L., Cairns, K., & Whelan, T. (2016) Enhancing reciprocal partner support to prevent perinatal depression and anxiety: a Delphi consensus study. *BMC Psychiatry, 16,* 23. https://doi.org/10.1186/s12888-016-0721-0

Sanchez, B. (2022). Postpartum depression in women of color. *McNair Research Journal SJSU, 18.* https://doi.org/10.31979/mrj.2022.1806

Soltani, M., Shairi, M. R., Roshan, R., & Rahimi, C. R. (2014). The impact of emotionally focused therapy on emotional distress in infertile couples. *International Journal of Fertility & Sterility,* 7(4), 337–344.

Stone, S. D., & Menken, A. E. (2008), *Perinatal and postpartum mood disorders: Perspectives and treatment guide for the health care practitioner.* Springer Publishing Co.

Taylor, J. K. (2020). Structural racism and maternal health among Black women. *Journal of Law, Medicine & Ethics, 48*(3), 506–517. https://doi.org/10.1177/1073110520958875

Van Rijn – Van Gelderen, L., Ellis-Davies, K., Huijzer-Engbrenghof, M., Jorgensen, T. D., Gross, M., Winstanley, A., Rubio, B., Vecho, O., Lamb, M. E., & Bos, H. M. (2020). Determinants of non-paid task division in gay-, lesbian-, and heterosexual-parent families with infants conceived using artificial reproductive techniques. *Frontiers in Psychology, 11.* https://doi.org/10.3389/fpsyg.2020.00914

30

YORUBA NIGERIAN AND EUROPEAN-AMERICAN COUPLES

International Considerations for Therapy

Rachael A. Dansby Olufowote

Global Migration and Intercultural Marriage

As recently as 2020, 281 million people lived outside their country of birth, migrating to other countries despite growing travel restrictions due to the Covid-19 pandemic (Natarajan et al., 2022). Globalization and migration reveal increasing cases of international and interracial marriage around the world (International Organization for Migration, 2020), as well as more research into understanding international migration and global coupling (Moses & Woesthoff, 2019). Couple therapists can expect to work more often with intercultural couples as globalization and migration continue (Rastogi & Thomas, 2009). Among many international migrants are Nigerians, and upwards of 45% of whom reported plans to leave Nigeria permanently between 2018 and 2023 (Connor & Gonzalez-Barerra, 2022). Additionally, recent international migration trends showed the United States received the largest number of migrants in 2020, the most popular immigration destination that year (Natarajan et al., 2022). In the United States, the cultural landscape has shifted dramatically over the past few decades, and intermarriage has increased between interracial couples (Bialik, 2017). Numbers of intermarriages specifically between Africans and Americans have also risen with many unions being between West African men and American women (Burdin Asuni & Asuni, 1987; Durodoye & Coker, 2008). United States census data support the conclusion that African immigrants to the United States are more likely to be males (Burdin Asuni & Asuni, 1987; Durodoye & Coker, 2008) who often migrate to other countries in search of educational and economic opportunities (Adeagbo, 2013).

While the body of interracial relationship literature has been increasing in recent years, particularly focusing on Black-White couples despite their low intermarriage rates (e.g., Dunleavy, 2004; Foeman & Nance, 2002; Karis, 2003; Killian, 2001a), there is remarkably little research examining African/White couples and even less on Yoruba Nigerian and European-American coupling, marriage, relationship dynamics, or difficulties and

DOI: 10.4324/9781003297871-33

intervention strategies. These trends lead this chapter to focus primarily on Yoruba Nigerian men married to or in an intimate partnership with European American women to highlight the unique cultural and gendered dynamics that shape their relationships. The goal of this chapter is also to synthesize what we know about Yoruba Nigerian/European American couples and to expand that knowledge with a case example of a male Yoruba Nigerian/ female European American couple. Due to the sparse available literature specifically examining Nigerians in international relationships with Americans, all available literature has been included here, even those that appear outdated, to establish a foundation of knowledge about this population.

Background on Nigerian/European American Couples

Migration and Residence of Nigerian/European American Couples

Nigerian migration around the world and to the United States (U.S.) has been primarily marked by the Nigerian male's pursuit of education and stable economic opportunities that can increase one's sense of relevance to society in the ever-expanding global community (Oyebamiji & Adekoye, 2019). Globally, the U.S. has the third largest Nigerian population, following only Nigeria and the United Kingdom (Migration Policy Institute [MPI], 2015). Nigerian Americans reside across the 50 states but tend to cluster in major metropolitan areas offering economic and educational opportunities (MPI, 2015). Around 49% percent of Nigerian immigrants came into the U.S. after 2000 (MPI, 2015; American Community Survey [ACS], 2021), and as of 2021, there were about 348,000 Nigerian immigrants living in the U.S., making Nigeria the top birthplace among African immigrants in the country (ACS, 2021; Budiman et al., 2020).

The U.S. is a land ripe with educational opportunities, and if Nigerians can acquire visa sponsorship, many decide to make their migration to the U.S. permanent (Bangura, 2004), as it Is economically advantageous to returning to Nigeria. While some Nigerians may prefer to couple with other Nigerians, others are open to international relationships with people of varying racial and cultural backgrounds including South Africans (Adeagbo, 2013), African Americans (Durodoye & Coker, 2008), and European Americans (Imamura, 1986). Though recent numbers are not readily available, some estimate the number of Nigerian men married to international wives are in the thousands (Burdin Asuni & Asuni, 1987).

Determining an exact number of U.S. citizens living in Nigeria proves difficult, due to multiple factors, including no obligation for U.S. citizens to check in with the U.S. Embassy on arrival or exit and patterns of bribery and corruption that undermine Nigerian census efforts (Goodman, 2019). That said, a member of the U.S. State Department delegation to Nigeria in 2018 reported the U.S. Consulate in Lagos estimated 100,000 U.S. citizens lived and worked in Nigeria (Goodman, 2019). For the purposes of this chapter, consider that some of these may include U.S. wives of Nigerian husbands. As this chapter discusses other elements of these intercultural/international relationships, it is important to keep in mind these couples could be living either in the U.S. or in Nigeria. Some of the realities of being in a Nigerian/European American relationship will be similar regardless of country of residency, but in other cases, the dominant culture where the couple resides will affect these couples differently.

Cultural Bases for Expectations of Partners

Cultural Similarities

Religion and Spirituality. There are few, broad cultural similarities between Nigerians and European Americans. Elements such as spirituality, a strong African value, may or may not be shared by European Americans. In cases where it is a shared value, however, it can be a point of attraction between partners and a major influence on couple dynamics. Yoruba Nigerian culture is intensely spiritual, expressed in both religious practice (e.g., Christian, Catholic, or forms of indigenous worship; Falola, 2001) and art and music. Nigeria is a deeply religious and spiritual nation with its population almost evenly split between Muslims (50%) and Christians (48.1%) as of 2015 (Falola, 2001; Gramlich, 2020), and religion holds a preeminent place in Nigerian culture (Falola, 2001). The southern part of Nigeria, where the Yoruba reside is predominantly Christian (Falola, 2001; Gramlich, 2020). Currently, both Nigerian religious views and worldviews are an amalgamation of indigenous and Western/Eastern faith, education, political ideologies, and customs, and are a heavy influence on how millions of Nigerians understand reality and culture, how they relate with others, and how they respond to change and events (Falola, 2001). So powerful an influence is religion that Nigerians may turn to their spiritual doctrines, communities, and practices to navigate insecurity, suffering, sickness, and death (Falola, 2001). Across Nigerian subcultures, a widespread belief is that evil forces cause negative experiences such as illness, moral decay, relationship problems, poverty, and failure of the country; likewise, "Healing can come through religion by destroying all evil and negative forces. One way to know that evil has been conquered is to receive abundant blessings in wealth, property, advancement, and health" (Falola, 2001, p. 32). From this, professionals and European American partners could expect that in times of relational distress and insecurity, Yoruba Nigerian partners may privilege counsel from church and spiritual leaders over professional therapists and turn to their faith for solutions. Examinations of the religious landscape in the U.S. in 2014 show around 80% of European Americans say they believe in God and around 67% endorse Christianity (Pew Research Center, 2014), which on the surface aligns with religious trends among the Yoruba.

Education. Additionally, Nigerians and Americans tend to align in valuing higher education. Education is one of the most dominant values in Nigerian culture, and unlike some patriarchal societies, they value the education of women also, seeing an educated and professional wife as bringing status and respect to the family (Falola, 2001). Various polls have found about half of Americans value higher education (Marken, 2019; Jackson et al., 2021), with more favoring professional degree programs (e.g., medical school or law school; [Ipsos, 2021]), though this value is decreasing (down from 70% of Americans in 2013; Gallup, 2019). However, women and people of the global majority in the U.S. tend to report higher education as more important than do white males (Gallup, 2019).

Family Preferences for a Mate. One specific area Nigerian and European American couples may have in common are the preferences and views of their families for a mate. Most Nigerian parents "still prefer that their children marry a member of the same ethnic group as themselves" (Falola, 2001, p. 120). Likewise, European American parents and family may express resistance when interracial/intercultural couples announce their engagement (Killian, 2001b), even though attitudes toward interracial and intercultural relationships in the U.S. have improved in recent years, with a majority of Americans endorsing neutral to positive views (Bialik, 2017; Parker, et al., 2019). Nigerian parents tend to place value upon the partner's ethnicity, religion, city or town of origin, education, and occupation to ensure a good fit (Falola, 2001). Falola (2001) corroborates Imamura's (1986) study with international wives married to Nigerians in which the partners' own families expressed value-laden concerns and considerations about them getting married. These ranged from concerns about cultural differences (including religion), children, living internationally or far from home, and (Nigerian) concerns that international relationships would not be stable and that the foreign wives would not be able to carry on her husband's culture and fulfill the role of a Nigerian wife (Imamura, 1986). Relevant to this chapter is a comment about this from one White American female married to a Yoruba Nigerian male (Imamura, 1986): "Their reservation was that I was not a Yoruba ... That I would not be able to carry on the culture for him and for his grandchildren as another Yoruba person would do" (White American). European American parents will likewise be interested in whether the Nigerian partner shares enough values to be a good match. This may then mean that Yoruba Nigerian/European American couples must take additional steps to garner the support of their families.

Cultural Differences

There are arguably more cultural differences than similarities among American and African cultures, chief of which is the communal (Nigerian) versus individual (Western) worldview. Other significant value differences could include patriarchy/feminism and religious worldview. Additional cultural differences extend to marriage and family structures and gender role expectations.

Collectivism vs. Individualism. The community-oriented Nigerian society and the individual-oriented, western American society stand in direct contrast and can pose major challenges for Yoruba Nigerian and European American couples. The individualism that marks Western countries such as the U.S. has been associated with traits such as an independent rather than interdependent view of self, self-reliance, privileging self-interest, and using personal attitudes rather than social norms to regulate behavior (Hofstede, 1991; Triandis, 1995; as cited by Bazzi et al., 2020). In the U.S., Bazzi et al. (2020) tracked the history of "rugged individualism" that developed as people migrated to the frontier. Historical accounts support how families often lived in isolation on the frontier, and survival depended on their ability to be self-reliant, independent, and fostered a "self-first" mentality (Bazzi et al., 2020). Though the "frontier" in the U.S. has long since been populated, the individualistic survival strategy survived and has persisted and been inherited by many U.S.-born people (Bazzi et al., 2020). In contrast, in Nigerian society, survival of the community and the individual rely on collectivism that creates a "community first" mentality (Falola, 2001). For example, "Where public services do not exist or are minimal, the family organizes and distributes resources to help its members. The family is equally a social organization" (Falola, 2001, p. 117). With the community-orientation, people are expected to help extended family members and others in the community; the Yoruba, specifically, are fond of using the proverb, "It takes a whole village to raise a child" to emphasize community responsibility (Falola, 2001). Nigerians value community and kinship so much they actively reject individualism. They work to prevent people from considering themselves solely as individuals who do whatever they want without thought of the family, clan, or community, and they socialize children into this communal ethos (Falola, 2001). This is an old survival strategy where group commitment ensured collective survival (Falola, 2001).

European-American and Yoruba Nigerian couples are then tasked with reconciling these survival strategies that have been passed down intergenerationally. Increasingly popular in western countries, attachment theory and attachment-based couples therapy research have been supportive of the collectivist approach to human connection, highlighting the human need for interdependence and the connection that comes with it (e.g., Cassidy & Shaver, 2016; Johnson, 2019). This body of research has been breaking down western myths that dependence on others is inherently dangerous. Despite how nice it sounds to move towards a model of interdependence, this may be quite complex and difficult for European-American partners who have been intergenerationally socialized to consider self before others even in the most benign of ways.

Patriarchy vs. Feminism. Two major worldviews that shape family life and couple dynamics internationally are patriarchy and feminism. Many cultures around the world use a patriarchal structure, including Nigeria (e.g., Nigerian partners will be familiar with the practice of the family defining roles based on generation, gender, and age, and as a patriarchy, family and society give more power to men; Falola, 2001). This would translate into older partners and male partners holding more power than younger partners and female partners. Nigerian male partners may also expect a female partner would take her husband's name in marriage. Additionally, the extended family norms in Nigerian families also mean "the children will treat their father's cousins as brothers and sisters and may refer to them as such" (Falola, 2001, p. 119). This is important for European-Americans to understand, as it widely differs from the western concept of family, where the concept of siblings tends to be limited to biological, step, and adoptive relationships.

Historically the U.S. has been a patriarchal society as well (Ruggles, 2015). Though patriarchy began to collapse in the 19th century, patriarchal gender norms remained well-entrenched through the mid-twentieth century (Ruggles, 2015) and continued to influence concepts of family structures and gender norms (e.g., via United States Census labels for heads of household) through the 1970s. However, since the 1920s, the feminist movements have been challenging patriarchal ideas and pushing for more gender neutral and egalitarian relationship structures. As of 2020, 6 in 10 U.S. women identified as feminists and believe feminism has brought positive changes to the U.S. (Mesasce Horowitz & Igielnik, 2020). This data puts American women on par with the global rate (58%) of women who identify with feminism (Morris, 2019). With Yoruba Nigerian/European American couples most likely to be Nigerian Males and European American females (Burdin Asuni & Asuni, 1987; Durodoye & Coker, 2008), these couples are likely to bring differing worldviews into the relationship, and for the relationship to succeed, they must find ways to reconcile these differences.

Marriage and Gender Role and Expectations. With collectivism and individualism differences in mind for the Nigerian/American couple, we may also see cascading cultural differences in marriage beliefs and views of gender roles between partners. In contrast to the average American monogamous conjugal or nuclear family, Nigerian family structures have historically been large, often polygamous (Falola, 2001), and extended with in-laws closely involved. While most Nigerians still cherish children, the "educated elite" are increasingly favoring monogamous marriages with fewer children (Falola, 2001), which is becoming more like trends in Western countries. Additionally, if a couple lives close to relatives in

Nigeria, it is not uncommon for a wife's in-laws to involve themselves in the couple's issues (Falola, 2001).

Despite some Nigerian families moving toward Western conjugal and familial models, other values appear to remain as they were before. Marriage is still an important social custom that confers so much status and respect that young people are often pressured to marry, and married women will tolerate repeated infidelities by her husband to remain married (Falola, 2001). Nigerian marriage values also intersect with indigenous spiritual beliefs and Christianity to interpret relational problems and solutions; for example, "When marriages are in trouble...someone in the community may be suspected of being a witch. So strong is the desire for marriages to endure" (Falola, 2001, p. 119).

Aligning with traditional biblical values, younger family members are expected to honor and respect older members, old age is revered and celebrated, and wives are guided to obey their husbands (Falola, 2001). Christian Yoruba Nigerian families teach children to be silent while older members are speaking, believing younger members have nothing to teach older members but have everything to learn from them (Falola, 2001; J. Olufowote, personal communication, November 22, 2022). The Nigerian practice of associating age with wisdom and showing deep respect for elders extends also to the marital relationship where a younger spouse is expected to approach the older spouse with deference and humility, assuming the older knows better and is wiser simply because they have lived longer (Falola, 2001; J. Olufowote, personal communication, November 22, 2022).

Historically in Nigeria, even when the couple relationship is struggling, the stigma of divorce was often stronger than stigma associated with putting up with a bad marriage, leading many traditional Nigerians to refrain from divorcing their spouses and enlist the help of extended family to mediate conflict (Falola, 2001). Western influences have reduced the stigma of divorce and increased its prevalence (Falola, 2001). This is an additional possible area of value difference between Nigerians and European Americans, as American culture is more accepting of divorce, promoting personal happiness over unhappiness in marriage, and many European Americans will not tolerate repeated lapses in fidelity or necessarily blame evil spiritual forces for marital problems. Additionally, the worldview of the origin of marital problems as spiritual is not shared by many Western couples' therapists, which would likely be a barrier to successful cross-cultural therapy, but it should not be disregarded in treatment.

Closely related to patriarchy and feminism as well as the modernization of values that resulted from globalization are how gender roles are conceptualized and negotiated. In Nigeria (and sometimes the U.S.), patriarchal gender norms tend to dominate and result in women handling the majority of food preparation, household chores, and childcare (Falola, 2001). Feminism has challenged these ideas and where some Nigerian husbands are more willing to assist their wives with traditionally "female" tasks, many are still more traditional and may struggle if their wives ask them to start "helping out" around the house.

Interracial Romantic Attraction and Partner Selection

With all the aforementioned differences, one may wonder how any Yoruba Nigerian and European American couple could be attracted to each other and choose to stay together. Many theories exist attempting to explain interracial attraction and coupling. For example, similarity, familiarity, and a multicultural ideology have all been proposed as related to attraction in general. We are all drawn to those with whom we share some similarity of values, disposition, interests, race, etc. (Miller et al., 2007), and meta-analytic research showed participants' perceptions of similarity had a moderate effect on romantic attraction (Montoya et al., 2008). In contrast, increased familiarity with diverse cultures and racial groups may lessen the tendency to be more attracted to someone of our own race (Brooks & Neville, 2016). Additionally, among Black and White male college students, endorsing a multicultural ideology was positively associated with preference for females of a different race, and increased interracial contact among White males led to increased interracial attraction and decreased same-race attraction (Brooks & Neville, 2016).

Initial Attraction

Using the Stimulus, Value, and Role theory (SVR; Murstein, 1973) with 21 international wives married to Nigerian husbands living in Nigeria, Imamura (1986) qualitatively examined interracial mate selection from a multi-stage perspective. During the Stimulus stage, which describes how couples met and formed a relationship, results indicate five themes that describe international wives' differing stances at the beginning of the relationship: (1) she was attracted by first appearances/impressions with little to no knowledge of Africa; (2) she was already involved in activities in Africa when they met; (3) she had already considered dating a foreigner; (4) she did not consider the relationship permanent and the proposal came as a surprise; and (5) she disliked him at first but was persuaded by his persistence (Imamura, 1986).

A potential point of attraction to European Americans, Nigerians are expressive and dynamic in language, dress, customs, and interpersonal communication (Falola, 2001). Though quiet, reserved personalities exist in Nigerian society, in general, Nigerian communication styles could be described as "big and loud," where intrigued, joyful, and excited reactions on the positive hand, and upset, frustrated, or angry responses on the negative hand are both typically grand expressions, accompanied by high energy, vivid facial and body language expression, and exclamatory language (Falola, 2001). In fact, for some Nigerian men, one indicator of interpersonal interest is conveyed by extroverted, loud, and even over-the-top expressions of interest, whereas more shy, softer, or introverted responses can be interpreted as non-interest (J. Olufowote, personal communication, November 20, 2022). Similarly, when a Nigerian male feels comfortable and safe with another person (be it family, friend, or romantic partner), they may adopt an unbridled and free way of being and communication style (J. Olufowote, personal communication, November 20, 2022). For example, this may look like intense displays of anger and use of harsh and/or profane language when upset, but this is also accompanied by the expectation that one can always apologize and repair afterward (J. Olufowote, personal communication, November 22, 2022). To have the safety to freely express oneself positively or negatively and deal with the consequences later is often preferred over communicating more carefully or measuredly on the front end.

Courtship and Value Comparison

In courtship (and later in marriage) traditionally, Nigerians express love differently than Americans. For example, "A couple in love may not go to movies, eat out, hold hands in public, or kiss one another time and again" (Falola, 2001, p. 120). Rather, Yoruba Nigerians tend to emphasize mutual respect and responsibility, the moral raising and education of children, fidelity in the couple relationship, and caring for extended families (Falola, 2001). At the courtship phase of the relationship, then, Yoruba Nigerian and European American couples must navigate these differences and evaluate if they are a good match. However, during this stage, partners may not be fully aware of the differences between them. For example, Imamura (1986) found that almost half of the 21 female international participants never considered values might be different in Nigeria than what they had grown up with. The other half of the sample did consider value differences, and only sometimes did partners initiate conversations about these differences. Husbands in this study were concerned about their (future) wives' abilities to fit into Nigerian society and with husbands' friends and advised their future wives on what to do, sometimes meeting resistance. The wives who considered the impact of value differences varied as well—some disregarded that value differences were important because they held the liberal view that "the marriage should work, because people are people regardless of background or race" (Imamura, 1986, p. 39), but later learned value differences played an important role in their relationship dynamics.

There were many discrepancies in Imamura's (1986) study between expectations and reality, which is an important consideration regarding mate selection. The researcher noted that few foreign wives passed through the value comparison stage with any real understanding of Nigerian lifestyles or of Nigerian values. According to Imamura (1986), two independent processes seem to occur with Nigerian men and foreign women that are important for clinicians working with male Nigerian and female European American couples:

> The husband's family's greatest concern is with value differences, but they are not usually in direct communication with the wife. The husband is at the time either concealing these differences from the wife, ignoring them as not really important, or unaware himself that they exist and will affect their marriage. The wife in most cases is ignorant of these differences and assumes life in Nigeria will be similar to life abroad. She, therefore, goes through the value stage as she would, were she considering marrying someone from her own society. (p. 41)

A theme from this research that might still be true today is one or both partners underestimating the importance of both similar and different values in a marriage. Imamura's (1986) findings showed couples emphasizing similarities over nationality or ethnicity differences during courtship and wives viewing their future Nigerian husbands as they would anyone from their own culture. Couples may assume certain shared background characteristics, such as both being from conservative Christian families, means there are no value differences to contend with, only to find after getting married there are numerous nuances in beliefs within various conservative Christian traditions. Emphasizing similarities and giving less consideration to differences certainly helps couples justify being together and moving toward marriage but does little to help them prepare to manage differences once married.

Marriage and Role Adjustments

During the Role stage, while living in the wives' countries of origin, Imamura (1986) notes that couples went through role adjustments just like any other couple, international or otherwise. It was when they moved to Nigeria after being married that the wives had to go through the role stage again and readjust to environmental and cultural expectations. For Yoruba Nigerian and European American couples living in the U.S., the culture shock experienced by the couples in Imamura's research may not apply, but assessing for and understanding how smoothly marital role adjustment is going for these couples is still critical.

Navigating Cultural Differences

Much of the past intercultural/interracial literature has focused on these relationships from a problem perspective (e.g., Bratter & King, 2008; Fu et al., 2001; Solsberry, 1994), though some researchers are approaching the topic from positive perspective, focusing on the interactional processes that lead to successful relationships (e.g., Cheng, 2005; Gaines & Agnew, 2003; Karis & Killian, 2009; Thomas et al., 2003; Troy et al., 2006; Seshadri & Knudson-Martin, 2013; Yancey & Lewis, 2009). With the extensive cultural differences and possible challenges facing Yoruba Nigerian/European American couples noted in this chapter, it is important to understand how interracial and intercultural couples navigate these differences successfully to create a strong relationship.

Two studies stand out that investigated processes intercultural couples use to deal with diversity within their relationships (Crippen & Brew, 2013; Seshadri & Knudson-Martin, 2013). In Crippen and Brew's analysis to find a typology of cross-cultural parenting in the U.S., they found couples used strategies of cultural adaption including cultural assimilation, cultural tourism, cultural transition, cultural amalgamation, and dual biculturalism. *Cultural assimilation* occurred when one partner unilaterally accommodated the cultural norms, traditions, and values of the other partner, typically from the dominant culture. *Cultural tourism* described an asymmetrical strategy of foreign husbands accommodating to the parenting values of U.S. wives. *Cultural transition* was another asymmetrical strategy involving wives primarily accommodating to their husbands' cultures. *Cultural amalgamation* was a fourth strategy used by intercultural couples that described a blended culture approach where couples tried to acknowledge differences and transcend them. These couples also demonstrated mutual acculturation to a third culture. Finally, *dual biculturalism* demonstrated a mutual acculturation process to the culture of both partners. These partners held a high commitment to biculturalism and to passing down both cultures, norms, values, and behaviors to their children.

Seshadri and Knudson-Martin (2013) also used grounded theory methodology to understand the process of managing cultural differences among interracial and intercultural couples of varying backgrounds. Using an ecological systems theory lens and the couple as the developmental unit to conceptualize the varying layers of systemic relationships and interactions to manage, Seshadri and Knudson-Martin identified four types of interracial/intercultural relationship structures: *Singularly Assimilating*, *Integrated*, *Coexisting*, and *Unresolved*. They found four especially important processes for couples managing cultural differences and the clinicians who work with them: (i) creating a "we," (ii) framing differences, (iii) emotional maintenance, and (iv) positioning themselves within familial and social contexts (Seshadri & Knudson-Martin, 2013, p. 53).

Some couples also found a way to transcend racial and cultural differences. Specifically, they created a coherent "we" through fostering friendship, finding common ground in shared values, and using common ground to develop similar goals around culture. When couples were able to find common ground and create similar goals over time, this strengthened their sense of shared identity as a unit. Clearly, intercultural/interracial couples need a way to make sense of their differences. Primary strategies across couples included decentralizing racial and cultural differences, seeing racial differences as an attraction, showing cultural flexibility and respect, curiosity and desire to learn about differences, and celebrating differences (Seshadri & Knudson-Martin, 2013).

It was also important for interracial/intercultural couples to deal with insecurities and emotions when difficult situations occurred. They used this strategy by communicating their emotions and insecurities to one another and considered this a source of strength (Seshadri & Knudson-Martin, 2013). Additionally, most couples were willing to make at least some adjustments around culture. Together, they leaned on those who supported their relationship (e.g., friends, therapy) in the face of not being accepted by family or society. Partners also navigated various social contexts, including experiences of discrimination and negative opinions from others. This involved couples presenting a united front to and setting boundaries with their families, communities, and society on racial discrimination and cultural prejudice (Seshadri & Knudson-Martin, 2013). They also had to adopt nonreactive communication, learn to speak constructively with others who were being prejudicial, and use appropriate humor to address cultural prejudice and discrimination. For couples whose families were not accepting of their partnership, couples had to give them time and space to hopefully accept their partner.

In the following section, I provide an example of a Yoruba Nigeria/European American couple (identifying details disguised for privacy) that illustrates the current status of knowledge about Yoruba Nigerian and European American couples, the struggles they face, and the strengths they possess.

Case Example

Dr. Emmanuel Olufemi Olukoju (age 38) and Dr. Rebecca (Stanley) Olukoju (age 33) have been married for five years and have two daughters under the age of 4. They met in the U.S. while Rebecca was in graduate school and Emmanuel had just begun his first tenure track faculty position. Rebecca is a U.S. citizen with English ancestry from the southwest, and Emmanuel is a Yoruba immigrant from Ibadan, Nigeria. Education is important to both families, and they obtained doctorate degrees in their respective areas of expertise before they married and now work in higher education as faculty and administrators. Both Rebecca and Emmanuel come from conservative Christian families but from different denominations. Rebecca was initially drawn to Emmanual's tall, strong physical presence and dark complexion, and Emmanual was attracted to Rebecca's "sweetness" and how she served at their church in "behind the scenes roles."

When they met, they described their connection as "palpable," but they did not begin dating until three years into their friendship. Their courtship was entirely long-distance, meeting up on the weekends twice a month. The weeks in-between were filled with long conversations where they would talk about life and their interests and pray together. Meeting at church and coming from conservative Christian families, they both assumed they shared similar core values, and early conversations supported these assumptions. However, they never thought to talk about differences in Emmanuel growing up in communal, patriarchal society versus Rebecca in an individualist, feminist-leaning society. During courtship, Rebecca tried to get Emmanuel to talk about his family and culture, but he did not have many answers to her questions, finding it hard to explain what he had grown up with in terms of social and relational dynamics and expectations. Her own research on Nigerian/ American couples yielded no results, and though she wanted to learn more about him and his culture, Rebecca felt limited and stuck.

Their first year of courtship was happy and peaceful. They dated for one year before Emmanuel proposed marriage and they got engaged with the blessing of Rebecca's family. Emmanuel had not yet told his family about Rebecca, because in his culture and family, Nigerian families only want to meet serious partners. Their year of engagement, however, took on more stress as they planned their wedding with no help from family, and Rebecca navigated completing her doctoral internship and dissertation. Emmanuel began to complain during this period that Rebecca was too self-focused and seemed to expect him to serve her whenever she visited him. This was a main topic of early arguments, as Rebecca perceived him to have unrealistic expectations of her. They sought out pastoral premarital counseling from Emmanuel's pastor, which was most comfortable for him, as he had never been to counseling or therapy due to cultural stigma. The couple found it difficult to meet with the pastor regularly, because sessions had to be scheduled around when Rebecca could travel amidst her educational responsibilities. The premarital sessions with the pastor felt helpful but were too infrequent to be of any real support or sources of cross-cultural learning; in fact, during their few sessions, the European American pastor never brought up race, culture, or sexual expectations.

Emmanuel grew increasingly but silently uncomfortable with how he felt his culture was being underrepresented at the wedding and in their relationship. Focusing primarily on learning about Rebecca and her background, Emmanuel withheld sharing about his culture in many areas and was unable to describe how his culture could be better represented in their wedding and marriage. Ultimately, however, they found a way to represent both cultures' food and clothing in their wedding. By the time the wedding date arrived, Emmanuel and Rebecca argued every time they were together. Rebecca assumed it was simply a side effect of the stress of the long-distance relationship, planning the wedding, and finishing her doctorate, though Emmanuel secretly began to wonder if it was a sign of incompatibility. However, they did not talk about why they were arguing so much or whether it was an indicator that they should not marry and proceeded toward the wedding day as planned. They recall their wedding as nice but feeling like a performance.

Shortly after getting married, they moved to the Midwest (U.S.) for Emmanuel's job change. They were thousands of miles away from both sides of the family, though Emmanuel had a few close college friends who lived nearby; otherwise, they were bereft of any social or marital support. It took time to establish a new church community, and as Emmanuel got lost in the demands of his new job, Rebecca felt even more isolated and alone. During courtship, their daily devotional and prayer time was the primary container for meaningful conversation and connection, which Rebecca loved, but their conversations tended to be quite lengthy, something that made Emmanuel feel increasingly anxious. Once married, they continued daily morning devotionals, though Emmanuel began cutting them shorter so he could get to work on time. Without any other connecting ritual, Rebecca became anxious and tried to keep the conversations going only for them to turn into arguments that made Emmanuel late for work. Devotional time quickly became a major source of tension and conflict.

They also struggled to adjust to their new roles as a married couple. Since getting married, Emmanuel increasingly expected Rebecca to learn how to prepare Nigerian dishes. Though she did occasionally, Rebecca found cooking generally stressful and wanted to also prepare dishes she grew up eating. Emmanuel preferred to eat the foods he had grown up with and had no desire to accommodate and develop a shared culture around food. Rebecca struggled with the tension of either accommodating completely to match her husband's preferences or prepare two meals every night for dinner.

In the isolation and stress of being newlyweds in a strange place, their conflict occurred more frequently and escalated more quickly in their first year of marriage, and both look back on that year as one of the worst of their lives. Rebecca believed Emmanuel was privileging his own needs and preferences above her own. On the other hand, Emmanuel experienced Rebecca as resisting his leadership, being wild, disrespectful, needing to be tamed, and being too individualistic. Rebecca suggested they find a couple's therapist, but Emmanuel refused, believing it was inappropriate to bring someone else into their private marital issues. To help manage the conflict, Emmanuel began pulling away and talking less about deeper issues, believing this would bring more peace to their relationship. This continued for the next two years of their marriage, until both began to feel so disconnected that they recently tried addressing a few deeper issues again. They both want to be closer but have found communication to be painfully slow and difficult. Emmanuel and Rebecca cautiously sought out couple therapy to help them navigate their differences and communication difficulties and reduce the stress they each experience in their marriage.

Cross-Cultural Clinical Applications

Therapist Cultural Awareness and Knowledge

With Yoruba Nigerian/European American couples, therapists should consider one's own cultural background, values, and beliefs and whether one has any racial prejudices against dark-skinned people or intercultural relationships. Emmanuel may be generally unfamiliar with the practice of counseling or therapy, as it is more traditional to use family members or faith leaders for help with personal matters (Falola, 2001), and may not be inclined to enter therapy. If he does, research suggests being flexible in one's approach or style is critical to developing an effective therapeutic alliance (Durodoye & Coker, 2008). Critical self-of-the-therapist examinations around race, relationship values, gender roles, and worldviews will also help therapists adopt a cross-cultural multidirectional partiality crucial in developing and maintaining rapport (Dansby Olufowote, et al., 2022). It is also critical for therapists to demonstrate cross-cultural knowledge about the dynamics of and unique issues facing Nigerian/European American couples. Durodoye and Coker (2008) recommend clinicians develop and maintain knowledge and skills in the following areas: acculturation and possible immigration issues, financial management, in-laws and privacy, child-rearing, language and communication, and food.

Assessing How Well Couples' "We" is Working

Using a tool such as the "Clinical Guide to Relational Strategies for Interracial and Intercultural Couples: An Ecological Perspective" (Seshadri & Knudson-Martin, 2013) or the "Multiple Heritage Couple Questionnaire" (Henriksen et al., 2007), a therapist can explore how Emmanuel and Rebecca organize around cultural differences and what ongoing strategies they use to manage differences. In this case, they were struggling to develop a "we" identity and could be described as somewhere between Singularly Assimilating and Unresolved. Additionally, couple therapists should gather an in-depth understanding of the couple's spiritual and religious backgrounds, beliefs, and any spiritually informed understanding of the problem(s) that brought them to therapy. If the therapist is unfamiliar with their religious views, curiosity and self-education will be paramount to the building of a safe therapeutic alliance. It could also be important for therapists to consult with couples' religious leaders, and if any individual care is indicated, consider referring them to pastoral care for individual support while they receive professional couple therapy.

Ongoing Navigation of Cultural Differences

Given Seshadri and Knudson-Martin's (2013) finding that shared values helped couples find common ground and create a sense of "we," couple therapists should assess how well they are reconciling any differences between collectivist/individualist and patriarchal/feminist values, beliefs, and expressions of such, and if needed, focus on helping the couple identify what a shared worldview could look like. Emmanuel and Rebecca have been struggling to find common ground and find a sense of unity within their relationship, particularly struggling with these worldview differences. If Yoruba Nigerian and European American couples are struggling to form a sense of "we," an accommodating partner may be grieving the loss of an important tradition or life transition ritual, and therapists should be prepared to help partners make space for this grief (Seshadri & Knudson-Martin, 2013). In various ways, both Emmanuel and Rebecca are grieving the loss of important cultural traditions and values as they attempt to find common ground. It could also be helpful for therapists to assist couples with navigating tangible differences in culture (e.g., food preferences and preparation expectations; Durodoye & Coker, 2008) to facilitate more transparent communication of expectations and needs and to help them mutually accommodate cultures.

As research shows, the ongoing management of cultural differences is a socially constructed and primarily language-based process (Brummet, 2017; Crippen & Brew, 2013; Gergen, 2009; Seshadri & Knudson-Martin, 2013). With couples such as Emmanuel and Rebecca who need help with the basics of forming a unified couple identity, conversations around language use, how they make meaning of their own and each other's cultural backgrounds and preferences will be important. This can also help when partners from collectivist cultures like Emmanuel may ignore or neglect hurt feelings or addressing deeper issues for the sake of "peace" in the relationship (Moghadam et al., 2009). Research has also shown that more structured processes such as cognitive restructuring and communication skills training work well with African populations when addressing language and communication issues (Okwun, 2011).

Finally, Seshadri and Knudson-Martin (2013) suggest therapists make visible how partners are supporting one another around racial and cultural differences and emphasize *mutual* support over one-sided support. Both Emmanuel and Rebecca could benefit from this conversation to better recognize where each other is experiencing cultural and racial difficulties within the relationship and society and learn how they can support each other amidst isolation.

Safety and Conflict Escalation

As with all new couples to therapy, it is critical to assess for intimate partner violence (IPV), and if the perpetrating partner is Nigerian, to assess the nature and magnitude of the violence and if they are ready to take accountability or if they are using African culture as a rationalization for their behavior. With the conflict escalation and intense emotion Emmanuel and Rebecca experienced early in their marriage, psychoeducation about forms of violence and its effects on mental health may also be helpful (WHO, 2022). This is also an opportunity to explore and help each partner understand underlying cultural meaning and emotions that can trigger conflict escalation.

Future Research

Future research needs to explore more in-depth how Nigerian/European American couples negotiate and navigate cultural and racial differences and build a strong connection. While one study has explored this general phenomenon amongst a variety of interracial and intercultural couples (Seshadri & Knudson-Martin, 2013) and this chapter has drawn on those results, future research needs to confirm if their results hold true for Nigerian/European American couples or whether there are any important, unique strategies or conditions of successful negotiations. Due to the lack of research in this area, this is particularly well suited to qualitative methodologies.

A topic not covered here due to lack of clear, conclusive research is how Nigerians and European Americans may hold different conceptualizations of what constitutes intimate partner violence and/or appropriate negative emotional expression. Western clinicians and researchers need to better understand how Nigerians distinguish between appropriate, culturally based emotional expression and unsafe emotional escalation, controlling behaviors and other expressions of violence.

Finally, though not limited to Nigerian and European American couples, as globalization, migration, and intercultural relationships continue, we need to develop clearer strategies for helping partners from collectivist and individualist societies find ways to reconcile value and worldview differences. One thing intercultural literature has made clear is that successful couples share more core values than not (e.g., Crippen & Brew, 2013; Seshadri & Knudson-Martin, 2013). For couples who marry without a full understanding of their value differences or whose values may shift in marriage, therapists need better tools for helping them find common ground. These issues can be explored qualitatively to gather in-depth lived experiences of couples from collectivist and individualist societies who have reconciled these differences successfully.

Resources and Recommended Reading

- "The Multiple Heritage Couple Questionnaire" (Henriksen et al., 2007)
- "A Clinical Guide to Relational Strategies for Interracial and Intercultural Couples: An Ecological Perspective" (Table 1 within Seshadri & Knudson-Martin, 2013)
- Durodoye, B. A., & Coker, A. D. (2008). Crossing cultures in marriage: Implications for counseling African American/African couples. *International Journal for the Advancement of Counselling, 30*, 25–37. https://doi.org/10.1007/s10447-007-9042-9
- Falola, T. (2001). *Culture and customs in Nigeria.* Greenwood Press. ISBN: 0-313-31338-5
- Rastogi, M., & Thomas, V. (2009). *Multicultural couple therapy.* Sage Publications.

- Seshadri, G., & Knudson-Martin, C. (2013). How couples manage interracial and intercultural differences: Implications for clinical practice. *Journal of Marital and Family Therapy, 39*(1), 43–58. https://doi.org/10.1111/j.1752-0606.2011.00262.x
- Crippen, C., & Brew, L. (2013). Strategies of cultural adaption in intercultural parenting. *The Family Journal, 21*(3), 263–271.

Key Points

1. It is important to help Yoruba Nigerian/European American couples manage their differences well. Focusing on strengths, creating a "we," and helping them share emotions and cultural meaning with each other are useful strategies with intercultural couples (Seshadri & Knudson-Martin, 2013).
2. Despite the number of possible cultural and value differences Yoruba Nigerian and European American couples have, they also possess many strengths, and approaching treatment from a strengths-based perspective can be more helpful and hopeful than taking a problem-focused approach.
3. Having awareness of one's cultural background and experiences that may produce racial or cultural biases is paramount in the development and maintenance of good rapport with intercultural couples (Dansby Olufowote et al., 2022). It is also critical to develop skill in the use of cross-cultural multidirectional partiality (Butler et al., 2011).

References

Adeagbo, O. A. (2013). 'We are not criminals, we are just victims of circumstances': An exploration of experiences of Nigerian immigrant men that married South African women in Johannesburg. *National Identities, 15*(3), 277–296. https://doi.org/10.1080/14608944.2013.780016

American Community Survey (ACS). (2021). *Nigeria: S0201 Selected population profile in the United States* [Data Set]. United States Census Bureau. https://data.census.gov/table?q=Nigerians+in+the+U.S.+in+2021&tid=ACSSPP1Y2021.S0201

Bangura, A. K. (2004). African immigration and naturalization in the United States from 1960 to 2002: A quantitative determination of the Morris or the Takougang hypothesis. *Ìrìnkèrindò: A Journal of African Migration, 3*, 27–35. https://africamigration.com/issue/sep2004/september_2004_full_issue.pdf

Bazzi, S., Fiszbein, M., & Gebresilasse, M. (2020). Frontier culture: The roots and persistence of "rugged individualism" in the United States. *Econometrica, 88*, 2329–2368. https://doi.org/10.3982/ECTA16484

Bialik, K. (2017). Key facts about race and marriage, 50 years after Loving v. Virginia. From www.pewresearch.org/fact-tank/2017/06/12/key-facts-about-race-and-marriage-50-years-after-loving-v-virginia/

Brooks, J. E., & Neville, H. A. (2016). Interracial attraction among college men: The influence of ideologies, familiarity, and similarity. *Journal of Social and Personal Relationships, 34*(2), 166–183. https://doi.org/10.1177/0265407515562750

Brummett, E. A. (2017). "Race doesn't matter" A dialogic analysis of interracial romantic partners' stories about racial differences. *Journal of Social and Personal Relationships, 34*(5), 771–789. doi: 10.1177/0265407516658790

Budiman, A., Tamir, C., Mora, L., & Noe-Bustamante, L. (August 20, 2020). *Facts on U.S. immigration, 2018: Statistical portrait of the foreign-born population in the United States.* Pew Research Center. www.pewresearch.org/hispanic/2020/08/20/facts-on-u-s-immigrants-current-data/

Butler, M. H., Brimhall, A. S., & Harper, J. M. (2011). A primer on the evolution of therapeutic engagement in MFT: Understanding and resolving the dialectic tension of alliance and neutrality. Part 2-recommendations: Dynamic neutrality through multipartiality and enactments. *The American Journal of Family Therapy, 39*(3), 193–213. www.tandfonline.com/doi/abs/10.1080/01926187.2010.493112

Burdin Asuni, J., & Asuni, T. (1987). Towards the success of intercultural marriage: A Nigerian example. *Practicing Anthropology, 9*(3), 12–14. www.tandfonline.com/doi/abs/10.1080/01926187.2010.493112

Cassidy, J. & Shaver, P. R. (Eds.). (2016). *Handbook of attachment: Theory, research, and clinical applications* (3rd ed.). Guilford Press.

Cheng, S. (2005). The differences and similarities between biracial and monoracial couples: a sociodemographic sketch based on the census 2000. Paper presented at the meeting of the American Sociological Association, annual meeting, Philadelphia, PA.

Crippen, C., & Brew, L. (2013). Strategies of cultural adaption in intercultural parenting. *The Family Journal, 21*(3), 263–271. https://doi.org/10.1177/10664807134766

Connor, P., & Gonzalez-Barrera (March 27, 2019). Many Nigerians, Tunisians and Kenyans say they plan to leave their countries in the next five years. Pew Research Center. www.pewresearch.org/fact-tank/2019/03/27/many-nigerians-tunisians-and-kenyans-say-they-plan-to-leave-their-countr ies-in-the-next-five-years/

Dansby Olufowote, R. A., Seshadri, G., Samman, S. K. (July/Aug 2022). Why your interracial/multi-national couples might be dropping out: A self-of-the-therapist exploration of critical factors. *Family Therapy Magazine, 21*(4). https://ftm.aamft.org/why-your-interracial-multinational-coup les-might-be-dropping-out-a-self-of-the-therapist-exploration-of-critical-factors/

Durodoye, B. A., & Coker, A. D. (2008). Crossing cultures in marriage: Implications for counseling African American/African couples. *International Journal for the Advancement of Counselling, 30*, 25–37. https://doi.org/10.1007/s10447-007-9042-9

Dunleavy, V. O. (2004). Examining interracial marriage attitudes as value expressive attitudes. *Howard Journal of Communications, 15*(1), 21–38. https://doi.org/10.1080/10646170490275369

Falola, T. (2001). *Culture and customs in Nigeria.* Greenwood Press.

Foeman, A., & Nance, T. (2002). Building new cultures, reframing old images: Success strategies of interracial couples. *Howard Journal of Communications, 13*(3), 237–249. https://doi.org/10.1080/10646170290109716

Fu, X., Tora, J., & Kendall, H. (2001). Marital happiness and inter-racial marriage: A study in a multi-ethnic community in Hawaii. *Journal of Comparative Family Studies, 32*(1), 47–60. https://doi.org/10.3138/jcfs.32.1.47

Gaines, S. O., & Agnew, C. R. (2003). Relationship maintenance in intercultural couples: An interdepend-ence analysis. In D. J. Canary & M. Dainton (Eds.), Maintaining relationships through communica-tion: relational, contextual, and cultural variations (pp. 231–253). Lawrence Erlbaum Associates.

Gergen, K. (2009). *An invitation to social construction* (2nd ed.). Sage Publications.

Goodman, J. (2019). How many Americans live and work in Nigeria today? Quora.com. www.quora.com/How-many-Americans-live-and-work-in-Nigeria-today

Gramlich, J. (March, 3, 2020). *Fast facts about Nigeria and its immigrants as U.S. travel ban increases.* Pew Research Center. www.pewresearch.org/fact-tank/2020/02/03/fast-facts-about-nigeria-and-its-immigrants-as-u-s-travel-ban-expands/

Hofstede, G., (1991). *Cultures and organizations: Software of the mind.* McGraw-Hill.

Hud-Aleem, R., Countryman, J., & Gillig, P. M. (2008). Biracial identity development and recommendations in therapy. *Psychiatry, 5*(11), 37–44. www.ncbi.nlm.nih.gov/pmc/articles/PMC 2695719/

International Organization for Migration. (2020). *World migration report 2022.* IOM. https://publi cations.iom.int/books/world-migration-report-2022

Ipsos. (2021). *Hard truth higher education poll: Topline and methodology.* Ipsos. www.ipsos.com/sites/default/files/ct/news/documents/2021-08/Topline%20Hard%20Truth%20Civil%20Rig hts%20Studyv2.pdf

Imamura, A. E. (1986). Ordinary couples? Mate selection in international marriage in Nigeria. *Journal of Comparative Family Studies, 17*(1), 33–42. https://doi.org/10.3138/jcfs.17.1.33

Jackson, C., Newall, M., Lloyd, N. (August 21, 2021). *All Americans see the value of higher edu-cation, but race continues to be a partisan flashpoint.* Ipsos. www.ipsos.com/en-us/news-polls/all-americans-see-value-higher-education-race-continues-be-partisan-flashpoint

Johnson, S. M. (2019). *Attachment theory in practice: Emotionally focused therapy (EFT) with indi-viduals, couples, and families.* Guilford Press.

Karis, T. (2003). How race matters and does not matter for white women in relationships with black men. In V. Thomas, T. A. Karis & J. L. Wetchler (Eds.), Clinical issues with interracial couples: the-ories and research (pp. 23–40). Hawthorne Press.

Karis, T. A., & Killian, K. D. (Eds.) (2009). Intercultural couples: Exploring diversity in intimate relationships. Routledge, Taylor & Francis Group, LLC.

Killian, K. D. (2001a). Crossing borders: Race, gender, and their intersections in interracial couples. *Journal of Feminist Family Therapy*, 13(1), 1–31. https://doi.org/10.1300/J086v13n01_01

Killian, K. D. (2001b). Reconstituting racial histories and identities: The narratives of interracial couples. *Journal of Marital and Family Therapy*, 27(1), 27–42. https://doi.org/10.1111/j.1752-0606.2001.tb01137.x

Marken, S. (December 30, 2019). *Many in U.S. now consider college education very important*. Gallup. www.gallup.com/education/272228/half-consider-college-education-important.aspx

Mesasce Horowitz, J., & Igielnik, R. (2020). A century after women gained the right to vote, majority of Americans see work to do on gender equality: Methodology. Pew Research Center. www.pewresearch.org/social-trends/2020/07/07/methodology-36/

Migration Policy Institute (MPI). (June 2015). *The Nigerian diaspora in the United States*. [A report prepared for Rockefeller Foundation-Aspen Institute Diaspora Program (RAD)]. MPI. www.migrationpolicy.org/sites/default/files/publications/RAD-Nigeria.pdf

Miller, R, S., Perlman, D., & Brehm, S. S. (2007) *Intimate relationships*. McGraw-Hill.

Moghadam, S., & Knudson-Martin, C., Rankin Mahoney, A. (2009). Gendered power in cultural contexts part III: Couple relationships in Iran. *Family Process*, 48, 41–54. https://doi.org/10.1111/j.1545-5300.2009.01266.x

Montoya, R. M., Horton, R. S., & Kirchner, J. (2008). Is actual similarity necessary for attraction? A meta-analysis of actual and perceived similarity. *Journal of Social and Personal Relationships*, 25, 889–922. https://doi.org/doi:10.1177/0265407508096700

Morris, C. (November 25, 2019). Less than a third of American women identify as feminists. Ipsos. www.ipsos.com/en-us/american-women-and-feminism

Moses, J., & Woesthoff, J. (2019). Romantic relationships across boundaries: Global and comparative perspectives. *The History of the Family*, 24(3), 439–465. https://doi.org/10.1080/1081602X.2019.1634120

Murstein, B. I. (1973). A theory of marital choice applied to interracial marriage. In I. R. Stewart and L. E. Abt (Eds.), *Interracial marriage: Expectations and realities*, (pp.17–35). Grossman.

Natarajan, A., Moslimani, M., & Lopez, M. H. (December 16, 2022). *Key facts about recent trends in global migration*. Pew Research Center. www.pewresearch.org/fact-tank/2022/12/16/key-facts-about-recent-trends-in-global-migration/

Okwun, C. O. (2011). Effects of cognitive restructuring and communication skills training on conflict resolution among Nigerian couples. *International Journal of Peace and Development Studies*, 2(6), 179–189. http://www.academicjournals.org/IJPDS

Oyebamiji, S. I., & Adekoye, A. (2019). Nigerians' migration to the United States of America: A contemporary perspective. *Journal of African Foreign Affairs*, 6(1), 165–180. www.jstor.org/stable/26664092

Parker, K., Morin, R., & Menasce Horowitz, J. (March 2019). Views of demographic changes. In K. Parker, R. Morin, & J. Mesasce Horowitz (Eds.), *Looking to the future, public sees America in decline on many fronts*. From Pew Research Center, www.pewresearch.org/social-trends/2019/03/21/views-of-demographic-changes-in-america/

Pew Research Center. (May 30, 2014). *Religious landscape study: Whites*. Pew Research Center. www.pewresearch.org/religion/religious-landscape-study/racial-and-ethnic-composition/white/

Rastogi, M., & Thomas, V. (2009). *Multicultural couple therapy*. Sage Publications.

Ruggles, S. (2015). Patriarchy, power, and pay: The transformation of American families, 1800–2015. *Demography*, 52(6), 1797–1823. doi: 10.1007/s13524-015-0440-z

Seshadri, G., & KnudsonMartin, C. (2013). How couples manage interracial and intercultural differences: Implications for clinical practice. *Journal of Marital and Family Therapy*, 39(1), 43–58. https://doi.org/10.1111/j.1752-0606.2011.00262.x

Solsberry, P. W. (1994). Interracial couples in the United States of America: Implications for mental health counseling. *Journal of Mental Health Counseling*, 16(3), 304–317. https://psycnet.apa.org/record/1995-10522-001

Thomas, V., Karis, T. A., & Wetchler, J. L. (Eds.) (2003). Clinical issues with interracial couples: Theories and research. New York: Hawthorne Press.

Triandis, H. (1995). *Individualism & collectivism*. Westview Press.

Troy, A. B., Lewis-Smith, J., & Laurenceau, J. (2006). Interracial and intraracial romantic relationships: The search for differences in satisfaction, conflict, and attachment style. *Journal of Social and Personal Relationships*, 23(1), 65–80. https://doi.org/10.1177/026540750606017

WHO. (2022). *Preventing intimate partner violence improves mental health*. World Health Organization. www.who.int/news/item/06-10-2022-preventing-intimate-partner-violence-impro ves-mental-health

Yancey, G., & Lewis, R. (2009). *Interracial families: current concepts and controversies*. Routledge, Taylor and Francis Group.

31

PRACTICING COUPLE THERAPY IN THE MIDDLE EAST

Arab- and Muslim-Related Critiques and Clinical Considerations

Mona El Roby Saleh, Sarah K. Samman, and Rachael A. Dansby Olufowote

Introduction

For over 70 years in the western world, clinicians have devoted their attention to improving mental health (MH) for multiple members of a family system (Gehart, 2018; Nichols & Davis, 2021). This movement resulted in the significant development of various theoretical orientations, therapeutic modalities, and training in the treatment of couples and families. The discipline of marriage and family therapy, often referred to as couple and family therapy, has gradually expanded to a global audience, and the Middle East (ME) is no exception. This chapter focuses on synthesizing and expanding upon the nuance of the status of couple therapy in the ME, specifically focusing efforts on the experiences and therapeutic treatment of Arab Muslim couples.

This chapter is an attempt to help MH providers understand both similarities and differences that Middle Eastern Arabs and Muslims may experience in an attempt to identify, categorize, and acknowledge their heterogeneity. This is a significant area warranting interest as studies indicate many assume the terms Middle Eastern, Arab, and Muslim are interchangeable (see Sherif-Trask, 2011). Yet this is not the case, and MH clinicians must ensure they do not intentionally or unintentionally designate systems by any label, be it ethnic, racial, or religious. Doing so runs the risk of implying this is the main determinant of identification for these individuals, couples, and their families (see Sherif-Trask, 2011).

For this chapter, we hope to assist readers with describing and categorizing Middle Easterners, Arabs, and Muslims. We provide an overview of common linguistic, ethnic, racial, and religio-spiritual experiences for those who identify with all three categories and that often impact their unique struggles, socio-cultural and sacred perceptions of MH, and subsequent MH-seeking behaviors. We also provide a systemic application specific to this

DOI: 10.4324/9781003297871-34

underserved population as well as reflections on future research advances. We end our chapter with further reading resources as well as three key points for consideration.

Diverse Identities in the Middle East

Geographically, the term ME is used to differentiate between the Near East (e.g., East and Southeast Asia) and the Far East (e.g., Southeast Europe and North Africa) (Middle East, 2023). There have been varying descriptions of the ME. Because the label has changed over time, it is often difficult to obtain a consensus. For the purpose of this publication, the ME generally encompasses a majority of Western Asia (i.e., the Arabian Peninsula comprising Kuwait, Oman, Qatar, Saudi Arabia, United Arab Emirates, and Yemen; Bahrain; Iran; Iraq; Israel; Jordan; Lebanon; Palestine Liberation Organization; and Syria) and Northern Africa (i.e., Egypt).

There are various accounts of who initially used and coined the term. Nevertheless, a majority from the ME view it as a pejorative and discriminatory designation reflecting a western, Eurocentric, socio-political era rather than one that honors the inhabitants of the region (Hanafi, 2000). Moreover, many have largely coveted the region for geostrategic purposes (e.g., access to the Suez Canal and a significant percentage of global trade) and material resources (oil-rich reserves and historical artifacts; Amstrong, 2000). Due to these factors resulting in significant colonization and globalization processes, the region has experienced a significant change to its linguistic, ethnic, racial, and religio-spiritual identities. First, we will discuss linguistic identities in the region.

Linguistic Identities in the ME

With current beliefs in the social construction of language (Gergen, 2009), the way language is used matters. Systemic thinkers recognize that there is a relational, dialogical, and generative nature between language and knowledge (Gergen, 2009). Specifically, language that is both spoken and unspoken is the primary vehicle through which we gain knowledge and construct and make sense of the world. Language gains its meaning through its use and transforms past, present, and future experiences and results in the construction of knowledge. Because of this, systemic thinkers benefit greatly from understanding the importance of language and its use as the main dialogical tool to elicit therapeutic change (Chowdhury, 2010). Thus, recognizing the differences and complexities of language in the ME is critical for effective therapeutic relationships.

There are numerous languages spoken in the ME. The most common language in the region by population size is Arabic (Shoup, 2011). However, inhabitants use other languages such as Aramaic, Hebrew, Kurdish, and Persian (Horesh, 2019). On the same note, inhabitants may share a common linguistic and cultural background, though they may use their own dialects and cultural references that reflect their unique identities and understandings. These ethnic identities are further discussed in the following section.

Ethnic Identities in the ME

Specifically, the largest ethnic group in the ME are Arabs (Shoup, 2011), with a majority of the countries in the ME being members of the Arab League, otherwise known as the League of Arab States (Horesh, 2019). In 1942, there was a call to develop an official and shared linguistic identity for Arabs in the region due to socio-political and geostrategic processes that largely resulted in the subordination of the Arab identity. As a result of this effort, in 1944, five Arab countries signed the Alexandria Protocol lending formality to the official development of the League of Arab States in 1945 (Arab League 2023) and signed by seven Arab countries with the intent to develop and improve socio-cultural and socio-political relations (Arab League, 2023; Horesh, 2019). The number of States has waxed and waned over the years with a current membership of 22 States. These include Algeria, Bahrain, Comoros, Djibouti, Egypt, Iraq, Jordan, Kuwait, Lebanon, Libya, Mauritania, Morocco, Oman, State of Palestine (Palestine Liberation Organization), Qatar, Saudi Arabia, Somalia, Sudan, Syria (Syrian Arab Republic), Tunisia, United Arab Emirates, and Yemen (Arab League, 2023). However, clinicians must not exclude other ethnic groups in the ME region such as Druze, Jews, Kurds, Persians, and Turks.

Middle Eastern Arabs' Diverse Racial Identities. With Arabs internationally recognized as an ethnicity, there is still considerable variation in racial identity, despite evidence that race is a political and divisive social construct and which results in significant experiences with racial prejudice and bigotry globally, and in the Middle East and North Africa (MENA) specifically (Hilizah, 2022; King, 2021). For example, the Eastern parts of the ME such as Iran and Northern parts of the Arabian Peninsula are generally categorized as racially White. In comparison, northern parts of Egypt report racial diversity for various reasons, such as historical influences from the Greeks as well as European colonization from the Turks, French, and British Empire (see Daly, 2008; Petry, 1998). Moreover, in the southern parts of Egypt, Nubians physically present as well as identify strongly as Black (Moll, 2021). Nevertheless, for the sake of ease, the United States categorized native Europeans as well as Middle Easterners and North Africans as racially White (Management and Budget Office, 1997), despite not benifitting from this categorization. This often results in the erasure of their complex and intersectional identities and experiences and warrants respectful reevaluation of biases that perpetuate these stereotypes and subsequent clinical processes. To add further complexity to these identities, the following is a brief discussion of religio-spiritual (i.e., sacred) identities in the region.

Sacred Identities in the Middle East

Those inhabiting the region largely follow the Abrahamic religions (i.e., Judaism, Christianity, and Islam), essentially worshiping the same God. At the same time, clinicians could benefit from acknowledging the growing non-denominational, secular, as well as minority religions native to the region that often remain undeclared due to fears of censorship or marginalization.

Globally, Islam is the second largest religion after Christianity. There are currently over eight billion human inhabitants on earth. Of these individuals, more than two billion identify as Muslim. And it is expected that by 2050, the number of Global Muslims will exceed that of Christians (World Population Review, 2023). Approximately 27 countries adopt Islam as the state religion (Pew Research Center, 2017). Of those countries, the majority of Muslim born live in North and Central Africa, the ME, and Southeast Asia (World Population Review, 2023).

In contrast, Muslims in other regions, such as in Europe and North and South America, are Muslims that largely emigrated from those majority Muslim countries. In the United States, for example, many Muslims chose to emigrate from those countries in search of opportunities. Others, such as historic African Americans, were enslaved and forcibly removed from their homeland as part of the slave trade. And lastly, some Muslims in the United States identify as those that converted to Islam from groups such as European-Americans and Hispanic/Latinx populations (see Pew Research Center, 2007). Yet, how each person envisions and practices their religious beliefs differs.

Who are Muslims? Muslims are those who espouse Islam as their religion and believe that Prophet Muhammad (Peace Be Upon Him) is God's messenger. Islam requires the full submission to God (Allah) as well as peaceful behaviors and responsibilities towards Allah's creations, including the self (Hathout, 1995). There are two main denominations, Sunni and Shi'ite (Hathout, 1995), in addition to smaller sects such as Ahmadi, Bahai, and Sufi. Regardless of which sect one follows, Muslims largely report turning to their spiritual texts and interpretations for guidance and decision-making, particularly during relational conflict (Hathout, 1995, see also Mir-Hosseini, 2003).

Similar to Hathout (1995), Mir-Hosseini (2003) emphasized two essential terms that inform Muslim beliefs and behaviors. The terms *Shari'a* and *Fiqh* are often sources of confusion and conflict. *Shari'a* refers to the laws governing the Muslim experience (e.g., inheritance) and are constant and unchanging (Mir-Hosseini, 2003). On the other hand, *Fiqh* is the Islamic Jurisprudence or the task of seeking understanding of how to apply and implement *Shari'a Law* (Mir-Hosseini, 2003). This is possible through interpreting the sacred text (the Qur'an) and supplementing with Sunnah (i.e., confirmed verbal narrations and deeds that are "the second main source of Islamic Law;" Hathout, 1995, p. xv). As one could imagine, there are diverse and subjective interpretations and applications of sacred beliefs and practices within Islam. Because of the large geographical area of the region, one might presume diversity in racial identities as well.

Muslims' Diverse Racial Identities. The majority of global Muslims reside in East and Central Asian countries, and natives largely identify as racially Asian. Though small in size comparatively, these countries have the largest Muslim percentage of the total global Muslim population (The Pew Forum on Religion and Public Life, 2009). For example, Indonesia is the largest global Muslim-majority country representing 12.9% of Muslims globally, and has a Muslim majority of 88.2% of their total population (The Pew Forum on Religion and Public Life, 2009). Conversely, Saudi Arabia, represents approximately 2% of the world's Muslims despite approximately 97% identifying as Muslims from the total national population (The Pew Forum on Religion and Public Life, 2009). Saudi Arabia, a part of West Asia and much larger in size, is racially designated as White despite a diverse racial composition. From this, we surmise that geographical location in the Asian continent does not always equate with a politically and socially constructed Asian racial identity. Similarly, geographical locations in Northern Africa, such as Egypt, do not always correspond to Black racial identities. Regardless, reducing complex ethnic and racial experiences and identities to a category or label is superficial, detrimental, and a core reason why the teachings of Islam grounded much of its efforts to undermine and dismantle racial hierarchy (Hathout, 1995). Nevertheless, racial minorities in the ME often experience discrimination despite clear opposition from Islamic values and subsequent cannon (Hathout, 1995).

Racial Identities and Social Status. There still exists cases where racial identity and social standing directly impact relationships and coupling decisions and experiences (Hilizah, 2022). For example, interpersonal discrimination can be evident during the coupling process where cultural expectations often necessitate formal courting processes that involve the immediate and extended family. In addition to ethnic hierarchies such as those espoused by, for example, bedouins who adhere to strict ranks of social capital within and between their tribes, families may also espouse colorism (King, 2021). Clinicians in the ME have long shared observations of families reporting discomfort, balking at, or even refusing darker male suitors courting their lighter skinned daughters. For these reasons, it is critical for MH professionals, who may or may not possess those privileges, to advocate for clients using curiosity and culturally responsive and respectful clinical support when working with Middle Easterners, Arabs, and Muslims, and particularly during the coupling processes.

Mental Health Globally and in the ME with Arab Muslims

A global stigma around MH exists and those in the ME are no exception. Due to the prevalence and necessary treatment for legitimate MH concerns, the MH field expanded over the last few decades to include various international disciplines and careers. Examples from the World Health Organization (WHO, 2021) include social workers, psychologists, psychiatric nurses, and psychiatrists with an estimated workforce of 13 MH workers per 100,000 global inhabitants. Furthermore, only 31% of countries responding to the WHO survey and representing only 25% of WHO Members "reported the integration of mental health into primary health care" (p. 2) implying MH services as supplementary and beyond the scope of primary health care. Moreover, many use the terms clinician, psychotherapist, and therapist interchangeably. For the purpose of this chapter, therapists are clinicians utilizing a systemic lens in their treatment of individuals, couples, and families.

Furthermore, it appears that MH clinicians in the ME often practice at the undergraduate level under the umbrella of clinical psychologists. At this level, they often lack experience and training in treating contextually informed and complex MH concerns compared to their counterparts who choose to specialize and practice at the masters level. There also appears to be few international educational resources, certifications, and programs in the field of marriage or couple and family therapy in the language of origin or specific to the socio-cultural influences of the host country.

Meanwhile, the International Family Therapy Association (IFTA, n.d. [b]) invested efforts into marketing and amplifying the significant contributions of systemic thinkers. The Association offers an international designation as a certified family therapist (IFTA, n.d. [a]) to MH professionals, such as those above. With a changing clinical demographic, research on how to provide systemic informed clinical services for specific demographics and linguistic needs is lacking.

As previously established, discourses in the ME are vast and complex, largely due to the region's adherence to religio-cultural values, beliefs, and traditions. Inhabitants of the region often experience these values and beliefs as empowering and carry on the tradition within society and across generations. However, some discourses feel disempowering and can pose challenges to establishing and maintaining relationships, particularly intimate ones. Although listing them here is beyond the scope of this chapter, the following is a brief overview of MH services and experiences in the ME, including factors affecting MH-seeking behaviors.

Factors Affecting MH-Seeking Behaviors in the ME

There is increased attention devoted to examining the MH status and MH-seeking behaviors of those inhabiting the Muslim Arab world. Systems therapists often view MH struggles and dysfunction because of socio-religio-cultural beliefs. And like other cultures, there are problematic and prevalent stereotypes in the ME as well. We do not condone the misuse of these stereotypes and invite an attuned clinical approach that is anchored in curiosity and respect to positively influence this population and shift the cultural norm.

Confusing Shari'a and Fiqh. In many cases, Muslims may attend to strongly held and subjective religious understandings (i.e., Fiqh) that are believed to discourage MH-seeking behaviors. Smith (2011) pointed out that Islamic scriptures and prophetic narrations do not specifically indicate that seeking professional clinical help is disapproved religiously or rejected. However, some Muslims believe that sharing their problems with others is akin to complaining about God and rejecting His wisdom. They might also believe that complaining is a sign of weakness and lacks patience and religious endurance. Still, some believe "complaining to anyone other than God is a disgrace" (Dwairy & Van Sickle, 1996, p. 237). However, this quote appears decontextualized and is a regional and cultural saying that lacks support linking it directly to Prophet Muhammad (Peace Be Upon Him). Even so, the difficulty remains that lacking context and a nuanced understanding of this and other sayings and beliefs would create significant barriers to MH-seeking behaviors and services. This includes how seeking and accepting therapy might reflect poorly from and on the immediate and extended family system. Thus, engaging potential clients from this population is a critical endeavor.

MH Treatment Using Sacred Interventions. To add socio-religous complexity, Dwairy (2006) pointed out that in the Arabic language, the language of the Qur'an, the equivalent of the word mental illness is *jinnoon* (or *junoon* per Modern Standard Arabic). The root word is an indication of separation, for example, a separation of functioning from the mind. This word closely relates to the word *jin* (i.e., djin, genie, monster, or devil), a super-natural force that is seen as separate from the worldly plain. *Jinnoon* is also associated with other supernatural factors such as magic and the evil eye (envy) in addition to poor faith (Vally et al., 2018). Because some believe that psychological struggles such as depression and anxiety may be a result of supernatural forces, Dwairy (2006) reported that individuals often seek help from religious scholars and healers to exorcize the *"jin"* or to counter the evil eye through engaging in certain supplications or rituals.

However, seeking religiously informed interventions often prevents engaging in other means of evaluating their or their systems' experiences and limits options to treat minor psychological struggles as well as complex MH concerns or illnesses. Thus, ascribing mental illness to external factors results in limited beliefs in an internal locus of control thereby denying responsibility for problematic thoughts or behaviors (see Dwairy, 2006). By extension, some researchers such as Smith (2011) found that some Muslim Arabs believe that developing and maintaining a strong faith in a higher power protects them from evil. And though they may struggle, they see their struggles as a test and often choose to focus on strengthening their relationship with God, thereby viewing therapy as unimportant and unhelpful.

Furthermore, clinicians must consider contextual factors that may reinforce the choice to engage religious scholars or clergy who are often bound by moral obligations to maintain confidentiality. Conversely, some clients reported an understandable fear that MH professionals may not honor confidentiality (see Onsy, 2013; Tadros et al., 2022). Clients' doubts about therapists' legal and ethical responsibilities represent major barriers to MH-seeking behaviors.

MH Treatment Using MH Services

Conversely, Smith (2011) affirmed that Muslim-Arab-Americans in her study who decided to seek therapy predominantly did not view MH-seeking behaviors and services as incompatible with Islam or their religious values and beliefs. Smith reported they view therapists more positively as resources and helpers that work *with* them towards change. Moreover, Zolezzi et al. (2018) pointed out that Arabs' perceptions toward MH are shaped by several factors such as level of education, degree of awareness about mental MH, and gender.

A plethora of research confirmed that the higher one's educational level, the more positive the impact on one's MH (Kondirolli & Sunder, 2022) and the perceptions of MH treatment and services (Al-Kernawi et al., 2004; Onsy, 2013; Zolezzi et al., 2018). Further, an advanced education is often associated with an increased awareness level. And with education and awareness, there is often self-advocacy that results in challenging cultural and relational norms such as those that seem incompatible with MH needs and MH-seeking behaviors. In addition, Tadros et al. (2022) mentioned that women specifically may not engage in MH treatment as they are assumed to represent the family's honor. Thus, disclosing family matters to a therapist may be perceived as complaining about and shaming the family. Even worse, if a woman is diagnosed with a MH disorder, she may experience potential abuse, or in some cases, the husband may use his wife's MH status as an excuse to divorce her or abuse the practice of polygamy and marry a second wife (Al-Kernawi et al., 2004; see also Hathout, 1995).

Similar to Zolezzi et al. (2018), Kayrouz et al. (2018) found that Arabs often struggled with a lack of knowledge or understanding about what MH services were available or what constituted high quality therapy. Onsy (2013) punctuated this barrier in her report that one of the major hindrances preventing Egyptian couples from seeking therapy is the lack of awareness about the availability of professional couple therapists. Kayrouz et al. also identified another significant barrier to MH-seeking behavior, financial constraints. Though not specific to Arabs in the ME, this study explored the acceptability of seeking therapy among 503 Arabs in Egypt, Algeria, Yemen, Iraq, and Australia. Results of the online survey about therapy acceptability found that participants were unable to seek out therapeutic services because costs were prohibitive.

And lastly, it is prudent to discuss Smith's (2011) research on Muslim Arab Americans' attitudes toward therapy and how this information can be generalized to those in the ME. Smith reported that participants in her study were concerned about seeking therapeutic services due to worry or fear that: a) therapists may not uphold their responsibility to maintain confidentiality; b) therapists may lack knowledge about Islam and/or the Arab culture, and may provide inappropriate or incompatible interventions or treatment recommendations; and c) therapists may hold biases against them due to their religion, ethnicity, or culture. In addition to mirroring concerns held by Arab Muslims in their native countries about confidentiality (Onsy, 2013; see also Tadros et al., 2022), we can surmise that Arab Muslims in the ME may worry about how therapists might provide appropriate or compatible interventions as well as concerns that therapists may hold biases against them based on their religio-spiritual, cultural, or racial identities.

Factors Affecting Couple Relationships in the ME for Arab Muslims

Muslims families often view coupling processes as a sacred responsibility (Hathout, 1995). Similar to the western world, families often reinforce generational expectations of forming religious and legal unions through marriage. However, they often encourage couplehood and formal unions without providing necessary resources to set couples up for success in their relationships. Hassan (2005) reported on the Muslim experience and the high regard placed on marriage and the teachings that encourage men and women to create a religious union through marriage.

Marriage and Fulfilling Half of One's Religion

Haque and Kamil (2011) argued that different verses of the Qur'an clearly demonstrated that men and women were created from one soul, and that people's faith and deeds, not gender, determine their status. This is reflected in the following verses, "O humanity! Be mindful of your Lord Who created you from a single soul, and from it He created its mate, and through both He spread countless men and women" (Qur'an, 4:1). Scholars also reinforce the importance of becoming acquainted with others outside of the immediate family and social circle, particularly during the courting process, because God "made you into peoples and tribes so that you may come to know one another" (Qur'an 49:13).

Muslims promote this belief through the use of Prophet Muhammad's (Peace Be Upon Him) narration that when Muslims marry, they have "fulfilled half of their religion" (Hassan, 2005, p. 246). When considering a life partner, Hassan highlighted the basis of marriage in Islam as being on mutual affection and equality. The approximate translation of the Qur'anic verse (2:187) states: "Permitted to you on the night of the fasts is the approach to your wives. They are your garments. And ye are their garments." Many misunderstand this text to only reflect the physical and sexual nature of the union. This disregards the complex physical and psychological intent and function of a garment, one in which effort must be placed on compatibility to the temperament and personality of the wearer as well as to view each as protecting and adorning the other. In any union, there is an intimacy like no other and partners are more likely to commit to protecting and representing their union more favorably when there is a sense of respect, responsibility, engagement, all of which are partner positionings advocated by Knudson-Martin and Huenergardt (2015) and Samman and Knudson-Martin (2015). So in this mutually beneficial and reciprocal sense, the teachings of Islam favor justice and equity rather than stereotypical beliefs that place men in a position of power and privilege over women (Hassan, 2005; see also Hathout, 1995).

Gender Equity and Justice

Be that as it may, patriarchal biases and misinterpretations exist. As a result, some Muslims largely ignore the socio-cultural implications of narrations grounded in their responsibility to God's creations, including to be at peace with oneself as well as others; in this case, their life partners (Hathout, 1995). Some also overlook the rules and obligations required when forging this union that are established to protect each partner. For these and many other reasons, an increasing scholarly interest has developed over the last few decades to critically examine Islamic scriptures and its interpretive texts from the lens of gender justice. The goal of this scholarly interest is twofold: 1) criticizing religious interpretations that encourage patriarchy and sanction discrimination against women, and 2) to provide alternative interpretations that promote gender equality from the Islamic perspective (Al-Sharmani, 2014). This scholarly interest resulted in the emergence of Islamic feminism that primarily includes Muslim female scholars such as Amina Wadud (African-American), Ziba Mir-Husseini (Iranian), Asma Lamrabet (Moroccan), Omaima Abou-Bakr (Egyptian), and others.

Gender Equity and Rights Discourses. Mir-Husseini (2003) differentiated between three critical discourses on gender rights in the Muslim world. She identified the first as the predominant "traditionalist" discourse in which advocates espouse gender inequality and which is evident in Islamic legal scholars' (*fuqaha'*) depiction of marriage as an exchange contract (Mir-Husseini, 2003). In this discourse, a husband pays a dowry in return for sexual intercourse with his wife. Based on this discourse, the main purpose of marriage is sexual gratification and procreation, and the husband's obligation is to sustain the wife financially while the wife's duty is to meet his sexual needs. The man can unilaterally divorce (*talaq*) the wife without providing any grounds, while the wife can seek divorce through (*khul*) by returning the dowry or providing other materialistic compensation in return for the husband's consent for divorce (Mir-Husseini, 2003). If the husband refuses to consent, the wife resorts to the court in which the judge will force the husband to divorce her or the judge will initiate the divorce. Mir-Husseini (2003) argued that the traditionalist discourse reflects the predominant patriarchal values that places men in a superior position to women. This positioning expands to other areas such as depriving women of taking part in producing legal knowledge or being part of making and voting on laws that especially concern them. This contradicts Islamic tradition as Lady A'isha bint Abu Bakr, the Prophet's (Peace Be Upon Him) wife was heavily involved in religious discussions and played a critical role in leadership. She also countered prevalent patriarchal and oppressive discourses at the time (Mernissi, 1988). The *fuqaha* were shaped by the social and the legal contexts in which they lived when they interpreted the sacred religious text. However, some *fuqaha* are seen as absconding basic *Shari'a* principles of justice, freedom, and equality for personal gain.

The second discourse is the "neo-traditionalist discourse" and was developed in direct response to colonization and socio-political changes in the region (Mir-Husseini, 2003). Those that espouse this discourse did not perceive marriage as an exchange contract; however, they did not endorse gender equality either. Rather they believed that marriage is based on complementarity of roles between men and women (Mir-Husseini, 2003) such as those discussed by Knudson-Martin and Mahoney (2009).

Developers of the third discourse, the "Reformists," advocated for gender equality and emphasized that Islam not only accepts pluralism and democracy, but is also grounded in it (Mir-Husseini, 2003). Reformists call for gender equality and challenge the predominant patriarchal interpretations of religious texts that are not grounded in equality and fairness. Mir-Hosseini (2003) argued that the Reformists perceive *fiqh* as "reactive" because it reacts to the present social context and, therefore, can promote gender equality. Even within this discourse, there is a spectrum of radical and moderate reformists.

Gendered Responses to Marriage. With so many opinions about marriage, it is unsurprising when members of the community do not choose to marry. They often face scrutiny from others especially if they are of sound physical and mental health, financial status, and familial support (Hassan, 2005). The choice for lifelong celibacy and singlehood is especially problematic for women as they do not experience the same level of understanding or acceptance for their choices as do men (Hassan, 2005). In addition to gendered discourses reported by Mir-Husseini (2003), socio-cultural sanctions for polygamy in the Muslim faith create additional issues for women. Haque and Kamil (2011) reported that monogamy is the norm in Islam; however, in certain cases, polygamy is acceptable with the explicit condition that husbands treat their wives equitably. Yet gone are the days when polygamy served a humanitarian cause such as protecting the property of orphans, women, and the medically fragile, or whose caregivers died in battle (see Hassan, 2005). Thus, Haque and Kamil (2011), among many, emphasized how Islam demonstrates respect for women regardless of if members of the community espouse local traditions and cultures that violate their rights.

Family Involvement in Couple Relationships

With this said, families are commonly involved in coupling processes in the Arab Muslim world. Ali et al. (2004) reported that Muslim societies are generally collectivistic. Though the idea of collectivism is complex, what it implies is that members of a society or group are expected to show consideration, deference, and respect to parents and elders by seeking their consultation and approval prior to any critical decision-making processes. This deference and trust in families and elders often translates into the important roles they play in arranged marriages (Ali et al., 2004). Of course, these are not to be confused with forced marriages. Though consent from both parties is required, familial choices may cause contention between elders and their children when differences in opinions emerge while selecting the appropriate life partner (Ali et al., 2004). This is further exacerbated by the immediate, and sometimes extended, family's continued involvement in the marriage as couples might not be considered "a separate independent unit" (Abbott et al., 2012, p. 260).

Family Involvement During Conflict. Consequently, and through daily interactions, the union brings about a plethora of opportunities to experience and resolve conflict within the couple dyad and immediate and extended family system. The assumption for practicing Muslims is that couples will utilize the Qur'an and Sunnah as the map to spiritual and relational harmony and success (Hathout, 1995). When couples are unable to resolve issues between themselves and experience significant marital conflict, each partner may choose one arbiter from their respective family members to settle the conflict (Hassan, 2005). In this way, when conflict and distress occur, the extended family may invest significant effort to build harmony and save the marriage (Abbott et al., 2012).

Families Aren't Always the Best Arbiters. However, family members are often ill equipped to assist couples with transforming their relationships and may focus on who is right or wrong and what is religiously or culturally sanctioned or prohibited. This often results in exerting more blame and shame onto members of the couple system and into the relationship. For example, families adopt different, and sometimes conflicting, perceptions about gender roles and responsibilities in marriage and may have different ideas about how to resolve conflict (Haque & Kamil, 2011). Thus, seeking out services from a trained systems therapist can be critical in providing the appropriate therapeutic services to these couples. The following are specific clinical recommendations for the application of therapeutic services for this underserved population.

Clinical Considerations with Arab Muslim Populations in the ME

There is a MH crisis in the ME due to decades of socio-cultural and socio-political unrest resulting in significant individual and regional trauma and distress. Arab Muslims in the ME who legitimately could benefit from therapeutic services often lack adequate knowledge about the availability of therapeutic services (see Onsy, 2013), let alone actively seek out a MH specialist or vet therapists' scope of practice or competence. This leaves individuals, couples, and families feeling confused and less confident or likely to seek out MH services and effect change in their lives. Additionally, and unlike other countries with MH degree requirements and license oversight, potential clients in the ME might find themselves at a disadvantage when working with clinicians historically related to the field of psychology such as psychiatrists who are able to secure credentialing from medical licensing bodies. However, while these professionals provide services within their niche, they largely provide psychological services to individuals and, if working with couples and families, often use an individual assessment and intervention process rather than viewing the couple/family using a holistic and systemic lens and conceptualization approach.

Because some Muslim Arabs are reluctant to seek therapy, it is critical to promote MH services in the region that address their relational concerns. As mentioned, some of the reluctance is linked to barriers that include their belief that MH concerns are a result of external factors or poor faith, lack of and awareness of services, financial difficulties, and gendered differences.

Linguistic Considerations

MH professionals, and therapists specifically, could benefit greatly from investing in a social media and marketing presence that is linguistically attuned to their audience and attracts different clientele. They could use Modern Standard Arabic as well as regional dialects and cultural metaphors. They could also focus on recruiting fellow Arab professionals who are systemically trained and develop a think tank where they can develop linguistic and culturally appropriate interventions that reflect common factors specific to the culture as well as model specific techniques and interventions.

Ethnic, Racial, and Cultural Considerations

Therapists could also benefit from ensuring an ethnically, racially, and culturally responsive and attuned approach to their clients. Recognizing the population's heterogeneity is key to avoiding *ethnic gloss* (Boghosian, 2011). Trimble (1995) described ethnic gloss as a set of simple overgeneralizations and labels about certain ethnic groups that render invisible the unique cultural differences that exist within the members of these groups. In addition, attention to racial discourses and prejudices is critical for comprehensive case conceptualization and to ensure that therapists do not collude with socially constructed and disempowering racial discourses that privilege populations over others. Therapists have the opportunity to ensure they do not collude with implicit biases that harm clients and society at large. Another area of interest is culturally responsive clinical care and could include treating populations from different cultural backgrounds with curiosity and flexibility. Therapists need to validate the cultural experiences of this population (Tadros et al., 2022) in ways that make them feel understood and respected and create the steps necessary to be positively engaged in their treatment. Therapists' sensitivity to clients reflects a genuineness that matches clients' desire for understanding and compassion in their interactions with MH professionals.

Tadros et al. (2022) also argued for couple therapists to take into consideration the influence of the family in the lives of Muslim Arab couples when providing premarital or couple therapy sessions. And if unfamiliar with Muslim and Arab cultures, therapists must take the initiative to perform self-of-the-therapist reflections to challenge any biases or privileges they may have as well as seek out culturally informed training to broaden their understanding of the underserved and misunderstood population.

These are mirrored in Dwairy's (2006) recommendations that therapists treating Muslim Arabs show respect and acceptance and join and assess the positives of the family and how to evoke therapeutic change, in addition to the lesser discussed concern of therapists asserting privacy and confidentiality. All clients are entitled to private and confidential treatment. Tadros et al. (2022) recommended that therapists practice transparency and confirm their responsibility for maintaining privacy and confidentiality as a core therapeutic right and requirement. This is necessary to ensure clients feel confident that presenting issues will not be shared with others unrelated to the family system or treatment team. This is especially critical for Arab Muslims who may refrain from questioning cultural and sacred beliefs in therapy for fear that therapists may not only judge them, but may expose them to others resulting in significant and negative recourse.

Religious Considerations

Due to the inherent influence of sacred beliefs on Arab Muslims, therapists could benefit from comprehensively servicing this complex and heterogenous population. Though beyond the scope of this chapter, there is a plethora of research by established theorists and Middle Eastern and Muslim advocates on topics such as Muslims, Arab Muslims, Muslim Americans, Arab Muslim American, secular Muslims, and even cultural Muslims. For example, Daneshpour (2017) detailed how to provide culturally informed therapy to Muslims, though not "as a religious group, but a cultural group" (p. viii). However, due to our commitment to providing comprehensive care, we want to ensure that we do not render invisible many of this population's sacred beliefs that directly impact health-seeking behaviors such as those discussed previously.

For example, in addition to the importance of enhancing the literacy of MH in the Arab world, Zolezzi et al. (2018) emphasized the importance of challenging distorted perceptions about mental health as God's punishment or an act by supernatural forces. The authors recommended involving religious figures in marketing strategies and awareness campaigns that incorporate Islamic values and could encourage treatment-seeking behaviors. In the same vein, Tadros et al. (2022) recommended establishing MH awareness programs in schools, communities, and the workplace, in an effort to normalize MH concerns and services.

Moreover, Haque and Kamil (2011) argued that it is crucial that counselors and therapists be aware of the various misunderstandings about the Muslim faith and their effect on the MH of Muslims. It is believed that this would strengthen the therapeutic alliance between them and the clients, thereby positively affecting progress in therapy. The authors emphasized some important points that are significant for therapists to consider when treating Muslims. For example, therapists must understand that Muslims differ in their understanding of their religion as well as their degree of religiosity and commitment. Thus, therapists could benefit from assessing the types and influences of sacred beliefs during the intake process. Therapists could also benefit from explicitly assessing gendered beliefs that are grounded in sacred understandings (Haque & Kamil, 2011).

Gendered Considerations

Mir-Hosseini (2003) highlighted the influence of continually evolving cultural and legal contexts that shape the development of gender rights and equity within Islamic thought and interpretation. With this in mind, it is critical for MH specialists, particularly couple and family therapists, to consider the influences of equity and justice on couple relationships in addition to ethnic, racial, cultural, and other social locations. Therapists working with Muslim couples and families may benefit from learning more about the Islamic feminist movement. That is, Daneshpour (2017) pointed out that feminist therapy mainly focuses on promoting women's confidence, teaching them to express their needs, helping them to understand relationship dynamics with family members, and aiding the couple to understand the effect of the societal gender discourse on the distress in their relationships. For instance, the feminist therapist in couple therapy may highlight the major psychological stresses that a man experiences due to toxic masculinity that are imposed on them such as showing strength, hiding vulnerabilities, and lacking the display of empathy (Daneshpour, 2017). Thus, feminist family therapists' work with Muslim families can challenge the predominant patriarchal relationships within the family through advocating for the adoption of gender equality, mutual relationship, and respecting each other's emotions (Daneshpour, 2017). Thus, the feminist therapist can rely on the religious interpretations that are offered by the emerging Islamic feminists in their advocacy for gender equality.

In the same vein, Islamic feminist therapists may adopt Socio-Emotional Relationship Therapy (SERT; Knudson-Martin & Huenergardt, 2015) when working with Arab Muslim couples. According to Knudson-Martin and Huenergardt (2015), the SERT approach is based on the idea that therapists attune to the effect of the socio-cultural discourse on couples' relationships, their emotions, their thoughts, and their behaviors. They highlighted that the major premise of SERT is mutual and reciprocal support at the core of the relationship and reflected in the *Circle of Care* (Knudson-Martin & Huenergardt, 2015). This positioning is grounded in equality that is observed through sharing responsibilities for the relationship, showing mutual vulnerability, being attuned to each other's needs and perspectives, and exerting mutual influence on each other's thoughts, emotions, and behaviors (Knudson-Martin & Huenergardt, 2015). Thus, the feminist therapist may refer to Islamic feminists' interpretations of sacred texts to support that mutuality is aligned with Islamic values and can guide feminist therapists in how to promote and support the circle of care using SERT.

An example of sacred work related to the circle of care is the work of Esmiol Wilson (2015) who noted a parallel between individuals' relationships with God and their relationships with their partners. Individuals whose relationship with God is characterized as an obligation tend to have couple relationships that are devoid of mutuality. This is due to one partner having more influence on the relationship and also reflects the common lack of shared vulnerability. Conversely, individuals whose relationships are based on dialogue and sharing vulnerabilities with their God are more likely to carry that relational dynamic into their couple relationships through sharing their weaknesses and attuning to their partner's needs. These types of relationships are characterized by mutuality. Esmiol Wilson (2015) developed her model of mutuality based on the SERT circle of care (Knudson-Martin & Huenergardt, 2015) described previously. When there is a focus on developing a circle of care within couple relationships, couples learn to share responsibility for the successes or failures of their relationships, share their own vulnerabilities without worry of being judged, provide each other with mutual attention, and accept each others' influence on their behaviors, emotions, and thoughts (Knudson-Martin & Huenergardt, 2015). Esmiol Wilson (2015) recommended integrating spirituality into therapy and assessing religious beliefs that each partner and the couple as a whole may espouse. More importantly, she recommended that therapists pay close attention to the effect of religious discourses on couples' relationships and how potentially adopting a different level of spirituality by each member of the couple may affect their relational dynamics in positive ways (Esmiol Wilson, 2015).

Conversely, there are some attempts to incorporate Islamic values that, upon closer inspection, may have missed the mark. For instance, Menahal Begawala and David Penner (2016) published an Islamic reference to apply Gottman's *The Sound Relationship House Model* to couples with Muslim cultural backgrounds. The purpose of the book, as mentioned in the Introduction, is to provide the therapists with verses from the *Qur'an, Hadith,* and *Sunnah,* the last two of which are the statements and deeds of Prophet Muhammad (Peace be Upon Him), to help Muslim couples accept and apply the interventions proposed by the Gottman Model (Gottman, 2015). They emphasized that not all verses from the Qur'an or Hadith will be compatible with the Muslim readers' understanding of these religious sources. And in these cases, the readers can ignore them. Still, being told to ignore a fundamental issue could be interpreted as dismissive and does not afford the readers any additional considerations or alternatives. Furthermore, the authors provided their understsanding of the context and intent of verses of the Qur'an or Hadith and did not necessarily or precisely translate them into applicable therapeutic concepts. For this reason, it is critical that therapists who wish to publish on cultural and sacred interpretations do so based on a multitude of sources that honor the heterogeneity of the Muslim Arab population.

And lastly, Islamic feminist therapists believe it is critical to assess for power and control in couple and family relationships. Dwairy (2006) shared a critical intervention that is often left unshared. He recommended that therapists ensure that at the beginning of any couple session with powerful fathers or husbands, to express appreciation for them in spite of the stigma and potential financial hardship. In other words, Dwairy (2006) recommended that therapists first join with the powerful partner to listen to their experiences and opinions and speak to how important their contribution is to therapy. This directly corresponds with the works of Knudson-Martin and Huenergardt (2015) and Samman and Knudson-Martin (2015). Dwairy (2006) further highlighted that therapists can use verses from the Qur'an to restructure the clients' cognitions and help them acquire new meanings that can help facilitate therapeutic change. Dwairy also recommended that therapists seek consultation from religious scholars on issues that are out of their scope of practice or competence.Doing so ensures continued and genuine care as well as best therapeutic practices.

Reflection on Future Research

With the increase in globalization resulting in multilingual, interethnic, interracial, intercultural, and interreligious couple relationships, we believe researchers will expand on these topics in the immediate future. We also believe that couples will benefit greatly from therapists learned in areas related to maneuvering and negotiating relational goals around these topics, both as a couple and a family. We encourage therapists to invest in services that demonstrate advocacy for groups suffering from stigma and contextual issues that present as barriers to MH-seeking behaviors. Thus, therapists could benefit from advocating for client systems and invest in culturally diverse research related to marketing and destigmatizing MH services at a local and global level.

Resources and Further Reading

- Abul-Fadl, K. (2007). *The Great Theft: Wrestling Islam from the Extremists*. HarperOne.
- Amer, M. & Awad, G. (Eds.). (2016). *Handbook of Arab American Psychology*. Routledge.
- Amer, M. M. (2013). *Counseling and psychotherapy in Egypt: Ambiguous identity of a regional leader*. In R. Moodley, U. P. Gielen, & R. Wu, (Eds.), *Handbook of Counseling and Psychotherapy in an International Context* (pp. 19–29). Routledge.
- El Feki, S. (2014). *Sex and the Citadel: Intimate Life in a Changing Arab World*. Anchor Books.
- Farahzadi, Z. & Tasharrofi, Z. (2018). The effectiveness of empowerment of couples group therapy on marital satisfaction of couples referred to Better Life Counseling Centre, in Tehran, Iran. *World Family Medicine. 16*(1):156–161. https://doi: 10.5742/MEWFM.2018.93204
- Henry, H. M. (2015). Spiritual energy of Islamic prayers as a catalyst for psychotherapy. *Religion and Health, 54*, 387–398. https://doi: 10.1007/s10943-013-9780-4
- Henry, H. M. (2011). Egyptian women and empowerment: A cultural perspective. *Women's Studies International Forum, 34*, 251–259. https://doi.org/10.1016/j.wsif.2011.03.001
- International Family Therapy Association (IFTA). *Family Therapy Certification*. https://ifta-familytherapy.org/certifiedfamilytherapist.php
- Kholoussy, H. (2010). *For better, for worse: The marriage crisis that made modern Egypt*. Stanford University.
- Mir-Hosseini, Z., Al-Sharmani, M., Rumminger, J. & Marsso, S. (Eds.). (2022). *A feminist reader's guide to justice and beauty in Muslim marriage: Towards egalitarian ethics and laws*. Musawah.
- Journal of Muslim Mental Health. https://journals.publishing.umich.edu/jmmh/

Three Key Tasks

In summary, the following are three key tasks that therapists could benefit from attending in their work with Arab Muslims in the ME. These include an acknowledgement that language matters, spirituality matters, and there must be a serious attempt to develop appropriate and engaging marketing strategies in the region and for this specific population.

Language Matters

Although marriage and family therapy as a discipline originated in the west, therapists must acknowledge the seriousness of attuning to clients in the region using their language and metaphors. Therapists who speak English are in a privileged position rarely giving thought to the needs of non-English speakers. Just as Ken Hardy, an African American systemic therapist, spoke openly of being trained as an excellent White therapist (Wyatt, 2008), we too should acknowledge that our training is inherently biased and falls short of cultural responsivity. And a lack of advocacy is collusion with the status quo. Therefore, therapists could benefit from seeking out additional group processes/discussions and think tanks that identify nuanced and linguistically centered meanings, terminologies, and cultural references in a genuine attempt to engage clients from the region.

Sacred Beliefs Matter

Similarly, sacred beliefs in the region matter and therapy that honors this identity and belief system is likely to be more attuned to their needs and therapeutically successful. While complex and often daunting, it is critical for therapists to intentionally seek out spirituality-based therapeutic discussions with clients even if clients identify as "just Muslim." Attuning to their sacred relationship with their higher power can expose and explain relational dynamics that can directly affect the couple system (Esmiol Wilson, 2015). For this reason, it is essential to develop a knap-sack of appropriate and client-informed sacred assessments and interventions that encourage relational change. Conversely, avoiding these discussions can lead to reinforcing disempowering discourses and interactions contrary to the goals of couple therapy.

Therapists as Marketing Strategists and Advocates

Multiple sources of research indicate that there are significant barriers to MH-seeking behaviors, and poor MH marketing is one of them. The English language is the default when discussing systemic therapy and it is critical to consider how this specialty is marketed in non-English speaking countries. Marketing strategies must also address barriers to help seeking behaviors such as dismantling the stigma around MH, whether through misunderstanding sacred texts or adhering to disempowering cultural discourses. Marketing could include assurance that therapists are a specialized profession and have earned advanced training grounded in ethical practices. These include respect for linguistic, ethnic, racial, and sacred identities as well as a thorough understanding and adherence to consent, privacy, and confidentiality policies. And lastly, by expanding possibilities through marketing, therapists can encourage client access to otherwise financially prohibitive services by offering reduced cost sessions; group services such as group therapy, workshops, or webinars; or social media content such as free lectures or podcasts.

References

Abbott, D. A., Springer, P. R.., & Hollist, C. S. (2012). Therapy with immigrant Muslim couples: Applying culturally appropriate interventions and strategies. *Journal of Couple & Relationship Therapy*, 11(3), 254–266. www.doi/10.1080/15332691.2012.692946

Al-Kernawi, A., Graham, J., Dean, Y., & Eltaiba, N. (2004). Cross-national study of attitudes towards seeking professional help: Jordan, United Arab Emirates (UAE) and Arabs in Israel. *International Journal of Social Psychiatry*, 50, 102–114. www.doi/10.1177/0020764004040957

Al-Sharmani, M. (2014). Islamic feminism: Transnational and national reflections. *Approaching Religion*, 4(2), 83–94. https://doi.org/10.30664/ar.67552

Ali, S. R., Liu, W., & Humedian, M. (2004). Islam 101: Understanding the religion and therapy implications. *Professional Psychology: Research and Practice*, 35, 635–642. https://doi.org/10.1037/0735-7028. 35.6.635

Amstrong, K. (2000). *Islam: A short history*. The Modern Library.

Arab League. (2023, February 12). Britannica Online Encyclopedia. Retrieved February 27, 2023, from www.britannica.com/topic/Arab-League

Begawala, M. & Penner, D. (2016). *Islamic reference guide for the Gottman Method*. The Gottman Institute.

Boghosian, S. (2011). *Counseling and psychotherapy with clients of Middle Eastern descent: A Qualitative inquiry* [doctoral dissertation]. Utah State University.

Chowdhury, S. (2010). Is there a place for individual subjectivity within a social constructionist epistemology? *Journal of Family Therapy*, 32, 342–357. https://doi.org/10.1111/j.1467-6427.2010. 00496.x

Daly, M. W. (2008). *The Cambridge history of Egypt: Volume 2: Modern Egypt, from 1517 to the end of the twentieth century*. Cambridge University Press.

Daneshpour, M. (2012). Family systems therapy and postmodern approaches. In S. Ahmed and M. M. Amer (Eds.), *Counseling Muslims: Handbook of mental health issues and interventions* (pp.119–134). Taylor & Francis.

Daneshpour, M. (2017). *Family therapy with Muslims*. Routledge.

Dwairy, M. (2006). *Counselling and psychotherapy with Arab and Muslims: A culturally sensitive approach*. Teachers College Press.

Dwairy, M. & Van Sickle, T. D. (1996). Western psychotherapy in traditional Arabic societies. *Clinical Psychology Review*, 16(3), 231–249. https://doi.org/10.1016/S0272-7358(96)00011-6

Esmiol Wilson, E. (2015). Relational Spirituality, Gender, and Power: Applications to Couple Therapy. In C. Knudson-Martin, M. E. Wells, & S. K. Samman (Eds.), *Socio-emotional relationship therapy: Bridging emotion, societal context, and couple interaction* (pp. 133–144). Springer Series in Family Therapy.

Gehart, D. (2018). *Mastering competencies in family therapy* (2nd ed.). Brooks/Cole.

Gergen, K. J. (2009). *An invitation to social construction* (2nd ed.). Sage.

Gottman, J. (2015). *The seven principles for making marriage work: A practical guide from the country's foremost relationship expert*. Harmony.

Hanafi, H. (2000). The Middle East, in whose world? In B. Olav Utvik & K. S. Vikør (Eds.), *The Middle East in a globalized world* (pp. 1–9). Nordic Research on the Middle East 6.

Haque, A. & Kamil, N. (2011). Islam, Muslims and mental health. In S. Ahmed & M. M. Amer (Eds.), *Counseling Muslims: Handbook of mental health issues and interventions* (pp. 3–14). Taylor & Francis.

Hassan, R. (2005). Marriage: Islamic discourses. In S. Joseph (Ed.), *Encyclopedia of women and Islamic cultures* (pp. 246–249). Koninklijke Brill.

Hathout, H. (1995). *Reading the Muslim mind*. American Trust.

Hilizah (2022). *Racial discrimination and anti-Blackness in the Middle East*. Arab Barometer. www.arabbarometer.org/wp-content/uploads/ABVII_Racism_Report-ENG.p

Horesh, U. (2019). Languages of the Middle East and North Africa. In J. S. Damico & M. J. Ball (Eds.), *The SAGE encyclopedia of human communication sciences and disorders*. SAGE Publications Inc. http://dx.doi.org/10.4135/9781483380810.n349

IFTA. (n.d. [a]). *Certified family therapist*. International Family Therapist Association. https://ifta-familytherapy.org/certifiedfamilytherapist.php

IFTA. (n.d. [b]). *Family therapy associations*. International Family Therapist Association. www.ifta-familytherapy.org/linksassociations.php

Kayrouz, R., Dear, B. F., Karin, E., Fogliati, V. J., Gandy, M., Keyrouz, L., Nehme, E., Terides, M. D., & Titov, N. (2018). Acceptability of mental health services for anxiety and depression in an Arab Sample. *Community Mental Health Journal*, 54(6), 875–883. https://doi.org/10.1007/s10 597-018-0235-y

King, S. (2021). Anti-black racism and slavery in desert and non-desert zones of North Africa. *Racial formations in Africa and the Middle East: A transregional approach.* (pp. 35–40). Project on Middle East Political Science.

Knudson-Martin, C. & Huenergardt, D. (2015). Bridging emotion, societal discourse, and couple interaction in clinical practice. In C. Knudson-Martin, M. A. Wells & S. K. Samman (Eds.), *Socio-emotional relationship therapy: Bridging emotion, societal context, and couple interaction* (pp. 1–13). Springer.

Knudson-Martin, C., & Mahoney, A. (2009). *Couples, gender, and power: Creating change in intimate relationships*. Springer.

Kondirolli, F., & Sunder, N. (2022). Mental health effects of education. *Health Economics*, 31(Suppl 2), 22–39. https://doi.org/10.1002/hec.4565

Management and Budget Office. (1997). *Revisions to the standards for the classification of federal data on race and ethnicity*. www.whitehouse.gov/wp-content/uploads/2017/11/Revisions-to-the-Standards-for-the-Classification-of-Federal-Data-on-Race-and-Ethnicity-October30-1997.pdf

Mernissi, F. (1988). *The Veil and the male elite: A feminist interpretation of women's rights in Islam*. Basic Books.

Middle East. (2023, March 3). Britannica Online Encyclopedia. Retrieved March 4, 2023, from www.britannica.com/place/Middle-East

Mir-Hosseini, Z. (2003). The construction of gender in islamic legal thought and strategies for reform. *Hawwa*, 1(1), 1–26. www.doi.org/10.1163/156920803100420252

Moll, Y. (2021). Narrating Nubia: Between sentimentalism and solidarity. *Racial formations in Africa and the Middle East: A transregional approach.* (pp. 81–86). Project on Middle East Political Science.

Nichols, M. P. & Davis, S. D. (2021). *Family therapy: Concepts and methods* (12th edition). Pearson Education.

Onsy, E. (2013). *Attitudes toward seeking couples counseling among Egyptian couples: Towards a deeper understanding of common marital conflicts and marital satisfaction* [unpublished master's thesis]. The American University in Cairo.

Petry, C. F. (1998). *The Cambridge history of Egypt. Volume One: Islamic Egypt, 640–1517*. Cambridge University Press.

Pew Research Center. (October, 2007). *Muslim Americans: Middle class and mostly mainstream*. www.pewresearch.org/social-trends/2007/05/22/muslim-americans-middle-class-and-mostly-mainstream/#:~:text=Muslim%20Americans%3A%20Middle%20Class%20and%20Mostly%20Mainstream%20The,have%20divided%20Muslims%20and%20Westerners%20around%20the%20world

Pew Research Center. (October 3, 2017). *Many countries favor specific religions, officially or unofficially*. www.pewresearch.org/religion/2017/10/03/many-countries-favor-specific-religions-officially-or-unofficially/

Samman, S. K., & Knudson-Martin, C. (2015). Relational engagement in heterosexual couple therapy: Helping men move from "I" to "We." In C. Knudson-Martin, M. E. Wells, & S. K. Samman (Eds.), *Socio-emotional relationship therapy: Bridging emotion, societal context, and couple interaction* (pp. 79–91). Springer Series in Family Therapy.

Sherif-Trask, B. (2011). Muslim families in the United States. In M. Coleman & L. H. Ganong (Eds.), *Handbook of Contemporary Families: Considering the past, contemplating the future* (pp. 394–407) Sage Publications.

Shoup, J. (2011). *Ethnic groups of Africa and the Middle East: An encyclopedia*. ABC-CLIO.

Smith, J. (2011). *Removing barriers to therapy with Muslim-Arab-American clients* [Unpublished doctoral dissertation]. Antioch University.

Springer, P., Abbott, D., & Reisbig, A. (2009). Therapy with Muslim couples and families: Basic guidelines for effective practice. *The Family Journal, 17,* 229–335. https://doi.org/10.1177/10664 80709337798

Tadros, E., Ramadan, A. & Salman, M. (2022). The path we face: Clinical implications for destigmatizing therapy for Arab American couples. *Journal of Couple & Relationship therapy,* 1–17. https://doi.org/10.1080/15332691.2022.2086955

The Pew Forum on Religion and Public Life. (2009). *Mapping the global Muslim population: A report on the size and distribution of the world's Muslim population*. Pew Research. https://web.archive.org/web/20170205171040/http://www.pewforum.org/files/2009/10/Muslimpopulation.pdf

Trimble, J. (1995). Toward an understanding of ethnicity and ethnic identification and their relationship with drug use research. In G. Botvin, S. Schinke, and M.A. Orlandi (Eds.), *Drug abuse prevention with multiethnic youth* (pp.3–27). Sage.

Vally, Z., Cody, B. L., Albloshi, M. A., & Alsheraifi, S. N. M. (2018). Public stigma and attitudes toward psychological help-seeking in the United Arab Emirates: The media-tional role of self-stigma. *Perspectives in Psychiatric Care, 54*(4), 571–579. https://doi. org/10.1111/ppc.12282

World Health Organization. (2021). *Mental health atlas 2020*. World Health Organization. www.who.int/publications-detail-redirect/9789240036703

World Population Review. (2023). *Muslim population by country 2023*. https://worldpopulationreview.com/country-rankings/muslim-population-by-country

Wyatt, R. C. (2008). *Kenneth V. Hardy on multiculturalism and psychotherapy*. Psyhcotherapy.net. www.psychotherapy.net/interview/kenneth-hardy

Zolezzi, M., Alamri, M., Shaar, S. & Rainkie, D. (2018). Stigma associated with mental illness and its treatment in the Arab culture: A systematic review. *International Journal of Social Psychiatry, 64*(6), 597–609. https://doi.org/10.1177/0020764018789200

32

TOWARDS A BICULTURAL PARENTING MODEL FOR SOUTH ASIAN IMMIGRANT PARENTS

Rajeswari Natrajan-Tyagi and Shruti Singh Poulsen

Introduction

South Asians and specifically Indians from the South Asian diaspora have a long history of immigrating to the United States for higher education and professional development opportunities. Many remain in the United States to settle, raise families, and make the United States a long-term, permanent home while still maintaining their emotional, cultural, and physical ties to India. Raising their families, navigating the cultural challenges of living with multiple generations in the same household, and navigating the cross-cultural experiences that their US-born children are exposed to and part of, presents particular challenges to parents of South Asian-Indian descent and origin. Cultural hybridization is an inevitable process that families go through, merging old and new practices and creating new meanings (Sanagavarapu, 2010). In parenting practices too immigrant parents inevitably go through this hybridization process and try to make meaning of their old and new practices. Whether the new ascribed meanings are from a lens of deficit and fear or whether they are from a lens of empowerment and options can determine how immigrant parents are grappling with the hybridization process.

In this chapter, the authors first provide a contextual understanding of parenting practices from a South Asian perspective and a Western perspective. The experiences of South Asian parents and their children, their expectations, goals, and needs related to parenting will be discussed. This chapter will also present how these experiences compare to the experiences, expectations, goals, and needs related to parenting in the US context within the Western, majority culture. The authors will present the mental health and parenting concerns and challenges of South Asian parents for themselves and their children who are being raised in the United States. The chapter will also provide insight and guidance related to a "bicultural" approach to parenting for South Asian families in the context of US culture. The authors provide relevant resources and reading, as well as the main "takeaway" messages relevant to scholars and clinicians.

DOI: 10.4324/9781003297871-35

Contextual Understanding of South Asian Approaches to Parenting

While trying to describe and explain value-laden practices such as parenting, it is important to locate such practices within the social, economic, and cultural setting of these practices. The South Asian parenting practices, prior to globalization, have typically originated within an agrarian economy where occupations have been handed down generations from father to son. Families have resided in typically intergenerational households and in what is called the joint-family system, a system where the brothers and their families lived under the same roof. This means that generational hierarchy, homogeneity, and living in harmony with each other were values that ensured survival and prosperity of the family. The elders in the family were charged with the task of providing for the family, safe-guarding them, providing apprentice-ship for younger members, and taking care of the older and weaker members of the family. The philosophy of parenting in the South Asian cultures, within this socio-economic con-text, is deeply rooted in a psycho-spiritual realm (Singh, 2011). One of the central purposes of marriage and family is to ensure continuity of the family's cultural, spiritual, and eco-nomic lineage through children and to ensure their success (Das, 2018; Foner, 1997; Inman, Howard, Beaumont, & Walker, 2007; Segal, 1991; Viswanathan, Shah, & Ahad, 1997; Wakil, Siddique, & Wakil, 1981). Therefore, unlike Western cultures, the parent-child dyad is central in the South Asian family as opposed to the marital dyad, characterized by a deep, intense emotional bond between the mother and the child. The goals of parenting in a South Asian family are to socialize children to become more inter-related, inter-dependent and develop their familial and spiritual selves. To ensure the attainment of these goals, the organizing principles of duty, respect, and honor serve as powerful tools. The Asian family structure is patriarchal based on the principles of honor, humility, respect for elders and authority, pres-ervation of harmony, self-control, and dignity (Ho, Bluestein & Jenkins, 2008; Obeid, 1988). There is a definite hierarchical structure in the South Asian families with the parents wielding most of the power for decision making (Segal, 1991). While on one hand, a very indulgent and protective parenting style is utilized, the use of controlling parenting strategies such as shaming and strict discipline is also used to promote behaviors that conform to the trad-itional lifestyle of obedience and deferring to the parents' choices (Feghali, 1997). The values of obedience, self-restraint, deferred gratification, and focus on education are highly desired and inculcated across both genders, although socialization differs across gender lines when it comes to monitoring of unacceptable behaviors and upholding the honor of the family. Girls and women are more closely monitored and harshly punished for not following the norms of the family culture (Das & Kemp, 1997; Dasgupta,1998a; Ranganath & Ranganath; 1997).

Contextual Understanding of the Western Approaches to Parenting

Approaches to parenting in the United States can be contextually understood within the socio-economic context of neoliberalism. Neoliberalism, which originated as an economic theory, suggests that human life flourishes under the principles of free market. Free market economy calls for nurturing the values of individualism, competition, meritocracy and self-responsibility. In this context, families have privileged individualism over family solidarity. While the US culture is varied and diverse, and no one method to parenting is consistently or uniformly found across all families in the west, there are some overall generalities that can be applied to families and parenting in the United States. In the west and in particular in the United States, there is an expectation that children are to be raised to be independent, self-reliant, and to develop a sense of the "Self." The western model of childhood sets this life stage apart from adulthood. Children are not expected to continue the family trade but have career trajectories that may be outside of their parents' scope. This has tremendous consequences for parenting as parents are no longer called upon to ensure the economic security of their children or provide them apprenticeship in the family trade. Parents in the Western cultural context make big investments in their children's development and share power with them as a way of preparing them for a future and career in which the parents may not have expertise (Mariëtte de Haan, 2011). Parenting during earlier childhood often is based on authoritative styles that encourage children to make their own choices, experience consequences more directly, and engage with parents in ways that may be considered collaborative rather than authoritarian. Children are encouraged to speak up, have a voice, and input in their own choices and development, and to at times question or challenge the authority or expertise of older members of the family and within other systems such as schools. Developing a sense of mutual respect and cooperation between parents and children is a focus of western parenting. Children, within some developmental limitations, are treated as capable of making their own decisions; for example, decisions about their education, their social engagement with others, and their level of contribution and connection to their family system. Discipline is often administered using reasoning, discussion, explanation of rules, setting limits based on developmental stage of the child, and providing children with options and choices rather than unequivocal edicts and directives. When children violate cultural or societal norms, the consequences are typically meted out by the educational, legal, or economic systems rather than the family system. The socioeconomic context encourages individuals to question authority, disrupt the status quo, and make mistakes and learn from them.

South Asian Immigrants' Perceptions of American Parenting

While South Asian-Indians living in the United States might have limited exposure to families and parents outside of their own social, professional, and familial circles, they do develop perceptions of American parents based on their direct or indirect interactions through the media, observing them in public spaces, through systems such as schools, and through their own children who may be more fully exposed to and involved in the majority cultural context of the United States (Ochocka & Janzen, 2008). Based on these experiences and exposure, South Asian-Indians often view American parenting as permissive, lacking in authority with little or no moral guidance, and with no limits imposed on children regardless of age and development.

Perceptions of American families and parenting may include assuming that western parents "do not care" about their children enough or that they are not fully invested in their own children's future and welfare. This may lead to value-laden assumptions such as American parents and families have fewer values and beliefs about supporting togetherness, connection, and lack focus on the welfare of the family system across multiple generations. Other assumptions might include that in American families children can and are allowed to disrespect their parents, their elders, and that respect for a person's age, experience, and authority is not encouraged or expressed appropriately by parents. In a study conducted in Canada, immigrant parents had mixed feelings about how children in western countries were brought up. They seemed to think that the Canadian children were confident, friendly, and independent yet hedonistic and not always respectful (Ochocka & Janzen, 2008). American families may be viewed by immigrant parents as too separate within the family unit as well as across multiple generations, especially given that it is relatively rare in the United States for families to live in multi-generational households with grandparents,

parents, children, and sometimes extended family members such as uncles, aunts, and cousins. The perceived isolation of the nuclear family household in the United States, with elderly parents often in nursing homes or senior living communities, gives Asian-Indian parents the impression that Americans care little for intergenerational relationships and their value to children and other members of the family.

Grandparents and extended families were seen to be distant and uninvolved with children and child-rearing. This is perceived as a lack of kinship, familial obligation, filial piety, and unwillingness to fulfill familial responsibilities across generations. American parenting styles and approaches are often viewed as not honoring and supporting the continuity of family traditions, norms, and cultural values across generations. Whether fully accurate or not, South Asian-Indians often have a negative perspective of the abilities and priorities of American parenting practices and norms. South Asian parents may often view the western methods of parenting with suspicion, disdain, and dismiss these as inappropriate to their own cultural context of parenting. Given the often-negative perceptions of American parenting, and South Asian families own differing approaches to parenting their children, South Asian parents may experience cultural dissonance, and feel challenged in their abilities to parent in a different cultural and social context than their country-of-origin.

Parenting Experiences of South Asian Immigrants and Outcomes of Second-Generation Children

Literature on immigrant parenting has mostly focused on the negative aspects of parenting in a host culture that is vastly different in its culture and traditions than the culture of origin, especially the experiences of stress, loss of status (Perreira et al., 2006, Suárez-Orozco & Suárez-Orozco, 2001), and decrease in parental authority and control when children become translators or brokers of the language and the culture to their parents (Bush, Bohon, & Kim, 2010). For South Asian immigrant parents specifically, the most difficult part of raising children in a western society that has contradictory value systems is fighting to maintain their cultural identity in terms of language, customs and attitudes while at the same time encouraging their children to achieve educational and financial success in the new land (Dasgupta, 1998; Ranganath & Ranganath, 1997). Immigrant parents struggle to provide a cultural context for their children, especially due to lack of the extended family system in the United States. They fear losing their children to the American culture and are apprehensive of facing criticism from extended family back home if their children appear to become "too American." Some resort to extensive involvement in their cultural networks, which may in turn stunt the families' exploration into the new culture (Baptiste Jr., 1993). Some families react by becoming rigid, impose restrictions and enforce traditional values that may not be even followed in the home culture anymore.

The loss of parental authority becomes exaggerated during children's adolescence when conflicts and power struggles arise from their children's need for greater autonomy, power, and separation (Dasgupta, 1998). South Asian immigrant parents are better able to compromise and adapt to superficial cultural changes like music, movies, and food or to changes that align with their migratory aspirations, such as nurturing their daughters' career ambitions than to change their core parenting beliefs regarding family obligations, career choices, respect for elders, dating, sexuality, and marriage (Kar, Campbell, Jimenez, & Gupta, 1995; Patel, Power, & Bhavnagri, 1996; Srinivasan, 2001, Wakil, Siddique, & Wakil, 1981).

A review of studies conducted on outcomes of immigrant parenting among second-generation Asian children revealed that Asian teens had difficulty expressing their emotions and discussing problems with their parents (Rhee, Chang & Rhee, 2003) compared to Caucasian teens. Asian teens especially have difficulty communicating with their fathers and report difficulties in being assertive and authentic with their families. It was found that typically Asian adolescents experienced their immigrant parents as critical and insulting and being unable to listen and understand their issues. A study conducted in the UK on young South Asian adolescents revealed that teens, especially females, typically get into disciplinary arguments with their parents around issues of dating, cultural practices, and educational/employment choices that lead to great psychological distress (Khan & Waheed, 2009). Second-generation Indian-American teens and young adults report experiencing significant pressure to pursue careers in areas such as medicine and engineering that are familiar to their parents (Ranganath & Ranganath, 1997). Youth who choose more nontraditional career paths such as the arts and social sciences experience significant family conflicts that range from discouragement to threat of withdrawal of financial support in college. Thus, second-generation youth may cope with these expectations by leading different lives inside and outside their homes and going to great lengths to maintain secrecy around their activities such as dating, drinking, and sexual activities outside of their homes (Khandelwal, 2002; Maira, 2002). The credibility of the parental authority may be challenged by second-generation children who experience the traditional and conservative socializing messages sent by their immigrant parents as contradicting contemporary norms in their culture of origin. They may experience their parents' cultural norms to be frozen in a time warp while the culture has evolved in the 'natal' culture (Das, 2018). Overall, substantial research among South Asians and other Asian immigrants shows that second-generation children experience acute pressure to balance meeting social and academic expectations, and blending into the new society with demands for maintaining cultural identity from family (Das & Kemp, 1997; Farver, Bhadha, & Narang, 2002; Ibrahim et al., 1997) leading to negative mental health outcomes for immigrant youth.

Towards a Model of Bicultural Parenting

Biculturalism in parenting refers to adaptations made by immigrant parents in their parenting approaches and styles to incorporate new insights and strategies from the host culture while at the same time maintaining cultural parenting practices that are meaningful and functional from their ancestral culture. Children of many South Asian immigrants already show traits of biculturalism, which are manifested in low levels of family conflict, sound psychological functioning, good academic performance, and high-paid careers (Das, 2018). This shows that many immigrant parents are already believers in biculturalism. However, there are many who still fear the process of hybridized parenting, and even among the believers, there are many who struggle with managing conflict between the different parenting orientations. In this section, we try to provide an expanded understanding of biculturalism and bicultural parenting and steps to move towards biculturalism.

1. *Busting the myth that immigrants are proselytized into host parenting orientation*: The first task we undertake is to bust the idea for immigrant parents that they are passive receivers of the host culture and lack agency in the process. Papastergiadis (2000) used the concept of "cultural translation" to show that transformations in immigrant child-rearing practices is not a linear model. This concept does not see immigrant cultures as mindlessly adopting practices from the foreign culture or considering their own cultural practices as inferior and needing of correction. Instead, the translation process is a

dynamic interaction where the modified practices are neither like those of the country to origin nor like that of the host culture. They are new solutions that Papastergiadis (2000) states is a result of immigrant parents living in borderland of contradicting traditions. For example, immigrant parents allow for more autonomy in children while at the same time combine it with close-knit family ties.

2. *Moving away from fear of children "becoming confused" to confidence that children are "becoming culturally rich"*: Immigrant parenting styles that do not enforce traditional cultural norms are stereotypically seen as producing children who experience identity crisis. The term "ABCD" is a derogatory term that stands for "American Born Confused Desi (Indian)" and is characteristically used within the Indian community to describe the second-generation young adults who are conflicted within themselves. We believe that immigrant parents need to move away from fear-based parenting to adopting a confident approach with a belief that a balanced, bicultural approach to parenting provides opportunities for their children to learn cultural navigational skills, being able to access the strengths and resources of multiple cultures and contexts, and add a layer of developmental sophistication to the second-generation children and immigrant parents alike.

3. *Moving away from fear of "losing culture" to conviction of "gaining parenting options"*: Bicultural parenting provides immigrant parents additional tools and skills to their parenting "toolbox." Rather than viewing their exposure to new ways of being and parenting as something that drains their cultural reservoir, immigrant parents can reframe it as something that adds to their parenting repertoire. When immigrant parents incorporate more permissive styles of parenting, their children's self-esteem has been shown to improve (Driscoll et al, 2008). Research also shows that when immigrant parents add practices of listening and validating their children's ideas and involve them in decision making in developmentally appropriate ways, there is less parent-child conflict and children show willingness to see their parent's perspective (Benbassat & Priel, 2012, 2014; Deroma, Lassiter, & Davis, 2004; Grusec, 2011; Grusec et al., 2000; Hastings & Grusec, 1997). When faced with lack of social support from extended family, immigrant fathers were able to demonstrate role flexibility and become more actively involved in their children's lives (Abbott & Gupta, 2009), which led to positive outcomes in parent-child dynamics showing that biculturalism provides opportunities for gaining multiple parenting strategies and options.

4. *Taking steps to contain parental anxieties*: An important step towards a more bicultural approach to parenting is for South Asian parents to acknowledge, become aware of, and understand more clearly their own anxiety both about their parenting abilities and skills overall, as well as their abilities to navigate these skills and abilities in what they might perceive as a "foreign" or even "hostile" environment. Parenting is generally fraught with questions of one's own competence, adequacy, and skills at each development stage in a child's life. South Asian parents may benefit from first addressing these questions and anxieties so that they can more fully embrace the benefits and possibilities of bicultural parenting. One method to developing better understanding, awareness, and regulation of one's anxiety is to engage in one's own family-of-origin work that supports the understanding of one's experiences of being parented and raised by their own parents, exploring one's growing up experiences in a different cultural and social context, and learning about parenting practices and patterns from a multi-generational lens.

5. *Moving away from an attitude of resistance and tolerance of the host culture to an attitude of acceptance*: Another important step towards bicultural parenting is for South Asian parents to cultivate a sense of acceptance and openness to the idea that the acculturation

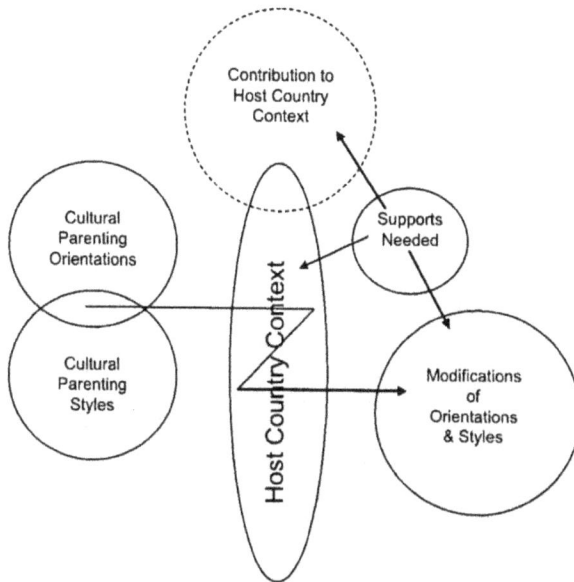

Figure 32.1   Bicultural Parenting Framework (Ochocka, J. & Janzen, R., 2008)

that children are experiencing is to their benefit and in support of improved functioning as they navigate life across multiple cultural contexts. When immigrant parents not only tolerate the host culture but open up to it, they find themselves more open to having dialogue with one's children about culture, identity, and different cultural norms and experiences. When parents are more transparent about their own challenges and experiences of acculturation and share their vulnerabilities, they can paradoxically influence their children to have a better understanding of where they come from, engender more ethnic affinity, and ultimately foster more feelings of connection and support.

6. *Moving away from a mindset of "adhering to what is cultural" to a mindset of "adhering to what is functional"*: As discussed in the beginning of this chapter, cultural practices originate and are embedded in socioeconomic contexts. Understanding the contextual origins of parenting practices can be extremely helpful to immigrant parents to evaluate whether their parenting practices are relevant in their current context. For example, implicit obedience, which was once a desired quality in children, was functional in an intergenerational family system with an agrarian economy. However, in nuclear family systems living in a meritocracy-based neoliberal societies, implicit obedience is no longer functional. Children need to be socialized to confront authority and challenge the status quo. These are qualities deemed necessary in the work setting to make disruption and innovation possible.

7. *Moving away from biculturalism being a unidirectional process to a multidirectional process*: Ochocka and Janzen (2008) present a new framework (Figure 32.1) for understanding immigrant parenting that was developed through a participatory action project involving 50 focus group interviews with 317 new immigrant parents (1–3 years of immigration) from 12 cultural-linguistic communities in Canada. The framework represents the idea that biculturalism is not a one-way-street, where immigrant parents shed their culture to take on the culture of the host country. The existing

conceptualization that acculturation is done just by the immigrant families to the host cultures has been challenged (Dominguez & Maya-Jariego, 2008) and evidence has been provided about how host individuals also acculturate into the immigrant culture. This shift in view from a unidirectional to a multidirectional model of acculturation can empower immigrants to view their process of seeking a bicultural style of operation as a give-and-take opportunity. Ochocka and Janzen's (2008) framework for immigrant parenting speaks to the concept of "parenting contributions," that is, the reciprocal ways in which the immigrants add to the understanding and practice of parenting in the host culture. Immigrant parents in this study shared that the contributions that they can make to the host cultures in terms of parenting orientation and style are as follows: a) placing greater value on showing respect to elders, b) inculcating the value of reciprocal care of parents by children when parents grow old, c) greater emphasis on education and monitoring of children's educational activities as part of parenting, and d) importance of directive parenting and staying connected with children at all stages of their life span. This give-and-take perspective can empower immigrant parents to have agency in the way they choose to modify their parenting practices.

Research Agenda & Implications: Reflections

With increased immigration from the South Asian diaspora and increased acceptance and openness to accessing mental health services, it is imperative that clinicians, and specifically family therapists, develop a better understanding of the experiences, challenges, and opportunities in immigrant parenting. The focus of this chapter was to present information and understanding of South Asian families and their needs, especially in the area of parenting in different cultural settings. Family therapists may be increasingly faced with clients, parents, children, and families of South Asian origin in their clinical practice seeking out support in issues such as parenting, raising children, and navigating cultural norms and experiences. It is imperative that clinicians enhance their knowledge and experience of these diverse families and their cultural experiences as parents and families, so that they can be supported in their goals to engage in parenting approaches that honor their own cultural experiences and values, while also benefitting from the use of bicultural approaches to parenting.

Resources and Further Reading

Additional resources and reading for understanding parenting, in general, and bicultural parenting, in specific, are as follows:

Parenting from the Inside Out: How a Deeper Self-Understanding can Help you Raise Children who Thrive. This book by Daniel J. Siegel and Mary Hartzell looks at how parents can support their developing child holistically by understanding themselves and their emotional/psychological needs and experiences. This book is very relevant in the context of bicultural parenting. Growing up Global: Raising Children to be at Home in the World. This book by Homa Sabet Tavangar gives many tips on how we can bring up children as global citizens who have an international perspective. From Old Roots to New Soil: Advice for South Asian Indians and other Immigrants on Home, Family, Marriage, Children and Navigating Life in a New Country. This book is a collection of short articles by Dr. Thomas Kulanjiyil addressing many issues that South Asian immigrants face in the North American cultural context. Building Cultural Intelligence (CQ): Nine Megaskills. This book by Richard, D. Bucher talks about the important of cultural intelligence that help promote cross-cultural understanding. The author details nine skills that are needed to be culturally intelligent and to succeed in an increasingly global community.

Three takeaways

- Understanding the experiences of South Asian-Indian families and parents – their challenges, concerns, expectations of themselves, and their families
- Understanding a bicultural approach to parenting, and how it can both honor and enhance South Asian-Indian parents' approach to parenting by increasing their openness to other cultural parenting practices
- Being able to support South Asian-Indian parents and families as they bridge the perceived gap and differences between their cultural norms around parenting and incorporating western approaches to parenting to provide a sense of balanced parenting.

Conflict of Interest

We have no conflicts of interest to disclose.

References

Abbott, D., & Gupta, P.M. (2009). Influence of American culture on East Indian immigrants' perceptions of marriage and family life. In R.L. Dalla, J. Defrain, J. Johnson, and D.A. Abbott (Eds.), *Strengths and challenges of new immigrant families* (pp. 93–116). New York: Lexington Books.

Baptiste Jr., D. A. (1993). Immigrant families, adolescents and acculturation: Insights for therapists. In B. H. Settles, D. E. Hanks III, & M. B. Sussman (Eds.), *Families on the move: Migration, immigration, emigration, and mobility* (pp. 341–363). New York: The Haworth Press, Inc.

Benbassat N., & Priel B., (2012). Parenting and adolescent adjustment: the role of parental reflective function. *Journal of Adolescence, 35*(1), 163–74. http/doi.org/10.1016/j.adolescence.2011.03.004. Epub 2011 Apr 16. PMID: 21497896.

Bhagwati, Jagdish, and T. N. Srinivasan. (2022). "Trade and Poverty in the Poor Countries." *The American Economic Review, 92*(2), 180–83. JSTOR, http://www.jstor.org/stable/3083398. Accessed 26 July 2023.

Bucher, R. D. (2008). *Building cultural intelligence (CQ): Nine megaskills*. Pearson.

Bush, K. & Muruthi, B., Bohon, S. & Kim, H. (2016). Adaptation Among Immigrant Families.

Das, A., & Kemp, S. F. (1997). Between two worlds: Counseling South Asian Americans. *Journal of Multicultural Counseling and Development, 25*(1), 23–33. https://doi.org/10.1002/j.2161-1912.1997.tb00313.x

Dasgupta, S. D. (1998). Gender roles and cultural continuity in the Asian Indian immigrant community in the U.S. *Sex Roles: A Journal of Research, 38*(11–12), 953–974. https://doi.org/10.1023/A:1018822525427

DeRoma V.M., Lassiter K.S., Davis V.A. (2004). Adolescent involvement in discipline decision making. *Behavior Modification* 2004 May;28(3):420–37. http://doi.org/10.1177/0145445503258993. PMID: 15104870.

Domínguez, S., & Maya-Jariego, I. (2008). Acculturation of host individuals: Immigrants and personal networks. *American Journal of Community Psychology, 42*(3–4), 309–327. https://doi.org/10.1007/s10464-008-9209-5

Farver, J. A. M., Narang, S. K., & Bhadha, B. R. (2002). East meets West: Ethnic identity, acculturation, and conflict in Asian Indian families. *Journal of Family Psychology, 16*(3), 338–350. https://doi.org/10.1037/0893-3200.16.3.338

Feghali, E. K. (1997). Arab cultural communication patterns. *International Journal of Intercultural Relations, 21*(3), 345–378. https://doi.org/10.1016/S0147-1767(97)00005-9

Foner, N. (1997). The immigrant family: Cultural legacies and cultural changes. *International Migration Review, 31*(4), 961–974. https://doi.org/10.1177/019791839703100407

Grusec J. E. (2011). Socialization processes in the family: social and emotional development. *Annual Review of Psychology, 62*, 243–69. doi: 10.1146/annurev.psych.121208.131650. PMID: 20731599.

Grusec JE, Goodnow JJ, Kuczynski L. (2000). New directions in analyses of parenting contributions to children's acquisition of values. *Child Development, 71*(1), 205–211. http://doi.org/10.1111/1467-8624.00135. PMID: 10836575.

Haan, M. de (2011). Immigrant Learning. In K. Symms Gallagher, R.K. Goodyear, D.J. Brewer & R. Rueda (Eds.), *Urban education: a model for leadership and policy* (pp. 328–341). New York: Routledge.

Hastings, P., & Grusec, J. E. (1997). Conflict outcome as a function of parental accuracy in perceiving child cognitions and affect. *Social Development, 6*(1), 76–90. https://doi.org/10.1111/j.1467-9507.1997.tb00095.x

Ho, C., Bluestein, D. N., & Jenkins, J. M. (2008). Cultural differences in the relationship between parenting and children's behavior. *Developmental Psychology, 44*(2), 507–522. https://doi.org/10.1037/0012-1649.44.2.507

Inman, A. G., Howard, E. E., Beaumont, R. L., & Walker, J. A. (2007). Cultural transmission: Influence of contextual factors in asian indian immigrant parents' experiences. *Journal of Counseling Psychology, 54*(1), 93–100. https://doi.org/10.1037/0022-0167.54.1.93

Kar, S. B., Campbell, K., Jimenez, A., & Gupta, S. (1995). Invisible Americans: An exploration of Indo-American quality of life. *Amerasia Journal, 21*(3), 1–26.

Kulanjiyil, T. (2023). *From old roots to new soil: Advice for South Asian Indians and other immigrants on home, family, marriage, children and navigating life in a new country.* Self-Published.

Obeid, R. A. (1988). An Islamic theory of human development. In T. R. Murray (Ed.), *Oriental theories of human development* (pp. 155–174). New York: Lang.

Obeid, R. A. (1988). An Islamic theory of human development. In T. R. Murray (Ed.), *Oriental theories of human development* (pp. 155–174). New York: Lang.

Ochocka, Joanna & Janzen, Rich. (2008). Immigrant parenting: A new framework of understanding. *Journal of Immigrant & Refugee Studies, 6.* 85–111. 10.1080/15362940802119286.

Papastergiadis, N., & Russell, S. S. (2001). The turbulence of migration: globalization, deterritorialization and hybridity [Review of The turbulence of migration: globalization, deterritorialization and hybridity]. *International Migration, 39*(1), 143–144.

Patel, N., Power, T. G., & Bhavnagri, N. P. (1996). Socialization values and practices of Indian immigrant parents: Correlates of modernity and acculturation. *Child Development, 67*(2), 302–313. https://doi.org/10.2307/1131815

Pereira T, Lock J, Oggins J. (2006). Role of therapeutic alliance in family therapy for adolescent anorexia nervosa. *International Journal of Eating Disorders,* 2006 Dec; *39*(8), 677–84. doi: 10.1002/eat.20303. PMID: 16937386.

Ranganath, V. M., & Ranganath, V. K. (1997). Asian Indian children. In G. Johnson-Powell, J. Yamamoto, G. E. Wyatt, & W. Arroyo (Eds.), *Transcultural child development: Psychological assessment and treatment* (pp. 103–125). John Wiley & Sons Inc.

Rehman, A. U., Khan, M. I. & Waheed, Z., (2019). School heads' perceptions about their leadership styles: A qualitative study. *Journal of Education and Educational Development, 6*(1), 138–153.

Rhee S, Chang J, Rhee J. (2003). Acculturation, communication patterns, and self-esteem among Asian and Caucasian American adolescents. *Adolescence.* 2003 Winter; 38(152): 749–68. PMID: 15053499.

Segal, U. A. (1991). Cultural Variables in Asian Indian Families. *Families in Society, 72*(4), 233–242. https://doi.org/10.1177/104438949107200406

Siegel, D. J., & Hartzell, M. (2013). *Parenting from the inside out: How a deeper self-understanding can help you raise children who thrive.* TarcherPerigee.

Srinivasan, S. (2001). "Being Indian," "being American": A balancing act or a creative blend? *Journal of Human Behavior in the Social Environment, 3*(3–4), 135–158. https://doi.org/10.1300/J137v03n03_10

Suárez-Orozco, C., & Suárez-Orozco, M. M. (2001). Children of immigration. Harvard University Press.

Tavangar, H. S. (2009). *Growing up global: Raising children to be at home in the world.* Ballantine Books.

Viswanathan, R., Shah, M. R., & Ahad, A. (1997). Asian-Indian Americans. In S. Friedman (Ed.), *Cultural Issues in the Treatment of Anxiety* (pp. 175–195). New York: Guilford.

Wakil, S. P., Siddique, C. M., & Wakil, F. A. (1981). Between two cultures: A study in socialization of children of immigrants. *Journal of Marriage and the Family, 43*(4), 929–940. https://doi.org/10.2307/351349

33

AN INTEGRATION OF COLLABORATIVE LANGUAGE SYSTEMS AND SYMBOLIC EXPERIENTIAL FAMILY THERAPY WITH TRANSNATIONAL FAMILIES

Nicole Sabatini Gutierrez and K. Loette Snead

Introduction

With increased travel mobility and globalization, the prevalence of transnational families across the globe continues to increase (Baldassar et al., 2014; Delgado, 2022; McNeil Walsh, 2023). Transnational families maintain a sense of togetherness, connection, and involvement even though they are separated by geographic distance, with some family members living at least part of the time, if not all of the time, in a different country (Bryceson & Vuorela, 2002). Typically, transnational families have some members that remain in the country of origin and some members that have migrated elsewhere. Transnational families can reside in more than two countries and can have generational differences in terms of which country is considered to be the *home* country. These families maintain a family identity that transcends geography and is referred to in the literature as a *copresence*, or *living apart together* (Baldassar et al., 2014). Transnational structure can be the result of migration, commuting between countries (fly-in-fly-out), military deployment, divorce/separation and subsequent relocation, etc. There are many reasons that families may become transnational, including push factors (complex, dangerous, and/or undesirable situations in country of origin that make it necessary to leave); pull factors (desirable conditions in the host country such as education resources, the perception of more political freedom, and/or employment opportunity); and globalization, which has led to increased number of international marriages, etc. (Sohleim & Ballard, 2016). In general, it is imperative for Couple and Family Therapists (CFTs) to consider that the traditional White/Western

DOI: 10.4324/9781003297871-36

cisheteronormative view of the nuclear family system that consists of two parents and one or more children is not representative of the true diversity of family experiences. In addition to the many different family structures that do exist (LGBTQIA+ families, families of choice, blended families, single-parent families, foster and adoptive families, etc.), more and more families across the world are identifying as transnational. And, while transnational families themselves are not monolithic and can intersect with the aforementioned diverse family dynamics, it is important for CFTs to be mindful of the common challenges and strengths that are unique to the transnational family experience.

Transnational families have members that are migrants to a new country with different cultural norms, customs, and systems, and members that remain in the country of origin who also have to adjust to new family roles and power dynamics with the absence of the migrant family members (Solheim et al., 2016). Ambiguous loss, which describes the loss associated with being either physically present but emotionally absent, or emotionally present but physically absent (Boss, 1999/2006/2010), is a common experience in transnational families both for members in the country of origin and migrant members. The length of the separation, whether it is voluntary or forced, and other concrete stressors experienced by the family can impact experiences of ambiguous loss in clinically relevant ways (Baldassar et al., 2014; Solheim et al., 2016). Concrete stressors include depleted financial resources for those in the country of origin and/or the country of migration, discriminatory immigration laws and acculturative stress for migrant members, and fear and worry about the safety of family members across locations (Baldassar et al., 2014; Delgado, 2022). Transnational families report higher quality of life and better mental health outcomes when they have more perceived control over their ability to travel and visit one another and can do so more freely, particularly during times of family crisis or transitional life stage milestones (Gerber & Ravazzini, 2022). Not being able to cross borders due to things such as the global COVID-19 pandemic, politically motivated xenophobic travel restrictions, or conflict and war can increase ambiguity and thus exacerbate the loss (Bravo, 2017; Galvan et al., 2022; Gerber & Ravazzini, 2022; Simola et al., 2023).

Transnational families have certain reciprocity of care expectations, much like other family structures (Baldassar et al., 2014). These care expectations are influenced by cultural gender norms (i.e., women in the system are expected to care for children, adult children are expected to care for elder adults, etc.). The challenge for transnational families is that traditional expectations of care giving may not be viable in the same ways simply due to geographic location. Families may have to re-negotiate these expectations and the power dynamics that follow. The ability for generations in a family system to appropriately care for one another consistent with transitional life stage needs is largely dependent on documentation status, laws, and politics around migration and travel. Transnational families from different countries are likely to have different levels of mobility (i.e., Global South typically has less mobility than the Global North due to systemic racism and xenophobia; Baldassar et al., 2014; Galvan et al., 2022). Visiting amongst transnational families can include migrant members returning to country of origin, members residing in the country of origin visiting the migrants in the new country, or both groups meeting in a third (often more neutral) country. The type of family meet-up can impact role negotiation when in-person contact is established, and the life stage of family members can also impact role negotiation and determine when/where/how the meetup occurs. For example, migrant members who have very young children may be temporarily less mobile than adult members residing in the country of origin. Transnational visiting impacts the relationships of those involved in many ways (McNeil Walsh, 2023).

Literature on transnational families tends to focus on the behaviors or practices that these families engage in to remain in contact with one another, and there is a need for more understanding of the sensory-emotional experiences and intimacy needs of such family members (Simola et al., 2023). Thus, a clinical approach that integrates postmodern ideas about the power of cultural discourse and the importance of language in co-constructing meaning, and an experiential process that centers intimacy and relational cohesion of the system may be ideal when working clinically with transnational families. For transnational families, ambiguous loss, disruption to family hierarchy, family role confusion, and barriers to maintaining cohesiveness and intimacy have many important clinical implications. A therapeutic approach such as Symbolic Experiential Family Therapy (SEFT) that attends specifically to transitional life stage positionality, family roles and hierarchies, negotiation of stress and conflict, and emotional intimacy (Napier & Whitaker, 1978; Whitaker & Ryan, 1989) seems very well-suited for working with this population. Likewise, the Collaborative Language Systems (CLS) emphasis on political discourse and client empowerment through the use of a co-created dialogical process (Anderson & Gehart, 2012) can help to support transnational families that have to navigate multiple political systems simultaneously just to maintain their relationships.

This chapter will briefly review clinical considerations for working with transnational families. The theoretical consistencies between and rationale for integrating Collaborative Language Systems and Symbolic Experiential Family Therapy when working with transnational families will then be discussed. Additionally, two case studies will be presented to demonstrate the application of this integrative approach with this population. Finally, key takeaways for working with transnational families from an integrative postmodern-experiential perspective will be identified.

Clinical Considerations with Transnational Families

Family separation is inherently a part of being a transnational family, and aspects of it can be voluntary and involuntary/forced. Forced family separation impacts the ambiguous loss process differently and can be very traumatizing (Galvan et al., 2022; Roy & Yumiseva, 2021; Tu, 2023). Documentation status also impacts the experience of family separation, because family members that are undocumented are essentially immobilized. Family separation has health implications and has deleterious effects on mental, emotional, and physical health, particularly when parents/caregivers are separated from their children and when family members are not able to be physically present during times of emergency or death (Galvan et al., 2022).

For migrant family members, the separation is not just from the people in the system, but also from the culture of origin. First, second, and third generations can experience a sense of *cultural homelessness* as a result of being disconnected from their culture (Henderson, 2016). Not having a sense of belonging to or ownership of either the culture of origin or the culture of migration is impacted by the migrant's level of access to a cultural community in the country of migration, their experiences of discrimination or racism in the host country, and their level of connection with family members who remain in the country of origin. Multi-lingual people may not identify a single language as their "primary language," which can further contribute to ambiguity of cultural identity (I am not either this or that, I am not exactly both, I am a third thing that is entirely different than either part on its own and different than my family members; Henderson, 2016). Transnational families that prioritize a high level of engagement and support can help those members that have migrated to maintain a sense of cultural identity and this can mitigate the grief and loss that they experience and support their cultural or ethnic identity development. Some theorists postulate that, because of differences in acculturation levels, transnational families may experience higher conflict between generations, but other research shows that there can actually be higher levels of generational solidarity in transnational families. From this perspective, intergenerational bonds between generations are strengthened by the family separation experience because it highlights the family's strength and resilience and produces a sense of gratitude and belonging (Albertini et al., 2019).

Ambiguous Loss

The focus of much of the literature on transnational families is on the ambiguous loss process experienced by all members of the system. Transnational families can experience both forms of ambiguous loss – they can experience psychological presence but physical absence when those who have migrated are physically distant from the family and country of origin, though both people and place remain psychologically present; Boss, 2006). Likewise, they can experience physical presence but psychological absence when visiting one another – family members have access to physical closeness but experience a sense of pronounced emotional disconnect as they become increasingly aware of the limitations of remaining connected primarily through telecommunications for long periods of time. Families that have infrequent visits for various reasons have less ability to share experience in the present and may have more challenges with physical intimacy, which becomes apparent when reunited. Distinct from the loss of a loved one that has a matter-of-fact nature, ambiguous loss is a concept that accounts for loss that is uncertain or unclear (Solheim & Ballard, 2016; Solheim et al., 2016). Most often death is accompanied by some sort of ritual that symbolizes the loss, where it is also possible to have family members that are physically absent but psychologically present and vice versa, which can result in grief symptoms associated with ambiguous loss (Solheim et al., 2016). There is no community recognition of ambiguous loss, and it often leaves family members stuck where large decision-making, problem-solving, or definitive family roles are nonexistent, thus extending the feeling of never-ending uncertainty for those involved. When recalling the experience of witnessing her parents struggles with ambiguous loss, Boss (1999) stated:

> The family that exists in people's minds is more important than the one recorded in the census taker's notebook, especially when family members are increasingly separated and on the move because of work demands, unemployment, domestic break-ups, war, or simply their own choices. (p.31)

Whether an individual is physically there and mentally unavailable or mentally present and gone physically, the loss can lead to a variety of symptoms, including those of depression and anxiety (Boss, 1999; Solheim & Ballard, 2016; Solheim et al., 2016). The greater amount of uncertainty and/or stressors involved in the ambiguous loss (i.e., unknown location of a loved one, fear for safety, etc.), the greater the impact on the well-being of the family (Boss, 1999; Solheim & Ballard, 2016). From a perspective that captures aspects of both CLS and SEFT, it has been urged that clinicians should be wary of assumptions about family life that are largely based on Western traditions (Baldassar et al., 2014). Ideas about the family and distance are socially constructed (Baldassar et al., 2014). Therefore, new meaning can be made through dialogic conversation and increased flexibility in understanding the here-and-now experience of the family. Clinicians can aid transnational families in exploring family roles to mitigate boundary ambiguity and expand on a flexible understanding of family identity (Solheim et al., 2016). Ambiguous loss thrives in uncertainty where questioning and mutual inquiry can serve to interrupt the monologue to shed light on new meaning and solutions as the problem continues to evolve.

There are several components of ambiguous loss that are unique to transnational families: chronic stress (Delgado, 2022; Galvan et al., 2022; Solheim et al., 2016), boundary ambiguity and role renegotiations (Roy & Yumiseva, 2021; Solheim & Ballard, 2016; Solheim et al., 2016; Tu, 2023), and resilience (Solheim & Ballard, 2016; Solheim et al., 2016). *Chronic stress* refers to the concrete stressors experienced continuously by family members at home and/or abroad and include acculturative stress and discrimination experienced by migrant family members, financial worry on both sides, separation during times of family emergency or crisis (such as deaths or serious illnesses of family members), and chronic worry about the safety and security of family members from afar. *Boundary Ambiguity* refers to the difficulty maintaining or confusion around family roles and responsibilities post-migration of some family members (Solheim et al., 2016). Various people in the system may theoretically have more structural power (such as older adults or males in patriarchal systems), but may be so far removed from the day to day interactions of other family members that roles must shift out of necessity (e.g., caregiver roles need to be adopted by those in closer proximity to members that need cared for). Sometimes caregiver roles have to be sourced out to extended family members or even people outside the family system, as is the case when elderly family members need round the clock care but there is no longer any younger generations remaining in the country of origin to care for them (Baldassar et al., 2014; Tu, 2023) Sometimes with language barriers in the host country, and the need for translation, younger generations (second or third) can be put in positions outside of the norm for the cultural hierarchy, further contributing to role ambiguity (Solheim & Ballard, 2016). Perceptions about the migration process, level of boundary ambiguity, and level of agency family members have in the migration or separation process interact with migration related trauma and chronic stressors. When people feel more connected to transnational family members, are able to maintain a sense of cultural connection and proximity, can establish clear and flexible family roles, and have access to the financial and/or legal resources needed to maintain hope for reunification, they are better able to cope with ambiguous loss (Solheim & Ballard, 2016). Transnational migration can result in loss of status and threat to gender identity for some family members (Roy & Yumiseva, 2021). For example, in families where the father has migrated to increase financial opportunity for the family, children may form bonds with other male family members that are more accessible in the country of origin. The fathers and children in these transnational families, particularly those that are forcibly separated, can experience PTSD as a result (Roy & Yumiseva, 2021). It can be difficult to share trauma narratives and communication challenges can exacerbate this difficulty. Consistent contact at a distance does improve transnational relationships, but there are still challenges to emotional intimacy and ambiguous loss still prevails (Galvan et al., 2022; Solheim et al., 2016; Roy & Yumiseva, 2021).

In spite of the many structural and emotional challenges that transnational families experience, increased awareness of family resilience is often part of the ambiguous loss process that can be emphasized in the therapeutic relationship. For example, Solheim et al. (2016) found that resilience increased when family members received social support from extended family in both Mexico and in the United States because it helped family members to maintain hope for reunification and focused on the goals for migration. Participants in this study reportedly refrained from sharing their troubles because they did not want to worry other family members. Some participants reported that not knowing the extent of hardship experienced on the other side actually did make it easier to cope with their ambiguous loss, while other participants reported that they would have preferred more authenticity in their conversations. Meaning-making was also very important for the ambiguous loss process of participants in this study. When participants were able to make meaning of the family separations, they were better able to cope with the loss. If families can make meaning of the loss that they experience through a strength-based empowered lens, then they can better cope with the loss and reconstruct a new resilient transnational family identity (Boss, 2010).

Advances in technology and access to internet-based chat and video applications like WhatsApp, Zoom, and Facebook Messenger that cut down on international telephone charges have made communicating in real time much more accessible for transnational families (Baldassar et al., 2014; Francisco, 2015). This increased availability of communication can help families cope with ambiguous loss and can help migrant family members stay connected to their cultural identity (Francisco, 2015). However, when families already have cultural difficulties addressing conflict and establishing emotional intimacy, the quality of the virtual contact may not be as strong as it could be. Systemic clinicians that are willing to engage in the here-and-now experiential process of the therapeutic relationship can help transnational families bridge communication gaps, cope with ambiguous loss, and deepen cohesion and intimacy between members.

Acculturative Stress & Ambiguous Loss

Acculturation has often been used as a measure or marker to represent how well immigration populations are adjusting or adapting to the new cultural environment (Falicov, 2019). This view of acculturation assumes that high degrees of assimilation (i.e., less use of native languages, ethnic foods, etc.) are adaptive, however, the process of moving to a new country or navigating between many places can contribute to a lack of clarity regarding cultural values in migrant family members. In the case of transnational families, managing bicultural identity can be difficult and isolating. It can be extremely helpful for there to be flexibility in the family system and compassion regarding the often survival-based need to acculturate because of racist discourses and discrimination in the host country (Falicov, 2019). Acculturative stress can lead to anxiety, depression, feelings of alienation, and suicidality (Tineo et al., 2021). Acculturative stress is the result of rigid dominant discourse in society that requires immigrants to change or give up aspects of their cultural identity to be accepted within another. Clinicians can aid transnational families in deepening their connection and their identity as a transnational family by highlighting the different socio-political pressures and often real safety concerns that all members face in different ways.

Transgenerational Transmission and Racial Trauma

Research on various immigrant populations (i.e., Latinx, Asian, & Muslim) has shown that the experience of discrimination is a predictor for acculturative stress (Falicov, 2019; Tineo et al., 2021). Discrimination and resulting racial trauma are further exacerbated by aspects of intersectionality such as gender, sexual orientation, age, and microaggressions based in xenophobia (Comas-Diaz, 2019). Given the continuous nature (i.e., potential for daily encounters) of racial-ethnic discrimination and systemic racism, healing these compounded wounds can be challenging (Comas-Diaz, 2019). Moreover, racism shows up in three forms: institutional (e.g., immigration laws & racial assimilation); individual (e.g., exposure to discrimination and/or microaggressions); and cultural (e.g., generational White supremacy; Liu & Modir, 2020). The United States, for example, has a long history of scapegoating certain racial-ethnic groups when a large catastrophe occurs like that of the 9/11 terrorist attacks or the most recent COVID-19 pandemic where countless Muslim and Asian individuals have been targeted (Liu & Modir, 2020). The historical trauma experienced by marginalized populations, including transnational families, involves colonization, enslavement, genocide, the destruction of Native tribal lands, the use of internment camps during World War II, and living as a political refugee (Comas-Díaz et al., 2019; Harrell, 2000). Through acts of socialization like storytelling and observing the long-term effects on elders, historical trauma is passed down generationally (Harrell, 2000). Studies on racial trauma tend to focus on explicit events and do not account for transgenerational experiences (Kirkinis et al., 2018). It is important for clinicians to consider that racial trauma includes both direct racist encounters daily throughout life, along with experiencing transgenerational vicarious traumatization through association with a particular ethnocultural group (Comas-Díaz et al., 2019; Kirkinis et al., 2018). It should be noted that some transnational families may all reside in Western/Euro-Centric countries and, particularly those that are White/Caucasian, may not experience generational trauma associated with racism like other transnational families. Even these families, depending upon the political associations between the countries that they are collectively residing in, may experience acculturative stress and discrimination related to a nationalist culture in one or more of the countries in question.

Like other instances of traumatic exposure, safety and consent become priorities within the therapeutic setting as well as in the outside world. While clinicians cannot protect clients from the microaggressions and/or racism they may face in larger society, particularly in countries that have a culture of nationalism, it is important to validate client's experiences of discrimination and explore resources for other safe avenues of culturally appropriate support. Clinicians can also aid families through the exploration of racial-ethnic socialization practices to build coping skills as well as resilience in the face of discrimination and racism, as increasing a sense of belonging has been shown to reduce race-based traumatic stress (Liu & Modir, 2020). As those in transnational families are multicultural, the experience of discrimination and racial trauma experienced amongst members may be very nuanced. For example, a transnational family may also be a multi-racial or intercultural family. It is the systemic therapist's job to open conversation surrounding race and culture while remaining aware of the inevitability of their personal bias.

Theoretical Foundation – An Integrative Postmodern Experiential Approach

So far, we have highlighted a few of the most common complex experiences that transnational families may bring into the therapeutic relationship. We believe that an integration of Collaborative Language Systems and Symbolic Experiential Family therapy is well-suited for transnational families for many reasons, which we will expound upon in this section. It seems important to first describe the theoretical consistencies between the two models and our reasons for integrating them prior to discussing the application of the integrative approach to working with transnational families. Both of us practice clinically from a trauma-informed, social justice-oriented perspective, and we deeply value the importance of the therapeutic relationship with all clients. The process of integrating CLS and SEFT was not one that was borne out of working solely with transnational families, but rather is the approach that best fits our personal theories of change when working with clients of all social locations and presenting concerns.

CLS and SEFT are both models that emphasize a theoretical stance or worldview on human relationships rather than a set of interventions or therapist-prescribed goals for therapy (Anderson, 1997; Anderson & Gehart, 2012; Whitaker & Bumberry, 1988; Whitaker & Ryan, 1989). In both models, the client is viewed as the expert on their lives and both are rooted in client empowerment and increasing self-agency by focusing on process over content and the co-created here-and-now experience of the therapeutic relationship (Anderson, 1997; Whitaker & Ryan, 1989). Whitaker's belief that truth cannot be known aligns with a postmodern perspective of subjective truth (Smith, 1998). Likewise, both models posit that the therapist is isomorphically changed by the process of therapy just as the client is. What Anderson (1997) called the *dialogical space* between client and therapist, Whitaker (Whitaker & Ryan, 1989) referred to as the *therapeutic encounter*: a place where mutual puzzling and curiosity can occur, and the therapist and the client are able to consider new possibilities in the process of making meaning of experiences. Whitaker referred to this as the *language of options* (Connel et al., 1993), which includes a collaborative exploration of the subconscious of both therapist and client. The SEFT focus on experience and symbolism, which are both subjective, makes the model well aligned with the postmodern social constructivist paradigms of CLS (Smith, 1998). The dialogical technique of *appropriately unusual comments* in CLS can be likened at least in part to *psychotherapy of the absurd* (Anderson, 1997; Whitaker & Bumberry, 1988), where the therapist introduces possibilities that the client would never imagine considering in order to encourage their own creativity of thought to identify alternative meanings to problems that are most often developed in response to rigid and uncompromising discourses that stigmatize, pathologize, or otherwise oppress the client family system.

The focus on language in CLS is rooted in the social constructivist perspective that reality is constructed through the use of language, and people and systems that have the most structural power often dictate how discourse is used to shape a collective experience (Anderson, 1997; Anderson & Gehart, 2012). SEFT also focuses largely on language, specifically the *language of pain and impotence*, the *language of inference*, and the aforementioned *language of options* (Whitaker & Ryan, 1989). The language of pain and impotence is the point through which the therapist enters the family's realm of experience, where the therapist expresses empathy and validation for the client's presenting concerns and joins the system. Whitaker posited that people often use metaphor and symbolism to disguise their true thoughts and feelings because it is too risky and vulnerable to speak directly. Through the *language of inference* the therapist uses their intuition to make the covert more overt, which is similar to the CLS concept of *being public* (Anderson & Goolishian, 1988). The *language of options* is perhaps the most congruent with the CLS change theory, where the client and therapist expand the client's perspective to find alternative meanings for their experiences that are more supportive of the change that the clients desire.

The philosophical consistencies between the model abound, but there is one fundamental limitation of each model that prompted the integration of the two. While SEFT has been said to be compatible with postmodernism (Smith, 1998), the theory does not explicitly address power, gender, politics, and broader systemic inequities that marginalize clients and contribute to problem formation. While the stance of the SEFT therapist is not that of an "expert," there is an interpretive nature of the model, as it is also largely informed by psychodynamic and Gestalt theories and encourages the use of bilateral transference (both transference of the client and countertransference of the therapist; Neill & Kniskern, 1982). The CLS postmodern attention to the influence of power structures on the ways in which not only the client but also the therapist makes meaning of experiences addresses this limitation quite well (Goolishian & Anderson, 1987). The emphasis for family therapy in managed care is on measurable behavior outcomes, which can be a form of colonization of mental health as it prioritizes the dominant discourse (the most privileged and usually White, Western, cisheterosexual perspectives) of mental and relational wellness and can also privilege the beliefs of the therapist instead of the wishes of the clients (Aducci, 2012). Therapists working with families that have had negative experiences with the healthcare field and/or other larger sociopolitical systems (e.g., immigration, child protective services, the legal system, etc.) must recognize how oppression may be impacting the client system (Aducci, 2012). From a CLS perspective, knowledge is constructed through language and it is transformed over time contingent upon the "knower." Therapists are transparent about their knowledge and biases and the emphasis is on the co-creation of meaning in the here and now of the therapeutic relationship (Anderson & Gehart, 2012; Goolishian & Anderson, 1987). In SEFT, the therapist's authentic use of self is the most important intervention in therapy – we believe that the experiential therapist needs to be particularly mindful of their positionality. The therapist's social location (their race/ethnicity, socio-economic status, level of education, sexual orientation, gender expression, ability, culture, etc.) undoubtedly informs their case conceptualization and thus also the therapeutic relationship.

The primary limitation of CLS is that the theory of change does not adequately emphasize the corrective emotional experiences that occur in the context of the therapeutic relationship. Goolishian and Anderson (1987) proposed that change is not a result of a structural shift but a process of creating new meaning through conversational exchange. Whitaker much agreed that structural shifts are not enough to produce second-order change, but the SEFT change theory also proposes that insight and awareness are not enough to produce change either (Napier & Whitaker, 1978; Whitaker & Bumberry, 1988; Whitaker & Ryan, 1989). Change happens in the intimate experience of the existential encounter in the process of therapy. What that means is that there is an emotional shift, rather than purely a cognitive one. This SEFT change process is actually supported by recent neuroscience findings (Bailey, 2022; Roberts & Chafin, 2020). It is thought that appropriate (non-distressing) anxiety activates the right brain/emotion center (limbic system) of the brain and allows for a spontaneous relational interaction that can help to rewire neural pathways, supporting Whitaker's idea that the change that occurs in the process of therapy is nonconscious and thus not a cognitive process (Roberts & Chafin, 2020). For transnational families that are negotiating many structural and cultural challenges, different forms of ambiguous loss, and often also trauma (i.e., traumatic migration or war/political conflict in the country of origin), helping the family to restore a sense of emotional intimacy and cohesion can be extremely healing.

Application with Transnational Families

In addition to the opportunity to increase intimacy and connectedness in transnational families, an integration of SEFT and CLS can support these diverse family structures in other important ways. Research shows that changing relational dynamics, power imbalances, and role ambiguity are a part of the ambiguous loss experience in transnational families (Baldassar et al., 2014; Boss, 2010; Solheim & Ballard, 2016; Solheim et al., 2016). Identifying gendered cultural discourses about power and family role expectations can assist the family system in exploring the influence of such discourses on the distress experienced by individual members and the system as a whole (Anderson, 2014; Anderson & Goolishian, 1988). Engaging the family members that are able to be present in the therapy sessions in enactments of their role rigidity can assist the therapist in illuminating the rigidity of their assigned roles in an effort to expand the "symptom" (whatever the family's presenting concern is) to the broader system, thus depathologizing individual members and opening up the possibility for more fluidity in family roles (Whitaker & Ryan, 1989). The family members that might traditionally have the most structural power (based on age or generational position and gender) are often logistically not able to maintain the same sense of power when families are separated by geography (Baldassar et al., 2014; McNeil Walsh, 2023 Roy & Yumiseva, 2021). For example, Roy and Yumiseva (2021) found that fathers that migrate for financial gain and to increase opportunities for the family reported that they felt as though they were "providing from the shadows," as their position in the family was not as stable when they were separated from their families because they had little awareness of the day-to-day experiences of the family members that remained in the country of origin. Transnational migration can result in loss of status and threat to masculine gender identity. Children may form bonds with male family members that are more accessible in the country of origin, thus exacerbating the ambiguous loss experience for these fathers (Roy & Yumiseva, 2021). Exploring the ways that the father and other family members are all making meaning of the reasons for his migration can illuminate new possibilities that can foster empathy and understanding between family members and highlight the strengths and resiliencies in the system. Likewise, engaging a family like this in an experiential process that allows different family members to "try on" the burdens of the "provider from the shadows" and the other family roles (such as emotional caretaker, scapegoat, family hero, translator, cultural liaison, etc.) can encourage them all to be less rigid, and thus more flexible and adaptive.

The language of pain and impotence can help transnational families directly name the racism, xenophobia, and/or nationalism that they may experience through the migration process. Any acculturative stress that may be experienced can also be acknowledged and alternative meaning can be made of the family's experience, highlighting their strength and resilience through dialogical conversation, the use of symbolism and metaphor, mutual puzzling, and shared inquiry (dialogue between and within; Anderson & Goolishian, 1988). By identifying cultural discourse around intimacy, emotional expression, conflict resolution, etc., the family can be assisted in bridging the gap of physical absence in order to increase intimacy and cohesion.

Clinical Examples/Application of this Integrative Approach

We believe that the best way to make this integrative approach come alive is to share clinical examples of the work that we have done with transnational families. We will start by situating ourselves in the social context in an effort to be more transparent about the power and privilege that we hold. We have different social locations and cultural backgrounds, and so we naturally interpret and apply this integrative approach somewhat differently. We are hopeful that showcasing two different family systems from two different self-of-the-therapist lenses will highlight the flexibility of this collaborative experiential approach.

Nicole's Experience

I am a White, cisgender, pansexual woman that passes as straight because I am currently in a heterosexual marriage with a straight cisgender man. I hold much privilege and power not only because of my gender expression and race, but also because I hold a doctorate and have been practicing as a therapist for more than 12 years. I am ethnically Italian and Polish. I do not identify as being a member of a transnational family, as I have had no contact with family members who still reside in Poland or Italy (my great grandparents migrated to the so-called United States by way of Ellis Island between the first and second World Wars). Though I have worked clinically with transnational families countless times, I have no direct experience with transnationalism. My partner is half Mexican-American and half German-American, and the majority of his paternal side of the family (including his father) are from and currently reside in Mexico. I have some experience with transnational family dynamics in that regard, but still very much consider myself to be an outsider of this phenomenon.

The family in question contacted me because I specialize in trauma and chemical dependency in the family. They were referred by a treatment center that Paul (16-year-old cisgender male) had been discharged from as part of his aftercare. Paul reportedly used marijuana and alcohol to cope and had been expelled from his high school because he had been found having marijuana in his backpack while on school grounds. Paul's mother Giovanna (50) reported that since Paul had discharged from treatment the family had been in high conflict, especially Paul and his siblings. Maria (21) and Giuliana (28) are Paul's half-siblings. Giovanna was previously married to their father and divorced when Maria was just under 4 and Giuliana was 10. Giovanna, Maria, and Giuliana are Italian immigrants that migrated to the United States within a year from the divorce, as Giovanna had met and quickly remarried Paul's father Jeremy (55), an American that was living in Italy for a short time for work. At the time that Giovanna reached out for services, she, Jeremy, Maria, and Paul lived together in California, and Giuliana had returned to live near her biological father, maternal and paternal grandparents, and extended family in Italy. Paul reportedly felt left out because he did not speak Italian, and when his sisters were together, they mostly spoke to one another in Italian. Paul was decidedly the scapegoat for the family system, Maria was stuck in the middle as the mediator, and Giovanna was the black sheep. When Giovanna requested family therapy, she described the relational dynamics between the siblings and Jeremy, and much of her conversation focused on the conflict between Giuliana and Jeremy, though she reportedly wanted to engage in family therapy to "support Paul's sobriety." Because Giovanna focused so much on Paul and Jeremy's conflict with Giuliana, I was very hesitant to see the family without Giuliana being present. I was concerned that leaving her out of therapy would further alienate her as the transnational family member, which would essentially collude with the system and perpetuate the family conflict. This was just prior to the world-changing COVID-19 pandemic and when I asked Giovanna what it would take to be able to get Giuliana in the therapy room, she shared that Giuliana would be traveling to California for the Christmas Holiday and would be in town for three weeks. Though that was two months from the time that Giovanna reached out, I told her that I would be happy to give her referrals for other family therapists if she wanted to begin treatment more immediately, but in order to win the *battle for structure* (Napier & Whitaker, 1978) I held firm that having Giuliana in therapy would be the best course of action. Giovanna agreed to wait, and we had sessions twice a week over the course of the three weeks that Giuliana was in town, totaling 6 two-hour family therapy sessions.

Throughout the course of therapy my initial assessment of the rigid family roles and ambiguous loss proved to be accurate. The whole family was grieving the loss of Giuliana, as she was not only physically absent when she returned to Italy, she had been emotionally absent from the system since the family immigrated to the United States. Giuliana was grieving the loss of the family that she felt alienated from, and reportedly did not find the sense of belonging that she was yearning for when she decided to return to her family in Italy. My intuition told me to align with her first, even though in doing so I took the risk of alienating other family members. The whole time she lived in California she felt as though Italy was her home, but after living in the United States between the ages of 12 and 23, she no longer felt as though she exactly fit in to the culture in Italy either. In my attempt to expand the symptoms (family conflict and Paul's substance misuse) to the broader system (the entire family system and the broader social structures that make it challenging for transnational families to interact), we revealed that Giuliana actually felt a lot of remorse for the way that she treated Jeremy when she was an adolescent. As a teenager she felt as though she would be betraying her loyalty to her biological father if she were to develop a relationship with Jeremy, and also held a lot of anger towards him because she blamed him for Giovanna's abrupt decision to migrate to the United States. Giovanna revealed that her relationship with Maria and Giuliana's father was very contentious and she left Italy because she had been shunned not only by his family but also her own, who were devout Catholics and did not believe in divorce. When she met Jeremy, he was the only person that did not seem to shame her for her life choices and she desperately needed that during a time when she felt like a "worthless failure." Jeremy was able to speak to the grief he felt about not knowing how to connect with Giuliana because she was so angry. In his family of origin conflict was avoided at all costs and when there were eventual blowouts, they would be swept under the rug and never discussed again.

Through appropriately unusual comments (Anderson, 1997; Anderson & Gehart, 2012) and heightening the constructive anxiety in the system (Napier & Whitaker, 1978; Whitaker & Bumberry, 1988), I was able to activate an experiential process in the course of the sessions where the family members began to express themselves more authentically than they had in the past ten years. Together, through the language of pain and impotence and mutual puzzling, we explored the cultural discourses about vulnerability and intimacy, gender roles, and conflict negotiation that had kept the family stuck in rigid and uncompromising roles for so many years. Paul was able to speak to his experience as the scapegoat, feeling as though he had been labeled as the "problem," when in reality he was the only one being brave enough to show how much pain he was in. We were subsequently able to rotate the scapegoat role to each member of the system as we discussed the ambiguous loss and explored alternative meanings for the family's identity as a transnational family. The family also explored the symbolic conflicts that they had continued to engage in because it was too difficult and confusing for them to directly address the many dialectical experiences of being a transnational blended family system. They could feel like a cohesive family system and also acknowledge that there were distinct subsystems of the family that had different cultural experiences, separate cultural identities, and different meaning making systems. The family were able to speak about a bicultural identity that Maria, Giovanna, and Giuliana shared in ways that Paul and Jeremy did not. It had often felt to them as though there were three distinct families rather than one cohesive family: Paul, Jeremy, and Giovanna; Giovanna, Giuliana, and Maria; and Maria, Paul, Jeremy, and Giovanna. One or two people were always on the outside of the system. The SEFT emphasis on intimacy and family cohesion aligned with the family's goals for therapy. Giuliana invited the family to come to Italy to visit her, to meet her partner, and see the life that she had begun to build. Paul and Maria had visited Italy several times throughout their childhood, but no one in the family had been since Giuliana moved back, which had confirmed her belief that they were glad that she was gone. Maria felt abandoned by Giuliana and obligated to stay in the United States with her younger brother. Her feelings of obligation became suffocating and she had abandoned her role as the mediator much in the way that Giuliana had abandoned her, which is why Maria and Paul had been in such conflict prior to entering therapy. The family were able to collaboratively explore familiar family stories and co-create new, yet-to-be-told stories (Anderson, 1997). I transparently shared my worries about the family's pattern of scapegoating the person who was brave enough to tell the truth about their pain (as evidenced first through Giuliana when she shared her anger and difficulty with immigration and divorce as a teen, and then through Paul's use of substances to cope with his grief about the family separation). We addressed Giuliana's sense of obligation to care for her elderly grandparents in her mother's place because she was the only one who was physically able to do so given the geographic challenges, and identified ways to increase role flexibility there as well as they negotiated what it meant to be in a transnational family.

During the pandemic, Giovanna reached out for individual support. She had just lost her mother to COVID19, only two months after losing her father to it. We met through Zoom, as the shelter-in-place orders were still active in California. She was devastated that travel restrictions between the United States and Italy prohibited her from going to Italy to see her parents before they passed. She expressed guilt for not visiting more prior to the pandemic and reported that she still had not been able to travel to Italy since Giuliana had moved back there. Her burden of guilt was greatest because Giuliana had to be the one to care for her grandparents prior to their hospitalizations and she was living alone in their house at the time of my session with Giovanna. We cried together and I shared that I felt impotent: there are no therapeutic words or interventions for grief that can soothe the pain she was feeling in those moments. She acknowledged that she had been grieving in one form or another since she decided to immigrate to the United States, stating that she had always intended to go back to Italy when she and her parents entered the stage of life where she would become the caretaker and they would need her care. I reminded her of my worry from our family therapy sessions: that the family would scapegoat the person who was brave enough to tell the truth about their pain. I asked her who she thought the scapegoat would be this time, and she said that she would rather it be her than one of her children, so she made a commitment to tell them about her pain before she found some symbolic way to avoid it. I encouraged the family to make the best use of technology that they could and engage in more regular contact with one another to strengthen the bonds between members, and to increase cohesiveness as a whole. They started a group chat on WhatsApp that allowed them to communicate internationally with Giuliana in real-time when she returned to Italy.

I was able to move through my own ambiguous loss process regarding self-of-the-therapist cultural identity challenges when working alongside this family system. It is important to note that this family was privileged in that their country of origin is Italy, and aside from travel restrictions related to the COVID19 pandemic, they did not experience any political barriers that impacted their ability to travel between countries. They had more financial resources at some times more than others and were able to travel more when they had the resources to do so. Giovanna, Maria, and Giuliana also spoke English prior to immigration and came from a European country, and so did not experience the marginalization and xenophobia that many immigrants to the United States do. As a result, their ambiguous loss process was not compounded by experiences of racism, though Giovanna reported that when her uncle and aunt had migrated several decades prior, their experience as Italian migrants was much different than hers.

Loette's Experience

As a multiracial (i.e., African and White) cis-gendered Woman, when working with clients I aim to keep my own intersectionality in mind and the impact it may have when having the privilege to hear the deepest parts of individuals' lives. While I am not directly from a transnational family, my grandmother is from the United Kingdom and upon moving to the United States when marrying my grandfather, she had the experience of transitioning between two home countries and trying to keep in touch with family for a time. I have very brief memories of family from the UK. I cannot claim to truly understand transnationalism from my own experiences, but with clients as the experts of their life, my aim is to provide a space for curiosity as we grow together.

Martha (age 32) and Luciana (age 30) are sisters who help their mom support extended family living in Guatemala. Martha and Luciana both identify as cis-gendered women and Guatemalan American. The sisters sought treatment to improve their connection with each other but also gain a better understanding of family roles and generational trauma because of acculturation challenges. Martha and Luciana are the middle siblings of four with an older and younger brother. Additionally, the family works together to help Martha raise her 10-year-old son. At the beginning of treatment, they all lived in the same house household, along with their mom and younger brother. Newly engaged, Luciana recently moved into her own apartment with her fiancé about two hours away from the family home. She commutes to the family home on weekends to help manage finances and connect with extended family during the weekly virtual Zoom call with their dad and grandparents in Guatemala. Often, they are also conversing with their mother on the other side of the screen as she travels to Guatemala whenever possible to manage her parents' healthcare. As Luciana has just moved out of the family home, Martha has taken on added responsibility in supporting her younger brother and son, especially when their mom is out of the country. Symbolically speaking Luciana has often served as the mediator in the family, while Martha who has been in recovery from alcohol abuse for 12 years is labeled as the scapegoat. Ambiguous family roles make it challenging for Martha to know how to best support the family when their mom is present and away. Both sisters have not been in the physical presence of their father in about 11 years since he was last able to visit and fear for his safety on a regular basis due to the level of violence in Guatemala. Technology has vastly increased the amount of contact between the family; however, money challenges still limit contact.

In considering therapeutic intervention, most time was spent establishing safety, increasing efforts toward connection outside of therapy, determining how to talk about different aspects of trauma, and increasing understanding of family roles. Sessions began with an open stance regarding what would be brought up for conversation. This process was labeled as "check-in" within the therapeutic system that started with whoever took initiative that day where the therapist prioritized the language of pain and impotence to connect with aspect of human suffering. Over time the family moved from having more closed dialogue between two people (i.e., one client and therapist) to open dialogue between all involved in therapy. Questioning was also utilized throughout the therapeutic journey to engage in mutual inquiry regarding how each member is experiencing the problem here-and-now. The symbolic world of each family member was achieved using the language of inference and curiosity to explore the meaning of each problem as it dissolved into the next.

Areas for Future Research and Clinical Consideration

Overall, research that prioritizes the experience of transnational families is lacking. It has been urged that acculturation is an unpredictable measure of adaption or assimilation in that the use of a variety of cultural customs are in a state of flux (Falicov, 2019). Future studies that focus on the potential multicultural essence of transnational families and acculturative stress may offer insight to the factors that empower and foster resiliency. In considering ambiguous loss, Boss (2006) related that this type of grief does not show up in the same way for all families where some may not experience any adverse effects. Investigation into the different experiences within the context of ambiguous loss and transnational families could shed light on the factors that impact why some experience the phenomenon more strongly than others. As previously discussed, transgenerational transmission of trauma, and racial trauma specifically, is largely left unaccounted for in any study let alone those on transnational families.

Like all other healthcare disciplines (Rene et al., 2022), the COVID-19 pandemic has impacted the field of CFT in many ways. At the onset of the pandemic, the vast majority of therapists quickly shifted from delivering services in-person in an office, agency, or hospital setting to delivering services entirely or almost entirely via telehealth through the use of videoconference platforms or even telephone (Hertlein et al., 2021). Even after health restrictions were lifted, many therapists continue to practice via telehealth, with some practitioners moving their therapy practices entirely online, and preliminary research shows that telehealth can be as viable as traditional in-person therapy (Greenwood et al., 2022). Families that were forced to shelter in place remained without contact from one another for long periods of time, and this particularly affected transnational families that were no longer able to travel across borders to see one another. The ambiguous loss process typically experienced by transnational families was exacerbated by the impossibility of connection for families that strongly desired physical proximity in a time of collective trauma, death, and illness that made the reality of geographic separation all too tangible, thus minimizing the benefits of connecting virtually (Simola et al., 2023). Like other forms of forced separation (Galvan et al., 2022; Roy & Yumiseva, 2021), it may take time to fully understand the implications of the pandemic on transnational families. For many transnational families, the licensure restrictions on interjurisdictional practice are likely to be confusing. These families will understandably wonder: *If we can Zoom, Skype, WhatsApp, or FaceTime with one another, then why can't we conduct family therapy sessions in that way?* It is important for systemically trained relational therapists to be increasing their clinical competency with online delivery methods and continually engaged in advocacy efforts to expand service delivery methods to meet the growing needs of a global population of exponentially increasing transnational families.

Three Key Takeaways

- Transnational families often experience sociopolitical challenges that can impact their mental and relational health. Therapists need to be mindful of and assess for the influences of such challenges (and experiences of racism, nationalism, xenophobia, etc.) on the family's ability to remain cohesive and their presenting concerns.
- All members of a transnational system are likely to be experiencing ambiguous loss and role ambiguity. Therapists should normalize ambivalence and assist the family in identifying realistic ways to remain connected to one another and their culture of origin.
- An integrative approach of Collaborative Language Systems and Symbolic Experiential Family Therapy can be beneficial for assisting transnational families in making new meaning of their experiences as a family as they re-negotiate more flexible family roles.

Resources and Further Reading

Anderson, H. (1997). *Conversation, language, and possibilities: A postmodern approach to therapy.* Basic Books.

Anderson, H., & Gehart, D. (Eds.), (2012). *Collaborative therapy: Relationships and conversations that make a difference.* Routledge.

Falicov, C. J. (2019). Transnational journeys. In M. McGoldrick & K. V. Hardy (Eds.), *Re-visioning family therapy: Addressing diversity in clinical practice., 3rd ed.* (pp. 108–122). The Guilford Press.

Whitaker, C. A., & Bumberry, W. M. (1988). *Dancing with the family: A symbolic-experiential approach.* Philadelphia: Brunner/Mazel.

Whitaker, C., & Ryan, M. O. (1989). *Midnight musings of a family therapist.* New York: W. W. Norton & Co.

References

Aducci, C. J. (2012). "Ask the person that lived it. that would be me." A discursive therapy approach to countering social inequalities in a couple's therapy session. *Journal of Feminist Family Therapy*, 24(4), 340–356. https://doi.org/10.1080/08952833.2012.710817

Albertini, M., Mantovani, D., & Gasperoni, G. (2019). Intergenerational relations among immigrants in Europe: the role of ethnic differences, migration and acculturation. *Journal of Ethnic & Migration Studies*, 45(10), 1693–1706. https://doi.org/10.1080/1369183X.2018.1485202

Anderson, H. (1997). *Conversation, language, and possibilities: A postmodern approach to therapy.* Basic Books.

Anderson, H. (2001). Postmodern collaborative and person-centered therapies: what would Carl Rogers say?. *Journal of Family Therapy*, 23(4), 339–360.

Anderson, H. (2014). Collaborative-dialogue based research as everyday practice: Questioning our myths. *Systemic Inquiry: Innovations in Reflexive Practice Research*, 60–73.

Anderson, H., & Gehart, D. (Eds.), (2012). *Collaborative therapy: Relationships and conversations that make a difference*. Routledge.

Anderson, H., & Goolishian, H. A. (1988). Human systems as linguistic systems: Preliminary and evolving ideas about the implications for clinical theory. *Family Process*, 27(4), 371–393.

Anderson, H., & Goolishian, H. (1992). The client is the expert: A not-knowing approach to therapy. *Therapy As Social Construction*, 25, 39.

Bailey, M. E. (2022). Science catching up: Experiential family therapy and neuroscience. *Journal of Marital and Family Therapy*, 48(4), 1095–1110. https://doi.org/10.1111/jmft.12582

Baldassar, L. (2007). Transnational Families and Aged Care: The Mobility of Care and the Migrancy of Ageing. *Journal of Ethnic & Migration Studies*, 33(2), 275–297. https://doi.org/10.1080/13691830601154252

Baldassar, L., Kilkey, M., Merla, L., & Wilding, R. (2014). Transnational families. In J. Treas, J. Scott, & M. Richards (Eds.), *The Wiley Blackwell companion to the sociology of families* (pp. 155–175). John Wiley & Sons. https://doi.org/10.1002/9781118374085.ch8

Berry, J. W. (2001). A psychology of immigration. *Journal of Social Issues*, 57(3), 615–631. https://doi.org/10.1111/0022-4537.00231

Berry, J. W., Kim, U., Minde, T., & Mok, D. (1987). Comparative studies of acculturative stress. *International Migration Review*, 21(3), 491–511. doi:10.2307/2546607

Boss, P. (1999). *Ambiguous loss: Learning to live with unresolved grief*. Harvard University Press.

Boss, P. (2006). Loss, trauma, and resilience: Therapeutic work with ambiguous loss. New York: W. W. Norton & Co.

Boss, P. (2010). The trauma and complicated grief of ambiguous loss. *Pastoral Psychology*, 59(2), 137–145. doi:10.1007/s11089-009-0264-0.

Bravo, V. (2017). Coping with dying and deaths at home: How undocumented migrants in the United States experience the process of transnational grieving. Mortality, 22, 33–44. https://doi.org/10.1080/13576275.2016.1192590

Bryceson, D., & Vuorela, U. (Eds.), (2002). The Transnational Family: New European Frontiers and Global Networks. Oxford: Berg.

Cheon, H.S., & Murphy, M. J. (2007). The self-of-the-therapist awakened: Postmodern approaches to the use of self in marriage and family therapy. *Journal of Feminist Family Therapy*, 19(1), 1–16. https://doi.org/10.1300/J086v19n01_01

Comas-Díaz, L., Hall, G. N., & Neville, H. A. (2019). Racial trauma: Theory, research, and healing: Introduction to the special issue. *American Psychologist*, 74(1), 1. http://dx.doi.org/10.1037/amp0000442

Connell, G. M., Mitten, T. J., & Whitaker, C. A. (1993). Reshaping family symbols: A symbolic-experiential perspective. *Journal of Marital and Family Therapy*, 19(3), 243–251. https:// doi. org/ 10. 1111/ j. 1752-0606. 1993. tb00985. x.

Delgado, V. (2022). Family formation under the law: How immigration laws construct contemporary Latino/a immigrant families in the U.S. *Sociology Compass*, 16(9), 1–13. https://doi.org/10.1111/soc4.13027

Falicov, C.J. (2019) Transnational Journeys. In M. McGoldrick & K. Hardy (Eds.), *Revisioning culture, race and class in family therapy* (pp. 108–122). New York: Guilford Press.

Francisco, V. (2015). 'The Internet Is Magic': Technology, intimacy and transnational families *Critical Sociology*, 173–190. http://dx.doi.org/10.1177/0896920513484602

Galvan, T., Rusch, D., Domenech Rodríguez, M. M., & Garcini, L. M. (2022). Familias Divididas [divided families]: Transnational family separation and undocumented Latinx immigrant health. *Journal of Family Psychology*, 36(4), 513–522. https://doi.org/10.1037/fam0000975

Gehart-Brooks, D. R., & Lyle, R. R. (1999). Client and therapist perspectives of change in collaborative language systems: An interpretive ethnography. *Journal of Systemic Therapies*, 18(4), 58–77. https://doi.org/10.1521/jsyt.1999.18.4.58

Gehart, D. R., & Tuttle, A. R. (2003). *Theory-based treatment planning for marriage and family therapists: Integrating theory and practice*. Brooks/Cole, Cengage Learning.

Gerber, R., & Ravazzini, L. (2022). Life satisfaction among skilled transnational families before and during the COVID-19 outbreak. *Population Space & Place*, 28(6), 1–32. https://doi.org/10.1002/psp.2557

Goolishian, H. A., & Anderson, H. (1987). Language systems and therapy: An evolving idea. *Psychotherapy: Theory, Research, Practice, Training*, 24(3S), 529.

Greenwood, H., Krzyzaniak, N., Peiris, R., Clark, J., Scott, A. M., Cardona, M., Griffith, R., Glasziou, P. (2022). Telehealth versus face-to-face psychotherapy for less common mental health conditions: Systematic review and meta-analysis of randomized controlled trials. *JMIR Mental Health*, 2022 Mar 11; 9(3):e31780. doi: 10.2196/31780. PMID: 35275081; PMCID: PMC8956990.

Haagsman, K., Mazzucato, M. & Dito, B. D. (2015). Transnational families and the subjective well-being of migrant parents: Angolan and Nigerian parents in the Netherlands. *Ethnic and Racial Studies*, 38(15), 2652–2671, DOI: 10.1080/01419870.2015.1037743

Hansen, H. R., Shneyderman, Y., McNamara, G. S., & Grace, L. (2018). Assessing acculturative stress of International Students at a U.S. Community College. *Journal of International Students*, 8(1), 215–232.

Harrell, S. P. (2000). A multidimensional conceptualization of racismrelated stress: Implications for the wellbeing of people of color. *American Journal of Orthopsychiatry*, 70(1), 42–57. https://doi.org/10.1037/h0087722

Henderson, D. (2016). Cultural homelessness: A challenge to theory and practice. *Psychodynamic Practice: Individuals, Groups and Organisations*, 22(2), 165–172. https://doi.org/10.1080/14753634.2016.1145388

Hertlein, K. M., Drude, K., & Jordan, S. S. (2021). "What Next?": Toward telebehavioral health sustainability in couple and family therapy. *Journal of Marital and Family Therapy*, 47(3), 551–565. https://doi.org/10.1111/jmft.12510

Kilkey, M., & Merla, L. (2014). Situating transnational families' care-giving arrangements: the role of institutional contexts. *Global Networks*, 14(2), 210–229. https://doi.org/10.1111/glob.12034

Kirkinis, K., Pieterse, A. L., Martin, C., Agiliga, A., & Brownell, A. (2018). Racism, racial discrimination, and trauma: A systematic review of the social science literature. *Ethnicity & Health*, 26(3), 392–412. https://doi.org/10.1080/13557858.2018.1514453

Liu, S. R., & Modir, S. (2020). The outbreak that was always here: Racial trauma in the context of COVID-19 and implications for mental health providers. *Psychological Trauma: Theory, Research, Practice, and Policy*, 12(5), 439. https://doi.org/10.1037/tra0000784

Mazzucato V., Schans, D. (2011). Transnational Families and the Well-Being of Children: Conceptual and methodological challenges. *Journal of Marriage and Family*, 73(4), 704–712. doi: 10.1111/j.1741-3737.2011.00840.x.

McNeil, W. C. E. (2023). Visiting here, there, and somewhere: Multi-locality and the geographies of transnational family visiting. *Global Networks*, 23(1), 277–290. https://doi.org/10.1111/glob.12419

Muruthi, B. A., Nasis, T., Jordan, L. S., McCoy, M., Grogan, C., & Farnham, A. (2015). Collaborative therapy approach: Implications for working with Afro-Caribbean families coping with infidelity. *Journal of Systemic Therapies*, 34(3), 26–43. https://doi.org/10.1521/jsyt.2015.34.3.26

Napier, A., & Whitaker, C. (1978). *The family crucible: The intense experience of family therapy*. New York: HarperCollins.

Neill, J. R., & Kniskern, D. P. (1982). *From psyche to system: The evolving therapy of Carl Whitaker*. New York: Guilford Press.

Peters, H. C., & Das, B. (2021). SEFT: A Critical Review and Call to Action. *Journal of Professional Counseling: Practice, Theory & Research*, 48(1), 1–14. https://doi.org/10.1080/15566382.2020.1871259

Rene, R., Cherson, M., Rannazzisi, A., Felter, J., Silverio, A., & Cunningham, A. T. (2022). Transitioning from In-Person to Telemedicine Within Primary Care Behavioral Health During COVID-19. *Population Health Management*, 25(4), 455–461. https://doi.org/10.1089/pop.2021.0292

Roberts, T. W., & Chafin, M. L. (2020). Neuroscience and symbolic-experiential family therapy: Roots of [Contemporary] psychotherapy. *The Family Journal*, 28(2), 138–145. https://doi.org/10.1177/1066480719894944

Roy, K., & Yumiseva, M. (2021). Family separation and transnational fathering practices for immigrant Northern Triangle families. *Journal of Family Theory & Review*, 13(3), 283–299. https://doi.org/10.1111/jftr.12404

Simola, A., May, V., Olakivi, A., & Wrede, S. (2023). On not "being there": Making sense of the potent urge for physical proximity in transnational families at the outbreak of the COVID19 pandemic. *Global Networks*, 23(1), 45–58. https://doi.org/10.1111/glob.12382

Smith, G. L. (1998). The present state and future of symbolic-experiential familytherapy: A postmodern analysis. *Contemporary Family Therapy*, 20(2), 147–161. https://doi.org/10.1023/A:1025073324868

Solheim, C. A., & Ballard, J. (2016). Ambiguous loss due to separation in voluntary transnational families. *Journal of Family Theory & Review*, 8(3), 341–359. https://doi.org/10.1111/jftr.12160

Solheim, C., Zaid, S., & Ballard, J. (2016). Ambiguous Loss Experienced by Transnational Mexican Immigrant Families. *Family Process*, 55(2), 338–353. https://doi.org/10.1111/famp.12130

Tineo, P., Lowe, S. R., Reyes-Portillo, J. A., & Fuentes, M. A. (2021). Impact of perceived discrimination on depression and anxiety among Muslim college students: The role of acculturative stress, religious support, and Muslim identity. *American Journal of Orthopsychiatry*, 91(4), 454. https://doi.org/10.1037/ort0000545

Tu, M. (2023). Ageing, migration infrastructure and multigenerational care dynamics in transnational families. *Global Networks*, 23(2), 347–361. https://doi.org/10.1111/glob.12390

Whitaker, C. A., & Bumberry, W. M. (1988). *Dancing with the family: A symbolic-experiential approach*. Philadelphia: Brunner/Mazel.

Whitaker, C. A., & Malone, T. P. (1953). The therapist as a person. In *The roots of psychotherapy* (pp. 135–158). Philadelphia: Blakiston. https:// doi. org/ 10. 1037/ 14553-012

Whitaker, C., & Ryan, M. O. (1989). *Midnight musings of a family therapist*. New York: W. W. Norton & Co.

34

RELATIONAL RESILIENCY IN AN AGE OF DIGITAL CHAOS

Collective Strategies for Prevention and Healing in an Electronic World

Katherine M. Hertlein

Introduction

Resiliency has been defined as "the capacity of a dynamic, malleable system to withstand challenges to its stability, viability, or development" (Mehta et al., 2016, p. 604). The term "relational resiliency" in couple and family scholarship has been used to describe individual resilience in a relational setting – that is, how to be resilient as an individual and bring those skills to bear in a relational context. Its applications have been limited to recovery from intimate partner violence (Neustifter & Powell, 2015), children in foster care (Lynch, 2011), and childhood cancer (Brody & Simmons, 2007).

Few authors in the field of couple and family therapy have advocated for the role of the systems approach in resiliency; those who have discussed relational resiliency have not attended to the issues related to today's relational technological concerns. This is particularly surprising since relationships are a primary context in which resiliency occurs (Walsh, 2003). In the early 2000s, when the concept of relational resiliency was introduced, technology was not as pervasive as it is in our culture and families as is it today and, therefore, not included in the application of the framework. Yet technology's presence in our lives has increased. Today there are an estimated 3.5 billion Internet users worldwide, with that number increasing annually (Internet Live Stats, 2016). The effects of the increased presence for individuals can be both physiological and psychological. For example, studies indicate texters experience changes in heart rate, respiration, and comfort, including tension in the upper extremities and shallow breathing, particularly for ethnic minorities (Lin & Peper, 2009) and increased musculoskeletal symptoms (Chang et al., 2007). High-frequency cell phone users show a decline in cardiorespiratory fitness and an increase in sedentary behavior (Lepp et al., 2013) and increase in headaches (Acharya et al., 2013). Researchers have also found a link between anxiety and Internet usage when controlling for depression, noting that those with higher degrees of social anxiety will be more likely to have used the

DOI: 10.4324/9781003297871-37

Internet in problematic ways than those without such symptomology (Lee & Stapinski, 2012). Such ill effects may also be true for children who use cell phones (Sudan et al., 2013).

Resiliency Toward Technology

Composed of individuals, couples and families also continue to be plagued with serious problems related to technologies including online gaming addiction, online sex addiction, infidelity, cyberbullying, cyberstalking, sexting, and sexually charged information in places easily accessible to youth (Hertlein & Blumer, 2013). For example, online gaming addiction and sex addiction have a host of associated behavioral symptoms, including impulse issues, which can have prominent implications for one's relationship (Blinka et al., 2016). Cyberbullying can have deleterious effects on the family, including impairment in academic or work performance, increased conflict with family and peers, and in severe cases, self-harm. Online infidelity has been demonstrated to have the same effects on an individual's self-perception, the experience of betrayal and trauma, the organization of the couple relationship, and the other relational outcomes (e.g., Cravens & Whiting, 2016). Exchanging sexually explicit texts has been associated with other personal risks such as increasing engagement in casual sex with unknown partners (Davis et al. 2016; Dir & Cyders, 2015; Dir et al., 2013), particularly for women, which can subsequently increase the likelihood of contracting STIs or other negative outcomes. Other relational issues include increased opportunities for infidelity, interruptions to emotional intimacy, impaired trust, and lack of clarity in communication (Hertlein & Ancheta, 2014a).

As serious as these issues are, it is surprising that technology continues to be omitted from writings about resilience. For example, a recent volume addressing the issue of family resilience (Becvar, 2013) included chapters addressing resilience when working with a variety of ethnic populations, applying resiliency to clinically address loss, sexual violence, and issues surrounding at-risk youth, but had no mention of technology's presence and influence in these areas. Walsh (2003) argued that the development of relational resiliency occurs in the context of how a family is *organized*, how a system *solves problems*, and how families are influenced by *belief systems*. This framework can be applied to today's digitally embedded relationships. Considering technology and families, research has shown that 1) technology has implications for the organization of families (Hertlein, 2012); 2) technology has the power to assist systems in problem-solving (Hertlein & Blumer, 2013); and 3) couples and families are affected, in part, by their beliefs about technology usage (Ortiz et al., 2011).

The field of couple and family therapy is at a crossroads. We bear a pronounced responsibility in helping families successfully navigate issues as they emerge in our society, particularly in the context of technology, as it now pervades every aspect of our lives. Though we are the most appropriate discipline to examine the effects on the family and related systems, relatively little has been addressed by our profession. The trend in technology publications have been inconsistent in the field of couple and family studies. Some of the early research dealt with general problems related to technology such as online sexual activities, online infidelity, and impact on offline relationships (Hertlein & Webster, 2008). In a content analysis of technology articles in couple and family journals, there were only 79 articles published out of 13,274 across a 15-year period in 17 journals whose focus was technology-related issues (Blumer et al., 2014). Types of articles represented in this group were those focused on clinical practice (how to use technology in one's clinical practice regarding effectiveness for certain conditions and special considerations for therapy), cybersex and couples, education and training, online support and resources, teen and child use, administrative side of therapy, and cyber addiction. Within the cybersex and couples category, most of the articles (n = 18; 24% of the total number of cyber articles) discussed recovery from infidelity and sexual concerns, but nothing was included from a strength-based approach. The few articles (n = 4, 5% of the 79 evaluated, 0.003% of all articles published in that time) dedicated to teen and child use centered on assessing problems related to technology for youth, such as monitoring internet use and talking to youth about sex. In a field whose dedication is to families, the fact that there were only four articles in 15 years across 17 journals displays a clear gap in the literature. This is especially problematic because youth who engage in sexting are also not often able to adequately recognize the emotional and psychological consequences which result from sexting, including increased opportunity for cyberbullying, depression, and riskier sexual behavior (Ahern & Mechling, 2013; Van Ouytsel et al., 2015). In addition, no article tied how computers or other forms of technology could be used in conjunction with resiliency.

Purpose

The topic of technology's role in couple and family life is of acute importance to family therapy's advancement because how individuals use technology and technology's contribution to the development and maintenance of maladaptive relationship dynamics is now a predominate feature in treatment settings with only the Couple and Family Technology Framework (Hertlein, 2012) describing how to manage its effects. Furthermore, the interventions generally employed by therapists for Internet or social media-related problems involve simply removing the computer/device from the interactions (Hertlein & Piercy, 2008). In a world where we are surrounded by these technologies, it is not a realistic solution. Learning about the effect of technology on individuals and relational systems will also inform how we solve the problems driven by these very same technologies.

This chapter supports Barnard's (1994) call for moving away from pathologizing and better attending to the role of resilience in the practice of couple and family therapy. It has two primary objectives: First, I will expand the definition of relational resiliency by including the collective component and introduce a new term into the literature: *collective relational resiliency*. Second, I will describe how to use the *Couple and Family Technology* framework to foster engagement in collective relational resiliency in a digital world.

Collective Relational Resiliency Defined

As mentioned above, relational resiliency is a known term in the literature. We as therapists see it every day: in the families who are supporting their youth in coming out; in family members who are supporting other children through academic trauma. Yet the global problems in the world, relational resiliency is not enough. We need to come together in ways that connect us not only to our family subsystem, but to those of the families around us. Bronfenbrenner (1977) underscored this point with the ecological systemic approach, demonstrating that we are all individual affected without our microsystems by larger systems, including the time period in which we live and the context of our governance structure. At present, we as a civilization have significantly more global issues to remedy impacting all the world's citizens. From global war, a population-indiscriminate virus, natural disasters, climate change, and marginalization of segments of our fellow human beings, the challenges in our present day extend beyond what the family and our immediate microsystem relationships can resolve or even reasonably handle. As DeFrain (2022) in citing Olson noted: "All the problems in the world either begin in families or end up in families." (p. 1). We also have more people who share our global concerns. For example, the pandemic was a worldwide problem that crossed any border walls, separating oceans, and international borders. It was an equal opportunity destroyer in some ways as everyone was vulnerable yet provided us with a window in how we are all human, no matter the origin of one's passport.

Thus, the concept of collective resiliency was borne out of the concept of relational resiliency on a global scale. It means cultivating new ways to support each other and demonstrate resilience in broader ways across more distant regions and populations. Collective relational resiliency means developing ways to bring our relational resiliencies (i.e., the strengths problem-solving skills, and we share as a couple or family) and bringing those strategies to positively affect our community and the global collective. It assumes that individuals have some level of resiliency that they bring to the relationships and the resiliency skills cultivated within the relationship are then shared with others to support the collective.

Collective relational resiliency also holds true to the foundational concepts in family therapy. It provides for positive feedback loops (von Bertalanffy, 1968) as those building relational resiliency will pass that on to their community. Von Bertalanffy was convinced that systems theory was becoming increasingly important in how to handle the increasing complexity of society's problems. The proposal here is that employing collective relational resiliency – especially via technology – is a reasonable strategy to address the complexities. Another concept in general systems theory is that there is a continuous flow (both in and out) of information (von Bertalanffy, 1968). As mentioned earlier, developments in technology keep us connected in a way where we can input information into the collective with touch on a screen and pull-down information in the same way. Third, the principle of equifinality posts that we can reach the same end point through various means (von Bertalanffy, 1968). This principle allows us to be creative in the way that we address the complicated problems facing us, which includes developing new ways to use technology.

Using Technology to Foster Collective Relational Resiliency

As much as the events and contextual circumstances serve to divide our humanity, there are many mechanisms that can bring us together. The mechanisms successful in bringing those relationships together and allowing us a way to solve these problems by coming together to one place, all having a voice at the table, are those to which we all have access. One prime example of this is using technology as a medium to support and foster collective relational resiliency. In fact, the use of technology has been described to bridge gaps in professional disciplines because segments of every discipline intersect with technology usage (see, for example, Drude et al., 2019). We also know that people use technology in every country in the world (Internet World Stats, 2023). While North America has the highest penetration of Internet users (94%), Asia has the highest number of Internet users at 3 billion. Further, the adoption of Internet technologies globally continues to steadily rise, making technology in our lives a staple, no matter one's nationality.

Collective relational resiliency strategies can be created through reliance on circumstances in which technology is advantageous to relationships. Such advantages include relationship initiation (such as meeting others through various technology mediums), using technologies for conflict management and gathering information as to how to manage a problem when it emerges in a relationship, demonstrating a commitment to one another, and using it to reduce one's own anxiety by way of checking in with a partner (Hertlein & Ancheta, 2014a). Other applications of technology to augment relationship development or repair include the treatment of sexual dysfunctions (Hertlein, 2010), intimacy building in couple relationships (Hertlein, 2016), and problem-solving and relationship development in a more comfortably paced environment (Hertlein & Ancheta, 2014b).

The *Couple and Family Technology Framework* (Hertlein, 2012; Hertlein & Blumer, 2013; Hertlein & Twist, 2019) identifies several key components of the Internet and technology that contribute to altering our relationship structure and processes. These elements include accessibility, affordability, acceptability, anonymity, ambiguity, accommodation, and approximation (Hertlein & Stevenson, 2010). Accessibility, acceptability, and affordability are the biggest drivers of the seven in their contribution to using technology for fostering collective relational resiliency. Acceptability refers to how acceptable these technologies are in our day-to-day lives. Examining Internet penetrations rates in various regions as notes above, the use of Internet technologies is highly acceptable worldwide. Accessibility refers to the access we as global citizens have not just to technology, but the software and apps embedded in technology. This means that we are connected to each other instantly and constantly accessing the Internet (PEW Research Center, 2022). It also means that we have access to know what is happening globally and be able to provide support, resources, or intervene. We can also do so in ways that are affordable. For example, both local and global disasters have found effective ways to use social media to support their crisis management strategies (Mitcham et al., 2021). To provide support in this way did not require travel to those areas, but instead provide support in ways that were within everyone's financial means and abilities.

Approximation is also important to the fostering of collective relational resiliency. Rooted in social presence theory (Short et al., 1976) and media richness theory (Daft & Lengel, 1984), approximation means that technology that is most impactful to us are those types that best approximate real-world situations (Ross & Kauth, 2002). Further, the strategies that feel the most supportive to the recipient are synchronous communication strategies (Hertlein & Twist, 2019). Taken together, this means that collective resilience can be fostered more effectively by technologies that best mimic the conditions of in person relationships such as apps using synchronous communication in settings where we can best approximate in person relationships. This includes being highly responsive to those who are suffering via quickly delivered communications, just as we would in in-person interactions; creating a setting either through words or background that conveys the spirit of approximation. This might include developing methods by which we might provide more self-disclosure to one another to convey the non-verbal cues we would miss in text-based interactions.

Future Directions

As mentioned, the framework was originally developed from examining data-based publications and other scholarly literature in education, family studies, and communication studies. Therefore, expansion of the model depends on multidisciplinary interaction and education, whose sources include a learning environment with scholars who specialize in computer science, technology, media studies, and information systems. This will allow scholars to develop a comprehensive understanding of the ways in which technology can be applied to increase collective relational resilience strategies in couples and families for issues related to technology as well as issues globally that might be better resolved or managed through using technology in ways to cultivate resilience. Interaction with those who specialize in technology would keep us as family therapy scholars abreast of changes and advances in technology so they might influence how we refine our current models or develop our own.

Further, a key characteristic of the *Couple and Family Technology* framework is its ability to be applied to couples and families of diverse backgrounds. The framework does not advocate for a specific way of using the Internet and new media. The framework references the notion that technology affects process and structure; in some ways, the effect is positive and in other ways is negative. In this model, the therapist reserves judgment about how the family should proceed with technology in their lives and instead assists the family with the implications and interventions congruent with their own beliefs and value system. In some families, for example, appropriate interventions may center around creating more rigid boundaries between parents and their teens; in some cultures/family systems, it may be more appropriate to make boundaries more diffuse. Interaction with scholars for varied backgrounds would assist in expanding the current interventive options described to be more widely applicable.

Another future direction would include how collective relational resiliency is affected by the state of social justice and marginalized populations. Power is often a culturally bound issue, and in some cultures or families, parents have more power within a family system than in others. Parents from an authoritarian parenting perspective tend to raise children who are less emotionally intelligent because the discipline relied on shame, guilt, is punitive, and relies on seeking approval of others (Sung, 2010). In families who have access to technology, the roles may be flipped; the adolescent has more power in this context because they have more expertise using technology than their parents (Thomas, 2011). Thus, adolescents may have more power in their relationship with their parents because of their technological knowledge. At the same time, this increased knowledge is not always protective; adolescents who have more knowledge about technology but who have parents less knowledgeable may be more prone to cyberbullying victimization because their parents may be unaware of what is happening to them or aware about how to stop it. Therefore, interactions with scholars who interact with youth and study teen behavior, especially regarding teen risk-taking, are critical.

Communication patterns are also key to further developing and refining the model. Secrecy, for example, is one problematic communication frequently cited in relationships (Gobin & Freyd, 2014; Jang, 2008). It is also becoming a widespread issue in relationships because of the individual and personal design of technology (Zitzman & Butler, 2009). Because cell phones are independent (as opposed to shared) devices, users have a certain amount of privacy regarding how they use the phone. Adolescents may opt to use the phone as one method of interacting with their peers in secret. As they become more secretive, they may use the Internet more frequently and engage in riskier behavior online, resulting in greater likelihood of being victims of cyberbullying (Kowalski et al., 2014).

Three Key Takeaways

1. Use technology to bridge us, not divide us.

2. Because technology can introduce global problems, it can be one (of many) global solutions.
3. Technology can be a resource to solve other global problems, not just the ones associated with technology itself.

References

Acharya, I. P., Acharya, I., & Waghrey, D. (2013). A study on some psychological health effects of cell phone usage. *International Journal of Medical Research and Health Sciences, 2*(3), 388–394. https://doi.org/10.5958/j.2319-5886.2.3.068

Ahern, N. R., & Mechling, B. (2013). Sexting: Serious problems for youth. *Journal of Psychosocial Nursing and Mental Health Services, 51*(7), 22–30. https://doi.org/10.3928/02793695-20130 503-02

Barnard, C. P. (1994). Resiliency: A shift in our perception? *The American Journal of Family Therapy, 22*(2), 135–144. https://doi.org/10.1080/01926189408251307

Becvar, D. S. (2013). *Handbook of family resilience*. New York: Springer.

Blinka, L., Škařupová, K., & Mitterova, K. (2016). Dysfunctional impulsivity in online gaming addiction and engagement. *Cyberpsychology: Journal of Psychosocial Research on Cyberspace, 10*(3), article 1. https://doi.org/10.5817/CP2016-3-5

Blumer, M., Hertlein, K. M., Smith, J., & Allen, H. (2014). How many bytes does it take?: A content analysis of cyber issues in couple and family therapy journals. *Journal of Marital and Family Therapy, 40*(1), 34–48. https://doi.org/10.1111/j.1752-0606.2012.00332.x

Brody, A. C., & Simmons, L. A. (2007). Family resiliency during childhood cancer: The father's perspective. *Journal of Pediatric Oncology Nursing, 24*(3), 152–165. https://doi.org/10.1177/10434 54206298844

Bronfenbrenner, U. (1977). Toward an experimental ecology of human development. *American Psychologist, 32*(7), 513–531. https://doi.org/10.1037/0003-066X.32.7.513

Chang, C. J., Amick, E., Benjamin, C., Menendez, C. C., Katz, J. N., Johnson, P. W., Dennerlein, J. T. (2007). Daily computer usage correlated with undergraduate students' musculoskeletal symptoms. *American Journal of Industrial Medicine, 50*(6), 481–488. https://doi.org/10.1002/ajim.20461

Cravens, J. D., & Whiting, J. B. (2016). Fooling around on Facebook: The perceptions of infidelity behavior on social networking sites. *Journal of Couple & Relationship Therapy, 15*(3), 213–231. https://doi.org/10.1080/15332691.2014.1003670

Daft, R. L., & Lengel, R. H. (1984). Information richness: A new approach to managerial behavior and organizational design. In L. L. Cummings & B. M. Staw's (Eds.), *Research in organizational behavior 6* (pp. 191–233). Homewood, IL: JAI Press.

Davis, M. J., Powell, A., Gordon, D., & Kershaw, T. (2016). I want your sext: Sexting and sexual risk in emerging adult minority men. *AIDS Education and Prevention, 28*(2), 138–152. https://doi.org/10.1521/aeap.2016.28.2.138

DeFrain, J. (2022). All the problems in the world either begin in families or end up in families. *Journal of Problem-Based Learning, 9*(1), 1–3. https://doi.org/10.24313/jpbl.2022.00129

Dir, A. L., & Cyders, M. A. (2015). Risks, risk factors, and outcomes associated with phone and internet sexting among university students in the United States. *Archives of Sexual Behavior, 44*(6), 1675–1684. https://doi.org/10.1007/s10508-014-0370-7

Dir, A. L., Cyders, M. A., & Coskunpinar, A. (2013). From the bar to the bed via mobile phone: A first test of the role of problematic alcohol use, sexting, and impulsivity-related traits in sexual hookups. *Computers in Human Behavior, 29*, 1664–1670. https://doi.org/10.1016/j.chb.2013.01.039

Drude, K., Hertlein, K. M., Hilty, D., & Maheu, M. (2019). Telebehavioral health competencies in interprofessional education and training: A pathway to interprofessional practice. *Journal of Technology in the Behavioral Sciences, 1–10.*

Gobin, R. L., & Freyd, J. J. (2014). The impact of betrayal trauma on the tendency to trust. *Psychological Trauma: Theory, Research, Practice, and Policy, 6*(5), 505–511. https://doi.org/10.1037/a0032452

Hertlein, K. M. (2010). The integration of technology into sex therapy. *Journal of Family Psychotherapy, 21*(2), 117–131. https://doi.org/10.1080/08975350902967333

Hertlein, K. M. (2012). Digital dwelling: Technology in couple and family relationships. *Family Relations, 61*(3), 374–387. http://dx.doi.org/10.1111/j.1741-3729.2012.00702.x

Hertlein, K. M. (2016). "Your cyberplace or mine?": Electronic fantasy dates". In G. R. Weeks, S. T. Fife, and C. M. Peterson's (Eds.), *Techniques for the couple therapist: Essential interventions from the experts*. New York: Routledge.

Hertlein, K. M., & Ancheta, K. (2014a). Advantages and disadvantages of technology in relationships: Findings from an open-ended survey. *The Qualitative Report, 19* (article 22), 1–11. https://doi.org/10.1080/00224499.2011.604748

Hertlein, K. M., & Ancheta, K. (2014b). Clinical application of the pros and cons of technology in couple and family therapy. *American Journal of Family Therapy, 42*(4), 313–324. https://doi.org/10.1080/01926187.2013.866511

Hertlein, K. M., & Blumer, M. L. C. (2013). *The Couple and Family Technology Framework: Intimate relationships in a digital age*. New York: Routledge.

Hertlein, K. M., & Piercy, F. P. (2008). Treatment and assessment of Internet infidelity cases. *Journal of Marital and Family Therapy, 34*(4), 481–497. https://doi.org/10.1111/j.1752-0606.2008.00090.x

Hertlein, K. M., & Stevenson, A. J. (2010). The seven "As" contributing to Internet-related intimacy problems: A literature review. *Cyberpsychology: Journal of Psychosocial Research on Cyberspace, 4*(1), article 1. Retrieved from: www.cyberpsychology.eu/view.php?cisloclanku=2010050202

Hertlein, K. M., & Twist, M. (2019). *The Internet Family: Technology in couple and family relationships*. New York: Routledge.

Hertlein, K. M., & Webster, M. (2008). A systemic research synthesis of the impact of technology on couples and families. *Journal of Marital and Family Therapy. 34*(4), 445–460. https://doi.org/10.1111/j.1752-0606.2008.00087.x

Iliardi, S. (2010). *The depression cure*. New York: De Capo Lifelong Books.

Internet Live Stats (2016). *Internet users*. Retrieved November 24, 2016, from: www.internetlivestats.com/internet-users/

Internet World Stats (2023). World Internet Users and 2023 Population Stats. Retrieved February 2, 2023, from: www.internetworldstats.com/stats.htm

Jang, S. A. (2008). The effects of attachment styles and efficacy of communication on avoidance following a relational partner's deception. *Communication Research Reports, 25*(4), 300–311. https://doi.org/10.1080/08824090802440220

Kowalski, R. M., Giumetti, G. W., Schroeder, A. N., & Lattanner, M. R. (2014). Bullying in the digital age: A critical review and meta-analysis of cyberbullying research among youth. *Psychological Bulletin, 140*(4), 1073–1137. https://doi.org/10.1037/a0035618

Lee, B. W., & Stapinski, L. A. (2012). Seeking safety on the Internet: Relationship between social anxiety and problematic Internet use. *Journal of Anxiety Disorders, 26*, 197–205. https://doi.org/10.1016/j.janxdis.2011.11.001

Lepp, A., Barkley, J. E., Sanders, G. J., Rebold, M., & Gates, P. (2013). The relationship between cell phone use, physical and sedentary activity, and cardiorespiratory fitness in a sample of U.S. college students. *International Journal of Behavioral Nutrition and Physical Activity, 10*, 79, 1–9. https://doi.org/10.1177/2158244015573169

Lin, I., & Peper, E. (2009). Psychophysiological patterns during cell phone text messaging: A preliminary study. *Applied Psychophysiology Biofeedback, 34*, 53–57. https://doi.org/10.1007/s10484-009-9078-1

Lynch, S. (2011). Challenging stereotypes of foster children: A study of relational resilience. *Journal of Public Child Welfare, 5*(1), 23–44. https://doi.org/10.1080/15548732.2010.526903

Mehta, D. H., Perez, G. K., Traeger, L., Park, E. R., Goldman, R. E., Haime, V., …Jackson, V. A. (2016). Building resiliency in a palliative care team: A pilot study. *Journal of Pain and Symptom Management, 51*(3), 604–608. https://doi.org/10.1016/j.jpainsymman.2015.10.013

Mitcham, D., Taylor, M., & Harris, C. (2021). Utilizing social media for information Ddspersal during local disasters: The communication hub framework for local emergency management. *International Journal of Environmental Research and Public Health, 18*(20), https://.doi.org/10.3390/ijerph182010784.

Neustifter, R., & Powell, L. (2015). Intimate partner violence survivors: Exploring relational resilience to long-term psychosocial consequences of abuse by previous partners. *Journal of Family Psychotherapy, 26*(4), 269. https://doi.org/10.1080/08975353.2015.1097240

Ortiz, R. W., Green, T., & Lim, H. (2011). Families and home computer use: Exploring parent perceptions of the importance of current technology. *Urban Education, 46*(2), 202–215. https://doi.org/10.1177/0042085910377433

PEW Research Center (2022). Teens, social media, and technology 2022. Retrieved September 18, 2022 from: www.pewresearch.org/internet/2022/08/10/teens-social-media-and-technology-2022/

Ross, M., & Kauth, M. (2002). Men who have sex with men, and the Internet: Emerging clinical issues and their management. In A. Cooper (Ed.), *Sex and the internet: A guidebook for clinicians.* New York: Brunner-Routledge.

Short, J., Williams, E., & Christie, B. (1976). *The social psychology of telecommunications.* Hoboken, NJ: John Wiley & Sons, Ltd.

Sudan, M., Khefiets, L., Arah, O. A., & Olsen, J. (2013). Cell phone exposures and hearing loss in children in the Danish National Birth Cohort. *Paediatric and Perinatal Epidemiology, 27,* 247–257. https://doi.org/10.1111/ppe.12036

Sung, H. Y. (2010). The influence of culture on parenting practices of east Asian families and emotional intelligence of older adolescents: A qualitative study. *School Psychology International, 31*(2), 199–214. https://doi.org/10.1177/0143034309352268

Thomas, M. (2011). *Deconstructing digital natives: Young people, technology, and the new literacies.* New York: Routledge.

Van Ouytsel, J., Walrave, M., Ponnet, K., & Heirman, W. (2015). The association between adolescent sexting, psychosocial difficulties, and risk behavior: Integrative review. *The Journal of School Nursing, 31*(1), 54–69. https://doi.org/10.1177/1059840514541964

von Bertalanffy, L. (1968). *General System Theory: Foundations, development, applications.* New York: George Braziller.

Walsh, F. (2003). Crisis, trauma, and challenge: A relational resilience approach for healing, transformation, and growth. *Smith College Studies in Social Work, 74*(1), 49–71. https://doi.org/10.1080/00377310309517704

Zitzman, S. T., & Butler, M. H. (2009). Wives' experience of husbands' pornography use and concomitant deception as an attachment threat in the adult pair-bond relationship. *Sexual Addiction & Compulsivity, 16*(3), 210–240. https://doi.org/10.1080/10720160903202679

AFTERWORD

To the therapists reading this text: if you hear the song I have sung in this text, you will understand. We hold the key to solving relational problems worldwide (since love and fear are part of the human condition) all in our well-trained hands. Just one key unlocks them both; it is there at our command to use to advance global compassion and understanding. It is my hope that this book provides avenues toward tolerance and diversity of perspective. Today, our work is more important than ever.

INDEX

For Product Safety Concerns and Information please contact our EU
representative GPSR@taylorandfrancis.com
Taylor & Francis Verlag GmbH, Kaufingerstraße 24, 80331 München, Germany

www.ingramcontent.com/pod-product-compliance
Lightning Source LLC
Chambersburg PA
CBHW081215220326
41598CB00037B/6781